Psychogenic Movement Disorders

Neurology and Neuropsychiatry

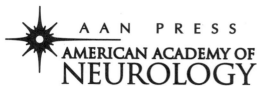

AMERICAN ACADEMY OF
NEUROLOGY

Psychogenic Movement Disorders

Neurology and Neuropsychiatry

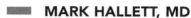

■■■ **MARK HALLETT, MD**
Chief, Human Motor Control Section
National Institute of Neurological Disorders and Stroke
National Institutes of Health
Bethesda, Maryland

■■■ **STANLEY FAHN, MD**
H. Houston Merritt Professor of Neurology
Director, Movement Disorders Group, Neurology
Columbia University, New York
Attending Physician
Neurology, NY Presbyterian Hospital
New York, New York

■■■ **JOSEPH JANKOVIC, MD**
Professor, Department of Neurology
Baylor College of Medicine
Department of Neurology
Faculty, Department of Neurology
The Methodist Hospital
Houston, Texas

■■■ **ANTHONY E. LANG, MD, FRCPC**
Professor, Department of Medicine (Neurology)
University of Toronto
Director, Movement Disorders Centre
Toronto Western Hospital
Ontario, Canada

■■■ **C. ROBERT CLONINGER, MD**
Wallace Renard Professor of Psychiatry
Washington University in St. Louis
St. Louis, Missouri

■■■ **STUART C. YUDOFSKY, MD**
D.C. and Irene Ellwood Professor and Chairman
Menninger Department of Psychiatry and Behavioral Sciences
Baylor College of Medicine
Director, Psychiatry Service
The Methodist Hospital
Houston, Texas

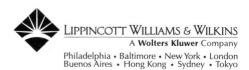

LIPPINCOTT WILLIAMS & WILKINS
A **Wolters Kluwer** Company
Philadelphia • Baltimore • New York • London
Buenos Aires • Hong Kong • Sydney • Tokyo

Acquisitions Editor: Frances DeStefano
Managing Editor: Scott Scheidt
Developmental Editor: Sarah M. Granlund
Project Manager: Fran Gunning
Manufacturing Manager: Ben Rivera
Marketing Manager: Adam Glazer
Design Coordinator: Holly Reid McLaughlin
Cover Designer: Christine Jenny
Production Services: Laserwords Pvt. Limited
Printer: Edwards Brothers

The American Academy of Neurology has endorsed this book series and has authorized AAN Enterprises, Inc., to display the AAN logo and the words *American Academy of Neurology* on each edition.

© 2006 by AAN Enterprises, Inc.
Published by
Lippincott Williams & Wilkins
530 Walnut Street
Philadelphia, PA 19106
LWW.com

Library of Congress Cataloging-in-Publication Data

Psychogenic movement disorders / editor-in-chief, Mark Hallett ; associate editors, C. Robert Cloninger ... [et al.].—1st ed.
        p. ; cm.
    Includes bibliographical references and index.
    ISBN 0-7817-9627-X (alk. paper)
    1. Psychomotor disorders. 2. Somatoform disorders. 3. Medicine, Psychosomatic. I. Hallett, Mark. II. Cloninger, C. Robert.
    [DNLM: 1. Psychomotor Disorders—Congresses. WM 197 P974 2005]
    RC376.5.P79 2005
    616.8'3—dc22
                        2005015079

Contents

Preface

Psychogenic movement disorders, sometimes also referred to as "functional" or "non-organic" movement disorders in contrast to "organic" movement disorders, fall into the category of medically unexplained symptoms and signs. Functional disorders are those that arise due to malfunction of the brain without any (obvious) brain lesion. Psychogenic movement disorders are a valuable model for all medically unexplained symptoms since they are easily measurable. This book is the proceedings of an international workshop on psychogenic movement disorders, which are common, but not well understood or treated by the medical community. Patients diagnosed with psychogenic movement disorders are typically referred to neurologists, particularly those who specialize in such movement disorders. While psychogenic movement disorders may include somatization, factitious disorder, and malingering, they are most commonly examples of conversion. They are psychiatric disorders that neurologists see. Neurologists have generally had limited knowledge or experience how to manage patients with psychogenic movement disorders, and psychiatrists often fail to recognize that the neurological symptoms and signs are a product of underlying psychological disturbance. The problem is common and the resulting symptoms are often chronic and very disabling. Given the large number of these patients and their disability, advances in understanding and treating these disorders are urgently needed.

The task of defining psychogenic disorders, advancing knowledge about their mechanisms and providing guidance for their treatment is difficult and requires a multidisciplinary effort. Neurologists and psychiatrists need to work together with the help of psychologists, physiatrists, and basic scientists. In October 2003, such a group gathered together to discuss the state of the art regarding psychogenic movement disorders. The effort was supported and sponsored by the Movement Disorder Society and the National Institute of Neurological Disorders and Stroke, with support from AstraZeneca, Bristol-Myers Squibb Company, Pfizer, Inc., GlaxoSmithKline, Allergan, Inc., Ortho-McNeil Pharmaceutical, Amarin Pharmaceuticals, Inc., UCB Pharma, and Wyeth. We are grateful to all of them.

Although neurologists and psychiatrists tend to speak different languages, the meeting showed the progress that could be made when the two groups work together. We were able to recruit most of the speakers at the meeting to provide chapters for this book. Additionally, there were some free communications, and the best of these are also in this book as abstracts.

This book represents a start. Any physician who sees these patients (or any patients with medically unexplained symptoms) should find it valuable. What often applies to the treatment of psychogenic movement disorders usually applies to other psychogenic neurological symptoms as well. Therefore, much of the discussion in this text can be extended beyond movement disorders. Questions are raised here that need answers. Hopefully, a future edition of a book like this will demonstrate progress that will reflect an improvement in our understanding of how the mind (brain) influences the body.

Mark Hallett, MD
Stanley Fahn, MD
Joseph Jankovic, MD
Anthony E. Lang, MD
C. Robert Cloninger, MD
Stuart C. Yudofsky, MD

Contributors

PETER ASHBY, MD, FRCP Professor Emeritus, Department of Medicine–Neurology, University of Toronto; Staff Physician, Department of Neurology, Toronto Western Hospital, Toronto, Canada

POLO ALBERTO BANUELOS, MD Medical Resident, Department of Internal Medicine, Baylor College of Medicine, Houston, Texas

JOHN J. BARRY, MD Associate Professor, Department of Psychiatry, Stanford University, Stanford Hospital, Stanford, California

CHRISTOPHER BASS, MA, MD, FRCPSYCH Honarary Senior Lecturer, University Department of Psychiatry, Warneford Hospital; Consultant in Liaison Psychiatry, Department of Psychological Medicine, John Radcliffe Hospital, Oxford, United Kingdom

KAILASH P. BHATIA, MD, DM, FRCP Reader in Clinical Neurology, Sobell Department of Movement Neuroscience, Institute of Neurology; Honary Consultant Neurologist, Department of Clinical Neurology, National Hospital for Neurology, London, United Kingdom

STEVEN BIELAMOWICZ, MD Professor and Chief, Division of Otolaryngology, The George Washington University, Washington, DC

FRÉDÉRIC BOURDAIN, MD Neurologist, Service de Neurologie, Hôpital Foch, Suresnes Cedex, France

RICHARD J. BROWN, PHD, CLINPSYD Lecturer in Clinical Psychology, Academic Division of Clinical Psychology, University of Manchester; Clinical Psychologist, Department of Clinical and Health Psychology, Manchester Mental Health and Social Care Trust, Manchester, United Kingdom

PETER BROWN, MBBCHIR, MA, MD, FRCP Professor, Sobell Department of Movement Neuroscience, Institute of Neurology; Honary Consultant Neurologist, National Hospital for Neurology, London, United Kingdom

MICHIKO KIMURA BRUNO, MD Clinical Assistant Professor, Department of Medicine, John A. Burns School of Medicine; Staff Neurologist, Department of Medicine, Kapiolani Medical Center at Pali Momi, Aiea, Hawaii

JOSÉ CHACÓN, MD Associate Professor of Neurology, Department of Neurology; Director, Movement Disorders Clinic, Hospital Universiterio Virgen Macarena, Sevilla, Spain

ROBERT CHEN, MA, MBBCHIR MSC, FRCPC Associate Professor, Department of Medicine, University of Toronto; Senior Scientist, Toronto Western Research Institute, University Health Network, Toronto, Canada

C. ROBERT CLONINGER, MD Wallace Renard Professor of Psychiatry, Washington University, St. Louis, Missouri

ESTHER CUBO, MD, PHD Visiting Assistant Professor, Department of Neurology, Rush University Medical Center, Chicago, Illinois; Attending Neurologist, Department of Neurology, Clinica de la Zarzuela, Sanatorio del Rosario, Madrid, Spain

GREGORY MARK DE MOORE, FRANZCP Clinical Lecturer, Psychological Medicine, University of Sydney, Sydney, Australia; Staff Specialist, Department of Psychiatry, Westmead Hospital, Westmead, Australia

JUSTO GARCIA DE YEBENES, MD Neurologist, Neurology Department Hospital Ramón y Cajal, Madrid, Spain

ALEXANDRA DEGENHARDT, MD Department of Neurology, Beth Israel Deaconess Medical Center, Boston, Massachusetts

JAVIER LÓPEZ DEL VAL, MD Neurologist, Neurology Department, Hospital Clinico Zaragoza, Zaragoza, Spain

GÜNTHER DEUSCHL, MD Professor, Department of Neurology, Christian-Albrechts-Universität; Head, Department of Neurology, Universitätsklinikum Schleswig-Holstein, Kiel, Germany

STEWART A. FACTOR, DO Professor of Neurology, Director, Movement Disorders, Department of Neurology, Emory University School of Medicine, Atlanta, Georgia

STANLEY FAHN, MD H. Houston Merritt Professor, Department of Neurology, Columbia University; Head, Division of Movement Disorders, Department of Neurology, Neurological Institute, New York Presbyterian Hospital, New York, New York

HUBERT H. FERNANDEZ, MD Co-Director, Movement Disorders Center; Co-Director, Residency Training Program, Department of Neurology, University of Florida, Gainesville, Florida

GEREON R. FINK, MD, PHD Full Professor, Department of Neurology—Cognitive Neurology, RWTH Aachen University; Chief, Department of Neurology—Cognitive Neurology, University Hospital Aachen, Aachen, Germany

KIMBERLY A. FINNEGAN, MS Clinical Research Speech Pathologist, Laryngeal and Speech Section, National Institutes of Health, Bethesda, Maryland

KELLY D. FOOTE, MD Assistant Professor, Department of Neurosurgery, University of Florida College of Medicine; Attending Physician, Department of Neurosurgery, Shands Hospital, Gainesville, Florida

BLAIR FORD, MD Associate Professor, Attending Neurologist, Columbia University Medical Center, New York, New York

PATRICIA FURER, PHD, CPSYCH Assistant Professor, Department of Clinical Health Psychology, University of Manitoba; Clinical Psychologist, Anxiety Disorders Program, Department of Clinical Health Psychology, St. Boniface General Hospital, Winnipeg, Canada

NESTOR GALVEZ-JIMENEZ, MD, MSC, FACP Clinical Associate Professor of Biomedical Science, Department of Biomedical Science, Charles E. Schmidt College of Science, Florida Atlantic University, Regional Campus of the University of Miami Miller School of Medicine, Boca Raton, Florida; Chief, Movement Disorders Program, Department of Neurology, Cleveland Clinic Florida, Weston, Florida

PAULA GERBER, MD Professor, Barrow Neurological Institute, Muhammad Ali Parkinson Research Center, Phoenix, Arizona

CHRISTOPHER G. GOETZ, MD Professor of Neurological Sciences, Professor of Pharmacology, Rush Medical College, Rush University Medical Center; Senior Attending Neurologist, Rush University Medical Center, Chicago, Illinois

ANDREW GOLDFINE, MD Resident, Department of Neurology, New York Presbyterian Hospital, New York, New York

R.B. GOVINDAN Professor, Department of Neurology, University of Kiel, Kiel, Germany

MARK HALLETT, MD Chief, Human Motor Control Section, National Institute of Neurological Disorders and Stroke, National Institutes of Health, Bethesda, Maryland

PETER W. HALLIGAN, PHD, DSC Professor of Cognitive Neuroscience, Department of Psychology, Cardiff University, Cardiff, United Kingdom

TAKASHI HANAKAWA, MD, PHD Assistant Professor, Human Brain Research Center, Kyoto University Graduate School of Medicine; Attending Physician, Department of Neurology, Kyoto University Hospital, Kyoto, Japan

NAZLI A. HAQ, MSCMA Research Psychologist, Behavioral Endocrinology, National Institute of Mental Health, Bethesda, Maryland

MELANIE J. HARGREAVE, RN Clinical Nurse Coordinator, Movement Disorders Program, Department of Neurology, Cleveland Clinic Hospital, Weston, Florida

MARIE HERBERSTEIN, PHD Senior Lecturer, Department of Biological Sciences, Macquarie University, North Ryde, Australia

DONALD S. HIGGINS, JR, MD Associate Professor, Department of Neurology, Albany Medical College, Parkinson Disease & Movement Disorder Center, Albany, New York

VANESSA K. HINSON, MD, PHD Assistant Professor, Department of Neurosciences, Medical University of South Carolina; Director of Movement Disorders, Department of Neurosciences, Medical University of South Carolina, Charleston, South Carolina

SERENA WAN-SI HUNG, MD Clinical Research Fellow, Movement Disorders Centre, Division of Neurology, University of Toronto, Ontario, Canada

JOSEPH JANKOVIC, MD Professor, Department of Neurology, Baylor College of Medicine; Faculty, Department of Neurology, The Methodist Hospital, Houston, Texas

KENJI KANSAKU, MD, PHD Assistant Professor, Division of Cerebral Integration, Okazaki, Japan

HANS-PETER KAPFHAMMER, MD, PHD Full Professor and Chairman, Psychiatric Department, Medical University Graz, Graz, Austria

H. FLORENCE KIM, MD Assistant Professor, Department of Psychiatry, Baylor College of Medicine, Houston, Texas

FLORIAN KOPPER, MD Professor, Department of Neurology, University of Kiel, Kiel, Germany

JERALD D. KRALIK, PHD Postdoctoral Fellow, Laboratory of Systems Neuroscience, National Institute of Mental Health, Bethesda, Maryland

ANTHONY E. LANG, MD, FRCPC Professor, Department of Medicine—Neurology, University of Toronto; Director, Movement Disorders Centre, Toronto Western Hospital, Toronto, Canada

RONALD P. LESSER, MD Professor, Departments of Neurology and Neurosurgery, The Johns Hopkins Medical Institutions, Baltimore, Maryland

SUE LEURGANS, PHD   Professor, Department of Neurological Sciences & Preventive Medicine, Rush University, Chicago, Illinois

JOEL K. LEVY, PHD   Adjunct Assistant Professor, Department of Family and Community Medicine, Baylor College of Medicine, Houston, Texas; Neuropsychologist, Houston, Texas

GURUTZ LINAZASORO, MD   Director, Centro de Investigación Parkinson, Policlínica Gipuzkoa, San Sebastián, Spain

CHRISTY L. LUDLOW, PHD   Senior Investigator, Medical Neurology Branch and Laryngeal and Speech Section, National Institute of Neurological Disorders and Stroke, Bethesda, Maryland

ZOLTAN MARI, MD   Clinical Fellow, Human Motor Control Section, National Institute of Neurological Disorders and Stroke, National Institutes of Health, Bethesda, Maryland

JOHN C. MARSHALL, PHD   Professor Emeritus, Department of Clinical Neurology, University of Oxford; Director, Neuropsychology Unit, Radcliffe Infirmary, Oxford, London

MARIA J. MARTI, MD, PHD   Associate Professor of Neurology, Department of Medicine, University of Barcelona; Consultor of Neurology, Servicio de Neurologia ICN, Hospital Clinic I Universitari, Barcelona, Spain

MICHAEL F. MAZUREK, MD, FRCP(C)   Professor, Department of Neurology, Psychiatry and Behavioural Neurosciences, McMaster University; Consultant Neurologist, Department of Neurology and Psychiatry, McMaster Medical Centre, Ontario, Canada

ERIC S. MOLHO, MD   Associate Professor, Department of Neurology, Albany Medical College, Parkinson's Disease and Movement Disorders Center, Albany Medical Center; Associate Professor, Department of Neurology, Albany Medical Center, Albany, New York

GREGORY F. MOLNAR, MSC   PhD Candidate, Institute of Medical Science, University of Toronto; Department of Medicine—Neurology, Toronto Western Hospital, Toronto, Canada

JOHN C. MORGAN, MD, PHD   Assistant Professor, Movement Disorders Program, Department of Neurology, Medical College of Georgia; Staff Neurologist, Department of Veterans Affairs Medical Center, Augusta, Georgia

JOHN G. MORRIS, MA, MD, FRACP, FRCP   Professor, University of Sydney; Head, Department of Neurology, Westhead Hospital, Westhead, Sydney

PHILIPPE NUSS   Research Fellow, Membrane Trafficking, INSERM U538; Head, Psychiatry Department, Psychosis First Episode and Dual Diagnosis Unit, Saint Antoine University Hospital, Paris, France

MICHAEL S. OKUN, MD   Assistant Professor, Departments of Neurology and Neurosurgery, and Co-Director Movement Disorders Center, Departments of Neurology and Neurosurgery, University of Florida McKnight Brain Institute, Gainesville, Florida

FRED OVSIEW, MD   Professor, Department of Psychiatry, University of Chicago; Chief, Clinical Neuropsychiatry and Medical Director, Adult Inpatient Psychiatry, University of Chicago, Chicago, Illinois

IAN P. PALMER, MB, CHB, MRCPSYCH   Professor of Military Psychiatry, Visiting Professor, Division of Psychological Medicine, Institute of Psychiatry, De Crespigny Park, King's College, London

MICHEL PANISSET, MD   Associate Professor, Department of Medicine, University of Montreal; Co-Director, André-Barbeau Movement Disorders Clinic, Hôtel-Dieu–CHUM, Montréal, Canada

LOUIS J. PTACEK, MD   Investigator, Department of Neurology, Howard Hughes Medical Institute, University of California; Coleman Distinguished Professor, Department of Neurology, University of California, San Francisco, California

FRANK PUTNAM, MD   Psychiatrist, Director of The Mayerson Center for Safe and Happy Children, Cincinnati Children's Hospital, Cincinnati, Ohio

NIALL P. QUINN, MD   Professor of Clinical Neurology, Sobell Department of Motor Neuroscience and Movement Disorders, Institute of Neurology; Honary Consultant Neurologist, Division of Clinical Neurology, National Hospital for Neurology and Neurosurgery, London, United Kingdom

JAN RAETHJEN, MD   Department of Neurology, University of Kiel, Kiel, Germany

MARIA C. RODRÍGUEZ-OROZ, MD, PHD   Associate Professor, Department of Neurology, University of Navarra; Consultant, Department of Neurology and Neuroscience, Clinica Universitaria de Navarra, Pamplona, Spain

P. ROSEBUSH, MSCN, MD, FRCP(C)   Associate Professor, Department of Psychiatry and Behavioural Neurosciences, McMaster University; Director, Inpatient Psychiatry, Hamilton Health Sciences–McMaster Site, Ontario, Canada

HANS-BERND ROTHENHÄUSLER, MD   Associate Clinical Professor of Psychiatry, Department of Psychiatry, University of Medicine of Graz; Director of the Division of Consultation Psychiatry Service, Universitätsklinik für Psychiatrie, LKH-Universitätsklinikum Graz, Graz, Austria

PEDRO J. GARCIA RUIZ, MD, PHD   Staff Neurologist, Department of Neurology, Fundacion Jimenez Diaz, Madrid, Spain

ANTHONY J. SANTIAGO, MD Section Head, Movement Disorders, Department of Neurology, Rockwood Clinic; Attending Physician, Department of Neurology, Sacred Heart Medical Center, Spokane, Washington

GHISLAINE SAVARD, MD, FRCP(C) Associate Professor, Department of Neurology, McGill University; Psychiatrist, Department of Neurology, Montreal Neurological Hospital, Montréal, Canada

RANDOLPH B. SCHIFFER, MD The Vernon and Elizabeth Haggerton Chair in Neurology; Chair, Department of Neuropsychiatry and Behavioral Science, Texas Tech University Health Sciences Center, Lubbock, Texas

SUSANNE A. SCHNEIDER, MD Research Fellow, Sobell Department of Motor Neuroscience and Movement Disorders, Institute of Neurology; Honary Clinical Consultant, National Hospital for Neurology and Neurosurgery, London, United Kingdom

ANETTE SCHRAG, MD, PHD Senior Lecturer, Clinical Neurosciences, Royal Free & University College Medical School; Consultant Neurologist, Department of Neurology, Royal Free Hospital and Luton and Dunstable Hospital, London, United Kingdom

KAPIL D. SETHI, MD, FRCP Professor, Department of Neurology, Medical College of Georgia, Augusta, Georgia

MICHAEL SHARPE, MA, MD Professor of Psychological Medicine, School of Molecular and Clinical Medicine, The University of Edinburgh, Royal Edinburgh Hospital, Edinburgh, United Kingdom

HOLLY A. SHILL, MD Neurologist, Movement Disorder Section, Barrow Neurological Institute, Phoenix, Arizona

SEAN A. SPENCE, MD, MRCPSYCH Reader in Psychiatry, Department of Academic Clinical Psychiatry, Division of Genomic Medicine, University of Sheffield; Consultant Psychiatrist, Homeless Assessment and Support Team, Sheffield Care Trust, Sheffield, United Kingdom

JON STONE, MB, CHB, MRCP Research Fellow in Neurology, School of Molecular and Clinical Medicine, University of Edinburgh; Specialist Registrar in Neurology, Department of Clinical Neurosciences, Western General Hospital, Edinburgh, United Kingdom

DANIEL TARSY, MD Associate Professor, Department of Neurology, Harvard Medical School; Director, Movement Disorders Center, Department of Neurology, Beth Israel Deaconess Medical Center, Boston, Massachusetts

MADHAVI THOMAS, MD Director, Movement Disorders Research Center, Texas Neurology PA; Neurologist, Associate Attending, Department of Internal Medicine, Baylor University Medical Center, Dallas, Texas

PHILIP D. THOMPSON, MBBS, PHD, FRACP Professor of Neurology, University Department of Medicine, University of Adelaide; Director of Neurology, Department of Neurology, Royal Adelaide Hospital, Adelaide, Australia

W. CRAIG TOMLINSON, MD Assistant Clinical Professor, Department of Psychiatry, Columbia University; Assistant Attending Psychiatrist, Department of Psychiatry, The New York Presbyterian Hospital, New York, New York

MICHAEL TRIMBLE Professor of Behavioral Neurology, Institute of Neurology, London, United Kingdom

JEAN-MARC TROCELLO, MD Department of Neurophysiology, Saint-Antoine Hospital, Paris, France

ANTONIO VAZQUEZ, MD Neurologist, Neurology Department, Hospital Clinico San Carlos, Madrid, Spain

MARIE VIDAILHET, MD Professor of Neurology, Salpêtrière Hospital, Paris; Professor of Neurology, Department of Neurology, Saint-Antoine Hospital, Paris, France

VALERIE VOON, MD Lecturer, Department of Psychiatry, University of Toronto; Staff Psychiatrist, Department of Psychiatry, Toronto Western Hospital, Toronto, Ontario

KEVIN DAT VUONG, MA Instructor, Department of Neurology, Baylor College of Medicine, Houston, Texas

JOHN R. WALKER, PHD Professor, Department of Clinical Health Psychology, University of Manitoba; Director, Anxiety Disorders Program, Clinical Health Psychology, St. Boniface General Hospital, Winnipeg, Canada

MICHAEL I. WEINTRAUB, MD, FACP, FAAN Clinical Professor of Neurology, Clinical Professor of Medicine, New York Medical College, Valhalla, New York; Adjunct Clinical Professor of Neurology, Mt. Sinai School of Medicine, New York, New York

DANIEL T. WILLIAMS, MD Clinical Professor of Psychiatry, Department of Psychiatry, Columbia University College of Physicians & Surgeons; Attending Physician, Department of Psychiatry, New York Presbyterian Hospital, New York, New York

DAVID R. WILLIAMS, MBBS, FRACP PhD Candidate, Reta Lila Weston Institute, University College London; Clinical Research Fellow, Movement Disorders, National Hospital for Neurology & Neurosurgery, London, United Kingdom

MARC WILLIAMS Department of Psychiatry, Columbia University College of Physicians & Surgeons; New York Presbyterian Hospital, New York, New York

STEVEN P. WISE, PHD Research Biologist, Laboratory of Systems Neuroscience, National Institute of Mental Health, Bethesda, Maryland

JOANNE WUU, SCM Instructor, Biostatistician, Department of Neurological Sciences, Rush University Medical Center, Chicago, Illinois

CINDY ZADIKOFF, MD Chief Resident, Department of Neurology, Harvard Beth Israel Deaconess Medical Center, Boston, Massachusetts

ADAM ZEMAN, MA, BM, BCH, MRCP, MD Senior Lecturer; Consultant, Neurologist, Clinical Neurosciences, University of Edinburgh, Western General Hospital, Edinburgh, United Kingdom

History

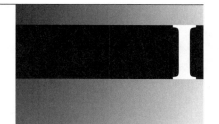

1

Charcot and Psychogenic Movement Disorders

Christopher G. Goetz

ABSTRACT

In his neurologic unit at the Hôpital de la Salpêtrière, the neurologist Jean-Martin Charcot studied many patients who today would likely be considered to have psychogenic movement disorders. Collectively diagnosed primarily under the designation hysteria, these patients had a variety of focal neurologic signs, sometimes static and sometimes fleeting. Tremors, dystonic postures, chorea, stereotypes, and complex, often bizarre, contortions were among the phenomena. Although Charcot's intense interest in hysteria has prompted some historians to label him incorrectly as a psychiatrist, his views remained entrenched in neuroanatomy and he never considered psychological stress as the primary cause of neurologic signs. His study methods and interpretation of hysteria were controversial and led to his serious loss of scientific credibility in the closing years of his career. Although these studies are largely forgotten, as the modern field of psychogenic neurology emerges as a new research arena, Charcot's controversial work on hysteria requires review as a primary historical foundation for contemporary work. Although many of the criticisms of Charcot's work on hysteria are justified, a reconsideration of primary source documents from his lectures, case histories, and notes emphasizes Charcot's views on anatomic, hereditary, and physiologic issues that reemerge in the modern study of psychogenic movement disorders.

INTRODUCTION

Jean-Martin Charcot (1825–1893) was the premier clinical neurologist of the 19th century (Fig. 1.1). Working in Paris at the Hôpital de la Salpêtrière, he converted the walled hospice-city into a world-famous neurologic service. He drew colleagues and students from around the world to study with him and to attend his lectures and classroom demonstrations. Studying with Charcot provided younger colleagues with the credentials to develop neurologic careers and return to their native cities or countries as neurological specialists (1).

Although Charcot contributed to many areas of neurology and medicine, his most important areas of research focused on three issues: the development of a nosology or classification system for neurology (2,3); the practical application of the anatomoclinical method whereby he correlated for the first time specific clinical neurologic signs with focal anatomic lesions (4); and, finally, the study of the neurologic disorder hysteria (5).

Modern readers may consider the topic of hysteria to be outside the realm of neurology and more suitable to the research career of a psychiatrist. In the 19th century, however, hysteria was a specific and, largely due to Charcot's work, well-defined neurologic diagnosis. Psychiatry dealt primarily with diseases causing insanity,

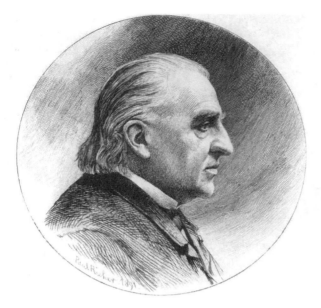

Figure 1.1 Jean-Martin Charcot. Engraving by P. Richer, 1892. (From Goetz CG. *Charcot, the clinician: the Tuesday lessons.* New York: Raven Press, 1987.)

and during this period French neurology and psychiatry were completely separate specialties (6). Neurology was linked to internal medicine, and in Charcot's case most specifically to geriatric medicine. In studying hysteria, Charcot approached the disorder categorically as a neurologist, firmly bound to the growing knowledge of neuroanatomy and without links to or active interactions with psychiatrists of his day. A member of many medical societies and groups that crossed the interface of neurology and allied fields, Charcot was never a member of any psychiatric association (1).

The topic of this volume, psychogenic movement disorders emphasizes an interface between neurology and psychiatry that Charcot never knew. Indeed, he dealt with the gamut of movement disorders, making pivotal observations that affect the history of Parkinson disease, Gilles de la Tourette syndrome, Huntington disease, dystonia, and tremors, but he worked exclusively within the context of neuroanatomy (2). Within Charcot's extensive work on hysteria, the modern movement disorder specialist will find cases that likely fit the current designation of psychogenic movement disorders. Nonetheless, in examining these entities within a very strictly neurologic context without a psychiatric focus, it is very reasonable to ask if Charcot can be legitimately viewed as a key figure in the study of this diagnostic domain. Is Charcot an appropriate starting point historically for an up-to-date consideration of psychogenic movement disorders?

This chapter will argue that Charcot contributed indirectly to the modern understanding of the topic of psychogenic movement disorders and provided a number of

pertinent observations and experimental approaches for studying patients who fit this diagnostic category. But throughout his career, in his nosologic analysis, anatomoclinical approach, and specific studies of hysteria, Charcot never dealt directly with the concept of psychological stress as a primary cause of neurologic diseases. To trace Charcot's contributions to psychogenic movement disorders, this chapter will examine Charcot's views on movement disorders as a nosologic classification, his concept of disease etiology, and the diagnosis of hysteria. With this background, the chapter will then explore Charcot's observations and conclusions on the role of suggestion, by self and outside persons, on neurologic function, specifically with reference to movement disorders. These analyses will help to place the topic of psychogenic movement disorders in the historical context of Charcot's contributions and provide a framework for the modern data and experimental approaches discussed in the remaining chapters of this volume.

MOVEMENT DISORDERS IN THE CHARCOT NOSOLOGY: THE *NÉVROSES*

Prior to Charcot, most neurologic disorders were described by large categories of symptoms and not by anatomical lesions. Motor disorders included weakness, spasms, and palsies. Multiple sclerosis and Parkinson disease were not differentiated, and cases with either diagnosis were coalesced because they both were marked by tremor. Charcot's clinical skills, discipline of a systematic method of examination, and large patient population allowed him to refine clinical categories, defining several disorders with both archetypal presentations as well as variants or *formes frustes* (1). With this clinical analysis, Charcot published the first major description of Parkinson disease (7), supervised the seminal article by Gilles de la Tourette on tic disorders (8), and wrote on chorea (9) and various forms of focal dystonia, termed occupational spasms (10). These reports remain neurologic anchors of clinical description, even in the 21st century.

The leitmotif of Charcot's approach was termed the "anatomoclinical method" or *méthode anatomoclinique*. On the basis of the model originally applied by Laennec, Charcot sought to identify the anatomical basis of neurological symptoms (4). In this two-part discipline, the first step involved the examination of thousands of patients and a careful description of their neurologic signs. Taking advantage of the vast population within the Salpêtrière wards, he culled the medical service to categorize patients by the signs they demonstrated and studied them to document symptom evolution over time. His hand-written notes and sketches of patients were kept in large patient files that can still be examined at the Bibliothèque Charcot within the modern Salpêtrière complex (Fig. 1.2).

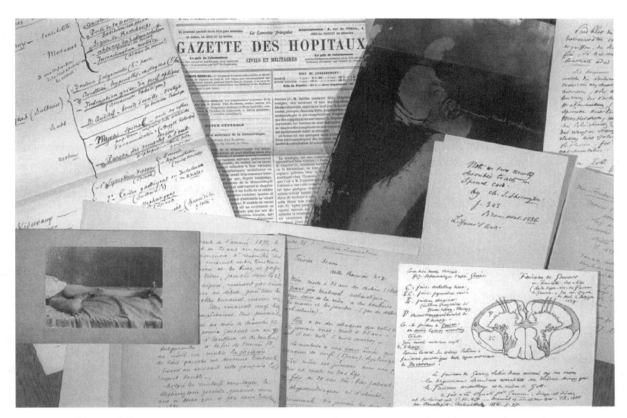

Figure 1.2 The anatomoclinical method. Charcot's file on a patient at the Salpêtrière, showing his hand-written notes, anatomical drawings, photographic documents, and accompanying articles pertinent to the case. (From Goetz CG, Bonduelle M, Gelfandt. *Charcot: constructing neurology.* New York: Oxford University Press, 1995.)

The second phase of the anatomoclinical method involved autopsy examinations. Because the Salpêtrière patients were wards of the state, when they died Charcot likely had automatic access to nervous system tissue. He developed a sophisticated neuropathology service and focused his postmortem studies on a systematic process that cross-referenced identified lesions to the clinical signs experienced during life. Charcot's crowning anatomoclinical research concerned the identification of amyotrophic lateral sclerosis, internationally still widely known as Charcot's disease. He demonstrated that spasticity and pseudobulbar effect related to upper motor neuron lesions of the lateral columns, whereas atrophy and fasciculations occurred in the body regions associated with anterior horn cell loss (11). Comparable anatomoclinical studies illuminated the pathologic basis of locomotor ataxia, myelopathies, and some of the early aphasia syndromes.

As dramatic as these discoveries were, the second phase of study was not always revealing. Numerous entities, including several movement disorders, Parkinson disease, choreas, tics, and dystonic spasms, were not associated with anatomic lesions that Charcot could identify. Charcot established a new category of neurologic disorders, the *névroses* or neuroses, to classify the numerous neurologic

conditions that were well-characterized clinically but still had no identifiable lesion (3). The term *neurosis* in English today applies to psychiatric conditions, although this newer usage dates to the 20th century. Because of the ambiguity of the English term, *névrose* will be used throughout this discussion. This category of *névroses* was intentionally tentative, as Charcot anticipated that future studies would identify the responsible structural lesions.

Other diagnoses that fell under the category of the *névroses* included paroxysmal disorders like epilepsies, migraines, and hysteria. In contrast to the *névroses* with static signs that Charcot believed could eventually be explained with more precise autopsy analyses, he contended that paroxysmal *névroses* did not have static lesions but related to transient or, in his terms, "dynamic" changes in physiologic function within very specific neuroanatomic regions (12). He deduced the involved brain regions by drawing parallels between focal signs seen during these paroxysmal episodes and anatomoclinical discoveries he had previously made with disorders showing similar, but static, signs and clear anatomical lesions. The focal signs that occurred in the midst of a focal epileptic spell, migraine attack, or hysterical episode therefore related to involvement of the same neuroanatomic regions affected in subjects with similar clinical signs due to strokes or abscesses. In this way, when he observed a focal seizure of the left hand with a residual postical paresis, Charcot concluded that the right motor cortex of the precentral gyrus was transiently affected, since he had seen this same area lesioned with tumors or strokes in cases of static left hand weakness. As a natural extension to hysteria, another *névrose*, he concluded similarly, arguing that in hysteria the signs of transient hemiparesis, blindness, contorted postures, and other focal signs had a specific neuroanatomic basis.

CHARCOT AND THE CAUSE OF NEUROLOGIC DISEASES

Charcot's observational skills and dispassionate evaluation of neurologic signs led him to see himself as "a photographer," and he was particularly conscious of the pitfalls of preconceived bias (10). Nonetheless, Charcot held to one primary preconception throughout his career and maintained that the underlying cause of all primary neurologic disease was hereditary (1). In his view, largely reflective of the 19th century as a whole, he adamantly held that patients with neurologic diseases inherited from prior generations a weakness, or *tache*, that predisposed them to neurologic disorders. Environmental factors, including cold, trauma, stress, and infections, influenced the underlying proclivity to disease and could provoke or exacerbate signs in affected subjects. The same environmental factors, however, would have no impact on subjects without the familial *tache*. Conversely, within a family with neurologic disease, the avoidance of unhealthy influences could protect subjects so that even with the hereditary condition some careful members could remain asymptomatic or only mildly affected (10).

Charcot constructed extensive family trees in support of his premise and showed that most neurologically impaired patients had obvious or hidden family members with neurologic diseases as well. He emphasized, however, that the actual neurologic manifestations of disease varied among family members. In one genealogy (Fig. 1.3) (10) the parents were afflicted with aphasia, hemiplegia, and epilepsy, whereas the children revealed their neurologic disorder in the form of locomotor ataxia and general paresis (dissimilar inheritance). More rarely, the same manifestations of neurologic impairment passed between generations (similar inheritance). Within Charcot's conceptual framework of the neuropathic family of diseases, disorders due to structural lesions and the *névroses* were equal in neurologic legitimacy, all being fundamentally hereditary and all intermingled within families.

Against this familial backdrop, the final clinical manifestations of the neurologic disorder depended largely on an array of environmental factors or *agents provocateurs*. For instance, in the case of locomotor ataxia or tabes dorsalis, Charcot held adamantly that syphilis was not the cause of the illness but was frequently associated with the disorder because syphilis weakened the body:

> There are conditions that relate to diseases as provocative agents. Trauma can unveil almost any illness to which a person is already predisposed. Syphilis too is undoubtedly important, and if we see many ataxics who were once syphilitic, we can reasonably ask whether ataxia would have ever developed without prior syphilis. Without syphilis, the tabes will not develop at all clinically, or, if it does, it will come later (2,10).

In a similar context, he noted that children with Sydenham chorea often had added cardiac disease, the latter causing a generalized weakening of the body and allowing the clinical expression of hereditary chorea. Other environmental precipitants, both acute and chronic, included cold, shock, and humidity, all seen as provoking or exacerbating influences that potentially unleashed neurologic syndromes, including Parkinson disease, chorea, tics, epilepsy, and hysteria among hereditarily predisposed subjects (7,10).

Charcot's views of multiple manifestations of a single hereditary disorder within a family may be viewed as particularly modern or painfully simplistic. On the one hand,

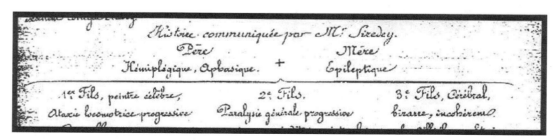

Figure 1.3 Genealogic tree of a patient showing Charcot's insistence on hereditary factors underlying neurologic disorders. A father with aphasia and hemiplegia and a mother with epilepsy had three children, one with locomotor ataxia, a second with general paresis, and a third with incoherent, bizarre behaviors. (From Goetz CG. *Charcot, the clinician: the Tuesday lessons.* New York: Raven Press, 1987.)

the Charcot view is supported directly by modern examples of spinocerebellar ataxias that show different phenotypic expressions of a single genotype. On the other hand, because all neurologic conditions were considered hereditary, Charcot completely overlooked the distinctive nature of such conditions as Huntington disease. In his view, the hereditary pattern in Huntington disease was more uniform (similar inheritance) than in other disorders where dissimilar inheritance predominated, but this characteristic was not distinctive enough to mark it as a particular entity separate from Sydenham chorea (2,10).

Given Charcot's unquestioned view of hereditary disease causation, the concept of primary "psychogenic" neurologic disorders and specifically psychogenic movement disorders is a non sequitur in the strict sense. Nowhere in Charcot's writing will the reader find arguments that a healthy person without a hereditary proclivity to disease could develop a neurologic disorder from any psychological influence, whether stress, trauma, excitement, or despair. On the other hand, as indicated previously, Charcot appreciated the roles of stress, emotional or minor physical trauma, and excitement as within the repertoire of *agents provocateurs*. These influences, although not restricted to one diagnosis, were particularly important when dealing with hysteria.

CHARCOT AND HYSTERIA

After 1870 and especially after 1880, Charcot devoted a particular effort to studying hysteria (1). The clinical features of hysteria were varied but specific, including characteristic focal neurologic signs such as hemiparesis, hemianesthesia, contractures of the extremities, or bizarre involuntary movements. These findings could be statically present but were often fleeting or intermittent. Men and women were affected, and, within the hysteric's family tree, Charcot was consistently comfortable that he could establish the hereditary mark of neurologic disease.

Several specific features helped Charcot to identify hysterics. In comparing the distribution of weakness, sensory loss, or postures of these hysterical patients, Charcot acknowledged that the pattern of neurologic impairment was similar to, but usually not exactly the same as those seen with classical structural lesions. Weakness was not necessarily accompanied by reflex changes, hemianesthesia tended to split the midline, and postures were more variable among hysterical subjects than the contractures he saw after strokes or other defined lesions (13). Furthermore, the degree of involvement was usually more extensive, more intense, and seemingly more disabling in hysteria than seen with a comparable lesion of structural origin. Similarly, multiple hysterical signs often occurred simultaneously or could be found in the past history—for example, a patient

with hysterical monoplegia often had accompanying hemianesthesia or a past history of hystero-epilepsy. Importantly as well, hysterical signs were very often linked historically to a minor physical injury affecting the involved body part. This injury occurred in close juxtaposition to the neurologic signs that developed quickly and fully, rather than showing a slow evolution. Finally, hysterical signs resolved under the influence of hypnosis and could in some cases be treated permanently with hypnotic suggestion. Collectively, these features helped Charcot in classifying hysteria as a unified entity, and because the presumed neurologic impairment was fundamentally dynamic and physiologic rather than static, the observed patterns validated the relationship between the *névroses* and the organic disorders. Commenting specifically on the dynamic lesion site in a case of hysterical upper extremity paralysis, Charcot drew his anatomic conclusions from parallels with structural lesions: "It is, I contend, in the gray matter of the cerebral hemisphere on the side opposite the paralysis and more precisely in the motor zone of the arm (12)."

As a group, the hysterics typically also showed an emotional effect of exotic elaboration, and though this feature aggravated the practical study of hysterics, in fact it helped to set them nosologically apart from subjects with other diagnoses. Speaking of his own Salpêtrière population, Charcot stated:

> But you must not forget that it is a characteristic of hysterical subjects to exaggerate their phenomena, and they are more prone to do so when they think they are observed and admired (14).

This observation made the detailed documentation of individual signs sometimes difficult without the added experimental tool of hypnosis, to be discussed below.

The issue of elaboration or exotic signs should not imply that Charcot considered hysteria as either neurasthenia or malingering. The focal neurologic presentation of hysteria distinguished the condition categorically from neurasthenia, where global fatigue and vague symptoms predominated the presentation. The transient nature of many hysterical spells and the patients' elaboration of signs always prompted Charcot's consideration of malingering or attempted deception on the part of the patient. In this context, Charcot was severe in his scrutiny, and he weeded out elements of conscious fabrication among hysterics through a number of physiologic studies to demonstrate that the specific hysterical signs were involuntary and unconscious. Speaking of simulation within the context of underlying hysteria, he warned of:

> … the slyness, cleverness and unexpected tenacity that women will show in trying to fool people in the midst of their hysteria, especially when the would-be victim is a doctor (15).

HYSTERIA AND MOVEMENT DISORDERS

Within the large category of hysterics, what movement disorders did Charcot find? The celebrated painting by Louis Brouillet, *A Clinical Lesson at the Salpêtrière* (Fig. 1.4), captures a young hysteric with a dystonic hand, showing a twisted, flexed wrist posture. Other forms of dystonic postures can be found among Charcot's cases of "contractures," and in these cases most developed static deformities, although some fluctuated (16). The pattern of activated muscles resembled, but was not identical to, the postures seen in organic lesions of the lateral corticospinal tracts or irritation of the peripheral nerves. Charcot emphasized the temporal relationship to an acute, but usually very minor, injury or emotional stress. The hand contracture in Figure 1.5A occurred immediately after the patient scraped her hand on a piece of broken glass, and the deformity seen in Figure 1.5B developed in a blacksmith who singed his hand and forearm. Other examples included arm spasms that occurred after throwing a stone or severe foot inversion deformities that occurred after kicking. Whereas these spasms resisted physical manipulation or electrical stimulation, they resolved with ease during hypnosis or other techniques of suggestion. Often they were accompanied by other signs of hysteria, including hystero-epileptic fits, hemianesthesia, and restricted visual fields, collectively termed "hysterical stigmata."

When uncertain whether a dystonic hand spasm was hysterical or due to simulation, Charcot applied a stress test in which he positioned the hand on a table with the hand attached to a weight (Fig. 1.6). He monitored the wrist contractions and the patient's respiratory movements over 30 to 60 minutes. Whereas the hysteric showed a maintained posture and steady, regular respiratory movements, a malingering or simulating subject quickly fatigued, as evidenced by irregular muscle contractions and erratic respiratory efforts.

In his formal lectures and his show-and-tell presentations, Charcot presented hysterical cases of tremor, tics, and chorea. Within the category of subjects with hysterical rest tremor, oscillations were usually more variable than in typical Parkinson disease, ranging between 3.5 and 6 cycles per sec, in contrast to the very strict characteristics of typical parkinsonian tremor, found to be 4 to 5 cycles per sec (9). Unusual tics that were complex in character and bizarre were termed hysterical when they were highly stimulus-sensitive or situationally based, for example, occurring only under exposure to bright light (17). A special form of chorea known as "rhythmic chorea" occurred in hysterics. In modern neurology, choreic disorders are unified by irregular and inconsistent movements as seen in Sydenham and Huntington disease, but Charcot only reluctantly accepted such movements in the nosology of chorea. He preferred to respect the strict epistemology of terms and

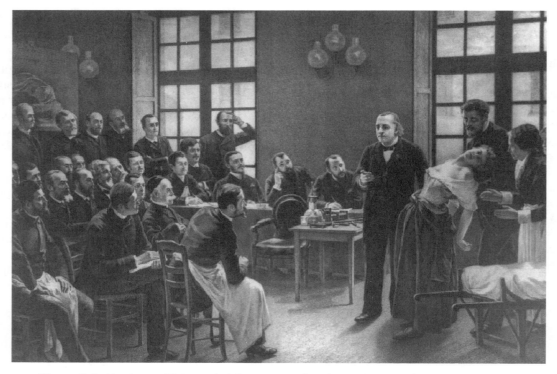

Figure 1.4 Une Leçon Clinique à la Salpêtrière (A Clinical Lesson at the Salpêtrière) by Brouillet, showing Charcot and a hysterical patient with a hand dystonia. (From Goetz CG, Bonduelle M, Gelford T. *Charcot: constructing neurology.* New York: Oxford University Press, 1995.)

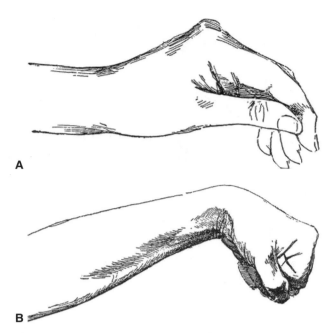

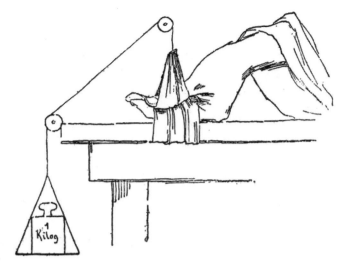

Figure 1.6 Differentiating hysterical contractures from simulation. Charcot used the experimental apparatus shown with respiratory monitoring attached to the chest to show that hysterical patients maintained their contractures in spite of a weighted stress without changing respirations whereas the simulating subjects fatigued and respirations became irregular.

Figure 1.5 Hand contractures and abnormal postures seen in hysteria. Charcot emphasized that the hand was held in a manner atypical of organic lesions **(A)** and often the fist was clenched intensely **(B)**. Drawings by P. Richer.

emphasized that *chorea* was derived from the Latin root for "dance" and therefore considered predictable cadence and rhythm to be the true hallmarks of chorea (2). In this context, rhythmic chorea of hysteria was the archetype of true chorea. Charcot found that patients with this diagnosis developed highly specific occupational movements, like swimming motions, hammering stereotypies, egg-whipping gyrations with the arm, or a rhythmic and alternating foot pattern that resembled gypsy dances as seen in the Andalusian region of southern Spain (Fig. 1.7). Some patients did incessant sit-ups or rhythmic movements that in other contexts would be normal, complex behaviors but that were clearly pathologic because of their intrusive and disabling nature (Fig. 1.8).

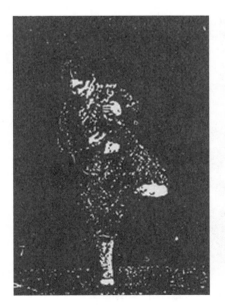
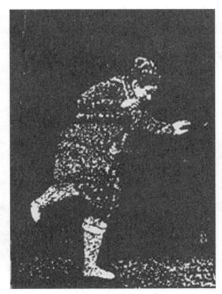
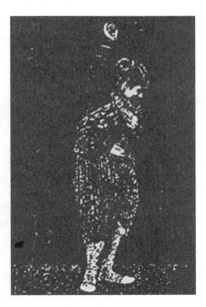

Figure 1.7 Hysterical rhythmical chorea. Time-lapse sequential photographs of a subject showing repetitive dancing movements that in Charcot's words resembled the patterns of Andalusian gypsies. Photographed by A. Londe. (From Charcot J-M. *De l'hystérie-épilepsie. Oeuvres complètes, t.1.* Paris: Bureaux du Prosres Medical, 1872:367–385.)

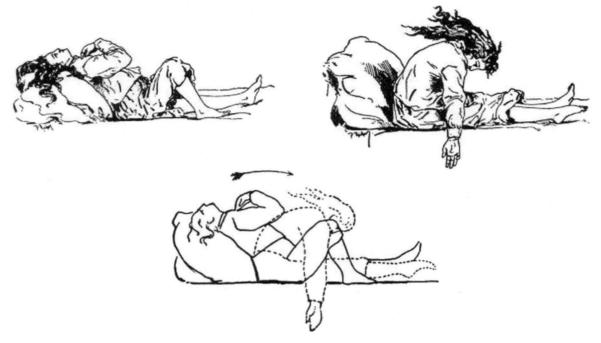

Figure 1.8 Hysterical rhythmical chorea. Incessant sit-up stereotypy of a patient with hysteria. Drawing by P. Richer. (From Charcot J-M. *De l'hystérie-épilepsie. Oeuvres complétes, t.1.* Paris: Bureaux du Prosres Medical, 1872:367–385.)

The most exotic of the movement disorders involved the celebrated *arc-en-cercle* opisthotonic posturing that occurred in the context of hystero-epileptic spells (10). Typically portrayed in images of women, the phenomenon occurred in men as well (Fig. 1.9). In contrast to many other forms of hysterical movement disorders, these exotic movements occurred as isolated episodes usually lasting minutes to hours and were so characteristic of hysteria as encountered at the Salpêtrière that the patient displaying this behavior was diagnosed hysterical without further consideration.

HYSTERIA AND PSYCHOLOGICAL INFLUENCES: THE ROLE OF SUGGESTION

To study hysteria in an experimental setting, Charcot invoked two previous observations: first, the close temporal link between hysterical signs and an event involving emotional stress or minor physical trauma; and second, the facility by which physicians could hypnotize hysterical patients. Whereas the emotional stresses recounted by hysterics were of a wide variety and included fear, abandonment,

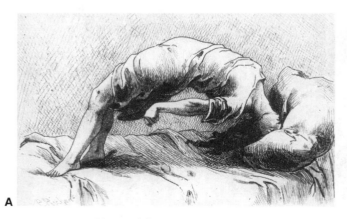
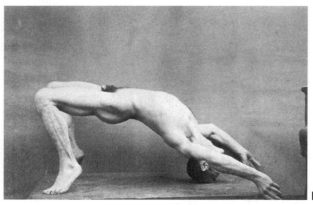

Figure 1.9 The celebrated, exotic opisthotonic posturing (*arc-en-cercle*) seen as part of hysteria and specifically hystero-epilepsy. Although most patients with this behavior were women **(A)**, the movement disorder syndrome also occurred in men **(B)**. (From Goetz CG, Bonduelle M, Gelfandt. *Charcot: constructing neurology.* New York: Oxford University Press, 1995.)

and intense passion (13), cases involving minor trauma were more homogeneous and became a particularly rich resource for study. Charcot was a consulting physician for the national railroad company and hence evaluated a large number of patients who endured injuries in the context of their work. Though there were many serious injuries, Charcot was impressed with the number of neurologic cases seen after seemingly inconsequential physical trauma (16). The neurologic signs among these latter railway workers included weakness, anesthesia, or spasms that fit best into the category of hysteria. Charcot dispelled the historical bias that hysteria occurred only in women and effeminate young men. Discussing this point in his classroom of predominantly male doctors, he stated:

Male hysteria is not at all rare, and just among us, if I can judge from what I see each day, these cases are often unrecognized by even distinguished doctors. One can concede that a young and effeminate man might develop hysterical findings after experiencing significant stress, sorrow or deep emotions. But that a strong and vital workman, for instance, a railway engineer, fully integrated into the society and never prone to emotional instability before, should become hysteric—just as a woman might—this seems to be beyond imagination. And yet, it is a fact—one that we must get used to. Such was the case with so many other ideas today so universally accepted because they are founded on demonstrable evidence; but for so long, they met only skepticism and sarcasm—it is only a matter of time (18).

Basing his diagnosis on the criteria for hysteria outlined above, Charcot considered the medical literature from England where railway accidents were of particular public and medical concern. He also discovered the writing of the Englishman J. Russell Reynolds (1826–1896), who greatly influenced Charcot with his 1869 article "Paralysis and other disorders of motion and sensation dependent on idea (19)." Charcot invariably cited this paper as the founding contribution for his own school's work on hysteria and emotional suggestion. On the basis of this writing, Charcot considered that emotional stress or a minor traumatic event could provoke focal neurophysiologic alterations in the brain with resultant neurologic impairments in hysterics. Repeated thoughts of the original inducing event could somehow unleash the same physiologic dysfunction that, repetitively, in Charcot's words, "for want of a better term, we designate *dynamic or functional lesions* (12)." Charcot's term for this latter construct was *autosuggestion*. Charcot's perspective, however, remained always founded in neuroanatomy:

I have lightly struck the man's shoulder. In his case, as with any particularly predisposed neurologic subject, this minor trauma, this focal jolt, is sufficient to induce throughout his entire arm, a feeling of numbness and heaviness, the essence of paralysis; by the means of autosuggestion, this trace paralysis rapidly becomes complete. It is within the center controlling psychologic processes, by that I mean within the cerebral hemispheres, that the phenomenon clearly takes place (10).

In parallel, with these ideas of autosuggestion Charcot had begun work on hypnotism at the Salpêtrière. He was impressed that hysterics were easily hypnotized and during a trance, the physician could induce or dissipate hysterical signs by suggestion (10). This construct integrated well with the observations of autosuggestion and led Charcot to propose that suggestion, whether internally or externally generated, must play a pivotal role as an *agent provocateur* for the unleashing of the dynamic, physiologic lesions underlying typical hysterical symptoms. Whereas original provoking forces may have been external in the form of stress or trauma and could still affect the patients as in an experimental setting of hypnosis, autosuggestion accounted for the spontaneous and self-perpetuating spells. (20). In the view of the Salpêtrière school, hysteria and a proclivity to hypnosis thereby became interchangeable. The Charcot classroom and hospital ward became an experimental laboratory where repeated hypnotic inductions allowed Charcot and his students to study the gamut of hysterical signs and their phases of development (1). Speaking of the most dramatic of episodes, termed hystero-epilepsy, characterized by a climax of opisthotonos posturing and often contractures (Fig 1.9), Charcot exclaimed to his students in the midst of a patient demonstration:

Now, here we have the epileptoid phase. Remember this sequence—epileptoid phase, arched back, then vocalizations. The arched back that you now see is rather pronounced. Now here comes the phase of emotional outbursts that fuses with the back arching, and now there is a contracture phase (17).

Charcot's work with hypnotism brought him both fame and condemnation (1). Many neurologists of the day dispelled these demonstrations as theatrical maneuvers of no scientific value and considered the exotic disorders seen at the Salpêtrière to be too frequent and too unusual to be independent of Charcot's own charisma. Disputes occurred over the requisite link between hysteria and hypnotism. Throughout this late period, covering the end of the 1880s up to his death in 1893, Charcot found his work on hysteria eroding on all fronts: the unquestioned acceptance of dynamic nervous system lesions, the categorical hereditary etiology of neurologic disorders, the role of autosuggestion to hysteria, and the pathognomonic hypnosis–hysteria link (21).

In the final years of Charcot's life he produced very limited writing to clarify his final stand on hysteria as a neurologic entity, but the few documents that do exist suggest considerable self-questioning and the recognition of the need to reformulate his thinking (22). The first is a passage written after Charcot's death by his late assistant Georges

Guinon in his reflective essay *Charcot Intime* (23). Describing his meeting with Charcot the night before his teacher left on the summer vacation from which he never returned, Guinon recounted that Charcot considered his original concept in need of full revision. No indication of the type of needed revamping is provided, but the passage clearly indicates that the topic of hysteria remained of intense interest to Charcot and that new work was envisioned. The second line of evidence is more valuable because it is written by Charcot himself and comes from a brief preface that he wrote for a monograph by his colleague A. Janet (24). Though he alludes to the idea casually, as if readers could find extensive documentation elsewhere in his writings, in fact the short passage is the only clear indication of Charcot's pivotally new consideration of mental or psychiatric links with hysteria:

> These works confirm a point of view that I have oftentimes expressed—which is that hysteria is for the most part a mental illness. This particular aspect of the disorder should not be neglected, if one wants to understand and treat hysteria (24).

Within Charcot's extensive publications and formal texts on hysteria, no statement alludes directly to a seminal shift toward mental or psychiatric causative roles of hysteria. Even though a number of Charcot's later lectures on hysteria approached topics that could be considered in the realm of mental disorders, double personalities, and, very unusually, forms of amnesias, he retained his neuroanatomic perspective (25). As a group, although the collective evidence suggests that Charcot may have been moving toward ideas that would today be considered closely linked to a true psychogenic cause of neurologic signs, documentation is insufficiently clear to establish a solid argument that Charcot's thinking ever fundamentally changed.

The last monograph that Charcot wrote was called *Faith-cure*, published originally in English and later translated back into French for publication as *La Foi qui Guérit* (26). In this essay Charcot considers the pilgrimages that took place annually at Lourdes and examines how patients whom the traditional medical system had failed to cure find within themselves the capacity to heal through faith. As a positivist and anticleric, Charcot spent no time on a discussion of divine intervention but approached these "miracles" medically as examples of cure through autosuggestion. It is not a treatise specifically on hysteria, but within the context of the continuing tradition of pilgrimages to Lourdes, many modern neurologists may consider cases healed of parkinsonism, tremors, tics, or dystonic contractures during such events at Lourdes to be psychogenic. The text is significant to Charcot's work on hysteria because, in this case, he deals with autosuggestion as a means of self-therapy and cure, not as a means to precipitate disease.

CHARCOT AND FREUD: THE MENTOR'S NEVER SATED OBSESSION

Much has been written about the relationship between Sigmund Freud's seminal psychoanalytic works on the causes of diseases and his mentorship by Charcot (6,21, 25). This relationship, however, should not be overinflated. Freud came to Paris for a short period in 1885 to study neuropathology with Charcot, and there he witnessed Charcot's demonstrations of hysteria, participated in hypnosis sessions, and interacted with the circle of collaborators working on hysteria. Freud's diaries clearly confirm that this period of study with Charcot was a turning point in his career, and the exposure was immeasurably important to his later development of psychoanalytic theory (1,25). Freud's pivotal identification that each patient's stress has symbolic importance and that this stress is actually at the origin of psychogenic neurologic or other signs may have indeed been inspired by these Salpêtrière experiences, but there is absolutely no indication that these conclusions originated with Charcot himself. Clearly, Charcot's neurologic emphasis precluded any particular concern over the type or nature of the provoking stimulus to hysterical spells. As such, because Freud's fundamental contributions are so related to the symbolic importance of stress, it is historically inaccurate to ascribe to Charcot the role of Freud's pivotal predecessor in this domain. As Gelfand points out:

> … it is simply anachronistic to assimilate Charcot to the genealogy of psychoanalysis constructed by Freud and dutifully repeated by generations of his followers where he tends to appear as a kind of John the Baptist figure announcing the coming of Freud (1).

Freud's novel focus on the meaning behind the stressful events related to hysteria launched him on an independent path, leaving Charcot still searching for neuroanatomic lesions. Charcot's student, Ballet, described his teacher as "haunted by the preoccupation (27)" to find the pathologic underpinnings of hysterical hemiplegia, as he continued to pose the question: "There is without doubt a lesion in the nervous centers, but where is it situated, and what is its nature (8)?" Modern specialists dealing with psychogenic movement disorders may ask if we are any closer than Charcot to answering these anatomical questions. New functional imaging techniques provide researchers with direct tools to examine Charcot's putative dynamic lesions and to test his hypothesis that physiologically based alterations, perhaps comparable to those associated with placebo-related improvements, in fact occur in psychogenic disorders (28). The studies described in the subsequent chapters of this volume will help to place Charcot in the modern context of research in psychogenic movement disorders and will consider issues developed by him and related to genetic predisposition and physiologic changes that underlie the manifestations unveiled by patients in this neurologic category of diseases.

REFERENCES

1. Goetz CG, Bonduelle M, Gelfand T. *Charcot: constructing neurology.* New York: Oxford University Press, 1995.
2. Goetz CG. *Charcot, the clinician: the Tuesday lessons.* New York: Raven Press, 1987.
3. Goetz CG. The father of us all—Jean-Martin Charcot: neurologist and teacher. In: Rose FC, ed. *Neuroscience across the centuries.* London: Smith-Gordon, 1989.
4. Charcot J-M. Leçon d'ouverture. *Oeuvres complètes, t.3.* Paris: Bureaux du Progrès Médical, 1887:1–22.
5. Micale M. Hysteria and its historiography: a review of past and present writings. *Hist Sci.* 1989;27:223–261,319–351.
6. Gelfand T. Sigmund-sur-Seine: fathers and brothers in Charcot's Paris. In: Gelfand T, Kerr J, eds. *Freud and the history of psychoanalysis.* Hillsdale, NJ: Analytic Press, 1992:29–57.
7. Charcot J-M. De la paralysie agitante. *Oeuvres complètes, t.1.* Paris: Bureaux du Progrès Médical, 1872:155–188.
8. Gilles de la Tourette. Étude sur une affection nerveuse caractérisée par l'incoordination motrice accompagnée d'écholalie et de copralalie. *Arch Neurol.* 1886;9:19–42,158–200.
9. Charcot J-M. Tremblements et mouvements choréiformes: chorée rhythmée. *Oeuvres complètes, t.3.* Paris: Bureaux du Progrès Médical, 1887:215–228.
10. Charcot J-M. *Leçons du mardi á la Salpêtrière.* Paris: Bureaux du Progrès Médical, 1887–1888.
11. Goetz CG. Amyotrophic lateral sclerosis: early contributions of Jean-Martin Charcot. *Muscle Nerve.* 2000;23:336–343.
12. Charcot J-M. Sur deux cas de monoplégie brachiale hystérique de nature traumatique chez l'homme. *Oeuvres complètes, t.3.* Paris: Bureaux du Progrès Médical, 1887:315–343.
13. Charcot J-M. De l'hystérie-épilepsie. *Oeuvres complètes, t.1.* Paris: Bureaux du Progrès Médical, 1872:367–385.
14. Charcot J-M. De l'influence des lésions traumatiques sur le développement des phénomènes d'hystérie local. *Presse Méd.* 1878;4:335–338.
15. Charcot J-M. De l'ischurie hystérique. *Oeuvres complètes, t.1.* Paris: Bureaux du Progrès Médical, 1872:275–299.
16. Charcot J-M. Deux cas de contracture hystérique d'origine traumatique. *Oeuvres complètes, t.3.* Paris: Bureaux du Progrès Médical, 1887:97–124.
17. Charcot J-M. Tic non-douloureux de la face chez une hystérique. *Oeuvres complètes, t.3.* Paris: Bureaux du Progrès Médical, 1887:47–50.
18. Charcot J-M. À propos de l'hystérie chez l'homme. *Oeuvres complètes, t.3.* Paris: Bureaux du Progrès Médical, 1887:253–280.
19. Russell JR. Certain forms of paralysis depending on idea. *BMJ.* 1869;2:378–379;6:483–485.
20. Charcot J-M. Deux nouveaux cas de paralysie hystéro-traumatique. *Oeuvres complètes, t.3.* Paris: Bureaux du Progrès Médical, 1887:441–463.
21. Widlocher D, Dantchev N. Charcot et l'hystérie. *Rev Neurol.* 1994;150:490–497.
22. Goetz CG. The prefaces of Charcot: leitmotifs of an international career. *Neurology.* 2003;60:1333–1340.
23. Guinon G. Charcot intime. *Paris Méd.* 1925;56:511–516.
24. Charcot J-M III. Préface. In: Janet P, ed. *État mental des hystériques: les stigmates mentaux.* Paris: Rueff, 1892.
25. Gelfand T. Becoming patrimony: when, how and why Charcot got into hysteria. In: Goetz CG, ed. *History of neurology: Jean-Martin Charcot.* Minneapolis, MN: American Academy of Neurology Publ. 1993:53–68.
26. Charcot J-M. Faith-cure. *New Review.* 1892;11:244–262.
27. Ballet G. La domaine de la psychiatrie. *Presse Méd.* 1911;10:377–380.
28. De la Fuente-Fernandez R, Ruth TJ, Sossi V, et al. Expectation and dopamine release: mechanism of the placebo effect in PD. *Science.* 2001;293:1164–1166.

2

Freud and Psychogenic Movement Disorders

W. Craig Tomlinson

ABSTRACT

Freud, a neurologist and neuroscientist by training, became interested in hysteria initially as a student of Jean-Martin Charcot in the 1880s. Although Freud was hardly alone among his contemporaries in his interest in the psychogenic nature of hysteria, through his contact and work with Josef Breuer in the 1880s and 1890s, he developed a theory that went far beyond the ideas of his contemporaries, specifying the mechanism of psychogenesis of hysterical symptoms. This paper sketches the development of Freud's notions about hysterical symptomatology, touching on developments in psychoanalysis since Freud. It will also suggest that the historical evolution of Freud's interest in psychogenic symptomatology—from the study, early in his career, of the more florid hysterical symptoms that characterize psychogenic movement disorders, to more subtle forms of neurotic conflict as his theory evolved—was in part responsible for a legacy of overreaching by psychoanalysts after Freud.

...there exists the fact, inaccessible through mechanical understanding, that simultaneously to the mechanically definable excited state of specific brain elements, specific states of consciousness, only accessible through introspection, *may* occur. The actual fact of the connection of changes in the material state of the brain with changes in the state of consciousness, even though [this fact is] mechanically incomprehensible, makes the b[rain] the organ of mental activity. Even if the nature of the connection is incomprehensible to us, it is itself not lawless, and, based upon combinations between experiences of the external senses on the one hand and internal introspection on the other hand, we are able to state something about these laws. If a specific change in the material state of a specific brain element connects with a change in the state of our consciousness, then the latter is entirely specific as well; however, it is not dependent on the change in the material state alone *whether* or not this connection occurs. [Freud, 1888, transl. (1,2)]

In the late nineteenth century, the ailments now classified by neurologists as psychogenic movement disorders and by psychiatrists as subtypes of conversion disorders were regarded as symptom complexes falling under the broader rubric of hysteria. Thought by many historians of psychiatry to have been a far more prevalent illness than now (3), hysteria was inarguably a topic of enormous medical and broad cultural interest at the time in Europe and North America. Freud, a neurologist and neuroscientist by training, became interested in hysteria initially as a student of Jean-Martin Charcot in the 1880s. Among his contemporaries, Freud was hardly alone in his interest in hysteria; Pierre Janet, among many others, was deeply interested in the subject (3–5). But it was through his contact and work with Josef Breuer in the 1880s and 1890s that Freud developed a theory that went far beyond the ideas of his contemporaries, specifying the mechanism of psychogenesis of hysterical symptoms. Although Freud's theory continued to evolve substantially over the next half century, some key notions in Freud's mature theory were concepts of unconscious conflict and fantasy, a dynamic unconscious, repression, defense, and the notion of infantile sexuality.

With the apparent epidemiologic decline of hysteria in the early decades of the 20th century, as well as the internal development of his own theory, Freud's focus on hysterical symptomatology also gradually shifted toward other forms of psychogenic symptomatology, primarily including inhibitions, anxiety, and character pathology. Freud and his followers, however, often continued to interpret hysterical motor symptoms in much the same way as they interpreted all psychogenic symptoms: as related to conflict and psychological defense.

This paper will briefly sketch the development of Freud's notions about hysterical symptomatology, commenting also on developments in psychoanalysis since Freud. I will also suggest that the historical evolution of Freud's interest in psychogenic symptomatology—from the study, early in his career, of the more florid hysterical symptoms that characterize psychogenic movement disorders to more subtle forms of neurotic conflict as his theory evolved—was in part responsible for a legacy of overreaching by psychoanalysts. This overreaching proceeded along at least two principal lines: In emulation of Freud's early interpretive style and the dramatic symptoms it addressed, 20th century psychoanalysts often presumed psychological causes for both psychogenic and organic disorders, and interpreted them in order to construct an apparently coherent illness narrative even without adequate data. Furthermore, they often assumed (in accordance with Freud's earliest, but later superseded, theories of psychotherapeutic action) that simple explication of a previously repressed experience by the physician ("making the unconscious conscious") would constitute an effective psychotherapeutic treatment. This double error contributed to both poor therapeutic results and widespread skepticism about psychoanalytic theory and practice.

The earliest unequivocal assertion that a patient's life history is the source of hysterical symptomatology is to be found as early as 1888 in Freud's article on hysteria for Villaret's medical encyclopedia (6). Shortly after returning from his studies with Charcot in Paris, Freud makes reference to the new method of Breuer in treating hysteria: to "lead the patient under hypnosis back to the psychical prehistory of the ailment and compel him to acknowledge the psychical occasion on which the disorder in question originated (7,8)." This new method of treatment, Freud stressed, not only produced "successful cures" otherwise unobtainable, but was the method most appropriate to hysteria because it "precisely imitates the mechanism of the origin and passing of these hysterical disorders (7,8)." This was a radical statement for this time, when hysteria was largely regarded (by Charcot and Janet, among others) as determined by hereditary degeneration. (Today we make essentially the same etiologic case when we assign responsibility to "genetic factors.")

In Freud's early studies of the 1890s, under the twin influences of Charcot and Breuer, he emphasized the role of trauma in hysteria. In asserting that psychical trauma was the basis of all hysteria, Freud was already departing from Charcot's notions of traumatic hysteria. Freud emphasized

that hysterical symptoms had to be explained in patients who had not suffered *physical* traumas at all (7,9). Making use of Breuer's earliest psychotherapeutic techniques at this point, such as questioning under hypnosis, Freud formulated his first crucial postulate:

> *There is a complete analogy between traumatic paralysis and common, non-traumatic hysteria.... In the latter there is seldom a single major event to be signaled, but rather a series of affective impressions—a whole story of suffering* (7,9).

But Freud went still further at this point, citing a number of case histories from his collaborative work with Breuer (*Studies on Hysteria*) to conclude that:

> ...the phenomena of common hysteria can safely be regarded as being on the same pattern as those of traumatic hysteria, and that accordingly every hysteria can be looked upon as traumatic hysteria in the sense of implying a psychical trauma, and that every hysterical phenomenon is determined by the nature of the trauma (7,9).

Furthermore, and interestingly always with the aid of hypnosis, once the traumatic event could be remembered and put into words *along with the accompanying affect,* the symptom would disappear. In clinical practice, Freud found that the memory would often be reproduced with extraordinary vividness, and the affect accompanying it was as intense as it had been during the original traumatic event.

Thus was born the famed cathartic cure, which was the basis of Freud and Breuer's work of the late 1880s and early 1890s. Of interest to the present audience, Freud addressed the question of how affective memory is created and either "worn away" or preserved intact:

> If a person experiences a psychical impression, something in his nervous system which we will for the moment call the sum of excitation is increased. Now in every individual there exists a tendency to diminish this sum of excitation once more, in order to preserve his health. The increase of the sum of excitation takes place along sensory paths, and its diminution along motor ones. So...it depends on this [motor] reaction how much of the initial psychical impression is left.... For quite slight increases in excitation, alterations in his own body may perhaps be enough: weeping, abusing, raging, and so on. The more intense the trauma, the greater is the adequate reaction.... If however, there is no reaction *whatever* to a psychical trauma, the memory of it retains the affect which it originally had.... We have found that in hysterical patients there are nothing but impressions which have not lost their affect and whose memory has remained vivid...observation shows that, in the case of all the events which have become determinants of hysterical phenomena, we are dealing with psychical traumas which have not been completely abreacted, or completely dealt with. Thus we may assert that hysterical *patients suffer from incompletely abreacted psychical traumas* (7,9).

For Freud, trauma involved an excess of stimulus. As he was to revise his theory over the next decade, that excess could be driven not only by external events but *by their interaction with inner experience*, including personality, fantasies, wishes, and fears. He was also to dramatically revise his theory of treatment: In the passages cited above, Freud held to the "abreaction" or cathartic cure. His clinical work, however, would gradually show him that more often, what patients require is more painstaking and time-consuming: namely, as he later put it, remembering, repeating, and working through of emotionally traumatic experience in therapeutic dialogue with another.

It is useful in this context to pause for a few moments on the topic of psychoanalytic clinical technique, which had powerful roots in 19th century hypnosis. Though the phenomenon of hypnosis was a topic of widespread public interest in the 18th century and its use was common in medical circles by the last decades of the 19th century, it was not until Hippolyte Bernheim that the phenomenon was decisively regarded as psychogenic in origin, as opposed to magnetic or physiologic (6). It was also Bernheim who proposed that hypnosis was *not* localizable to a particular brain function. It is easy to forget today that Freud used hypnosis and more active techniques extensively in his early work, not only hypnosis but directed concentration and focusing, active questioning, applying pressure to a patient's forehead, or even physical examination and the physical contact that went with it. Even the theoretical concept of "resistance," which in psychoanalysis would come to refer to a defensive operation by the patient, had its origins in patients who *resisted* hypnosis and suggestion. The actual clinical technique of Freud's early work was a far cry from the cold, detached, and silent stereotype of the Freudian analyst that later developed.

Freud and Breuer's technique did evolve during the time they treated the patients mentioned in the *Studies on Hysteria* to include one history-making innovation: the technique of free association, or asking patients to rigorously say whatever comes to mind, however silly, unrelated, embarrassing, or shameful. By eschewing hypnosis, directed questioning, and the distractions of suggestion that both entailed, Freud and Breuer's new technique of free association introduced a way of allowing patients to share their inner experience more intimately, and offered doctors a way to listen to patients more profoundly, than ever before. For one thing, even the shifts and transitions are often clues: Freud's work on dreams, among other things, led him to the notion that emotional processes in human beings are governed by a form of thinking and a language that does not function in the way that governs ordinary adult language and most of our logical, orderly conscious thought. Emotions, after all, develop richly in infancy and childhood, long before we have all of these adult cognitive abilities. What he called "primary process," the language of dreams and unconscious fantasy, involved thinking by affect-linked association, and assemblage of narratives—like a dream sequence—based on these associations. Hence, for Freud, a dream does tell a coherent story, if you read it as a rebus of associations to thoughts, feelings, and wishes. And what drives dream formation is the same kind of thinking that structures much of the waking emotional experience of human beings as well, normal and pathologic alike.

Freud would considerably refine these concepts in dealing with hysterical and other psychiatric symptoms he encountered in the following decades. But by the period between the first and second World Wars, analysts were already noting a shift in the symptomatology they were seeing. In place of the more dramatic symptoms of hysteria, they were seeing patients with more complex and subtle character problems: inhibitions in work, chronic problems in relations with others, emotional volatility or coldness, feelings of worthlessness and inferiority, and so forth (10). In part as a logical further development of Freud's theory, in part to meet this challenge, psychoanalysis also evolved its theoretical underpinnings. Beginning in the teens, Freud became much more interested in what we would today regard as character and personality formation: identifications with crucial figures in a person's life, responses to loss, or a person's strategies for warding off anxiety, depression, and other painful feelings.

These evolving clinical concerns drove the momentous shift inaugurated by Freud's introduction of his second or structural theory in the 1920s. That theory, which focused on the ego and its defenses against both internal and external threats, remains the cornerstone of modern psychoanalytic practice. Freud's new interests went hand in hand, however, with a dramatic shift of attention *away* from conversion disorders. In fact, Freud wrote essentially nothing about hysteria after 1910 (11). His interests in the final three decades of his life simply lay elsewhere. When we reflect that most of Freud's theoretical and clinical development and the bulk of his major writings came after this point, we have a startling development indeed: Since psychoanalysts in the following decades tended to rely overwhelmingly on the chapter and verse of Freud's writings, when they dealt with hysteria they clung to Freud's earliest theoretical formulations.

So if psychoanalysts did not abandon hysteria and psychosomatic illness altogether in the early decades of the 20th century, they tended to rely on some of Freud's earliest theoretical models when approaching it. Their springboard, following *early* Freudian theory, was a psychoanalytic theory in its initial stages and one that lacked much of the subtlety and clinical refinement of later psychoanalytic treatment. An example is Georg Groddeck, the self-styled "wild analyst" (he was really something more like the court jester in Freud's early circles), who began asserting in the early 1920s that *all* organic illnesses were physical expressions of unconscious emotional conflict (5). This is perhaps the clearest early pure expression that we have of psychoanalytic grandiosity in dealing with somatic disorders, such as the psychogenic movement disorders that are the subject of the conference on which this book is based. Groddeck's stance was unfortunately somewhat fateful, for some of the later history of psychosomatic medicine followed in his footsteps, interpreting wildly whether the illnesses were psychosomatic or organic. It is useful in this context to recall the later commentary of the psychoanalyst Sandor Rado, who noted that the oft-cited fear of Freud and other psychoanalysts of becoming simply the "handmaidens of psychiatry" actually represented the reverse: a grandiose wish on the part of psychoanalysis to swallow up all of the rest of medicine (12).

The impact of Freudian notions on concepts about psychogenic somatic disorders from this point, however, is also part of the larger history of psychosomatic medicine in the 20th century. That history has been succinctly summarized by the historian Theodore Brown as "the rise and fall of American psychosomatic medicine (13)." Perhaps the most crucial figure in setting the stage for this story would likely give an ambivalent wince to be so defined; Adolf Meyer was an enormously important figure in the history of the relationship between psychoanalysis and American medicine. Meyer, installed as chair of psychiatry in the newly founded Johns Hopkins Medical School, was the pre-eminent American academic psychiatrist in the first half of the 20th century and enormously successful in promoting the cause of psychiatry in the United States. As an outspoken advocate of what he termed "psychobiology," he campaigned stridently to erase false distinctions between the mental and physical, integrating psychiatry with other medical disciplines and with research in a way no one had before him (13,14).

Although he remained throughout his life an interested skeptic and never altogether accepted psychoanalysis, Meyer was also a crucial figure in the introduction of psychoanalysis in America and a keen observer and commentator on its development (14). Meyer's trainees would run departments throughout the country, and some, like Macfie Campbell and Franklin Ebaugh, sought actively to increase the role of psychiatry in the practice of internal medicine. Already with powerful advocates within medicine like Lewellys Barker, who was William Osler's successor at Hopkins and took a prominent interest in reviving the study of functional nervous disorders, the Meyerian enterprise and interest in psychogenic factors in medical illness exploded during the 1920s and 1930s (13). Walter Cannon, the eminent American physiologist, became absorbed in the study of how profoundly emotions affect physiology and organic functioning. Cannon published his *Bodily Changes in Fear, Hunger, Pain and Rage* in 1934, and two years later delivered the lead address to the American College of Physicians on "The Role of Emotion in Disease (13,14)." Flanders Dunbar's seminal work in the emerging psychosomatic field, *Emotions and Bodily Changes*, was also published in 1935 (13). As Theodore Brown has argued, these developments also coincided with an enormous move in American medical education (in part as a rebellion against Osler) to put the "whole person as a patient," including humanism and psychology, firmly back into the center of medical education, culminating in George Canby Robinson's efforts in the 1930s at Johns Hopkins (13).

With this powerful beginning, then, what happened to American psychosomatic medicine? It has been argued that its decline was precipitated by the explosion of biologic research and its fragmentation into specialized biologic fields, coupled with a decline in the interest and influence of psychoanalysis (13). But it is also arguable that from within the psychosomatic school itself, a heady enthusiasm that turned into arrogance was equally responsible for its decline. It is my belief that the developments of this period are one of the most important roots of the widespread disaffection with psychoanalysis within medicine (and a good deal of psychiatry) today. For in their naiveté and enthusiasm, the pioneers of psychosomatic medicine committed some of the most egregious overreaching in the history of psychiatry. Beginning in the 1920s with Groddeck, analysts began interpreting symbolic meaning to "visceral" illnesses, developing a theory of what they called "pregenital conversion" and interpreting unconscious mental conflicts at the source of virtually any physical symptom: ulcers, asthma, cardiac disease, and even the common cold (10). As the pre-eminent historian of American psychoanalysis, Nathan Hale, has observed, "the rhetoric of psychoanalytic psychosomatic medicine moved from diffidence to dogmatism" over the course of the 1930s and 1940s (10). Whereas Freud by and large had restricted himself, when interpreting a symbolic meaning, to the more dramatic somatic symptoms found in hysteria—like gait disturbances in the Dora case [see (15)]—his followers did not. At the same time, they managed to distance themselves from medicine and most importantly, from the research enterprise as well as their neighboring fields in the social sciences.

This kind of psychosomatic dogmatism coincided with a period of extreme theoretical dogmatism in American psychoanalysis itself, and by the 1950s American psychoanalysis was firmly in the grip of an orthodoxy that tolerated no dissent, even internally (14). Where there is no dissent in a field in which by its very nature data collection is subjective, problematic, and open to manipulation, there are no controls on overreaching and presumption, and social control of the professional and scientific organizations responsible tend to be reduced to oligarchy. This unfortunate history, particularly in its organizational ramifications, has recently been richly documented by Douglas Kirsner (16).

Otto Fenichels' enormously influential *Psychoanalytic Theory of Neurosis*, for example, published in 1945, was relatively cautious in its treatment of psychosomatics. However, its tone is telling. Fenichel treated the subject with flat decrees: not only (following Freud) that "motor paralysis is a defense against action," but "a spasm is a means of securing suppression of action, and simultaneously a tonic substitute for action"; or, a "contracture is a displacing substitute for an intended but inhibited muscular innervation. It usually represents the tonic rigidity which is the result of a struggle between opposing impulses (17)." Fenichel boasted confidently that "the prognosis of psychoanalysis in cases of conversion neuroses is favorable. In typical cases, the course of the treatment is especially satisfactory, in so far as the patients react immediately to interpretations with alterations in transference and symptomatology (17)." Would that it were that simple. In hindsight, Fenichel would be regarded by analysts today as adhering to absolute models of drive theory and symbolization.

These developments had another source arising from internal political struggles within American psychoanalysis itself. For roughly the first half of the 20th century, American psychiatry and psychoanalysis continued to distinguish themselves from their European counterparts by building and retaining a strong connection with each other. This began to change around mid-century as the result of a ferocious political struggle within organized psychoanalysis. The faction of psychoanalysis that saw its future as allied with medicine, research, and integration into a university setting lost this internal power struggle decisively and, arguably, disastrously. So today it is the task of historians to resurrect, for example, Franz Alexander's clear and full insistence on a complete biopsychosocial model of psychiatric illness in 1938 (decades before Engel, credited as the modern creator of that model). To quote Alexander from 1938:

> …instead of remaining an isolated discipline, with a specific object, method, and way of thinking which were shunned by all the other sciences, psychoanalysis has become more and more a part of medicine in so far as it is a therapy, and a part of social science in so far as it deals with human interrelationships. At the same time psychoanalysis has assumed a more scientific character…the interest in the theoretical superstructure of psychoanalysis has gradually given place to an emphasis upon the observational foundations of our field. The need for detailed and reliable records of analytical material to facilitate the rechecking of the findings by other observers and also to make possible a careful comparative microscopic study of this recorded material, has been clearly recognized…. The number of men in different fields of science who thoroughly understand the fundamental principles of psychoanalysis and who at the same time feel the need for more precise and even quantitative tests of psychodynamic formulations is growing steadily. Such a critical attitude is fundamentally different from the former uncritical prejudice which was definitely destructive because it rejected scientific evidence (18).

As I have argued elsewhere (14), some of the consequences of an inadequate integration of psychoanalytic organizations into academic medical and university-based research institutions, to the detriment of both, were predicted almost a half century ago by Sandor Rado, a psychoanalyst who had been powerfully influenced by Adolf Meyer. Rado, with Meyer's backing, had founded the first psychoanalytic institute within a university department and academic medical center at Columbia in 1945; he and his colleagues, however, remained somewhat ostracized within the politics of mainstream American psychoanalysis. The post-Meyerian viewpoint they represented all but vanished in a ferocious political controversy within American psychoanalysis (14).

To return to the topic at hand: Freudian theory is clearly now in a period of relative decline, not only within medicine and neurology but within our culture at large; this decline certainly also has reflected powerfully on the way that clinicians and researchers regard psychogenic movement disorders. I have tried to suggest some of the background leading to a situation in which some of the highly useful, even irreplaceable tools we have for understanding psychogenic disorders have been mishandled, misunderstood even by their practitioners, and isolated from research in neighboring disciplines like neurology and neuroscience. True, this decline has recently been offset by some recent examples of neuroscience research incorporating modern psychoanalytically informed theory and practice more than a century after Freud and Breuer's initial discoveries. And whether we know it or not, we subscribe to the one truly fundamental Freudian principle whenever we actually seek to *listen* profoundly to these patients and attempt to understand their experience and suffering. Freudian theory at its core assumes that a patient's experience and symptoms have either primary or at least secondary meaning, and that this can only be discovered by listening. I have argued both here and elsewhere that Freudians themselves share the blame for their loss of stature and for the fact that "Freudian theory" remains in the minds of many equated with the long-outmoded and non-essential hypotheses of a bygone era. Arguably, this history is one source of our continuing lack of understanding of psychogenic syndromes; for if we want to understand and provide help to patients with these complex, bedeviling, and frustrating afflictions, we will need to avail ourselves of all the tools at our disposal—and integrate them—when we seek to understand not only these disorders themselves, but the individuals who suffer from them in all their human complexity.

REFERENCES

1. Freud S. "Gehirn." [Brain]. Article in A. Villaret, *Handwörterbuch der gesamten medezin.* Stuttgart: Enke Verlag, 1990:1888–1891 (2 vols.); transl. Solms and Saling. London: The Hogarth Press, 1962.
2. Solms M, Saling M. *A moment of transition: two neuroscientific articles by Sigmund Freud.* Translated and edited by Solms M, Saling M. London: Institute of Psychoanalysis. London and New York: Karnac Books. 1990.
3. Micale MS. *Approaching hysteria: disease and its interpretations.* Princeton: Princeton Univ. Press, 1995.

4. Ellenberger H. *The discovery of the unconscious.* New York: Basic Books, 1970.

5. Gay P. *Freud: a life for our time.* New York: W.W. Norton & Company, 1988.

6. Reicheneder JG. *Zum konstitutionsprozess der psychoanalyse.* Stuttgart: Frommann-Holzboog, 1990.

7. Freud S. *The standard edition of the complete psychological works of Sigmund Freud.* London: The Hogarth Press, 1962.

8. Freud S. The neuro-pyschoses of defence. *Standard edition.* London: The Hogarth Press, 1962:1894:45–61.

9. Freud S. On the psychical mechanisms of historical phenomena: a lecture. *Standard edition.* 1893:27–39.

10. Hale NG, Jr. *The rise and crisis of psychoanalysis in the United States.* New York: Oxford University Press, 1995.

11. Freud S. The psycho-analytic view of psychogenic disturbance of vision (1910). *The standard edition of the complete psychological works of Sigmund Freud.* London: The Hogarth Press; 11: 209–218.

12. Roazen P, Swerdloff B. *Heresy: Sandor Rado and the psychoanalytic movement.* Northvale, New Jersey and London: Jason Aronson Inc, 1995. Edited from interviews with Rado, 1964.

13. Brown T. "The rise and fall of American psychosomatic medicine," lecture given at the New York Academy of Medicine, November 29, 2000. Available at http://human-nature.com/free-associations/riseandfall.html. Accessed 6/10/04.

14. Tomlinson WC. Sandor Rado and Adolf Meyer: a nodal point in American psychiatry and psychoanalysis. *Int J Psychoanal.* 1996; 77:963–982.

15. Gottlieb R. Psychosomatic medicine: the divergent legacies of Freud and Janet. *J Am Psychoanalytic Assoc.* 2003;51:857–881.

16. Kirsner D. *Unfree associations: inside psychoanalytic institutes.* London: Process Press, 2000.

17. Fenichel O. *The psychoanalytic theory of neurosis.* New York: W.W. Norton & Company, 1945.

18. Alexander F. Psychoanalysis comes of age. *Psychoanal Q.* 1938; 7:299–306.

Military and Mass Hysteria

3

Ian P. Palmer

ABSTRACT

Hysteria and mass hysteria are as old as war itself. Debate about their origins has been informed by conflict through the ages. Hysteria may be described as an unconscious symptom or symptom complex that exists in a social system for personal gain at a primary, secondary, or tertiary level. Given the implication of gain, and the fear of "contagion," hysteria is an anathema to all armies given the ubiquitous issues of medically unexplained symptoms, illness deception, and malingering. It will interfere with an army's ability to undertake its mission and may put others' lives at risk, especially during conflict when individual needs must be subordinated to the needs of the group. At times, however, it is possible that hysteria, or dissociative phenomena, may lead to acts of great self-sacrifice and heroism. The study of military psychiatry highlights the importance of contextualizing any presentations in social and cultural terms.

BACKGROUND

Armies exist to fight, not go to the hospital. Since military medical officers are primarily occupational physicians, they are required to view hysteria from both the individual and sociocultural perspective, particularly during military operations when group needs outweigh those of the individual; if it were otherwise, no army could fight (1).

Becoming ill is a social process that requires confirmation by others (2). Sick roles are a negotiation among the individual, doctors, employers, and society. These roles conform to cultural mores and norms, and are shaped by issues of class, gender, and the language of distress (e.g., the post-trauma dialectic). Issues of genuineness are also part of this negotiation and soldiers' illness behavior is open to differing interpretations. Within the strictures of military life and law, commanders are frequently presented with "misbehavior" and must question whether individuals are responsible for their actions. Commanders will contextualize the timing of a soldier's behavior, that is, why now? What has precipitated it? What will be the impact of this behavior in the individual and the unit? However, when civilians examine military cases, it should be remembered that they will view the case from a civilian paradigm, often in retrospect, from safety and without knowledge of military culture, or understanding or consideration of the responsibility the individuals have for their peers, subordinates, and superiors at the time of their initial presentation.

Objective signs of mental illness or disease may be stigmatized, especially those thought to be disingenuous, or when no organic cause can be found, for example, medically unexplained symptoms which may be diffuse [fatigue, muscle, and joint pains, sweats, memory difficulties, illness, (mis)behavior], or specific symptoms such as paresis, blindness, aphonia, amnesia, or fugue states (3). In a fashion similar to shellshock, the mental condition of posttraumatic stress disorder (PTSD) is currently not stigmatized (4).

Military commanders frequently feel doctors encourage soldiers to seek their discharge through "delinquency and avoiding responsibility for their actions" (5), or by "aiding" or encouraging malingering through their shameful use of "battle fatigue" (includes hysteria, shellshock, neurasthenia, etc.) as an excuse for cowardice (6,7).

Thus, the study of hysteria in a military culture requires attention be paid to its bedfellows: medically unexplained symptoms, illness deception, and malingering (8). Military psychiatry tells us that attention must be paid to the socio-cultural aspects of these diagnoses which lie at the borderline between many boundaries, for example: self/group/society; biological/psychological/social/cultural; disease/illness; neurological/psychiatric; real/imagined; objective/subjective (9). Without understanding and training in military psychiatry, disentangling malingering from shellshock, hysteria, and organic conditions has proven problematic, more so the closer the observer is to any combat action (10). Acute mental illness and malingering are most likely to appear at times of great social upheaval and stress. They are thus commonest in armies that are losing. At such times, group integrity and preservation is of paramount importance and internal threats are more feared than are external ones (11).

Whatever triggers hysteria, it is different in times of peace and war. Like courage, military commanders believe fear and mental breakdown are contagious. During the First World War, the pioneering English psychologist/doctor W.H.R. Rivers (12) believed that the process of enlistment, acculturation, and rigid discipline heightened suggestibility among soldiers, thereby predisposing recruits to hysterical breakdown. Any mental breakdown is an anathema to military culture, ethos, values, and norms, as it interferes with the mission and can put others at risk, both physically and psychologically. Individuals' failure to discharge the duties in accordance with their given rank is rightly judged harshly by peers, superiors, and perhaps most importantly, by subordinates. Such failure is likely to be seen as self-seeking, shameful, and selfish, given the acculturation involved in enlistment. Opprobrium is more likely when individuals do not "fit in" or have not "pulled their weight." Breakdowns must be earned. Furthermore, individuals inappropriately labelled and/or managed may be at risk of long-term incapacity and disability, particularly if a pension is granted.

Armies naturally cultivate the warrior paradigm based on concepts of chivalry and maleness in which self-control, comradeship, altruism, endurance, courage, and stoicism are valued as nowhere else in Western societies. Maleness is fostered and shaped through the use of shame sanctions (13) and where failure to function, and to do one's duty (social role), at whatever level, is a severe stigma due to which all ranks go to great lengths to avoid being seen to fail. At the outset of the First World War, such failure could lead a British soldier to either a court-marshal or lunatic asylum, possibly forever.

COMBAT

The first mention of the link between combat and hysteria is from the Battle of Marathon in 490 BC, where brave behavior on the battlefield was followed by a permanent symptom without physical explanation (14).

The Russo-Japanese War of 1904–1905 produced the first clear records that mental breakdown could occur during and after combat. That such breakdowns had a substantial social component to them was revealed by the observation that soldiers who remained close to the front line and to their units recovered better than those evacuated back to Moscow, a journey of about two weeks. Hysterical symptoms following gassing from Japanese grenades were noted and the thread of this remains in "modern" mass hysteria and societal anxieties triggered by foul smells. The debate in Continental Europe was furthered in 1907 and 1911 when examination of survivors and rescuers involved in explosions on the French vessels *Iéna* and *Liberté* revealed emotional change (nervous disturbance). Before World War I, the debate about the unconscious mind was predominantly Continental, involving Charcot, Janet, Freud, Babinski, and Pavlov. In Britain and the United States, this dialectic was anathema for many, given its sexual content (15).

The history of hysteria is a microcosm of the history of military psychiatry. The history of military psychiatry is one of amnesia, of lessons forgotten. The study of hysteria in soldiers in the First World War became a major catalyst in the widening debate in Britain about the unconscious mind and intra-psychic sequelae of external, traumatic events. Before the First World War, hysterical cases presenting with physical symptoms were seen in all wars and were treated as organic. Psychological breakdown was unheard of outside the psychoses; indeed, to label a soldier as "mad" meant permanent incarceration under the Lunacy Act. Psychological symptoms were either socially constructed or genetic (inherited degeneracy); the debate is not new.

The historic records reveal inconsistent disease classifications; idiosyncratic definitions and medical practice; varying psychological-mindedness; and understanding and empathy in doctors leading to diagnostic confusion and differing conclusions (16,17). Care must therefore be taken with this history as the variations of symptoms reported are due to the personalities of the observers, the places of observation, the variability of material, and so forth. In combat, few minor casualties reach base hospital and gross disorders often develop only in the safety of the hospital (18). Furthermore, First and Second World War data take no account of those with learning difficulties, which were common in the generally unselected conscripts.

Cases of hysteria were occurring from August 1914. In December 1914, one doctor wrote that his soldiers were "at risk of being diagnosed hysterical;" after all, hysteria was a disease of women or "foreigners," not true "Brits," particularly the British volunteer soldier. How, then, were they to be dealt with? Given the lack of psychological understanding and education, and the development of neurology as a new medical subspecialty, cases of hysteria with gross motor and sensory deficits were viewed as organic, treated as such, and evacuated to the U.K. with other medical and surgical cases. Although less stigmatizing, it was not long before doctors and patients were joined in a battle of wills in their management.

World War I was the first "industrial war." It was a war of stasis in which conscript soldiers were herded together and subjected to intense, inescapable bombardment including shockwaves, shrapnel, and entombment, unless, that is, a doctor was willing to evacuate them. While an organic label may allow collusion between doctor and soldier in order to protect the soldier from the stigma of a psychiatric label, it runs the risk of creating iatrogenic damage or valetudinarianism. We must also remember that many medical diseases are not stigma-free, for example, cancer, HIV/AIDS, tuberculosis, and skin diseases. By 1916, the doctors of the Royal Army Medical Corps had become, by default, the moral arbiters of whether a soldier was mad or bad, but only during and after the Battle of the Somme was psychiatric input clearly sanctioned, breakdowns having reached epidemic proportions.

The treatment of mental breakdowns before 1916 was thus organic in nature, involving evacuation to U.K. investigation, rest, and sympathy. After 1916, most cases were kept in France as close to the front as safe and treated by "suggestion." An individual of high social standing, for example, a doctor in a white coat, would attempt to persuade the soldier to return to duty by appeals to his loyalty, culture, duty, and so on, possibly augmenting it with hypnotism or faradism.

WHAT ARE THE COSTS OF DIAGNOSING HYSTERIA?

My fear is that excessive effort expended in the search for an organic cause may create iatrogenic harm. Before we see patients, we must consider what has happened to them and seek out their beliefs. What problems have they encountered with doctors and others before this referral? What do they want and what is an acceptable outcome for all parties? Doctors should undertake a developmental history with focus on childhood deficits, abuses, and neglects, including illness perceptions and behaviors in the individuals, their parents, and siblings. Military psychiatry shows us that we must contextualize our patients' presentations and be aware of the role played by politicians, the law, and media, for both good and evil.

Feigning illness is behavior indulged in by all ranks in all armed forces of all nations. It is one method soldiers have of trying to control their environment; results may be positive or negative for the individuals or their groups (19). With advances in medical science, it is more difficult to feign physical conditions, and while individuals still shoot themselves in the foot, they are more likely to present vague multisystem, nonspecific, subjective symptoms.

In addition, there is less stigma attached to mental illness—hence the tendency to feign psychiatric disorders. In the U.S. Veterans Administration system, malingering of PTSD is now believed to be common (20).

The financial cost to the nation may be measured in pensions. The most common cause of medical separation from the British and U.S. armies in the First and Second World Wars was mental illness, and in 1938, the pension bill for such was still rising in the United Kingdom. The current debate (21,22) about pensions for combat-related mental illness contains many of the elements of the debates about hysteria, that is, the belief that mental symptoms are increasingly easy to feign and either the patient is malingering or the psychiatrist has been duped, or, worse still, they are in collusion. Substantial and long-term financial costs will emanate from the medicalization of distress. Costs to the individual include the stigma of a psychiatric label and becoming a pawn in media/political activity.

If hysteria were to be destigmatized in society (23,24), would the army follow suit? I believe not. Enlistment and acculturation is a complex and dynamic process in the profession of arms, where group membership requires an extensive psychological investment from individuals if the benefits of the group are to be gained; to "fit in" is all, and exclusion a most powerful sanction. Given the mutual interdependency of fighting groups, those who break down in circumstances where others do not are unlikely to be trusted in future tight spots. This is true even if hysteria is found to be organic in nature; an individual would not be employable as a soldier. Furthermore, how will soldiers' responsibility for their actions be negotiated if hysteria is diagnosed?

MASS HYSTERIA

Contagion may be positive or negative, and is the key issue in mass hysteria. Contagion is a major threat to an army, as it may increase individuals' and an entire unit's risk of annihilation, and will diminish a unit's ability to complete its mission.

Hysteria may reveal itself covertly through refusal of vaccinations, with the attendant health risks, or more overtly, as happened in the First World War, when fear of chemical attack produced "gas hysteria" in frontline troops. The positive aspects of contagion are, however, nurtured in armies, namely, leading by example, courage, altruism, and the like. For those interested, there is a sociopolitical science of contagion and minority influence (25,26) that aims to quantify how determined individuals influence larger groups.

Instances of epidemic or mass hysteria have been recorded throughout history (27) and can affect all classes and age groups, although the young are felt to be more vulnerable. Historically, they have occurred after disasters such as plagues, famines, war, and civil disturbance. Mass hysteria is culturally specific behavior in which a whole group expresses exaggerated emotions in concert and in response to societal dilemmas. Themes change with time and have included "possession," poisoning (food, air), environmental toxins (miasmas, sick buildings), and vaccinations. Olfaction is a potent trigger in releasing powerful emotions, linked as it is to the paleoencephalon.

Episodes are more likely where there is an "institutional" atmosphere of constraint or stress in which a number of dissatisfied individuals act as a nidus in the process. Such individuals are usually of a higher status, real or imagined, than the majority and often have a background of emotional disturbance. Contagion spreads from high- to low-status individuals, particularly in closed and tightly knit groups. The beliefs expressed by the instigators are acceptable to the group and are further reinforced by acceptance. Generally, those most dissatisfied in any group are more likely to be affected.

Episodes of epidemic hysteria in industrial environments occur in situations where the nature of work is repetitive, boring, or routine, or where the physical environment is uncomfortable, noisy, smelly, dirty, too hot, or too cold, and the air quality is poor. In addition, psychological stressors such as poor management and pressure of targets add to the predisposing factors. Negative reactions to physical and social environments seem to be the most important factors in the genesis of this hysteria (28).

Simon Wessely (29) has proposed that such hysterical episodes may be divided into mass motor and anxiety hysterias. In the motor variety, any age group may be affected; prior tension is present, spread is gradual, and the outbreak may be prolonged. Abnormalities in personalities and environments are common. In the anxiety variety, spread is visual and rapid, occurs in schoolchildren, and resolution is equally rapid when individuals are separated from the source of contagion.

We may, therefore, predict that epidemic hysteria is more likely to occur in situations where there is (i) homogeneity of population, perhaps unified by circumstance and threat; (ii) isolated small groups with shared belief systems; (iii) younger individuals, for example, recruits; and (iv) some sort of predisposition in group members of higher status.

Epidemic hysteria may be easier to manage than an individual case. Management includes the discouragement of alarm and is achieved through the action of leading by example, quarantining those involved, reassurance through the provision of information from those of status in the community affected, and wherever possible, media control (30).

REFERENCES

1. Palmer I. War based hysteria—the military perspective. In: Halligan P, Bass C, Marshall JC, eds. *Contemporary approaches to the study of hysteria—clinical and theoretical perspectives.* Oxford: Oxford University Press, 2001.
2. Helman CG. *Culture, health and illness.* London: Wright, 1990:94.
3. Gilman S. *Disease and representations: from madness to AIDS.* Chichester: Wiley, 1982.
4. Devine PG. Stereotypes and prejudice: their automatic and controlled components. *J Pers Soc Psychol.* 1989;56:5–18.
5. Ahrenfeldt RH. *Psychiatry in the British army in the Second World War.* London: Routledge & Keegan Paul, 1958:103.
6. Patton GS. *War as I knew it.* Boston, MA: Houghton Mifflin, 1947:381–382.
7. Townsend JM. Stereotypes and mental illness: a comparison with ethnic stereotypes. *Cult Med Soc.* 1979;3:205–230.
8. Cooter R. Malingering and modernity: psychological scripts and adversarial encounters during the First World War. In: Cooter R, Harrison M, Sturdy S, eds. *War, medicine & modernity.* Stroud: Sutton Publishing, 1998:125–148.
9. Palmer I. Malingering, shirking & self-inflicted injuries in the military. In: Halligan P, Bass C, Oakley D, eds. *Malingering and illness deception.* Oxford: Oxford University Press, 2003.
10. O'Connell BA. Amnesia and homicide. *Br J Delinquency.* 1960; 10:262–276.
11. Flicker DJ. Sedition: a case report. *Psychiatr Q Suppl.* 1947;2(22): 187–199.
12. Rivers WHR. War neurosis & military training. *Ment Hyg.* 1918; 4(2):513–533.
13. Miller WI. *The mystery of courage.* Cambridge, MA: Harvard University Press, 2000.
14. Merskey H. Combat hysteria. In: *The analysis of hysteria. Understanding conversion and dissociation.* London: Gaskell, 1995.
15. Binneveld H. *From shellshock to combat stress. A comparative history of military psychiatry.* Amsterdam: Amsterdam University Press, 1997.
16. Myers CS. *Shellshock in France.* Cambridge: Cambridge University Press, 1940.
17. Whitehead IR. The British medical officer on the western front: the training of doctors for war. In: Cooter R, Harrison M, Sturdy S, eds. *Medicine and modern warfare* (Clio Medica S). Amsterdam/Atlanta, GA: Editions Rodopi B.V, 1999:163–184.
18. Ritchie RD. *One history of shellshock.* PhD Dissertation. San Diego: University of California, 1986.
19. Harrison M. Disease, discipline and dissent: the Indian army in France and England, 1914–1915. In: Cooter R, Harrison M, Sturdy S, eds *Medicine and modern warfare.* (Clio Medica S). Amsterdam/Atlanta, GA: Editions Rodopi B.V., 1999:185–203.
20. Carroll MF. Deceptions in military psychiatry. *Am J Forensic Psychiatry.* 2001;1(22):53–62.
21. Owen J. *Multiple Claimants v MoD. 21 May 2003. Copies available from Royal Courts of Justice, Mechanical Recordings Dept. Send/fax request on headed paper and copy [free of charge] will be forwarded.* Fax. 0207 947 6662; Tel. 0207 947 6362.
22. Braidwood A, ed. Psychological injury. Understanding and supporting. *Proceedings of the Department of Social Security. War Pensions Conference 2001.* London: The Stationary Office, 2001.
23. Mehta S, Farina A. Is being sick really better? Effect of the disease view of mental disorder on stigma. *J Soc Clin Psychol.* 1997; 4(6):405–419.
24. Porter R. Can the stigma of mental illness be changed? *Lancet.* 1998;352:1049–1050.
25. Penrose LS. *On the objective study of crowd behaviour.* London: H.K. Lewis, 1952.
26. Moscovici S, Mugny G, van Avermaet E, eds. *Perspectives on minority influence.* Cambridge: Cambridge University Press, 1985.
27. Merskey H. Epidemic or communicable hysteria. In: *The analysis of hysteria. Understanding conversion and dissociation,* London: Gaskell, 1995.
28. Colligan MJ, Murphy LR. A review of mass psychogenic illness in work settings. In: Colligan MJ, Pennebaker JW, Murphy LR, eds. *Mass psychogenic illness: a social psychological analysis.* Hillsdale, NJ: Lawrence Erlbaum Associates, 1982:33–55.
29. Wessely S. Mass hysteria: two syndromes? *Psychol Med.* 1987; 7:109–120.
30. Kelman HC, Hovland CI. Reinstatement of the communication in delayed measurement of attitude change. *J Abnorm Soc Psychol.* 1953;48:327–335.

The History of Psychogenic Movement Disorders

4

Stanley Fahn

ABSTRACT

Psychogenic movement disorders are part of the spectrum of a host of psychogenic neurologic disorders. Originally referring to these disorders as hysteria, neurologists began describing the various clinical phenomenological appearances of such disorders. Early on, tremors, convulsions, paralysis, and sensory complaints were recognized as sometimes being due to hysteria. Hysterical spasms and contractures were also recognized, and today these could be interpreted as manifestations of psychogenic dystonia. For about 100 years, from the mid-19th century until the mid-20th century, hysteria was a common feature in neurological textbooks. Not only were there discussions on etiology, but also extremely important were details on how neurologists could recognize which symptoms and signs were due to hysteria. By the mid-20th century, there was little written about psychogenic disorders in neurology textbooks as a discrete topic. Rather, these would be discussed in the specific section in which each neurologic disorder was covered, so, for example, psychogenic seizures would be covered in the section dealing with epilepsy.

After torsion dystonia was recognized as a neurological entity almost 100 years ago, different etiologies of dystonia were recognized, but eventually many cases of both generalized and focal dystonias were thought to be psychogenic. Then the pendulum swung, and it was thought that psychogenic dystonia rarely occurred. We are probably shifting into better awareness that psychogenicity can be a cause of all varieties of movement disorders. We need to learn how to recognize these disorders, because mistaking an organic disorder as a psychogenic one, and vice versa, sets back the appropriate treatment for patients.

INTRODUCTION

The term "hysteria" was the commonly used name for all psychogenic disorders, both neurologic and nonneurologic manifestations, until only recently, when terms such as "functional," "nonorganic," "psychogenic," and several others began to be used. Perhaps the switch was because "hysteria" became a pejorative word, and terms more acceptable to patients were desired. Whether "psychogenic" should be the preferred term is debatable, and is the subject of subsequent discussions in this book. Its use has the advantage that it emphasizes an etiologic cause of the disorder, one coming from the psyche.

The term "functional" might be more acceptable to patients, as well as to neurologists and psychiatrists who are evaluating the patient and prefer not to confront the patient and family members with the etiologic term psychogenic. But "functional" had been used by early neurologists and psychiatrists not only to refer to a psychogenic disorder, but also to one due to abnormal physiology rather than physical structural deficits, such as those that might come from trauma, tumors, and infection. For example, Putzel's monograph dedicated solely to common functional nervous diseases (1) has chapters on chorea, epilepsy, neuralgias, and peripheral paralysis. Bastian, an English neurologist at the National Hospital in London and slightly older than Gowers, condemned the practice of using the terms "hysterical" and "functional" synonymously (2). Bastian maintained that "if hysteria were defined as a neurosis in accordance with the views of Charcot and Briquet, then all cases of functional spinal paralysis should be placed in some other category" (30). Thus, the term "functional" could result in ambiguity, at least in terms of trying to distinguish between its current and past meanings. If the objection to using "psychogenic" is because of concern that the patient and family would react negatively to this term, then perhaps explaining that the symptoms are due to an altered brain physiology and not to a structural problem of the nervous system would satisfy. At a later time, when the clinician feels more comfortable, the term "psychogenic" can be introduced to emphasize the etiologic nature of the symptoms.

"Medically unexplained symptoms" as a substitute term has a vagueness that implies the clinician could not come up with an acceptable diagnosis. There are certainly medical conditions that are difficult to classify or in which there is considerable controversy on their etiology—reflex sympathetic dystrophy and chronic fatigue syndrome are two examples—and these could be listed as medically unexplained symptoms. But if psychogenesis is the etiology, why not use the term "psychogenic," even though there remains unexplained the physiology in the brain that underlies most cases?

In reviewing the history of psychogenic movement disorders, one needs to look back and determine what early neurologists and psychiatrists were referring to when they discussed hysteria. Hysterical paralysis and sensory loss (including blindness) have been known probably back in antiquity, and had been discussed before the era of Charcot and Freud, two well-recognized neurologists who gave considerable thought to the study of hysteria. In this review we will obtain an understanding of psychogenic movement disorders by studying neurology textbooks written in the 19th and early 20th centuries. This review is limited to English-language books. This is unfortunate because some of the great scholars of hysteria were French, such as Charcot and Briquet. Nevertheless, the Anglophones do offer us a perspective on the evolving thoughts of neurologic manifestations due to a psychogenic etiology. Thus, such a review provides us a perspective as to how today's views of psychogenic movement disorders came to be.

Topics to be discussed in this chapter will seek to answer the following questions. When were psychogenic abnormal movement phenomenologies first recognized? Were any movement disorders that are now recognized as organic at one time considered to be psychogenic? When were psychogenic movement disorders fully appreciated as a major differential diagnosis to be considered when evaluating

patients with a movement disorder? After reviewing 19th and early 20th century English-language neurology textbooks to learn what clinical features were considered hysterical and how the diagnosis was made, I will review more modern texts, but those that were published before the field of movement disorders evolved into a subspecialty. Finally, I will review developments in psychogenic movement disorders after the field became a subspecialty. One should keep in mind that many neurologists until the mid-20th century were both neurologists and psychiatrists, a feature of the close relationship between these two specialties in the early development of both fields. These neuropsychiatrists had considerable interest in hysteria, and the textbooks up to about 60 years ago elaborated considerably on their ideas of the causation of hysteria.

DESCRIPTIONS OF HYSTERIA IN 19TH CENTURY TEXTBOOKS OF NEUROLOGY

In one of the earliest textbooks of clinical neurology translated into English, Romberg (3) comments mainly on ideas of etiology, and does not provide much on the description of the clinical neurologic features seen in hysteria. He briefly mentions paroxysms, spasms of different body parts (including globus hystericus and trismus), and movements ranging from tremor to convulsions. Thus, seizures, tremor, and sustained muscle contractions (i.e., dystonia) were recognized by him to occur in patients with hysteria.

In "the first textbook on nervous diseases in the English language" (4), Hammond (5) devoted a full chapter to the topic of hysteria and presented several references, including that of Briquet (6), whose writings were influential to the field. The particular neurologic phenomena mentioned by Hammond can be divided into (a) sensory (hyperesthesia, anesthesia, pain), (b) motor weakness (paralysis, paraplegia, aphonia); and (c) abnormal movements (clonic spasms simulating chorea, tonic spasms, convulsions, globus hystericus, and tetanoid paroxysms). Hammond did not mention hysterical tremor. Although Hammond states that clonic spasms simulated chorea, today one would probably consider such clonic spasms to more likely be classified as dystonia with patterned movements of the spasms.

Hysteria as a cause of neurologic symptoms must have become fairly common because subsequent 19th century neurology texts also have chapters exclusively covering hysteria in varying degrees of detail. Wilks (7) has a fairly extensive section, but deals mainly with his ideas on etiology and behavior, and presents only anecdotal descriptions of some of his cases. He does mention pain, analgesia, and seizures. An English translation of Duchenne (8) devotes a small chapter to hysterical paralysis, concentrating on faradic stimulation of the affected muscles.

In his book covering lectures on localization of signs and symptoms of neurologic problems, Gowers (9) mentions in discussing hysteria, "there are few organic diseases of the brain that the great mimetic neurosis may not simulate." He emphasizes that one must not make a diagnosis of hysteria without first excluding organic disease. He also provides some general principles characteristic of hysteria, such as onset after emotion, increase on attention, grave symptoms of one type that will cease suddenly and be replaced by others which could not result from the same organic cause as the first, and differences in the symptoms of hysterical origin from the corresponding symptoms of organic disease. In this short section on hysteria, Gowers gives some "pearls" relating to hemiplegia, contractures, reflexes, spurious clonus, ocular convergence, hemianesthesia, ptosis, aphonia, and convulsions.

In a neurology textbook with chapters written by American authors and edited by Pepper and Starr, there is a very large chapter on hysteria written by Mills (10), followed by a second chapter by him on "Hystero-Epilepsy." Mills wrote a very thorough review, including a discussion of the historical development on the concept of hysteria. He mentions that the Catalog of the Surgeon-General's Library of 1885 lists up to 318 books and 914 journal articles on hysteria, dating back to references from Hippocrates. Mills states that the greatest work on the subject is that of Briquet (6), and in America the most prominent authority was Weir Mitchell. Mills gives a marvelous historical treatise on hysteria in his chapter. Dancing mania occurred in various mass hysterical outbreaks affecting children in Europe in 1237, 1278, 1374, and 1418. The last occurred in the chapel of St. Vitus in Strasburg. The name St. Vitus' dance was given to this condition, which later got transposed to the choreic disorder described by Sydenham, now known as Sydenham chorea. Dancing mania has continued into more modern times. Mills mentions that the New England "witchcraft" incidences were considered to be episodes of epidemic hysteria and hystero-epilepsy. Mills considered hysterical symptoms to be of four categories: (i) symptoms that are involuntary; (ii) symptoms that are artificially induced and then become involuntary; (iii) symptoms that are acted or simulated, but because of impaired mental power, are irresistibly performed; and (iv) symptoms that are purely acts of deception under the control of the patient. Neurologic hysterical phenomena described by Mills are convulsions, paralysis, aphonia, gait ataxia, chorea, rhythmical chorea, tremor, contractures, local spasms, and sensory phenomena, especially anesthesia. What he was describing as rhythmical chorea is not clear, for chorea today is considered as random brief contractions that tend to flow from one body part to another.

Gowers (11) had a large section devoted to hysteria in his textbook, which I will describe in some detail. He divided the clinical manifestations into the continuous and the paroxysmal. He gave descriptions of a number of clinical phenomena, including globus hystericus (a feeling of something suddenly closing the throat and stopping the

breath), which when intense may have the pharynx in spasm; hysterical convulsions; a range of sensory symptoms; and motor symptoms. Of the last, paralysis was most common, and can involve limbs and cranial muscles, including the larynx (mutism and aphonia). In terms of movement disorders, he mentioned ataxia of gait, as previously described by Briquet, and jerky voluntary movements. He mentioned spasmodic contractures that can even persist in sleep, that relax only with chloroform narcosis, and if continued over years, can lead to permanent contractures that are no longer responsive to chloroform. Today, these would be considered true contractures, whereas the use of the term in earlier textbooks would be considered sustained contractions. Trismus, paroxysmal rigidity, and tremor are other motoric features that would fit with psychogenic dystonia, paroxysmal dyskinesias, and tremor in today's classification. Gowers pointed out that hysterical tremor is rarely constant, but is usually evoked by movement and excitement, and tends not to appear on the initiation of the movement. He pointed out that such tremor differs from that of paralysis agitans (today known as Parkinson disease), while the fineness of the tremor differs from tremor of disseminated sclerosis, but not always. Hysterical tremor can involve the arms, legs, and head. Gowers also mentioned hysterical chorea and rhythmical movements. He further described symptoms that can involve the digestive, respiratory, urinary, and circulatory systems. In terms of diagnosis, Gowers emphasized that the most important diagnostic consideration is the absence of any unequivocal symptom of organic disease. The element of second importance is age and gender of the patient, for it was known from the work of Briquet (6) and Landouzy (68) that hysteria is most common in women, generally between the ages of 10 and 40, particularly in the teens.

Lloyd (12) wrote a large chapter on hysteria in the neurology textbook edited by Dercum that was filled with American authors. Much of Lloyd's efforts are similar to those discussed by prior authors. But Lloyd elaborates more on tremor, stating it is one of the most important motor stigmata of hysteria. But Lloyd associates it to trauma, alcohol, lead, and mercury, so it is not clear if he had distinguished between organic and psychogenic tremor. Lloyd also describes hysterical ataxia under the term of astasia-abasia, a term first attributed to Blocq.

Sachs (13), in his textbook on pediatric neurology, mentioned that hysteria is rare in adults and even rarer in children. He also stated hysteria is much less common in the United States, England, and Germany than in France and Russia. He divided clinical manifestations into three categories: (i) psychic (e.g., hysterical mania, epilepsy, and trances), (ii) motor (paralysis and spasms) and (iii) sensory (hyperesthesia and anesthesia). Like Gowers, Sachs emphasized that the diagnosis should be made only in case an organic affection can be positively excluded and if the symptoms are well recognized to fit that of hysteria.

Dana's textbook (14) also contains a chapter on hysteria. He divides the condition into hysteria minor and hysteria major. The former is characterized by the interparoxysmal state of emotional weakness, nervousness, hyperesthesia, and pains. There is no anesthesia or paralysis, and no convulsions. Hysteria major is characterized by the interparoxysmal manifestations of anesthesia, paralysis, contractures, tremors, peculiar mental conditions, and by paroxysms of an emotional, convulsive, or other serious nature. He includes prolonged attacks of coughing, hiccoughing, sneezing, and rapid breathing. Photographs of patients with so-called hysterical "contractures" resemble dystonia of the limbs. One cannot be certain that in these years prior to the first major description of organic dystonia (15,16), the condition as recognized today was not mistaken for a psychogenic spasm disorder.

DESCRIPTIONS OF HYSTERIA IN EARLY 20TH CENTURY TEXTBOOKS OF NEUROLOGY

Chapters on hysteria continued to be included in neurology textbooks published in the early part of the 20th century. In the chapter on hysteria in their textbook, Church and Peterson (17) describe the hysterical motor stigmata as being retarded, maladroit, and uncoordinated, with the inability to perform several acts simultaneously, weakness, and a tendency to rigidity and contractures. They also cover the sensory and convulsive phenomena. Of particular interest in this chapter are the reproductions of Richer's drawings of the various postures of hysterical seizures and movements; some of the tonic ones could be considered dystonia today (18).

Pearce (19) devotes a small section to hysteria in his textbook. It contains a helpful table comparing different features of organic and psychogenic seizures, but otherwise is rather scanty in its coverage of other phenomena of hysteria.

Ziehen (20), like a number of his predecessors, linked the etiology of hysteria for the most part to hereditary factors. It should be mentioned that Lloyd (12) was opposed to this view, and related hysteria to social factors. Ziehen elaborated on paralysis, contractures, and clonic spasms. But it appears that Ziehen did consider hemifacial spasms and facial tics as features of hysteria. This appears to be another example in which diseases recognized today as being organic could have been mistaken for hysteria a century or more ago. Ziehen expands on hysterical tremor and states that hysteria can take on any form of tremor, including rest and action tremor. Other motoric aspects covered in this chapter are hysterical chorea and incoordination.

Jelliffe (21) wrote a large chapter on hysteria for Osler's textbook of medicine. He reviews the history of hysteria from the time of Hippocrates, Pliny, Willis, and Sydenham up to his own time. Besides discussing views on etiology

(his own and those of others) of hysteria, Jelliffe describes clinical features, including rhythmic (e.g., tremor and coordinated impulsive movements) and arrhythmic movements (e.g., chorea and tetany). This is a thorough chapter, with coverage of epilepsy, weakness, and sensory disturbances.

In Oppenheim's English translation of the fifth edition of his textbook (22), he offers a fairly extensive coverage of hysteria, from etiology to clinical recognition to treatment. He describes rhythmically repeated stereotyped movements, including tremor, as well as hysterical contractures with fixed postures. He offers an interesting photographic contrast of the eyebrows in a patient with organic ptosis versus one with hysterical ptosis. He also reproduces drawings from Richer depicting various hysterical contractures. Oppenheim does seem to err in stating that blepharospasm is not an uncommon form of (hysterical) spasm and that torticollis may also appear on the basis of hysteria. He shows a photograph of a man with scoliosis when he is standing, but a straight back when he is lying prone. Oppenheim gives this as an example of hysterical scoliosis, but truncal dystonia characteristically can be present only in certain postures, particularly on standing and walking, while being absent when sitting or lying down. It is interesting that the "father" of dystonia (15) erred in depicting some symptoms as hysteria, when in fact they could be interpreted as organic dystonia today.

All in all, however, Oppenheim delivers a fairly elaborate clinical description of the types of hysterical manifestations that can be encountered in different parts of the body.

In the textbook of neurology by Starr (23), his chapter on hysteria continues to emphasize the hysterical temperament in some of the writings of earlier authors. Starr points out that the key to successful treatment is the susceptibility of these patients to suggestion. He also points out that if the physician is met by a spirit of opposition or doubt by the patient, the efforts will be useless. These observations continue to hold in today's climate, also. He recommended hypnotic suggestion treatment.

In the two-volume textbook on nervous and mental disease by White and Jelliffe, the British psychiatrist Jones (24) wrote a chapter on neurosis, in which he covered hysteria. There is little neurologic phenomenology in this chapter, and the emphasis is on the psychiatric aspects of neuroses and hysteria. Jones reviewed the treatment of hysteria, starting with the suggestion of the neurologist Weir Mitchell, who had promoted adherence to a specific diet. Jones emphasizes psychotherapy. Under the heading of suggestion, Jones expounds on hypnosis, suggestion during sleeping, persuasion, and side-tracking (diverting patients' attention as far as possible away from their symptoms and stimulating their interest in healthy activities). Jones, being a psychiatrist, covers many other aspects of psychiatric treatment including psychoanalysis.

In his textbook, Bing (25) devotes a chapter on the various neurologic manifestations of hysteria. He covers sensory, vasomotor, motor, and visceral symptoms, with larger sections on seizures, paralysis, and contractures. He makes valuable clinical points that the reflexes are never lost in the paralytic form, that ankle clonus is not present, but there could be pseudoclonus. He credits Oppenheim for pointing out that by holding a hysterically paralyzed extremity for some time in one's hand, sometimes the examiner can perceive occasional innervation impulses in the muscles, and if the limb is suddenly let loose, it is able to maintain a position for some time. Bing also brings to our attention the phenomenon of self-injury as a feature of hysteria.

Stewart (26), in his book, brings his experience as a World War neurologist to his extensive chapter on the "neuroses," mainly meaning psychogenic disorders. He emphasized that excluding an organic disease is insufficient to diagnose a neurosis, and that a secure diagnosis depends on finding characteristic positive phenomena. Another important point he makes is that hysteria is not willful and is "unconscious," in contrast to malingering. He also points out that hysteria and organic disease can coexist. In his chapter he equates neurasthenia to nervous exhaustion. He refers to hysteria as a suggestion neurosis, a disorder whereby symptoms can be reproduced by suggestion and can disappear by persuasion and suggestion. These are techniques used today in treating psychogenic disorders. Stewart amplifies his chapter with many photographs of hysterical motor features, including abnormal postures, astasia-abasia, paralysis, and spasms. Yet, one cannot be certain that the photo of "hysterical contractures of the left foot" is due to a psychogenic or an organic dystonia. The chapter provides extensive coverage of the examination of hysterical features and how to recognize many of them. Stewart has a separate chapter on war-neuroses. It is in this chapter that he mentions hysterical tremor.

The final chapter in the textbook of Wexler (27) is devoted to the neuroses. He covers ideas on mental mechanisms, etiology, and classification. Much of the clinical description is about personality and a number of neurologic phenomena, but not much on how to distinguish signs that are psychogenic from organic. He does not mention psychogenic tremor.

By the middle of the 20th century, neurology textbooks became less likely to have chapters devoted to hysteria. The large tome by Ford (28) on childhood neurology and the two- and three-volume epics of Wilson (29,30) do not contain chapters on hysteria, neuroses, or psychogenic disorders. The 1951 textbook of Nielsen (31) has a small chapter on hysteria, but Merritt's textbook of 1955 (32) and later editions through 2005 (33) do not. Hysteria and psychogenic neurologic disorders are largely restricted to the neurological examination and to the differential diagnoses of different neurological signs in today's teaching of neurology. The multivolume, multiauthored texts, for example, Bradley et al. (34), give only a few paragraphs on the topic of hysteria. The emphasis today is on organic diseases,

including molecular and genetic aspects of neurology. Yet, psychogenic neurology, including movement disorders, continues to be a common presenting problem, and is likely not diminished in frequency over time. Possibly patients have more sophisticated symptoms as they have more access to medical writings and viewing of patients with organic diseases.

SPECIFIC PSYCHOGENIC MOVEMENT DISORDERS BEFORE MOVEMENT DISORDERS BECAME A SUBSPECIALTY

Some specific movement disorders were the focus of certain clinical publications emphasizing that these disorders could be due to a psychogenic etiology. For example, Leszynsky (35) wrote a paper on hysterical gaits, and as seen in the above discussion of neurology textbook chapters, gait disorders are prominent in the discussion of hysteria. Even today, psychogenic gaits are a common manifestation of psychogenic movement disorders (36). Tics, on the other hand, were clearly felt by Meige and Feindel (37) not to be due to hysteria. Although the overwhelming numbers of patients with tics are not considered psychogenic in origin, Williams et al. (36) reported two patients with psychogenic tics. Dooley et al. (38) described two children with Tourette syndrome who also had pseudotics, and in whom the psychogenic movements resolved when the stressful issues in their lives were addressed.

Psychogenic tremors, which have been described from ancient times, were the subject of what the author described as the world's shortest paper. Campbell (39) emphasized that psychogenic tremor is most pronounced when attention is paid to it, and is least when the patient is diverted to another subject (i.e., distraction).

Torsion dystonia may be the most common organic movement disorder that has been misdiagnosed—both before and after the term was first used by Oppenheim (15)—as being psychogenic, whereas most cases are organic (40). Although it might be understandable why the bizarre movements in the children in a family reported by Schwalbe (41) in his medical thesis would be called hysterical, even after torsion dystonia was later described as an organic disease (16), cases with dystonia were being called psychogenic. For example, it was not uncommon for patients with torticollis to be considered to have their symptom due to a psychiatric problem and to be treated with behavioral therapy (42–44). Cooper and his colleagues (45) reviewed their series of 226 patients with torsion dystonia and found that 56 (25%) had a diagnosis of psychogenic etiology at some time during their illness. Lesser and Fahn (46) reviewed the records of 84 patients with idiopathic dystonia seen at Presbyterian Hospital in New York from 1969 to 1974 and found that 37 (44%) had been diagnosed previously that their movement

TABLE 4.1
REPORTS ON THE MISDIAGNOSIS OF DYSTONIA AS BEING PSYCHOGENIC

Marsden and Harrison, 1974 (47)	18/42 (43%)
Eldridge et al., 1969 (48)	23/44 (52%)
Cooper et al., 1976 (45)	56/226 (25%)
Lesser and Fahn, 1978 (46)	37/84 (44%)

abnormalities were due to an emotional disorder. These 37 patients consisted of 11 with generalized dystonia, 14 with segmental dystonia, and 19 with focal dystonia (14 with torticollis, 2 with oromandibular dystonia, and 3 with blepharospasm). Table 4.1 reveals the percentage of dystonic patients seen by several groups who had previously been misdiagnosed as being psychogenic. Somewhere between 25% and 52% of dystonic patients at one time or other had been mistaken for having a psychiatric condition.

On the obverse side, some psychogenic movement disorders are probably misdiagnosed as organic disorders. Probably the movement disorders with the highest prevalence rate of a psychogenic origin are the nonfamilial, so-called idiopathic, nonkinesigenic paroxysmal dyskinesias, as surveyed by Bressman et al. (49). They found that of 18 patients with paroxysmal dystonias, and with no known symptomatic etiology or positive family history for a paroxysmal dyskinesia, 11 were due to psychogenic causes. This represents 61% of such cases. The age at onset in these patients ranged from 11 to 49 years; 8 of the 11 were women. Thus, unless accompanied by a clear-cut family history, these paroxysmal dystonias are particularly commonly psychogenic, and their diagnosis is extremely difficult to make by virtue that between paroxysmal attacks, the patients are normal so that improvement with suggestion, placebo, or psychotherapy cannot be used to document the psychogenic etiology (40).

HISTORY OF PSYCHOGENIC MOVEMENT DISORDERS AFTER THE FIELD OF MOVEMENT DISORDERS BECAME A SUBSPECIALTY

As seen from the above review, psychogenic tremor, psychogenic gait disorders, psychogenic spasms, and psychogenic contractures were well-recognized more than 150 years ago. But otherwise, patients had movement disorders that were rarely considered to be of psychogenic origin. As late as 1975, at the First International Dystonia Symposium, Fahn and Eldridge (50) were not able to find a proven case of psychogenic dystonia. By 1978, a case I had suspected of being a factitious disorder while at the University of Pennsylvania in 1972 was eventually

documented as being psychogenic. This was the first case of 85 dystonia patients seen by this time point and was reported by Lesser and Fahn (46). By January 1983, I had seen five proven cases of psychogenic dystonia, and, with my colleagues, submitted an abstract to the American Academy of Neurology (AAN) meeting of 1983 (51). By the time of the meeting in April, the count had grown to 10 documented cases of psychogenic dystonia.

In the following year, Peter Whitehouse consulted me by telephone to describe a case he and his colleagues had seen at Johns Hopkins and wanted an opinion if this patient could possibly have psychogenic dystonia. I supported the idea, and the case report was subsequently published as the first proven case of Munchausen syndrome simulating torsion dystonia (52).

In 1986, at the Second International Dystonia Symposium held at Arden House in New York State, Fahn and Williams (40) presented 21 cases of documented or clinically established psychogenic dystonia. In the discussion that followed, David Marsden stated that he had trouble accepting the diagnosis, saying he had yet to encounter a case of psychogenic dystonia. This remark emphasizes how rare or even nonexistent psychogenic dystonia was thought to be in those early years when psychogenic movement disorders were beginning to be recognized and reported. In addition to presenting 21 cases of documented and clinically definite cases of psychogenic dystonia, Fahn and Williams presented a scale delineating the degree of certainty of the diagnosis of a psychogenic movement disorder. The scale lists the definitions as possible, probable, clinical definite, and documented, in order of certainty of the diagnosis.

In the last dozen years there have been numerous publications on specific psychogenic movement disorders such as gait (53–55), parkinsonism (56), tremors (57–59), myoclonus (60,61), and startle (62).

There continues to be uncertainty and debate as to whether the causalgia-dystonia syndrome (63) (causalgia-dystonia is akin to reflex sympathetic dystrophy and both are now often called complex regional pain syndrome) is an organic or a psychogenic disorder (64,65). A more satisfactory way of documenting psychogenic movement disorders other than reversing the signs and symptoms needs to be developed.

Within the classification of psychogenic movement disorders are the three psychiatric classifications of (i) somatoform disorder (including conversion disorder and somatization disorder), (ii) factitious disorder (including Munchausen syndrome), and (iii) malingering (66). Technically, malingering is not a psychiatric disorder, but it is listed in the psychogenic classification because it is not always possible to distinguish it from somatoform or factitious disorders. Thus, from a clinical point of view, malingering is in the differential diagnosis when one encounters a nonorganic movement disorder. Therefore, it seems appropriate to list malingering within the psychogenic categorization.

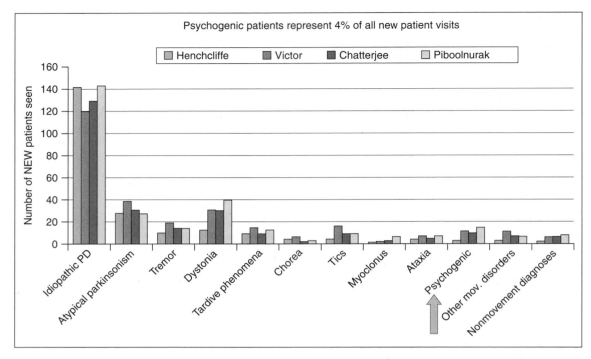

Figure 4.1 Psychogenic patients (arrow) represent 10% of all non-parkinsonian new patient visits (40/391) encountered by the movement disorder fellows over a two-year period in the movement disorder clinic at Columbia University Medical Center in New York City. The bars of different shades represent the new patient encounters seen by four movement disorder fellows during their two-year fellowship. [From Portera-Cailliau C, Victor D, Frucht SJ, et al. Designing the ideal movement disorders fellowship training program: the Columbia University experience 2001–2002. *Neurology.* 2004;62(Suppl. 5):A80, with permission.]

Psychogenic movement disorders appear to be more common than once thought, but perhaps clinicians are getting better at recognizing and diagnosing these disorders. At the present time, about 10% of newly encountered non-parkinsonian movement disorder cases being seen in our movement disorder subspecialty clinic are psychogenic in etiology (Fig. 4.1) (67). If all parkinsonian disorders are included in the new encounters, then psychogenic movement disorders are diagnosed in about 4% of all new patients in this specialty clinic. This symposium and its resulting monograph of the proceedings are the first to focus on the topic of psychogenic movement disorders.

REFERENCES

1. Putzel L. *A treatise on common forms of functional nervous diseases.* New York: William Wood & Co, 1880.
2. Kalinowsky LB. Henry Charlton Bastian (1837–1915). In Haymaker W, ed. *The founders of neurology. One hundred and thirty-three biographical sketches.* Springfield, IL: Charles C Thomas, 1953;242.
3. Romberg MH. *A manual on the nervous diseases of man.* Vol. II. Translated by Sieveking EH. London: Sydenham Society, 1853: 81–99.
4. Haymaker W. William Alexander Hammond (1825–1900). In Haymaker, W, ed. *The founders of neurology. One hundred and thirty-three biographical sketches.* Springfield, IL: Charles C Thomas, 1953;297.
5. Hammond WA. *A treatise on diseases of the nervous system.* New York: D. Appleton, 1871:619–636.
6. Briquet P. *Traité clinique et thérapeutique de l'hystérie.* 1859.
7. Wilks S. *Lectures on diseases of the nervous system delivered at Guy's Hospital.* Philadelphia, PA: Lindsay and Blakiston, 1878:361–380.
8. Duchenne BA. *Selections from the clinical works.* Translated by Poore GV. London: New Sydenham Society, 1883:349–353.
9. Gowers WR. *Diagnosis of diseases of the brain and of the spinal cord.* New York: William Wood & Co, 1885:200–203.
10. Mills CK. Hysteria. In: Pepper W, Starr L, eds. *A system of practical medicine.* Philadelphia, PA: Lea Brothers & Co, 1886:205–287.
11. Gowers WR. *A manual of diseases of the nervous system,* 2nd ed. Vol. II. Philadelphia, PA: Blakiston, 1893:984–1030.
12. Lloyd JH. Hysteria. In: Dercum FX, ed. *A textbook on nervous diseases.* Philadelphia, PA: Lea Brothers & Co, 1895:87–134.
13. Sachs B. *A treatise on the nervous diseases of children for physicians and students.* New York: William Wood & Company, 1895:85–108.
14. Dana CL. *Text-book of nervous diseases: being a compendium for the use of students and practitioners of medicine.* New York: William Wood & Company, 1897:476–496.
15. Oppenheim H. Über ein eigenartige Krampfkrankheit des kindlichen und jugendlichen Alters (dysbasia lordotica progressiva, dystonia musculorum deformans). *Neurol Centrabl.* 1911a; 30:1090–1107.
16. Flatau E, Sterling W. Progressiver torsionspasms bie kindern. *Z Gesamte Neurol Psychiatr.* 1911;7:586–612.
17. Church A, Peterson F. *Nervous and mental diseases,* 4th ed. Philadelphia, PA: WB Saunders, 1904:574–602.
18. Richer P. *Etudes cliniques sur la grande hysterie ou l'hystéroépilepsie.* Paris: Delahaye et LeCrosnier, 1885.
19. Pearce FS. *A practical treatise on nervous diseases for the medical student and general practitioner.* New York: D. Appleton and Co, 1904:302–312.

20. Ziehen T. Hysteria. In: Church A, ed. *Diseases of the nervous system.* New York: D. Appleton and Co, 1909:1045–1097.

21. Jelliffe SE. Hysteria. In: Osler W, ed. *Modern medicine. Its theory and practice.* Vol. VII. Philadelphia, PA: Lea & Febiger, 1910:811–867.

22. Oppenheim H. *Textbook of nervous diseases for physicians and students,* 5th ed., Translated by Bruce H. Edinburgh: Otto Schulzle, 1911b:1053–1111.

23. Starr MA. *Organic and functional nervous diseases. A text-book of neurology.* New York: Lea & Febiger, 1913:878–897.

24. Jones E. The treatment of the neuroses, including the psychoneuroses. In: White WA, Jelliffe SE, eds. *The modern treatment of nervous and mental diseases by American and British authors.* Philadelphia, PA: Lea & Febiger, 1913:331–416.

25. Bing R. *A textbook of nervous diseases for students and practising physicians in thirty lectures.* Translated by Allen CL. New York: Rebman Co, 1915:436–453.

26. Stewart JP. *The diagnosis of nervous diseases.* London: Edward Arnold, 1920:358–399.

27. Wexler IS. *A text-book of clinical neurology,* 2nd ed. Philadelphia, PA: WB Saunders, 1932.

28. Ford FR. *Diseases of the nervous system in infancy, childhood and adolescence.* Springfield, IL: Charles C Thomas, 1937.

29. Wilson SAK. *Neurology.* Vols. I & II. Baltimore, MD: Williams & Wilkins, 1940.

30. Wilson SAK. *Neurology.* Vols. 1, 2 & 3. Baltimore, MD: Williams & Wilkins, 1955.

31. Nielsen JM. *A textbook of clinical neurology.* New York: Paul B. Hoeber, 1951.

32. Merritt HH. *A textbook of neurology.* Philadelphia, PA: Lea & Febiger, 1955.

33. Rowland LP, ed. *Merritt's neurology,* 11th ed. Philadelphia, PA: Lippincott Williams & Wilkins, 2005.

34. Bradley WG, Daroff RB, Fenichel GM et al., eds. *Neurology in clinical practice.* Boston, MA: Butterworth-Heinemann, 1991.

35. Leszynsky W. Hysterical gait. *Nerv Ment Dis.* 1903;30:33–34.

36. Williams DT, Ford B, Fahn S. Phenomenology and psychopathology related to psychogenic movement disorders. *Adv Neurol.* 1995;65:231–257.

37. Meige H, Feindel E. *Tics and their treatment.* Translated from the French by Wilson SAK. London: Appleton, 1907:246.

38. Dooley JM, Stokes A, Gordon KE. Pseudo-tics in Tourette syndrome. *J Child Neurol.* 1994;9:50–51.

39. Campbell J. The shortest paper. *Neurology.* 1979;29:1633.

40. Fahn S, Williams DT. Psychogenic dystonia. *Adv Neurol.* 1988;50:431–455.

41. Schwalbe W. *Eine eigentumliche tonische Krampfform mit hysterischen Symptomen.* Inaug Diss, G. Schade, Berlin: 1908.

42. Brierly H. The treatment of hysterical spasmodic torticollis by behavior therapy. *Behav Res Ther.* 1967;5:139.

43. Meares R. Features which distinguish groups of spasmodic torticollis. *J Psychosom Res.* 1971;15:1–11.

44. Tibbets RW. Spasmodic torticollis. *J Psychosom Res.* 1971;15:461–469.

45. Cooper IS, Cullinan T, Riklan M. The natural history of dystonia. *Adv Neurol.* 1976;14:157–169.

46. Lesser RP, Fahn S. Dystonia: a disorder often misdiagnosed as a conversion reaction. *Am J Psychiatry.* 1978;153:349–452.

47. Marsden CD, Harrison MJG. Idiopathic torsion dystonia. *Brain.* 1974;97:793–810.

48. Eldridge R, Riklan M, Cooper IS. The limited role of psychotherapy in torsion dystonia. Experience with 44 cases. *JAMA.* 1969; 210:705–708.

49. Bressman SB, Fahn S, Burke RE. Paroxysmal non-kinesigenic dystonia. *Adv Neurol.* 1988;50:403–413.

50. Fahn S, Eldridge R. Definition of dystonia and classification of the dystonic states. *Adv Neurol.* 1976;14:1–5.

51. Fahn S, Williams D, Reches A, et al. Hysterical dystonia, a rare disorder: report of five documented cases. *Neurology.* 1983; 33(Suppl. 2):161.

52. Batshaw ML, Wachtel RC, Deckel AW, et al. Munchausen's syndrome simulating torsion dystonia. *N Eng J Med.* 1985;312:1437–1439.

53. Keane JR. Hysterical gait disorders: 60 cases. *Neurology.* 1989;39:586–589.

54. Vecht CJ, Meerwaldt JD, Lees AJ, et al. What Is It? Case 1, 1991. Unusual tremor, myoclonus and a limping gait. *Mov Disord.* 1991;6:371–375.

55. Lempert T, Brandt T, Dieterich M, et al. How to identify psychogenic disorders of stance and gait. A video study in 37 patients. *J Neurol.* 1991;238:140–146.

56. Lang AE, Koller WG, Fahn S. Psychogenic parkinsonism. *Arch Neurol.* 1995;52:802–810.

57. Fahn S. Atypical tremors, rare tremors and unclassified tremors. In PE: Findley LJ, Capildeo R, eds. *Movement disorders: tremor.* New York: Oxford University Press, 1984;431–443.

58. Koller W, Lang A, Vetere-Overfield B, et al. Psychogenic tremors. *Neurology.* 1989;39:1094–1099.

59. Deuschl G, Koster B, Lucking CH, et al. Diagnostic and pathophysiological aspects of psychogenic tremors. *Mov Disord.* 1998;13:294–302.

60. Monday K, Jankovic J. Psychogenic myoclonus. *Neurology.* 1993; 43:349–352.

61. Terada K, Ikeda A, Van Ness PC, et al. Presence of bereitschaftspotential preceding psychogenic myoclonus: clinical application of jerk-locked back averaging. *J Neurol Neurosurg Psychiatry.* 1995; 58:745–747.

62. Thompson PD, Colebatch JG, Brown P, et al. Voluntary stimulus-sensitive jerks and jumps mimicking myoclonus or pathological startle syndromes. *Mov Disord.* 1992;7:257–262.

63. Bhatia KP, Bhatt MH, Marsden CD. The causalgia-dystonia syndrome. *Brain.* 1993;116:843–851.

64. Lang A, Fahn S. Movement disorder of RSD. *Neurology.* 1990;40:1476–1477.

65. Kurlan R, Brin MF, Fahn S. Movement disorder in reflex sympathetic dystrophy: a case proven to be psychogenic by surveillance video monitoring. *Mov Disord.* 1997;12:243–245.

66. Fahn S. Psychogenic movement disorders. In: Marsden CD, Fahn S, eds. *Movement disorders 3.* Oxford: Butterworth-Heinemann, 1994:359–372.

67. Portera-Cailliau C, Victor D, Frucht SJ, et al. Designing the ideal movement disorders fellowship training program: the Columbia University experience 2001–2002. *Neurology.* 2004; 62(Suppl. 5):A80.

68. Landouzy H. *Traité complet de l'hystérie.* Paris, 1846.

Phenomenology: Neurology

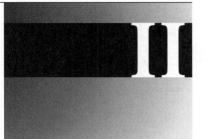

III

General Overview of Psychogenic Movement Disorders: Epidemiology, Diagnosis, and Prognosis

5

Anthony E. Lang

ABSTRACT

Epidemiologic studies of "medically unexplained symptoms" are fraught with problems. Despite numerous confounding issues, it is clear that conversion disorders are probably as common as other disabling conditions such as multiple sclerosis and schizophrenia. Little is known about the frequency of movement disorders as a manifestation of conversion disorders. Reports from subspecialty clinics all suffer from ascertainment as well as selection/referral biases with an underrepresentation of acute or transient cases and overrepresentation of chronic or refractory problems. Although underlying neurologic diseases need to be carefully excluded when dealing with such patients, the diagnosis itself is not one of exclusion. Certain historical features are common to many different types of psychogenic movement disorders (PMDs), including abrupt onset (often triggered by a minor injury for which litigation or compensation is sought), rapid progression to maximum disability or peak severity shortly after onset, static course, previous remissions, and paroxysmal exacerbations. Clinical features common to most PMDs are the incongruity with their organic counterparts and inconsistencies during the examination, over time or with historical information provided.

Additional "nonorganic" neurologic disturbances are also common, including give-way weakness, nonanatomic sensory disturbances, atypical pain syndromes, and extreme slowness of movement. Investigations may not be helpful (except for excluding specific underlying organic disorders), although electrophysiologic testing may be particularly useful in confirming the diagnosis in some PMDs, especially myoclonus and tremor. The diagnosis should not be made or refuted by physicians inexperienced in the investigation and management of both organic and psychogenic movement disorders. In the presence of clear positive confirmatory clinical features, the diagnosis should not be excluded on the basis of the screening psychiatric assessment failing to define the presence of underlying psychopathology. The natural history of PMDs is poorly defined, but often patients remain disabled over prolonged periods of time. Review of the appropriate literature highlights the need for considerable future research to establish a better understanding of all facets of PMDs including epidemiologic features, diagnostic methodologies, pathogenetic mechanisms, and, particularly, more effective treatment strategies.

In this chapter, I will provide an introductory discussion of several issues common to all psychogenic movement disorders. Specifics related to individual types of movement disorders will be covered in more detail in subsequent chapters. At the outset, it must be admitted that there is no consensus on diagnostic terminology. A variety of terms including hysterical conversion, somatoform disorders, "functional" symptoms, medically unexplained symptoms, and so on, have been applied. Although the term "psychogenic" is common in the movement disorder literature, it obviously has negative connotations for patients. The term "medically unexplained" is similarly considered pejorative, and Stone et al. have argued for a return to the use of "functional" to describe these problems (1). Another point that should be mentioned briefly is the fact that the term "movement disorders" is not necessarily widely recognized outside the field of neurology, and therefore it is quite uncommon for such patients to be distinguished or separated from the larger group of patients with "unexplained motor symptoms," where absence of motor function (e.g., hemiplegia, paraplegia) predominates. In fact, some follow-up studies have purposely excluded patients with abnormal motor activity "because of the risk of including patients whose symptoms might have an organic cause" (2). Another major problem in studies involving psychogenic movement disorders is the general lack of a gold standard by which a diagnosis can be established. In fact, a large proportion of movement disorders (particularly those designated as "idiopathic") lack any defining laboratory, electrophysiological, or imaging abnormalities. A relatively high proportion of patients seen by movement disorder experts do not fulfill the criteria for a "documented" psychogenic movement disorder, but instead are categorized as "clinically established" largely based on a variety of features that are felt by the clinician to be incongruent with established organic disorders or variably inconsistent by history and examination (3). Recognizing this, Williams et al. suggested that these two categories be combined to form the category of "clinically definite" (4). In the absence of defining diagnostic measures (aside from clinical features), a number of studies have characterized the frequency of the historical and clinical features in various psychogenic movement disorders which were diagnosed in large part on the basis of the presence of these features (i.e., a problem of self-fulfilling prophecy). This especially creates problems when some investigators feel that specific clinical features support a psychogenic origin, while others feel that the same features are characteristic of an established organic syndrome. The best example of this is the case of posttraumatic dystonia with or without associated complex regional pain syndrome (see Chapter 8).

PREVALENCE

There are numerous studies evaluating the epidemiology of somatoform disorders. As pointed out by Akagi and House (5), these are generally fraught with a variety of problems which these authors have subdivided into questions of case definition, case ascertainment, and selection of a suitable population to study. As mentioned above, specifically with respect to psychogenic movement disorders, the lack of confirmatory diagnostic testing compromises case definition even when the clinical criteria are adequate and rigidly applied. Case ascertainment is particularly confounded by the wide range of medical practices assayed (e.g., general practice, emergency room, neurology, or psychiatry in- or outpatient services, etc.) and the inclusion of acute versus chronic cases. Finally, applying the usual epidemiologic approach of defining a target population from which the study population is chosen and then taking an appropriate sample is generally not possible from the available literature, although one recent small study from Florence did attempt to utilize this format (6). Despite these confounding issues, it is clear that somatoform disorders or medically unexplained symptoms are probably as common as other disabling conditions such as multiple sclerosis and schizophrenia (5). It has been suggested that up to 50% of patients seen in specialty clinics or seeking secondary medical care can be classified as such (7–9) and as many as 30% to 40% of patients attending general neurology clinics have symptoms that are either not at all explained or only somewhat explained by organic disease (8,10–12). In patients who most frequently attend outpatient services, one study found that 27% had one or more consultation episodes in which the condition was medically unexplained, and 21% of all consultations were medically unexplained (13).

Epidemiologic studies of psychogenic movement disorders are lacking. All available reports originate from tertiary academic movement disorder clinics, and therefore it is impossible to say how common these disorders are in the community at large or even how common they are with respect to neurological conversion disorders in general. In the only series that divided medically unexplained motor symptoms into "absence of motor function" and "presence of abnormal motor activity," 48% had index symptoms in the former category, while 52% had symptoms such as tremor, dystonia, and ataxia (14). However, these figures may have been influenced by referral bias since Professor C. David Marsden was one of the senior authors. Factor et al. found that 28 of 842 (3.3%) consecutive movement disorder patients seen over a 71-month period were diagnosed as having a documented or clinically established psychogenic movement disorder (15). [A recent update of these numbers gave an almost identical figure: 135 of 3,826 (3.5%); S. Factor, *personal communication*, 2003.] Most other studies have described either the relative frequencies of specific subtypes of psychogenic movement disorders or have only indicated the proportion of patients with a specific subtype of movement disorder phenotype diagnosed as psychogenic (e.g., the proportion of all patients presenting with dystonia diagnosed as psychogenic). Obviously, even here, referral biases will have a great influence on the results. Tertiary care movement disorder clinics tend to see the more complex or difficult-to-diagnose cases. These clinics will also tend to accumulate more chronic or refractory cases, while patients with acute and short-lived symptoms (which typically have a better prognosis as outlined below) are less likely to be seen. In addition, the caseload of certain clinics may be influenced by their research interests. For example,

the designation of Columbia Presbyterian Medical Center as a Dystonia Medical Research Foundation Center of Excellence may have partially accounted for the higher proportion of patients with psychogenic dystonia (54%) (4) compared to most other centers (25% to 28%) (Table 5.1). Considering all of these possible biases, Table 5.1 provides a summary of the relative frequencies of various psychogenic movement disorders as seen in several subspecialty clinics. A noncomprehensive review of the database from the Toronto Western Hospital Movement Disorders Clinic found a high likelihood of the psychogenic etiology (i.e., "clinically definite") in 154/1,115 (13.8%) patients with tremor (excluding Parkinson disease), 91/1,078 (8.4%) with dystonia, 65/209 (31.1%) with myoclonus, 6/218 (2.8%) with chorea, 8/44 (18.2%) with nonspecified gait disturbance and 16/2,845 (0.6%) with parkinsonism.

TABLE 5.1

COMBINED DATA ON PSYCHOGENIC MOVEMENT DISORDERS SEEN AT SEVERAL MOVEMENT DISORDER CENTERS[a]

Psychogenic Movement Disorder	Toronto (Toronto Western Hospital)[b]	New York (Columbia Presbyterian Medical Center)[c]	Cleveland Clinic Florida[d]	Albany Clinic[e]	Paris[f]	Chicago (Rush Medical College)[g]	8 Spanish University Centers[g]	Baylor College of Medicine	Total
	(%)	(%)	(%)	(%)	(%)	(%)	(%)	(%)	(%)
Dystonia	91 (27)	82 (54)	14 (25)	30 (24)	20 (27)	25 (28)	14 (29)	89 (39)	365 (31)
Tremor	154 (45)	21 (14)	18 (32)	60 (47)	22 (29)	42 (48)[h]	23 (48)[h]	127 (56)	467 (40)
Myoclonus	65 (19)	11 (7)	4 (7)	17 (13)	0	11 (12)	8 (17)	30 (13)	146 (13)
Parkinsonism	16 (5)	3 (2)	0	11 (9)	9 (12)	12 (14)[i]	3 (6)[i]	6 (3)	60 (5)
Gait disorder	8 (2)	14 (9)	1 (2)	0	19 (25)	41 (47)[j]	24 (50)[j]	7 (3)	114 (10)
Tics	0	2 (1)	2 (4)	3 (2)	1 (1)	6 (7)	0	15 (7)	29 (2)
Other	6 (2)	19 (13)	17 (30)	6 (5)	4 (5)	10 (11)	1 (2)	1 (0.4)	64 (5)[k]
Total	340	152	56	127	75	147	73	275	1,245

[a]Various approaches have been used in the collection of this data. Some centers (see g) have listed all movements evident (therefore, the combination of the numbers of patients demonstrating movement disorder subtypes will be larger than the total number of patients seen) and others (b–f) have listed only the dominant movement disorder syndrome demonstrated by the patient. These numbers are combined only to provide a very rough estimate of the frequency of the different movement disorder phenotypes seen in patients with psychogenic movement disorders.
[b]Toronto Western Hospital (listed only predominant movement) (AE Lang, *personal observations*, 2003).
[c]Columbia Presbyterian Medical Center (listed all types of movement; 131 patients) (4); patients' symptoms were classified as dystonia (rather than placed in another category) if any dystonic features were present. In most other series, patients were classified according to the predominant movement disorder.
[d]Cleveland Clinic Florida (listed only the predominant movement, 1998–2002) (N Galvez Jiminez, *personal observations*).
[e]Albany Clinic—updated from Factor SA, Podskalny GD, Molho ES. Psychogenic movement disorders: frequency, clinical profile, and characteristics. *J Neurol Neurosurg Psychiatry*. 1995;59(4):406–412, with permission; S. Factor, *personal communication*, see this volume; listed only the predominant movement—83 definite, 39 probable, 5 possible.
[f]M. Vidailet, *personal communication*; listed only the predominant movement; seen over six years from a database of 4,400 patients with various movement disorders.
[g]See E. Cubo et al. in this volume; listed all movements present.
[h]Action tremor only included here (rest tremor also listed in data presented, overlapped with action tremor).
[i]Listed as "bradykinesia."
[j]Any gait disorder, not necessarily the primary problem.
[k]Others (n): chorea (11), blepharospasm/facial movements (8), "cerebellar" (4), "dyskinesias" (3), "stereotypies" (1), ballism (1), athetosis (1), stiff person (1), other (34).

DIAGNOSIS: GENERAL HISTORICAL AND CLINICAL CLUES

A number of important historical and clinical clues are applicable to all forms of psychogenic movement disorders. Table 5.2 provides a list of some of these. Clues specific to various subtypes of psychogenic movement disorder will be discussed in subsequent chapters. Taken individually, most of these "clues" are no more than that. Considerably more substantive evidence is required before a diagnosis of a psychogenic disorder can be confirmed. Examples of organic disorders demonstrating many of these features readily come to mind, and several of these are listed in Table 5.2.

There are numerous studies evaluating the misdiagnosis rate on long-term follow-up of patients originally believed to have a conversion disorder. Older studies, as exemplified by the influential work of Slater (17,18), which reported a high mis-diagnosis rate (61%), are criticized as flawed. More recent studies, including detailed neurologic assessments, and modern imaging and other investigations report that 5% to 10% of patients are later found to have symptoms that could have been accounted for by an underlying organic disorder (2,14,19,20). Interestingly, in

the series reported by Crimlisk et al., all three of the patients who were later diagnosed as having a definite organic neurologic condition were in the "abnormal motor activity" group (14). In a series reported by Moene et al. (21), ten of 85 patients were later found to be misdiagnosed and five of these ten had a movement disorder. The importance of careful neurologic assessment by a clinician experienced in the field of movement disorders is further emphasized by the fact that four of these five patients received their final diagnosis on the basis of a neurologic examination.

Various factors have been demonstrated to correlate with the accuracy of the diagnosis (on long-term follow-up) or with the occurrence of a misdiagnosis. These have varied from study to study. For example, supportive factors have included prior conversion disorders, recurrent somatic complaints, the presence of a model for symptoms, prior remission with conflict resolution, the number of physical symptoms [although the number of physical signs has correlated with a misdiagnosis (20)], extent of body pain, impairment of social function, the association with depression and anxiety, an earlier age of onset, and a nonprogressive course (10,21,22). It is clear from the literature that there are a number of characteristics that conventional wisdom often considers important in supporting a diagnosis

TABLE 5.2

GENERAL CLUES SUGGESTING THAT A MOVEMENT DISORDER MAY BE PSYCHOGENIC

A) Historical
1. Abrupt onset [stroke, Wilson, rapid-onset dystonia-parkinsonism, encephalitis]
2. Static course [several types of dystonia]
3. Spontaneous remissions (inconsistency over time) [idiopathic dystonias, tics, drug-induced MDs]
4. Precipitated by minor trauma [problem of peripheral trauma-induced MDs]
5. Obvious psychiatric disturbance [many organic MDs]
6. Multiple somatizations/undiagnosed conditions [coincidental association possible]
7. Employed in a health profession [coincidental]
8. Pending litigation or compensation [valid legal claim]
9. Presence of secondary gain [unreliable predictor of a conversion disorder]
10. Young female [males also affected; organic MDs obviously occur in young women]

B) Clinical
1. Inconsistent character of the movement (amplitude, frequency, distribution, selective disability) [embellishment]
2. Paroxysmal movement disorder [organic paroxysmal MDs]
3. Movements increase with attention or decrease with distraction [tics, some tremors, embellishment]
4. Ability to trigger or relieve the abnormal movements with unusual or nonphysiological interventions (e.g., trigger points on the body, tuning fork) [suggestibility in a patient with an organic MD]
5. False weakness [embellishment]
6. False sensory complaints [embellishment]
7. Self-inflicted injuries [Tourette syndrome]
8. Deliberate slowness of movements [basal ganglia-frontal lesions: obsessional slowness]
9. Functional disability out of proportion to exam findings [some forms of dystonia]
10. Movement abnormality that is bizarre, multiple, or difficult to classify [Wilson, thalamic lesions, certain hereditary dystonias, others]

C) Therapeutic responses
1. Unresponsive to appropriate medications [many organic MDs are treatment-resistant, e.g., tremors, dystonia]
2. Response to placebos [possible with organic MDs; (16)]
3. Remission with psychotherapy

MD, movement disorder.
Note: Comments in [ ] relate to the occurrence of these "clues" in examples of organic movement disorders.

that are not at all predictive or are, in fact, misleading. These include certain behavioral characteristics such as anxiety, la belle indifférence, overdramatization, evident secondary gain, improvement by suggestion or sedation (22), and atypical physical signs (20,23). Indeed, Mace and Trimble (20) found that a "psychiatric history" had been noted in nine of the 11 (82%) patients whose diagnosis had changed to an organic disorder compared to 26 of the 62 (42%) who remained classified as a conversion disorder at follow-up, suggesting that this history may have prejudiced the original diagnosis. Although some studies have shown that patients with a longer duration of symptoms may be more likely to fall in the misdiagnosis category (e.g., 21), it is clear that neither the duration of symptoms nor the severity of physical dysfunction is useful in separating psychogenic from organic disorders (10). In fact, disability may be more pronounced in patients with conversion symptoms since these patients are said to spend 1.3 to 4.9 days in bed per month compared to an average of one day or less for patients with major medical problems (24,25).

DIAGNOSIS

Several important general guidelines should be followed in considering a diagnosis of a psychogenic movement disorder. As will be outlined in subsequent chapters, there are a number of unequivocal positive features that should be used to support the diagnosis. Therefore, in cases that can be classified as "clinically definite," these characteristic positive features are consistent and reproducible, and the diagnosis is not one of exclusion. At present, in most cases of a psychogenic movement disorder these positive diagnostic features are largely clinical, but they may also include more objective investigations such as electrophysiologic testing. Future developments in the field will hopefully provide further reliable objective diagnostic tests.

The diagnosis should not be made on the basis of a suspicion of nonorganic illness without the involvement of appropriate neurologic, and preferably movement disorders, clinical expertise. For example, in one study (10) 28/300 patients were referred to a general neurology clinic "to reinforce my opinion of no neurological disease." Eleven (39%) of these were subsequently considered by the consultant neurologist to have symptoms that were largely or completely explained by organic disease.

The diagnosis is not made on the basis of the presence of concomitant psychopathology in the absence of unequivocal clinical evidence. As outlined above, there are several "suspicious" behavioral characteristics that have been shown to correlate poorly with the diagnosis of a conversion disorder. In addition, there are numerous examples of organic movement disorders associated with psychological and psychiatric disturbances such as depression,

obsessive–compulsive behavior, body image distortion, and so on. Patients with organic movement disorders may also suffer from coincident, unrelated psychopathology or may embellish their signs and symptoms. For this reason, I would disagree with the categorization of patients demonstrating clinical features consistent or congruent with organic disease but accompanied by false neurologic features or multiple somatizations as having a "probable" psychogenic movement disorder (3). A challenging variation on this latter theme is the occurrence of a distinct psychogenic movement disorder combined with an underlying organic one (26). Although this combination clearly does occur, in my experience it is less common than the embellishment of established symptoms and seems to be considerably less common than the association between pseudoseizures and organic epilepsy.

Just as the diagnosis is not made on the basis of the presence of concomitant psychopathology, the diagnosis should not be refuted in the absence of overt psychological disturbances when unequivocal positive clinical evidence for a psychogenic origin of the movement disorder is present. This should encourage a further, in-depth evaluation of the psychiatric status and consideration of an etiologic role for features that might not have been believed of sufficient severity or importance to have contributed to the clinical presentation.

PROGNOSIS

There is very little data in the literature specifically addressing the prognosis of psychogenic movement disorders. Considerably more information is available on the prognosis of conversion disorders in general. A better prognosis for subsequent improvement or remission in symptoms has been associated with a shorter duration of symptoms before assessment, a younger age of onset, the presence of definable psychiatric disorders such as depression or schizophrenia, and a change in marital status (2,14,20). In patients with short-lived symptoms (e.g., less than 3 months), a consistent finding is the strong relationship between a long-term good outcome and an early improvement in symptoms. For example, Binzer and Kullgren (2) found that 16 of 19 patients with total recovery at follow-up were already free of symptoms 6 months after diagnosis. In contrast, rates of complete recovery range from 25% to 28% in studies where the motor disorder was present for 18 months to 2 years before assessment (4,14), with the remaining patients reporting only partial or no improvement. Other factors associated with poor outcome have included the presence of an underlying personality disorder, the use of nonpsychotropic medications for the neurological symptoms (indicating the patients' success in obtaining prescribed medication despite diagnostic doubts), and the ongoing receipt of financial benefits or pending litigation (14,20). Although most studies have found that somatization disorder (SD) is an uncommon cause of conversion symptoms, this may change over time. Mace and Trimble (20) found that only three of their 73 patients (4%) received a diagnosis of "probable Briquet syndrome" on presentation (based on the chronicity of the history and the presence of multiple complaints across many organ systems). However, 36 of 56 patients interviewed 10 years later met DSM-III-R criteria for SD of two symptoms from a screening checklist and 23 (41%) reported three or more, and these scores were higher in patients whose symptoms did not improve and who sought more frequent consultations.

There have been only a small number of studies that have attempted to specifically address the prognosis of psychogenic movement disorders. Feinstein and colleagues interviewed 42 patients from a group of 88 subjects with "clinically definite" psychogenic movement disorders seen in our unit in Toronto (27). After an average of 3.2 years following the initial assessment (which was generally many months to years after the onset of symptoms), all but four patients still had the abnormal movement (90.5%). Of these four patients, two had replaced the abnormal movement by a different somatoform disorder. Twenty-three of these patients agreed to a further detailed neurological examination 8.6 ± 8.5 years after symptom onset. The characteristics of the movement disorder phenomenology were essentially unchanged from their original evaluation. Activities of daily living such as eating, dressing, and hygiene were reported impaired in 19 of the examined patients (82.6%). Of the patients whose symptoms had improved or stabilized, two-thirds had experienced this change within the first year of illness (J. Fine, A. Nieves, and A. Lang, *unpublished observations*). A similar poor long-term prognosis was described by Deuschl and colleagues (28), who found that only six of 16 patients with psychogenic tremor, seen on average 60 months after initial assessment, had improved and were free of symptoms or had only marginal residual disability. Patients with residual symptoms continued to experience moderate (75%) or marked (25%) impairment, and seven of eight professionals had retired or obtained pensions due to the tremor.

Contrasting with this negative experience are the results described by Williams, Ford, and Fahn (4) in a select group of 21 patients followed for an average of 1.8 years (range: 6 weeks to 7 years). They found that age, gender, intelligence, chronicity of illness, and movement disorder symptomatology had no influence on outcome. Their rigorous approach, which included extended hospitalization involving intensive psychiatric evaluation, resulted in "complete and permanent relief" of movement disorder symptoms in six of 21 (25%), "permanent, considerable relief of symptoms" in five, and "permanent, moderate relief" in two. One patient with significant improvement and four with partial relief had a subsequent return of most symptoms

and three had no improvement whatsoever. Of the seven patients with poor outcomes (no improvement or a subsequent return of most symptoms), two had a factitious disorder and one was felt to be malingering. At follow-up, 30% of adults were said to be disabled. This experience emphasizes the need for ongoing active psychiatric care and support; however, the prolonged hospitalization necessary may be impractical or even impossible in the era of managed care, and long-term follow-up documenting sustained improvement once the patient left the intensive therapeutic milieu was not generally available. In another longitudinal study (29) of 228 patients (72.8% women) with psychogenic movement disorders (mean age 42.3 ± 14.3 years, mean duration of symptoms 4.7 ± 8.1 years) followed for a mean duration of 3.4 ± 2.8 years, improvement of symptoms was noted in 56.6% of patients, while 22.1% were worse, and 21.3% remained the same at the time of follow-up. In this study, indices of strong physical health, positive social life perceptions, patients' perceptions of effective treatment by the physician, elimination of stressors, and treatment with a specific medication contributed to a favorable outcome. While these results are promising, the extent of the disability resulting from psychogenic movement disorders has an important effect on society in terms of health care dollars, lost wages, and disability support. These studies provide preliminary data supporting the conclusion that psychogenic movement disorders represent an important public health problem and highlight the need for additional outcome data in patients receiving a spectrum of treatment approaches in appropriately designed controlled clinical trials. It is hoped that the information and interest generated by this symposium will serve as an incentive for the necessary advances in this field.

REFERENCES

1. Stone J, Wojcik W, Durrance D, et al. What should we say to patients with symptoms unexplained by disease? The "number needed to offend." *BMJ*. 2002;325(7378):1449–1450.
2. Binzer M, Kullgren G. Motor conversion disorder. A prospective 2- to 5-year follow-up study. *Psychosomatics*.1998;39(6):519–527.
3. Fahn S, Williams PJ. Psychogenic dystonia. *Adv Neurol*. 1988; 50:431–455.
4. Williams DT, Ford B, Fahn S. Phenomenology and psychopathology related to psychogenic movement disorders. *Adv Neurol*. 1995;65:231–258.
5. Akagi H, House A. The epidemiology of hysterical conversion. In: Halligan PW, Bass C, Marshall JC, eds. *Contemporary approaches to the study of hysteria: clinical and theoretical perspectives*. Oxford: Oxford University Press, 2001:73–87.
6. Faravelli C, Salvatori S, Galassi F, et al. Epidemiology of somatoform disorders: a community survey in Florence. *Soc Psychiatry Psychiatr Epidemiol*. 1997;32(1):24–29.
7. van Hemert AM, Hengeveld MW, Bolk JH, et al. Psychiatric disorders in relation to medical illness among patients of a general medical out-patient clinic. *Psychol Med*. 1993;23(1):167–173.
8. Hamilton J, Campos R, Creed F. Anxiety, depression and management of medically unexplained symptoms in medical clinics. *J R Coll Physicians Lond*. 1996;30(1):18–20.

9. Nimnuan C, Hotopf M, Wessely S. Medically unexplained symptoms: how often and why are they missed? *QJM.* 2000;93(1): 21–28.
10. Carson AJ, Ringbauer B, Stone J, et al. Do medically unexplained symptoms matter? A prospective cohort study of 300 new referrals to neurology outpatient clinics. *J Neurol Neurosurg Psychiatry.* 2000;68(2):207–210.
11. Perkin GD. An analysis of 7,836 successive new outpatient referrals. *J Neurol Neurosurg Psychiatry.* 1989;52(4):447–448.
12. Creed F, Firth D, Timol M, et al. Somatization and illness behaviour in a neurology ward. *J Psychosom Res.* 1990;34(4):427–437.
13. Reid S, Wessely S, Crayford T, et al. Medically unexplained symptoms in frequent attenders of secondary health care: retrospective cohort study. *BMJ.* 2001;322(7289):767.
14. Crimlisk HL, Bhatia K, Cope H, et al. Slater revisited: 6 year follow up study of patients with medically unexplained motor symptoms. *BMJ.* 1998;316(7131):582–586.
15. Factor SA, Podskalny GD, Molho ES. Psychogenic movement disorders: frequency, clinical profile, and characteristics. *J Neurol Neurosurg Psychiatry.* 1995;59(4):406–412.
16. de la Fuente-Fernandez R, Ruth TJ, Sossi V, et al. Expectation and dopamine release: mechanism of the placebo effect in Parkinson's disease. *Science.* 2001;293(5532):1164–1166.
17. Slater E. Diagnosis of "hysteria." *Brit Med J.* 1965;1:1395–1399.
18. Slater ET, Glithero E. A follow-up of patients diagnosed as suffering from "hysteria." *J Psychosom Res.* 1965;9(1):9–13.
19. Couprie W, Wijdicks EFM, Rooijmans HGM, et al. Outcome in conversion disorder: a follow up study. *J Neurol Neurosurg Psychiatry.* 1995;58:750–752.
20. Mace CJ, Trimble MR. Ten-year prognosis of conversion disorder. *Br J Psychiatry.* 1996;169(3):282–288.
21. Moene FC, Landberg EH, Hoogduin KA, et al. Organic syndromes diagnosed as conversion disorder: identification and frequency in a study of 85 patients. *J Psychosom Res.* 2000;49(1):7–12.
22. Cloninger CR. The origins of DSM and ICD criteria for conversion and somatization disorders. In: Halligan PW, Bass C, Marshall JC, eds. *Contemporary approaches to the study of hysteria: clinical and theoretical perspectives.* Oxford: Oxford University Press, 2001:49–62.
23. Gould R, Miller BL, Goldberg MA, et al. The validity of hysterical signs and symptoms. *J Nerv Ment Dis.* 1986;174(10):593–597.
24. Smith GR Jr, Monson RA, Ray DC. Patients with multiple unexplained symptoms. Their characteristics, functional health, and health care utilization. *Arch Intern Med.* 1986;146(1):69–72.
25. Wells KB, Stewart A, Hays RD, et al. The functioning and well-being of depressed patients. Results from the medical outcomes study. *JAMA.* 1989;262(7):914–919.
26. Ranawaya R, Riley D, Lang AE. Psychogenic dyskinesias in patients with organic movement disorders. *Mov Disord.* 1990;5:127–133.
27. Feinstein A, Stergiopoulos V, Fine J, et al. Psychiatric outcome in patients with a psychogenic movement disorder: a prospective study. *Neuropsychiatry Neuropsychol Behav Neurol.* 2001;14(3): 169–176.
28. Deuschl G, Köster B, Lücking CH, et al. Diagnostic and pathophysiological aspects of psychogenic tremors. *Mov Disord.* 1998; 13(2):294–302.
29. Thomas M, Jankovic J. Psychogenic movement disorders: diagnosis and management. *CNS Drugs.* 2004;18:437–452.

Psychogenic Tremor and Shaking

6

Joseph Jankovic   Madhavi Thomas

ABSTRACT

The accurate diagnosis of psychogenic movement disorders (PMDs) is based not only on exclusion of other causes, but also on positive clinical criteria. Psychogenic tremor (PT) is the most common of all PMDs. We were able to obtain clinical information on 228 (44.1%) of the patients with PMD, followed for a mean duration of 3.4 ± 2.8 years. Among the 127 patients diagnosed with PT, 92 (72.4%) were female, the mean age at initial evaluation was 43.7 ± 14.1 years, and the mean duration of symptoms was 4.6 ± 7.6 years. The following clinical features were considered to be characteristic of PT: abrupt onset (78.7%), distractibility (72.4%), variable amplitude and frequency (62.2%), intermittent occurrence (35.4%), inconsistent movement (29.9%), and variable direction (17.3%). Precipitants included personal life stress (33.9%), physical trauma (23.6%), major illness (13.4%), surgery (9.4%), or reaction to medical treatment or procedure (8.7%). About a third of the patients had a coexistent "organic" neurologic disorder, 50.7% had evidence of depression, and 30.7% had associated anxiety. Evidence of secondary gain was present in 32.3%, including maintenance of a disability status in 21.3%, pending compensation in 10.2%, and litigation in 9.4%. Improvement in tremor, reported on a global rating scale at last follow-up by 55.1%, was attributed chiefly to "effective treatment by physician" and "elimination of stressors." The findings from this largest longitudinal study of patients with PT are consistent with other series. We review the clinical features, natural history, prognosis, pathophysiology, and treatment of PT based on our own experience as well as that reported in the literature.

INTRODUCTION

Psychogenic movement disorders (PMDs) are increasingly encountered in specialty clinics. The annual incidence of PMD in the Baylor College of Medicine Movement Disorders Clinic has been increasing at an exponential rate (Fig. 6.1) (1). This apparent increase in the incidence of PMD is probably related to improved recognition of common movement disorders by practicing neurologists; more atypical and difficult to manage disorders, many of which are psychogenic, are now referred to movement disorder specialists. Another reason for the increase may be increased recognition of these disorders by movement disorder specialists.

PT is the most common of all PMDs, accounting for 4.1% of all patients evaluated in our movement disorders clinic at Baylor College of Medicine (Table 6.1).

DIAGNOSIS OF PSYCHOGENIC TREMOR

Many patients with PMD are initially seen by their primary care physicians, and because of associated somatic complaints, are diagnosed as having "functional," "hysterical," "conversion," or "medically unexplained" disorders (2,3). The term "psychogenic," introduced into the literature by Robert Sommer, a German psychiatrist in 1894, has undergone several mutations since then as reviewed by Lewis in 1972 (4). His definition of the term "psychogenic," meaning "originating in the mind or in mental or emotional processes; having a psychological rather than a physiologic

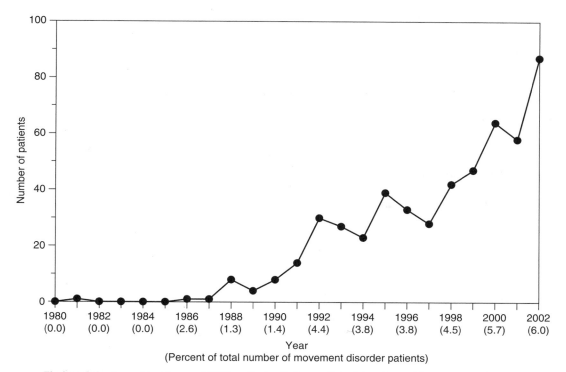

Figure 6.1 Annual incidence of PMD at Baylor College of Medicine. (From Thomas M, Jankovic J. Psychogenic movement disorders: diagnosis and management. *CNS Drugs*. 2004;18:437–452, with permission.)

origin," is used in this review (4). We use the term "psychogenic" rather than classify each patient into a specific diagnostic category, such as somatoform, factitious, malingering, or hypochondriacal disorder (5–7). Although exploration of the psychodynamic underpinning is important in understanding the basis of the PMD in each case, we find this information particularly useful in the management treatment rather than in the diagnostic phase of the evaluation.

It is important to emphasize that the accurate diagnosis of PT is based not only on exclusion of other causes, but is dependent on positive clinical criteria, the presence of which should prevent unnecessary investigation. The diagnostic process begins with a careful search in the patient's history for prior nonorganic disorders, surgeries without identifiable pathology, and excessive somatization. To understand more fully the underlying psychodynamic issues, it is essential to explore prior childhood adverse psychological, sexual, or physical experiences; personality factors; psychiatric history; drug dependence; evidence of a personal encounter or knowledge of a similar illness that could serve as a "model;" recent family life events; work-related or other injury; litigation; and possible secondary gain. We have adopted the following diagnostic classification, initially proposed by Fahn and Williams (8): (a) documented PMD (complete resolution with suggestion, physiotherapy, or placebo), (b) clinically established PMD (inconsistent over time or incongruent with the typical presentation of a classical movement disorder, such as additional atypical neurologic signs, multiple somatizations, obvious psychiatric disturbance, disappearance with distraction, and deliberate slowing), (c) probable PMD (incongruous and inconsistent movements in the absence of any of the other features listed in category b), and (d) possible PMD (clinical features of PMD occurring in the presence of an emotional disturbance).

TABLE 6.1

PSYCHOGENIC MOVEMENT DISORDERS (BAYLOR COLLEGE OF MEDICINE)

	N	%
N (1988–2002)	12,625	
Patients with diagnosis of PMD	517	4.1
Patients with follow-up	228	44.1
Duration of follow-up	3.4 ± 2.8 years	
Tremor	127	55.7
Dystonia	89	39.0
Myoclonus	30	13.2
Tics	15	6.6
Gait disorder	7	3.1
Parkinsonism	6	2.6

Psychogenic sensory and motor disorders, such as unexplained paralysis or blindness; false sensory loss; gait and balance problems; and pseudoseizures are well-recognized, but PMDs characterized by hypokinesia (slowness or paucity of movement), hyperkinesias (excessive movements), or ataxia (incoordination of movement) are among the most common forms of psychogenic neurologic disorders. The most common PMD is psychogenic tremor (PT), defined as tremor or shaking not fully explained by organic disease (negative or exclusionary criteria) and exhibiting characteristics, described later, that make the movement incongruous with any organic tremor (positive criteria).

The diagnosis of PT is facilitated by various clues based on historical information and examination. The phenomenology of PT ranges from rest, postural, and kinetic tremor to bizarre "shaking" or repetitive "jerking" resembling myoclonus (9) or seizures (pseudoseizures) (10,11). Although the tremor usually involves the limbs, some patients exhibit shaking of the head and face. When the facial movement is confined to only one side of the face, it may resemble hemifacial spasm (12). Most patients exhibit all three types of tremor—rest, postural, and kinetic—to a variable degree. The duration of the tremor varies considerably among and within patients. PT may be classified according to duration into three types: (i) long duration (either continuous or intermittent) tremor, (ii) short-lived or paroxysmal tremors lasting less than 30 seconds, and (iii) continuous tremor, with superimposed short paroxysmal episodes (13). Other clues to the diagnosis of PT include selective disability; spontaneous and intermittent remissions; trigger by injury, stress, loud noise, or other precipitants; poor response to medication; and recovery with psychotherapy.

On examination, PT is typically characterized by rhythmical shaking incongruous with known tremor types; variability of frequency, amplitude, direction, and location of movement; distractibility; entrainment; suppressibility; and deliberate slowing. In "the shortest paper," Campbell (14) pointed out that nonorganic tremors tend to decrease when attention is withdrawn from the affected area. Distractibility is defined as marked reduction, abolishment, or a change in amplitude or frequency of tremor when the patient is concentrating on other mental or motor tasks, such as repetitive alternating movements or a complex pattern of movements in the opposite limb. We often ask the patient to perform and repeat the following motor sequence of opposition of second, fifth, and third finger to the thumb of the contralateral hand. Entrainment is demonstrated when the original frequency (and amplitude) of tremor is changed in an attempt to match the frequency (and amplitude) of the repetitive movement performed by the patient volitionally or passively in the contralateral limb or tongue. In addition, we test for muscle tone, and specifically for evidence of active resistance against passive range of movement.

Some patients with PT may also have associated parkinsonism (15). In addition to rest tremor, patients with psychogenic parkinsonism demonstrate other tremor types; deliberate slowing; and resistance against passive movement, frequently varying with distraction. They may have a stiff gait and decreased arm swing when walking, often involving only one arm, which may or may not persist while running. Response to postural stability testing is often very inconsistent and many patients demonstrate an extreme response to even minor pull, flinging their arms, even though the arms may have been previously severely bradykinetic. Although they may retropulse, they almost never fall.

PT can affect any part of the body, but typically it causes shaking of the head, arms, and legs, often to a variable degree with changing anatomic distribution. Voice tremor may also be a manifestation of PT. Even palatal tremor has been reported to be a form of PT (16).

Physical examination of patients with PT may reveal other neurologic findings including false weakness, midline sensory split, lateralization of tuning fork, Hoover sign, pseudoclonus (clonus with irregular, variable amplitude), pseudoptosis (excessive contraction of orbicularis, with apparent weakness of frontalis), pseudo waxy flexibility (maintenance of limb in a set position, and inability to change this position), and convergence spasm (bilateral or unilateral spasm of near reflex, with intermittent episodes of convergence with miosis, and accommodation) (17). Another useful clue to the presence of PT is the apparent lack of concern, termed "la belle indifférence," with dissociation from the tremor and the "disability" it causes. Some patients even smile or laugh while they relate their history of the disability that the tremor causes, as well as during examination and videotaping. On the other hand, some patients demonstrate an inordinate amount of effort in performing manual tasks accompanied by sighing, facial grimacing, and exhaustion. They may also embellish or exaggerate the symptoms and show signs of panic, such as tachycardia, hyperventilation, and perspiration.

The clinical phenomenology of PT has been addressed by several authors (13,18,19). Koller et al. (18) described 24 (15 women) patients with PT, mean age 43.4 years (range: 15 to 78) and mean duration of symptoms 3.3 years (range: 1 week to 10 years). Although only five patients were described in detail, the authors noted that all patients exhibited variable amplitude and frequency; 92% changed direction of the tremor. Of the 24 patients, only six (25%) improved or resolved, but it was not clear over what period of time. In another series of PT, Deuschl et al. (19) described 25 (20 women) patients with "obvious nonorganic body shaking" in hands or legs (n = 20) or during stance (n = 5). The age at onset was 41.8 years (range: 15 to 77) and, similar to the other studies, 92% had an abrupt onset and 86.4% demonstrated distractibility. Of the 19 patients with formal psychiatric evaluation, depression was diagnosed in 63% and histrionic personality in 16%. Only six of 25 (24%) patients improved or "had only marginal residual disability." In a study by Kim et al. (13) of 70 (46 women) patients with PT, the mean age at onset was 36.1 years (range: 10 to 63) and mean duration of symptoms was 49.4 months. Fifty-one percent had some well-defined precipitant, such as physical injury in 23 and psychological insult in six. Although only ten of the 70 (14.3%) patients had a follow-up assessment (mean 19.4 months after the initial evaluation), the authors reported that the tremor spread in 38%, remained confined in 30%, and became generalized in 28%. The following features of PT were noted: variability, 88%; distractibility, 80%; abrupt onset, 73%; entrainment, 49%; and suggestibility, 33%.

Among 12,625 patients evaluated in the Baylor College of Medicine Movement Disorders Clinic between 1988 and 2002, 517 (4.1%) were diagnosed with a PMD. We were able to obtain clinical information on 228 of 517 (44.1%) patients with PMD, followed for a mean duration of 3.4 ± 2.8 years (20). Among the 127 patients diagnosed with PT, 92 (72.4%) were women, the mean age at initial evaluation was 43.7 ± 14.1 years, and the mean duration of symptoms was 4.6 ± 7.6 years. Of the 127 PT patients, 82 (64.4%) were categorized as having clinically established PT, 23 (18.1%) probable, 15 (11.8%) documented, and seven (5.5%) had possible PT. Table 6.2 lists clinical features in this population of PT patients.

Although many patients had a mixture of different movement disorders, PT was the predominant movement disorder in 55.7% of all PMD patients in whom follow-up data was available. Coexistent movement disorders included

dystonia (39%), myoclonus (13.2%), tics (6.6%), gait disorder (3.1%), parkinsonism (2.6%), and nonspecific dyskinesia (0.4%). In the majority of patients, some precipitating event could be identified prior to the onset of tremor, including personal life stress (33.9%), physical trauma (23.6%), major illness (13.4%), surgery (9.4%), or reaction to medical treatment or procedure (8.7%). Coexistent "organic" neurologic diagnoses that could not explain the manifested tremor or shaking, such as stroke, neuropathy, migraine headaches, fibromyalgia, seizure disorder, complex regional pain syndrome, multiple sclerosis, meningioma, and Parkinson disease, were present in 37% of PT patients. Coexistent organic movement disorder, present in 20 (15.7%) patients, included dystonia, parkinsonism, and organic tremor. Psychiatric comorbidities included depression in 50.7% and anxiety in 30.7%.

In some patients PT and other PMDs, particularly dystonia, may be manifested in the region of prior injury, and the PMD may be associated with complex regional pain syndrome, previously referred to as reflex sympathetic dystrophy (21–25). While the presence of posttraumatic, peripherally-induced movement disorders, particularly dystonia and tremor, is well-accepted, there appears to be a high frequency of associated psychiatric problems in this group of patients, particularly when associated with complex regional pain syndrome (26–28). There is, however, growing evidence from various physiologic and imaging studies suggesting that central reorganization follows this peripheral injury (29–33).

NATURAL HISTORY AND PROGNOSIS

Except for brief reports or abstracts (34), there are no published longitudinal studies of the natural history of PT. We have, therefore, designed a study that would provide data on prognosis and long-term outcome of PT. Patients diagnosed with PMD in our Movement Disorders Clinic between 1990 and 2003 with a follow-up for at least 3 years were included in this study. If lost to follow-up, the patients were contacted by letters or by phone and were administered structured interviews designed to assess current motor and psychological function. Evidence of secondary gain was present in 32.3%, including maintenance of a disability status in 21.3%, pending compensation in 10.2%, and litigation in 9.4%. In contrast to the other series (13,18,19) in which less than a third of the patients improved, the majority (58.7%) of the patients in our series rated themselves as "better" on a global self-rating scale. We identified the following poor prognostic risk factors: longer duration of PMD symptoms, history of smoking, precipitating event, secondary gain, psychiatric comorbidity, specific comorbidity of anxiety, neurologic comorbidity, other medical comorbidity, speech problems, positive family history of psychiatric/neurologic conditions,

TABLE 6.2

CLINICAL FEATURES OF PSYCHOGENIC TREMOR (N = 127)

Clinical Feature	n	%
Abrupt onset	100	78.7
Distractibility	92	72.4
Variable amplitude and frequency	79	62.2
Intermittent occurrence	45	35.4
Inconsistent movements	38	29.9
Variable direction	22	17.3
Irregular pattern	15	11.8
Suppressibility	15	11.8
Incongruous movements	14	11.0
La belle indifférence	14	11.0
Suggestibility	13	10.2
Sensory split	12	9.4
Entrainment	10	7.9
Active resistance to passive movement	9	7.1
Deliberate slowing	9	7.1
Nonpatterned	9	7.1
Position induced	8	6.3

somatizations of exhaustion, indices of social life perceptions, seeing some other physician/therapist, and dissatisfaction with the physician. Patients with poor or satisfactory social life perceptions were 118.51 (CI$_{95\%}$: 2.95, 4758.95; p <0.011) and 13.15 (CI$_{95\%}$: 1.19, 145.78; p <0.036) times more likely to report poorer outcomes than those with good social life perceptions, respectively. Furthermore, patients with any psychiatric comorbidity may be at greater risk for poorer outcome by a factor of 20.26 (CI$_{95\%}$: 0.94, 435.54; p = 0.055) and those who had an identifiable precipitating event were 10.03 (CI$_{95\%}$: 0.84, 120.15; p = 0.069) times more likely to have poorer outcomes.

PATHOPHYSIOLOGY OF PSYCHOGENIC TREMOR

In addition to clinical evaluation, the diagnosis of PT may be supported by physiological studies (35). Using quantitative accelerometry, Deuschl et al. (19) found that all 15 patients tested demonstrated the "coactivation sign," manifested by muscle activation in finger flexors and extensors about 300 msec before the onset of tremor. This finding is different from tremor recorded in patients with Parkinson disease, where the tremor bursts start immediately. In addition to the coactivation sign, absent finger tremor was the most consistent feature that separated Parkinson disease from organic tremor. In contrast to organic tremor, in which the amplitude dampens with loading (500 or 1,000 g), patients with PT had an increase in amplitude of their tremor with such loading. Future studies should employ such techniques to characterize PT further and to compare the clinical and physiologic features in patients with PT to those in organic tremor. For example, the technique of back-averaging electroencephalographic activity preceding electromyographic activity can be used to detect premovement potential in patients with PMD, not seen with organic involuntary movement (36). However, this technique is not very helpful in the case of tremor. Voluntary tapping of the contralateral limb usually results in either dissipation of the tremor or shifting of the tremor frequency to that of the metronome (37). Using accelerometry, Zeuner et al. (38) recently demonstrated that in contrast to essential and parkinsonian tremor, patients with PT showed larger tremor frequency changes and higher individual variability while tapping. A coherence entrainment test is another powerful electrophysiologic technique that has been found to differentiate psychogenic, dystonic, and other organic tremors (39).

TREATMENT OF PSYCHOGENIC TREMOR

In our longitudinal study, patients who reported improvement in their PT attributed the favorable outcome to a physician's prescribed treatment (48.7%), elimination of stressor(s) (19.5%), specific medication (14.6%), stress management (9.8%), biofeedback (7.3%), and psychotherapy (4.9%). Dissatisfaction with the physician appears to be the strongest prognostic risk factor of poor long-term outcome. Although there may be many reasons why PT patients become dissatisfied with their physicians, we suspect that the chief reason is the patient's unwillingness to accept the physician's diagnosis of PT and denial of any stressors (i.e., personal, family, or social) that may be contributing to the presenting condition. Therefore, gaining insight into underlying psychodynamic mechanisms of the PT is the first step toward effective treatment and favorable outcome.

Used effectively in diagnosing nonepileptic seizures (40), placebos may be useful in further defining PMD, including PT, and in carefully selected cases, the response to placebo may be used to support the reasons for the diagnosis during discussion with the patient (41). We do not use placebos as a treatment, but we take advantage of suggestibility in further defining the PMD. For example, applying a vibrating tuning fork to the affected limb, accompanied by a powerful suggestion that the vibration may either exacerbate or ameliorate the tremor, helps to characterize the phenomenology of the tremor. In some cases, we also ask the patients to hyperventilate to bring on the tremor, particularly when the tremor is paroxysmal. We find these maneuvers helpful in establishing and explaining the diagnosis. During our discussion of the diagnosis, we always fully disclose to the patient when and if placebos were used.

Although controlled trials in PT are lacking, we find the use of antidepressants particularly useful as ancillary measures to insight-oriented therapy, covered elsewhere in this volume (42). The choice is often dependent on whether there is an associated anxiety, in which case the selective serotonin reuptake inhibitors (SSRIs) are often beneficial; if insomnia is present, then the tricyclics may have some advantages. We also use mirtazapine, an antidepressant that enhances noradrenergic and serotonergic transmission and acts as a presynaptic α-2, 5HT2, and 5HT3 receptor antagonist. In contrast to the typical SSRIs, which can exacerbate tremor, mirtazapine has been reported to improve tremor in a small, open label study (43), although the drug has not been found to be effective in essential tremor in a double-blind, placebo-controlled trial (44). In addition to insight-oriented strategy and stress management, pharmacologic treatment of underlying depression and anxiety, psychological support, and physical and occupational therapy are critical in the comprehensive management of patients with PT.

REFERENCES

1. Thomas M, Jankovic J. Psychogenic movement disorders: diagnosis and management. *CNS Drugs.* 2004;18:437–452.
2. Crimlisk HL, Bhatia K, Cope H, et al. Slater revisited: 6-year follow-up study of patients with medically unexplained motor symptoms. *Br Med J.* 1998;31:582–586.

3. Sharpe M. Medically unexplained symptoms and syndromes. *Clin Med.* 2002;2:501–504.

4. Lewis A. "Psychogenic": a word and its mutations. *Psychological Medicine.* 1972;2:209–215.

5. Williams DT, Ford B, Fahn S. Phenomenology and psychopathology related to psychogenic movement disorders. *Adv Neurol.* 1995;65:231–257.

6. Abramowitz JS, Schwartz SA, Whiteside SP. A contemporary conceptual model of hypochondriasis. *Mayo Clin Proc.* 2002;77: 1323–1330.

7. Krahn LE, Li H, O'Connor MK. Patients who strive to be ill: factitious disorder with physical symptoms. *Am J Psychiatry.* 2003; 160:1163–1168.

8. Fahn S, Williams DT. Psychogenic dystonia. *Adv Neurol.* 1988; 50:431–455.

9. Monday K, Jankovic J. Psychogenic myoclonus. *Neurology.* 1993;43:349–352.

10. Reuber M, Pukrop R, Bauer J, et al. Outcome in psychogenic nonepileptic seizures: 1 to 10 year follow up in 164 patients. *Ann Neurol.* 2003;53:305–311.

11. Martin R, Burneo JG, Prasad A, et al. Frequency of epilepsy in patients with psychogenic seizures monitored by video-EEG. *Neurology.* 2003;61:1791–1792.

12. Tan EK, Jankovic J. Psychogenic hemifacial spasm. *J Neuropsychiatry Clin Neurosci.* 2001;13:380–384.

13. Kim YJ, Anthony S, Pakiam I, et al. Historical and clinical features of psychogenic tremor: a review of 70 cases. *Can J Neurol Sci.* 1999;26:190–195.

14. Campbell J. The shortest paper. *Neurology.* 1979;29:1633.

15. Lang AE, Koller WC, Fahn S. Psychogenic parkinsonism. *Arch Neurol.* 1995;52:802–810.

16. Williams DR. Psychogenic palatal tremor. *Mov Disord.* 2004; 19:333–335.

17. Chan RV, Trobe JD. Spasm of accommodation associated with closed head trauma. *J Neuroophthalmol.* 2002;22:15–17.

18. Koller WC, Lang AE, Vetere-Overfield B, et al. Psychogenic tremors. *Neurology.* 1989;39:1094–1099.

19. Deuschl G, Koster B, Lucking C, et al. Diagnostic and pathophysiological aspects of psychogenic tremors. *Mov Disord.* 1998;13:294–302.

20. Jankovic J, Thomas M, Vuong KD. Long-term outcome of psychogenic tremor. *Neurology.* 2004;62(Suppl. 5):A501.

21. Schwartzman RJ, Kerrigan J. The movement disorder of reflex sympathetic dystrophy. *Neurology.* 1990;40:57–61.

22. Bhatia KP, Bhatt MH, Marsden CD. The causalgia-dystonia syndrome. *Brain.* 1993;116:843–851.

23. Jankovic J. Post-traumatic movement disorders: central and peripheral mechanisms. *Neurology.* 1994;44:2008–2014.

24. Jankovic J. Can peripheral trauma induce dystonia and other movement disorders? Yes! *Mov Disord.* 2001;16:7–12.

25. Cardoso F, Jankovic J. Peripherally-induced tremor and parkinsonism. *Arch Neurol.* 1995;52:263–270.

26. Lang A, Fahn S. Movement disorder of RSD. *Neurology.* 1990; 40:1476–1477.

27. Verdugo RJ, Ochoa JL. Abnormal movements in complex regional pain syndrome: assessment of their nature. *Muscle Nerve.* 2000; 23:198–205.

28. Sa DS, Mailis-Gagnon A, Nicholson K, et al. Posttraumatic painful torticollis. *Mov Disord.* 2003;18:1482–1491.

29. Florence SL, Taub HB, Kaas JH. Large-scale sprouting of cortical connections after peripheral injury in adult macaque monkeys. *Science.* 1998;282:1117–1121.

30. Knecht S, Henningsen H, Höhling C, et al. Plasticity of plasticity? Changes in the pattern of perceptual correlates of reorganization after amputation. *Brain.* 1998;121:717–724.

31. Maihofner C, Handwerker HO, Neundorfer B, et al. Patterns of cortical reorganization in complex regional pain syndrome. *Neurology.* 2003;61:1707–1715.

32. Merzenich M. Long-term change of mind. *Science.* 1998;282: 1062–1117.

33. Schwenkreis P, Janssen F, Rommel O, et al. Bilateral motor cortex disinhibition in complex regional pain syndrome (CRPS) type I of the hand. *Neurology.* 2003;61:515–519.

34. Garza JA, Louis ED, Ford B. Long-term outcome of psychogenic movement disorders. *Neurology.* 2001;56:A120.

35. Ron M. Explaining the unexplained: understanding hysteria. *Brain.* 2001;124:1065–1066.

36. Brown P, Thompson PD. Electrophysiological aids to jerks, spasms and tremor. *Mov Disord.* 2001;16:595–599.

37. O'Sulleabhain PE, Matsumoto J. Time-frequency analysis of tremors. *Brain.* 1998;121:2127–2134.

38. Zeuner KE, Shoge RO, Goldstein SR, et al. Accelerometry to distinguish psychogenic from essential or parkinsonian tremor. *Neurology.* 2003;61:548–550.

39. McAuley J, Rothwell J. Identification of psychogenic, dystonic, and other organic tremors by a coherence entrainment test. *Mov Disord.* 2004;19:253–267.

40. Devinsky O, Fisher R. Ethical use of placebos and provocative testing in diagnosing nonepileptic seizures. *Neurology.* 1996;47: 866–870.

41. Levy R, Jankovic J. Placebo-induced conversion reaction: a neurobehavioral and EEG study of hysterical aphasia, seizure and coma. *J Abnorm Psychol.* 1983;92:243–249.

42. Jankovic J, Cloninger CR, Fahn S, et al. Therapeutic approaches to psychogenic movement disorders. In: Hallett M, Fahn S, Jankovic J et al., eds. *Psychogenic movement disorders: psychobiology and therapy of a functional disorder. Advances in neurology.* Philadelphia, PA: Lippincott Williams & Wilkins, 2005.

43. Pact V, Giduz T. Mirtazapine treats resting tremor, essential tremor, and levodopa-induced dyskinesias. *Neurology.* 1999;53:1154.

44. Pahwa R, Lyons KE. Mirtazapine in essential tremor: a double-blind, placebo-controlled pilot study. *Mov Disord.* 2003;18: 584–587.

The Phenomenology of Startle, Latah, and Related Conditions

7

Philip D. Thompson

ABSTRACT

Culture-bound startle syndromes, exemplified by latah, represent an exaggeration of the secondary component of the startle response. These syndromes differ from the "startle diseases," such as hyperekplexia, which represent exaggeration of the first or reflex component of the startle response, and psychogenic myoclonus. A distinctive feature of the culture-bound startle syndromes is the range of accompanying behavioral manifestations. This combination of a startle response and behavioral manifestations with vocalization, such as a simple noise or an expletive, following a fright or loud noise may be seen in Tourette syndrome and psychiatric illnesses. Similar responses can even be observed in otherwise normal subjects in some circumstances during everyday life. The propensity for such responses is enhanced by anxiety and the determinants of anxiety, such as fear. This link is mediated by connections between the amygdala and startle mechanisms.

THE STARTLE RESPONSE

The startle response provides the substrate for the commonest expression of generalized myoclonus. Sudden or unexpected visual, auditory, somatosensory, and vestibular stimuli elicit the startle response. The response may be augmented if these stimuli are accompanied by fright (1). The startle response consists of two components. The initial short latency component is a stereotyped reflex comprising a blink, a facial grimace, and brisk flexion of the neck, trunk, and upper limbs (2). Occasionally, limb extension is involved. The duration of this component is short and the responses habituate with repeated stimulation. The secondary component of the startle response occurs at a longer latency and is more variable in appearance and duration (1,3). The clinical manifestations of the secondary component are determined by the nature of the startling stimulus and the situation in which it occurs. This component is influenced by the state of arousal and attention (4). Accordingly, it contains emotional and voluntary behavioral responses to the startling stimulus. This part of the startle response has been described as an "orientating" response (3) in preparation for action towards the stimulus. The electrophysiologic characteristics of the second component of the startle response are less well-defined.

There are a number of clinical abnormalities of the startle reflex. These include pathologic enhancement of the earliest component of the reflex in familial hyperekplexia or startle disease (4,5), due to mutations of the glycine receptor gene (GLRA1) (6), and symptomatic hyperekplexia due to lesions in the region of the nucleus pontis caudalis of the brainstem reticular formation (2,7). Conversely, degeneration of this area of the brainstem in Steele–Richardson–Olszewski syndrome (8) results in loss of the early component of the startle response.

Exaggeration of startle responses have long been described in latah (9,10), Jumping Frenchmen of Maine (11,12), and related conditions referred to as "culture-bound startle syndromes" (13,14). More recently, exaggerated startle responses have been described in drug withdrawal, Tourette syndrome (15), and psychiatric conditions such as post-traumatic stress disorder (4,14). The nature of the startle response in the culture-bound startle syndromes will be considered further in this review.

LATAH

Latah was described by the British adventurer H.A. O'Brien in 1884 during his travels through the Malay Peninsula (9). The word "latah" refers to a nervous or ticklish disposition. In an eloquent account of the behavior of latah sufferers, O'Brien noted that it encompassed a degree of subservience, foreshadowing the importance of behavioral aspects of latah, particularly forced obedience. He declined to record the full expression of the behavioral aspects that have been detailed in more recent descriptions (10,13). In an attempt to put latah into some perspective today, it is helpful to review the original descriptions. The latah sufferer exhibited a prominent "start" in response to sound or a frightening stimulus. This was accompanied by a tendency to strike out at nearby persons and vocalizations with coprolalia. They appeared nervous and, in addition to the startle, were seemingly compelled to act in an impulsive manner in response to external stimuli. Words such as "tiger," "alligator" or "snake," particularly when shouted, evoked in "latahs" an exaggerated and fearful response such as cowering or behaviour such as jumping off a boat into the river. More complex behaviors were observed, including echolalia, echopraxia, and imitation behavior. O'Brien described imitation behavior in a man who copied O'Brien's waving and whistling, a woman who took off her clothes (despite his protestations) after a man removed his coat, and a cook on a river steamer who tossed a child in the air, then dropped the child, in response to a sailor performing the same actions with a piece of wood.

Many papers addressed the subject of latah over the next 100 years. All drew attention to the combination of a startle response and a variety of complex behaviors, especially echophenomena, vocalizations and coprolalia, and forced obedience. In the most recent article, Tanner and Chamberland presented a video demonstrating each of these behaviors in Indonesian Malays and concluded that the clinical picture had changed little since the original description (16).

THE JUMPING FRENCHMEN OF MAINE

At around the same time as O'Brien's description, George Beard reported his observations on the Jumping Frenchmen of Maine (11). These were French Canadian lumberjacks from adjacent Quebec who lived and worked in remote, isolated communities near Moosehead Lake in northwestern Maine. Beard's descriptions emphasize the behavioral aspects of the phenomenon, such as forced obedience and echolalia, as much as, if not more than, an exaggerated startle response (11). The social dimensions of the jumpers' behavior was also emphasized, and they appear to have been the source of entertainment. Beard observed, "When told to strike, he strikes, when told to throw it, he throws it, whatever he has in his hands." He examined echolalia by reciting Latin text (with which the lumberjacks would not have been familiar):

> …and he repeated or echoed the sound of the word as it came to him, in a quick sharp voice, at the same time he jumped, or struck, or threw, or raised his shoulders, or made some other violent muscular motion. They could not help repeating the word or sound that came from the person that ordered them any more than they could help striking, dropping, throwing, jumping or starting; all of these phenomena were indeed but parts of the general condition known as jumping (11).

Some of the behaviors observed in the lumberjacks, such as throwing knives, striking hot stoves, or jumping into fire or water, were potentially dangerous or injurious, further adding to the intrigue of the condition.

The jumpers were mainly men who were otherwise healthy. Beard emphasized the condition could be familial and begin in childhood. Subsequent reports of similar cases, all of French Canadian descent, shed little further light on this behavioral complex beyond the notion of a culturally determined and learned behavior as originally suggested by Beard (11). The recent examination of a small group of eight jumpers in the Beauce region of Quebec led to the conclusion that they exhibited situational behavior related to an isolated existence in a remote community, and that the phenomenon had diminished with the passage of time (12,17). Similar features were described in presumed descendants of the French Acadians from Nova Scotia, the "Ragin' Cajuns" of Louisiana (18), and others (19) who were possibly genetically related to the Jumping Frenchmen of Maine. Startle behavior was also described in other population groups (20).

MYRIACHIT

A short time after Beard's communications, Hammond reported the story told by two U.S. naval personnel of an unusual pattern of behavior in Eastern Siberia referred to as "myriachit" or "to act foolishly" (21). This report concerned one man who imitated the behavior of others. He also displayed echolalia, echopraxia, and perseveration. Hammond was impressed with the similarities of this behavior to the recently described Jumping Frenchmen of Maine. It is clear from the description that the patient found his behavior disturbing, though it entertained and amused onlookers.

CULTURE-BOUND STARTLE SYNDROMES

The "culture-bound startle syndromes" have been described in many cultures and societies (10,13,14). These syndromes are characterized by an exaggerated startle response to unexpected visual, auditory, and sensory stimuli associated with echolalia, vocalizations, coprolalia, echopraxia, and a range of prolonged and complex motor activities including forced obedience, imitation behavior, and environmentally dependent behaviors. In some cases the latter manifestations were initiated by external stimuli. Moreover, the behaviors were goal-directed and could be potentially harmful or injurious as observed in latah and the Jumping Frenchmen. These elements are clearly more complex and prolonged than the initial brief component of the startle reflex. From video observation of these responses (16,17), the onset latency lies within the range of voluntary reaction times. The prolonged response duration is consistent with these startle behaviors representing elaboration of the secondary or "orientating component" of the startle response intermixed with, and modified by, voluntary responses to the relevant stimulus.

Simons interviewed a series of American hyperstartlers ascertained through newspaper advertisements and found that these people reported behavioral accompaniments to the exaggerated startle response similar to those observed in latah (13). Throwing, vocalizations, and coprolalia were observed, but imitation behavior and forced obedience were not. The term "goosey" may also refer to similar behaviors (22).

TOURETTE SYNDROME AND STARTLE

The relationship with Tourette syndrome is of interest. Tourette was aware of the reports of latah and the Jumping Frenchmen at the time he described the condition that bears his name (23). Indeed, it seems likely that he was influenced by these descriptions in formulating his syndrome. There are several differences between Tourette syndrome and the culture-bound startle syndromes. The most obvious is the absence of motor tics in the culture-bound startle syndromes. However, reflex tics, stimulus-induced motor activity, and complex behaviors are well-recognized in Tourette syndrome. Motor tics typically occur after an internal premonitory sensation, but "reflex" tics may be triggered by external sounds such as coughing, sniffing, or particular words (24). Accordingly, stimulus-induced behaviors, complex motor activities, and vocalizations, with coprolalia and echolalia, occur in both Tourette syndrome and the culture-bound startle syndromes (25). Additional behavioral features such as echopraxia, obsessive–compulsive behaviors, touching, tapping, rituals, and other complex movements are common to both conditions. Late-onset startle-induced tics were examined electrophysiologically

and found to be variable in pattern, prolonged (duration up to 2 minutes), and occuring at long latency (120 to 160 ms) after the stimulus (26). These features clearly distinguish the responses from an exaggerated initial component of the startle reflex. However, the responses were not preceded by a premovement potential, suggesting they were not "voluntary" (26). An exaggerated startle response may occur in Tourette syndrome, though the frequency with which this occurs is debated (15,27). Tanner in her recent observations concluded on the basis of clinical observation that the behavior of latah differed from that seen in Tourette syndrome (16).

STARTLE IN PSYCHIATRY

There is an increasing amount of psychiatric literature concerning abnormalities of the startle response in relation to post-traumatic stress disorder, generalized anxiety disorder, schizophrenia, and drug withdrawal (4,14). Early psychiatric theories of the culture-bound startle syndromes were concerned with the relationship of the behavior to fright, fear, and trauma (13,14). Forced obedience, echopraxia, and coprolalia were interpreted as defensive behaviors occurring in the setting of overwhelming anxiety or fear that were elaborated according to the prevailing cultural customs (14). An exaggerated startle response has long been linked to "war neurosis," "shell shock," or "startle neurosis," (20) and is now an integral part of the diagnosis of posttraumatic stress disorder (4).

There is an expanding literature on the excitability of the startle response as a reflection of the level of arousal and emotional tone. From a neurophysiologic viewpoint, this linkage relates to the second component of the startle response, the "orientating" response (1,3), and must also be distinguished from voluntary stimulus contingent jumps and jerks (28).

ANATOMY OF THE STARTLE RESPONSES

The output of the first component of the startle response is generated within the nucleus pontis caudalis of the brainstem reticular formation in response to an auditory or trigeminal stimulus and transmitted to spinal motoneurons via the reticulospinal tracts (2).

The anatomic and physiologic substrates for the second component of the startle response are likely to be more widespread and are less understood. Central to these are connections between the amygdala, which mediates fear and influences the level of arousal, and other cortical and brainstem structures. Two main projection systems from the amygdala exist. Projections from the central and medial amygdala form part of the basal ganglia outputs through the bed nucleus of the stria terminalis to influence the hypothalamus, orbitofrontal cortex, and provide facilitatory projections to the pontine reticular formation (29,30). The amygdala also provides afferents to the nucleus basalis of Meynert, the cholinergic neurons of which have widespread projections to cerebral cortical areas and may be involved in cortical arousal. Ascending serotonergic raphe projections complete the network for arousal among the brainstem, amygdala, and limbic regions. Accordingly, there are many anatomical pathways to link the emotional tone or level of arousal of the organism and the startle response. This concept was emphasized in a recent case report of a young man with an amygdala lesion in whom the startle response was generally reduced but impaired contralaterally. Moreover, the startle response was not potentiated by aversive stimuli (31).

BEHAVIORAL PHENOMENA IN STARTLE

The neurologic significance of the behavioral phenomena described in these startle syndromes deserves further comment. It is widely recognized that a sudden startle response may be accompanied by a prolonged series of "orientating" movements and even vocalization, and that this response may be a normal phenomenon. Such responses often are evoked to provide a source of amusement for children and even adults. The more elaborate and complex behaviors described in the culture-bound startle syndromes can be interpreted from a neurologic viewpoint as environment-dependent behaviors. Such behaviors are observed in frontal lobe syndromes (32,33). These behaviors cannot be suppressed and may take the form of imitation behavior (33) or more complex utilization behavior (34). Such actions differ from the automatic impulsive imitation of echopraxia and the perseveration of simple movements. Lhermitte regarded these environment-dependent behaviors as representing the release of parietal lobe activity from frontal inhibition due to lesions of the inferior and mediobasal frontal lobes (35).

PSYCHOGENIC MYOCLONUS

Myoclonus accounts for 10% to 20% of psychogenic movement disorders (36–38). The clinical appearance is usually of segmental or generalized jerking, occurring at rest and during movement. An association with psychopathology, including other psychogenic neurologic signs, has been reported (36). Clinical examination typically reveals a reduction in the jerking during distraction. With mental tasks and instructions to perform repetitive movements, variability of the jerking is also evident. Although psychogenic generalized jerks may have a similar clinical appearance to responses in the culture-bound startle syndromes described above, psychogenic jerks are usually

described as occurring at rest. Moreover, the associated clinical features are of a psychogenic disorder. This is in contrast to the behavioral manifestations observed in the cultural syndromes.

Neurophysiologic methods are particularly useful in the analysis of myoclonus and can assist in distinguishing between voluntary jerking and cortical or brainstem myoclonus (28,39). The electromyographic pattern of voluntary jerks exhibits a triphasic pattern of activity between antagonist muscle pairs, similar to a voluntary movement. In contrast, cortical myoclonus typically consists of short-duration (25 to 50 ms) bursts of muscle activity, often cocontracting in antagonist muscles. Myoclonus of brainstem origin affects the upper body bilaterally and begins in the sternomastoid muscle at short latencies (less than 80 ms or so), depending on the stimulus. Demonstration of this pattern is particularly useful for diagnostic purposes (39).

When stimulus-induced jerks are present, measurement of the response will distinguish between reflex myoclonus and voluntary responses. The latency of cortical reflex myoclonus is very short and between 40 and 100 ms, depending on the limb involved and the height of the patient (28,39). In contrast, voluntary responses to a stimulus will occur around voluntary reaction times and may show considerable variation with distraction, for example, during the performance of dual tasks (see chapter 30).

REFERENCES

1. Wilkins D, Hallett M, Wess MM. Audiogenic startle reflex of man and its relationship to startle syndromes. *Brain.* 1986;109: 561–573.
2. Brown P, Rothwell JC, Thompson PD, et al. The hyperekplexias and their relationship to the normal startle reflex. *Brain.* 1991; 114:1903–1928.
3. Gogan P. The startle and orienting reactions in man. A study of their characteristics and habituation. *Brain Res.* 1970;18:117–135.
4. Grillon C, Baas J. A review of the modulation of the startle reflex by affective states and its application in psychiatry. *Clin Neurophysiol.* 2003;114:1557–1579.
5. Andermann F, Andermann E. Excessive startle syndromes: startle disease, jumping and startle epilepsy. *Adv Neurol.* 1986;43: 321–338.
6. Tijssen MAJ, Shiang R, Deutekom Jvan, et al. Molecular genetic re-evaluation of the Dutch hyperekplexia family. *Arch Neurol.* 1995;52:578–582.
7. Vidailhet M, Rothwell JC, Thompson PD, et al. The auditory startle response in the Steele-Richardson-Olszewski syndrome and Parkinson's disease. *Brain.* 1992;115(Pt 4):1181–1192.
8. Kimber TE, Thompson PD. Symptomatic hyperekplexia occurring as a result of pontine infarction. *Mov Disord.* 1997;12:814–816.
9. O'Brien HA. Latah. *J Straits Br Asiat Soc.* 1883;11:143–153.
10. Yap PM. The latah reaction: its pathodynamics and nosological position. *J Ment Sci.* 1952;98:515–564.
11. Beard G. Experiments with the "jumpers" or "jumping Frenchmen" of Maine. *J Nerv Ment Dis.* 1880;7:487–490.
12. Saint-Hilaire M-H, Saint-Hilaire J-M, Granger L. Jumping Frenchmen of Maine. *Neurology.* 1986;36:1269–1271.
13. Simons RC. The resolution of the latah paradox. *J Nerv Ment Dis.* 1980;168:195–206.

14. Howard R, Ford R. From the jumping Frenchmen of Maine to post-traumatic stress disorder: the startle response in neuropsychiatry. *Psychol Med.* 1992;22:695–707.
15. Stell R, Thickbroom GW, Mastaglia FL. The audiogenic startle response in Tourette's syndrome. *Mov Disord.* 1995;10:723–730.
16. Tanner CM, Chamberland J. Latah in Jakarta, Indonesia. *Mov Disord.* 2001;16:526–529.
17. Saint-Hilaire M-H, Saint-Hilaire J-M. Jumping Frenchmen of Maine. *Mov Disord.* 2001;16:530.
18. McFarling DA. The "ragin' Cajuns" of Louisiana. *Mov Disord.* 2001;16:531–532.
19. Stevens H. "Jumping Frenchmen of Maine." *Arch Neurol.* 1965;12:311–314.
20. Thorne FC. Startle neurosis. *Am J Psychiatry.* 1944;101:105–109.
21. Hammond WA. Miryachit, a newly described disease of the nervous system and its analogues. *NY State J Med.* 1884;39:191–192.
22. Hardison J. Are the jumping Frenchmen of Maine goosey? *JAMA.* 1980;244:70.
23. Goetz CG, Klawans HL. Gilles de la Tourette on Tourette syndrome. *Adv Neurol.* 1982;35:1–16.
24. Commander M, Corbett J, Prendergast M, et al. Reflex tics in two patients with Gilles de la Tourette syndrome. *Br J Psychiatry.* 1991;159:877–879.
25. Eapen V, Moriarty J, Robertson MM. Stimulus induced behaviours in Tourette's syndrome. *J Neurol Neurosurg Psychiatry.* 1994;57:853–855.
26. Tijssen MAJ, Brown P, Morris HR, et al. Late onset startle induced tics. *J Neurol Neurosurg Psychiatry.* 1999;67:782–784.
27. Sachdev PS, Chee KY, Aniss AM. The audiogenic startle reflex in Tourette's syndrome. *Biol Psychiatry.* 1997;41:796–803.
28. Thompson PD, Colebatch JG, Brown P, et al. Voluntary stimulus sensitive jerks and jumps mimicking myoclonus or pathological startle syndromes. *Mov Disord.* 1992;7:257–262.
29. Swanson LW, Petrovich GD. What is the amygdala? *Trends Neurosci.* 1998;21:3223–3331.
30. Hitchcock JM, Davis M. Efferent pathway of the amygdala involved in conditioned fear as measured with the fear-potentiated startle paradigm. *Behav Neurosci.* 2001;105:826–842.
31. Angrilli A, Mauri A, Palomba D, et al. Startle reflex and emotion modulation impairment after a right amygdala lesion. *Brain.* 1996;119:1991–2000.
32. Luria AR. *Higher cortical functions in man.* New York: Basic Books, 1980.
33. Lhermitte F. Utilization behaviour and its relation to lesions of the frontal lobes. *Brain.* 1983;106:237–255.
34. Lhermitte F. Human autonomy and the frontal lobes. Part II: patient behaviour in complex and social situations: the "environmental dependency syndrome." *Ann Neurol.* 1986;19:335–343.
35. Lhermitte F, Pillon B, Serdaru M. Autonomy and the frontal lobes. Part I: imitation and utilization behaviour: a neuropsychological study of 75 patients. *Ann Neurol.* 1986;19:326–334.
36. Monday K, Jankovic J. Psychogenic myoclonus. *Neurology.* 1993;43:349–352.
37. Williams DT, Ford B, Fahn S. Phenomenology and psychopathology related to psychogenic movement disorders. *Adv Neurol.* 1995;65:231–257.
38. Factor SA, Podskalny GD, Molho ES. Psychogenic movement disorders: frequency, clinical profile and characteristics. *J Neurol Neurosurg Psychiatry.* 1995;59:406–412.
39. Brown P, Thompson PD. Electrophysiological aids to the diagnosis of psychogenic jerks, spasms and tremor. *Mov Disord.* 2001;16:595–599.

Psychogenic Dystonia and Reflex Sympathetic Dystrophy

8

Anette Schrag

ABSTRACT

Dystonia was for many years misdiagnosed as a psychogenic condition, leading to inappropriate management strategies in a considerable number of patients. As a result, many neurologists are currently reluctant to make a diagnosis of psychogenic dystonia (PD), and this condition is now probably underrecognized. This is particularly so as dystonia largely remains a clinical diagnosis, and as unusual presentations can make the differentiation of neurologic disorders from PD very difficult. PD is typically classified as a secondary dystonia, but routine investigations are usually normal. Specialized neurophysiologic investigations show abnormalities in groups of patients with neurologic dystonia, but due to their insufficient sensitivity and specificity, these tests are not useful in the diagnosis of individual patients. However, in PD, careful psychiatric assessment and neurologic examination often reveal previous somatizations, psychiatric comorbidity, psychological stressors, and nonorganic signs. Furthermore, features of inconsistency over time or during examination, or of incongruency with typical presentations of dystonia (which should be judged by a neurologist with experience in movement disorders) are suggestive of this diagnosis, and allow PD to be diagnosed using defined criteria. Controversial patients are those with dystonia developing within days of a peripheral injury. Such dystonia is often fixed and may be associated with features of complex regional pain syndrome (CRPS) type I. Fixed dystonic postures are a common manifestation of PD and, although they can be seen following brain lesions, they are not seen in idiopathic dystonia. Controversy exists whether this syndrome of posttraumatic dystonia is due to abnormal cortical reorganization from a peripheral injury—akin to amputation stump movements—or whether at least a large proportion of these patients suffer from a psychogenic movement disorder, as suggested by the high proportion of nonorganic signs and associated clinical and psychiatric features.

INTRODUCTION

Although idiopathic torsion dystonia was considered an organic condition in its first descriptions (1,2), only in the last decades has it been universally considered a neurologic rather than a psychiatric disorder (3,4). Dystonias were, therefore, for many years attributed to psychological causes, resulting in unnecessary and unhelpful treatment strategies and considerable psychological consequences for sufferers and their families. As a result of this long history of misdiagnosis, there has been considerable reluctance among neurologists and psychiatrists in making a diagnosis of PD. However, the pendulum has perhaps swung the opposite way, and PD is now often underdiagnosed.

Overall, PD is a rare cause of dystonia and represents only approximately 5% of patients with dystonia, but among psychogenic movement disorders, dystonia accounts for approximately 20% to 50% of cases (5). While the term "psychogenic" is somewhat controversial, implying a psychological causation which cannot always be demonstrated, the term "psychogenic" contrasting with "organic" has been used in the literature to distinguish such patients from those with neurologic disorders. For the purpose of this chapter, I will refer to this perhaps overly simplified classification, which will be discussed elsewhere in this book.

DIAGNOSIS

Diagnostic Difficulties

The above diagnostic uncertainties reflect the considerable difficulties in making a diagnosis of PD. The definition of dystonia is not particularly helpful in making this diagnosis as it is descriptive, defining dystonia as "abnormal muscle contractions, often holding a body part in an abnormal position, that may be repetitive or tremulous" (6). This definition clearly encompasses PD as the cause for the abnormal muscle contraction. There is a plethora of conditions that can cause dystonia, and these have been classified by Fahn and others (6). The *primary dystonias* are those with no identifiable cause, and are often due to a genetic abnormality; *dystonia-plus* includes dystonias associated with other neurologic abnormalities such as myoclonus or parkinsonism; the *heredodegenerative dystonias* are heredodegenerative conditions in which dystonia may be part of the presentation; and *secondary dystonia* is due to a known symptomatic cause such as lesions in the basal ganglia. PD is classified in this last category.

There are a number of factors that contribute to the difficulties in differentiating psychogenic from other types of dystonia. The diagnosis relies almost entirely on clinical history, examination, and clinical judgment. There is no biologic marker or pathognomonic sign that in isolation allows an unequivocal diagnosis of PD, and, conversely, with the exception of a few available genetic tests for some types of dystonia, there is no biologic marker for primary dystonia. Even for secondary dystonia, a cause cannot always be found, and in at least two thirds of patients with organic dystonia, investigations are normal. It is true that an organic condition causing secondary dystonia must always be excluded by appropriate investigations, but the diagnosis of dystonia in the majority of cases remains a clinical one.

In addition, organic dystonia and PD both have a wide and overlapping spectrum of presentations, which often includes bizarre and unusual presentations that may appear inconsistent and be unique to individual patients. The differentiation of these conditions based on clinical features thus requires extensive experience with the wide spectrum of presentations of dystonia.

Finally, organic dystonia and PD can occur together, and a PD may have developed on top of an organic condition. Although this co-occurrence is probably not quite as frequent as the co-occurrence of epileptic and nonepileptic attacks [which is estimated to be up to 25% (7)], functional overlay in an underlying organic condition is always a possibility.

Despite these caveats, a diagnosis of PD is possible and can be made when (a) appropriate investigations have been negative, and (b) positive findings allow a diagnosis based on standardized diagnostic criteria (see below).

Clinical Clues

Characteristics of Dystonia

The characteristics of dystonia contribute to the confusion between organic dystonia and PD. Dystonia is often bizarre and may appear inconsistent, as it may be mild or absent at rest, worsen or only be present with action, and respond to sensory tricks (e.g., improvement of torticollis when the chin is touched—geste antagoniste); it may also only be apparent when *specific* actions are performed, for example, when walking forward but not when walking backward, when walking but not when running, when writing but not when using a knife and fork, or when playing an instrument but not during other actions involving the same muscles. However, primary dystonia, which is the main area of diagnostic difficulty, has characteristic patterns that help in the differentiation of primary dystonia from PD: whilst only some actions may trigger the dystonia, these actions will reliably do so; the pattern of abnormality is consistent over time with little change in its distribution and phenotype (although it may progress and spread); and the distribution and progression of primary dystonia is characteristic at different age groups. Thus, while childhood-onset primary dystonia typically starts in the lower limbs and slowly spreads to other body parts, primary dystonia with onset in adulthood does not usually affect the legs first, and typically remains restricted to the craniocervical region or the upper limbs. In addition, the onset of dystonia is usually gradual, and progression is slow over several months or years; there is not usually pain (with the exception of cervical dystonia, which can be painful), and it is typically mobile (and often absent at rest) and remains so until very late stages of advanced disease.

The most helpful features in making a diagnosis of PD are those that do not fit with these recognized patterns of primary dystonia, and are therefore incongruent with primary dystonia. Positive features for a PD thus include dystonic postures that start abruptly and progress rapidly to severe disability, often with a fixed dystonic posture without return to the neutral position at rest from the beginning. There may be marked fluctuations with exacerbations and (almost) complete remissions, which are rare in primary dystonia. The presentation may have been inconsistent over time, with a complete change in the nature of the abnormal movement or the development of other psychogenic movement disorders. Onset in the leg in an adult also suggests a PD once a symptomatic cause has been excluded, and so does a lack of sensory tricks and the presence of severe pain. However, none of these features are specific for PD. They can also occur in other secondary dystonias, and other secondary causes, such as a basal ganglia lesion, must be excluded before a diagnosis of PD is made.

Additional Medical History

The past medical history may also be revealing. Episodes of a different movement disorder in the same limb or another limb may have occurred with complete or partial remissions. There may also be a history of nonepileptic seizures or of other somatizations, putting the current presentation in the context of a wider somatoform illness. Previous somatizations may include other "functional" syndromes, such as fibromyalgia, atypical chest pain, irritable bowel syndromes (8), or other medically unexplained symptoms which may have resulted in a number of investigations and treatments, including operations (9). For example, inflammation may not have been found in an appendectomy performed for severe abdominal pain, or an episode of unexplained prolonged fatigue may have occurred previously. While patients with somatoform illness often report a number of previous diagnoses or complaints, the somatoform nature often only becomes apparent when patients or their general practitioners are specifically asked about the outcome of investigations (10).

The history may also be informative in other respects. It may reveal abnormal illness behavior, for example, noncompliance with treatment, "splitting" behavior among the health professionals involved in a patient's care, or "doctor-shopping." Litigation or a compensation claim may represent a maintaining factor, or there may be obvious secondary gain. There may have been an obvious psychological stressor before the onset of the PD, suggesting a diagnosis of conversion disorder, or psychological trauma in the past history. However, this type of information may be misleading as psychological conflicts are common in the population, and the coincidence between past psychological trauma and the presentation may be spurious.

Examination

The physical examination concentrates on four aspects.

1. *Absence of "hard" neurologic signs.* Most neurologists would be reluctant to make a diagnosis of a PD in the presence of "hard" neurologic signs. However, as mentioned above, psychogenic overlay may exist comorbidly with an underlying organic illness. This may occur for a variety of reasons, including the patient's wish to demonstrate the extent of his or her ailments (e.g. patients with Parkinson disease referred for stereotactic surgery) (Anthony Lang, *personal communication* in October 2003), or when patients have had previous experiences with doctors who were unconvinced of the seriousness of the problem. In addition, secondary physical changes may have occurred following a long-standing PD with prolonged immobilization, including wasting, trophic changes, or even osteoporosis. Furthermore, pseudoneurologic signs are not uncommon, including pseudoclonus, abnormal reflexes in a rigidly held limb, or pseudobabinski (often as a delayed, prolonged plantar extension), which can mislead the examiner. Although the interpretation of such findings is difficult, the recognition of the possibility of a pseudoneurologic sign facilitates the recognition of a psychogenic disorder.

2. *The presence of other nonorganic signs and findings,* such as nonorganic weakness, nonanatomical sensory loss, resistance to passive movements, bouts of whole-body shaking, or an excessive startle response. There may be extreme slowness, which, unlike bradykinesia, is not fatiguing and without a decrement in the amplitude of the movement. There may be consistent past-pointing in an otherwise normal (sometimes excessively slow) finger-nose test, and other tasks may simply not be completed (e.g., stopping two inches early in the finger-nose test). The most useful sign is probably the Hoover sign, which has been shown to quantitatively differentiate organic and nonorganic weakness (11) (see Chapter 13). However, caveats apply to all nonorganic signs. For example, give-way weakness may be seen if the movement causes pain, and sensory disturbance not following a nerve or radicular distribution is common in Parkinson disease and often predates the onset of motor symptoms. In addition, classical signs such as midline splitting, splitting of vibration sense, and la belle indifférence have poor specificity and are therefore of limited value in assessing these patients (12). There may also be a discrepancy between objective signs and disability (e.g., patients with mild unilateral weakness who are bed- or wheelchair-bound or, conversely, patients with no use of both arms who manage at home on their own). Similarly, there may be a

discrepancy between subjectively reported symptoms and investigations that exclude a pathophysiologic correlate (e.g., normal sensory evoked potentials in a patient reporting total loss of sensation in a limb).

3. *Features of a psychogenic movement disorder.* There are a number of specific, positive features which suggest the diagnosis of a psychogenic movement disorder, including PD (see Chapter 13). These include fluctuations during the examination, particularly an increase of the dystonia with attention and suggestion, and a decrease with distraction; a changing pattern of frequency, amplitude, or pattern; the ability to trigger movements with unusual or nonphysiologic interventions (e.g., trigger points on the body, passive movements of another limb); and the character of the dystonia may be incongruous with the presentation of an organic dystonia. The last is an important criterion in differentiating psychogenic and organic dystonia, but requires considerable experience with the presentation of dystonia, and it is therefore generally agreed that this diagnosis should only be made by a neurologist with experience in these disorders. The most reliable feature allowing a confident diagnosis of a PD (or other psychogenic movement disorder), however, is a marked and persistent improvement with psychotherapy, placebo, or suggestion. It is important that this response is significant and sustained, as placebo effects are well-recognized to improve movement disorders transiently up to 30% (13).

4. *Scars from multiple operations or self-inflicted injuries.* The physical examination may reveal multiple scars from multiple previous operations, which may be due to previous abnormal illness behavior or somatization, or self-inflicted injury, suggesting an underlying psychiatric disturbance.

Psychiatric Assessment

There are few studies assessing psychiatric aspects specifically in PD. However, psychiatric aspects of psychogenic movement disorders, which are discussed in detail elsewhere in this book, also apply to PD. In brief, "psychogenic movement disorders" summarize, from a neurologic point of view, a mixture of conversion disorders, somatoform disorders, factitious disorders, and malingering. While many patients with PD report an entirely normal mental state (and are often reluctant to see a psychiatrist), psychiatric assessment can provide useful information and potentially allow underlying psychological causes to be addressed. In particular, concurrent psychiatric comorbidity, which most commonly comprises depression, anxiety disorders, and personality disorders (5,14–16), may be diagnosed (and treated); previous episodes of psychiatric illness, behavioral abnormalities, and self-harm may be revealed; psychological stressors as precipitating or

maintaining factors identified and addressed, or a history of psychological trauma, including childhood sexual, physical, or emotional abuse, uncovered. Whilst these features may support a diagnosis of a psychogenic problem, none of them is specific for this and may be coincidental. Nevertheless, addressing these issues may improve patients' overall quality of life and lead to improvement of the physical presentation of a PD in a proportion of patients.

The differing characteristics of psychogenic and primary dystonia in the past medical history, history of dystonia, physical examination, and response to treatment are listed in Table 8.1, modified from Lang (17).

Diagnostic Criteria for PD

None of the features listed above is specific for PD. Not only does psychiatric comorbidity, a history of psychological stressors, or childhood abuse occur in a high proportion of people with neurologic illness or the general population, but psychogenic signs may occur in organic illness, and single episodes of somatization occur in a high proportion of people without reaching the diagnostic criteria for somatization disorder (18). However, some of these features of PD and psychogenic movement disorders in general are more suggestive of this diagnosis than are others, and the presence of several of these features increases the likelihood of this diagnosis. Based on these features, the diagnostic classification of psychogenic movement disorders, which reflects the degree of diagnostic certainty of this diagnosis, was modified for PD (19) (Table 8.2).

COURSE OF ILLNESS

As mentioned above, many patients with PD have a history of previous somatizations or other psychogenic movement disorders, which may have remitted spontaneously or with treatment. There may also have been paroxysmal exacerbations and remissions, but in others no fluctuations occur and the disorder remains stable over years. The prognosis is generally poor, with the majority of patients suffering long-term disability. However, outcome varies considerably, and while the PD remains stable in most patients, some develop other psychogenic movement disorders, replace the dystonia with a mental disorder, or experience complete remission of symptoms (14,17,20).

Investigations

Other than excluding causes for secondary dystonia, there are a few specific investigations that may contribute to the diagnosis of dystonia. Several abnormalities in spinal and motor cortical circuits have been reported in patients with

TABLE 8.1
DIFFERENCES BETWEEN PRIMARY DYSTONIA AND PSYCHOGENIC DYSTONIA

	Features Typical of Primary Dystonia	Features that *May* be Seen in Psychogenic Dystonia
Past medical history	Unremarkable for age	Previous somatizations
History of dystonia	Onset after injury rare	Onset after minor injury/operation common
	No clear association with psychological stressors	Psychological stressor before onset
	Onset in childhood (generalized dystonia)	Onset in adolescence or adulthood
	Gradual onset	Abrupt onset
	Spread slow	Rapid progression
	Leg onset only in childhood	Onset in legs common
	No or little fluctuation over time	Marked fluctuations in severity and exacerbations
	Pattern consistent over time	Movement disorder changes over time
	No pain (exception cervical dystonia)	Severe pain and secondary pain
	Remissions rare	Remissions common
Examination	Consistent action-specific pattern	Inconsistent activation pattern
	Recognized pattern of dystonia (can be deceptive)	Pattern incongruent with organic dystonia
	Mobile dystonia	Fixed dystonic posture
	Geste antagoniste	No sensory tricks
	Rarely modifiable	Distractablility/increase with attention/trigger points/ suggestibility
	Neurologic examination otherwise normal	Nonorganic signs and/or other psychogenic movement disorders
	Only mild or transient response to placebo, suggestion, or psychotherapy	Marked and persistent response to placebo, suggestion, or psychotherapy
		Scars indicating self-harm or previous somatizations
Psychiatric assessment	Mild depression or anxiety may coexist	Significant psychopathology, particularly depression, anxiety, personality disorders
		Past history of abuse
Social history		Secondary gain
		Compensation claim, litigation
		Abnormal illness behavior

From Lang AE. Psychogenic dystonia: a review of 18 cases. *Can J Neurol Sci.* 1995;22(2):136–143.

dystonia, including abnormalities of intracortical inhibition and of the cortical silent period (21), reduced reciprocal inhibition of H-reflexes in the forearm muscles (22), evidence of broad peak synchronization of motor units in antagonist muscles (23), and evidence for a new low frequency drive that is absent in controls but present in cervical dystonia (24). In addition, several imaging studies have demonstrated abnormal function on fMRI (25) or positron emission tomography (26). However, while all of these have helped the understanding of dystonia on a

TABLE 8.2
DIAGNOSTIC CRITERIA FOR PSYCHOGENIC DYSTONIA (14)

Documented[a]: Persistent relief by psychotherapy, suggestion, or placebo has been demonstrated, which may be helped by physiotherapy, or patients were seen without the dystonia when believing themselves unobserved.
Clinically Established[a]: The dystonia is incongruent with classical dystonia or there are inconsistencies in the examination, plus at least one of the following three: other psychogenic signs, multiple somatizations, or an obvious psychiatric disturbance.
Probable: The dystonia is incongruent or inconsistent with typical dystonia, or there are psychogenic signs or multiple somatizations.
Possible: Evidence of an emotional disturbance.

[a]As only the first two categories provide a clinically useful degree of diagnostic certainty, they have been combined to one category of "Clinically Definite."
From Williams DT, Ford B, Fahn S. Phenomenology and psychopathology related to psychogenic movement disorders. *Adv Neurol.* 1995;65:231–257.

group level, the sensitivity and specificity of these investigations are unknown, and it is not clear how useful these techniques are on an individual basis. In addition, they are only available in specialized centers and not in routine clinical practice. Therefore, these tests at present do not appear useful in the diagnosis of individual patients in clinical practice, but may become more important in distinguishing psychogenic and organic dystonia when further studies assessing the sensitivity and specificity of these tests become available.

REFLEX SYMPATHETIC DYSTROPHY

Reflex sympathetic dystrophy (RSD), now called complex regional pain syndrome (CRPS) type I, and dystonia with onset after peripheral trauma ("posttraumatic dystonia") (27) share many features of PD (Table 8.3). As a result, there has been a continuing controversy regarding the etiology of these conditions (28,29).

Posttraumatic dystonia usually occurs within hours or days after a minor injury, with a fixed dystonic posture, lack of a geste antagoniste, severe pain, and maximum disability soon after injury (27,30,31). Motor and sensory symptoms of posttraumatic dystonia overlap with those seen in CRPS type I (see below), but most reported cases of posttraumatic dystonia affected the neck and shoulders rather than the limbs, and were not accompanied by autonomic or trophic changes seen in CRPS. In a recent study (32), it has been argued that posttraumatic cervical dystonia may belong to the PDs rather than have an organic cause. Many patients had nonorganic signs, features suggestive of a psychogenic movement disorder, were involved in litigation (33), responded with improvement of posture and/or pain and sensory abnormalities to intravenous sodium-amytal tests, and had psychological conflicts on psychological testing. In another study of 103 patients with fixed (usually limb) dystonia, of whom the majority occurred after a minor injury, a substanial minority fulfilled strict criteria for PD or for somatization disorder, particularly when this history was specifically sought (34). However, others disagree and have disputed an association between CRPS and psychological disorders (28,35,36).

CRPS type I (or RSD) typically occurs after a minor peripheral injury and, in contrast to CRPS type II, is not associated with a nerve injury. Its features include autonomic dysfunction with edema, sudomotor and blood flow abnormalities, trophic changes (including osteoporosis),

TABLE 8.3

FEATURES OF POSTTRAUMATIC DYSTONIA, CRPS TYPE I, AND PSYCHOGENIC DYSTONIA

	Psychogenic Dystonia	CRPS Type I	Posttraumatic Dystonia
Injury before onset	+	+++	+++
Abrupt onset	+++	+++	+++
Rapid progression	++	+++	+++
Severe pain	++	++	++
Female preponderance	+++	+++	−?
Family history	−	−	−
Onset age (young) adulthood	++	++	++
Onset in lower limbs	+	+	+
Exacerbations	++	++	−?
Remissions	+	rare	−?
Fluctuations over time	++	−	−
Fixed posture	++	+++	+++
Autonomic changes	(−)	+++	(−)
Trophic changes	(+)	++	(+)
Nondermatomal sensory disturbances	++	++	+
Action-specific	−	−	−
Geste antagoniste	−	−	−
Distractible/suggestible	++	−	−
Nonorganic signs	++	+	+
Response to placebo, suggestion, or psychotherapy	++	−	−?
Psychological stressors evident	++	+	+
Significant psychopathology	++	+	−?
Abnormal illness behavior	++	+	−?
Response to anticholinergics	−	−	−
Response to botulinum toxin injections	+	+	+

+, occasionally; ++, commonly; +++, almost the rule; (−), minor temperature changes; (+), secondary when longstanding; −?, not known.

and sensory and motor abnormalities (37). Typically, there is severe pain, which is disproportionate to the inciting event, allodynia (an innocuous stimulus causing pain), hyper- or hypoalgesia not limited to the territory of a single peripheral nerve, or hyperaesthesia. Motor features of CRPS include a restricted range of movements, weakness, and stiffness. In addition, a proportion of patients have a movement disorder, particularly dystonia, which is typically fixed rather than mobile, but other movement disorders such as a jerky tremor and additional spasms also occur (38,39). This syndrome of dystonia combined with CRPS has been termed causalgia-dystonia (40). The frequency of movement disorders in CRPS varies among studies, and other features also vary among patients. The International Association for the Study of Pain (IASP) criteria for CRPS (see Table 8.4) therefore only include the core features of this disorder (41). It has been suggested that CRPS is a heterogeneous condition, not only because the clinical presentation of CRPS varies, but because a number of different causes can lead to a similar phenotype (37). Thus, while the majority of cases follow a peripheral injury, other causes, including stroke, heart disease, drugs, or pregnancy, can also lead to CRPS. In addition, there are patients who develop symptoms of CRPS without any obvious trigger.

The mechanism underlying posttraumatic dystonia and CRPS, type I or II, is poorly understood and is the subject of continued discussion. A plethora of studies on this subject has been published in the literature. The role of the sympathetic nervous system in CRPS type I, which is suggested by the name RSD, has latterly been questioned (42), and inflammation (43) or peripheral mechanisms such as sensitization of peripheral nociceptors, or ectopic or ephaptic transmission of nerve impulses have been suggested as possible mechanisms for CRPS and posttraumatic dystonia (27,37,44,45). Several features of CRPS,

such as contralateral spread and the occurrence of dystonia or tremor have also implicated central mechanisms (27). Impairment of interneuronal circuits at the spinal or brainstem level and maladaptive central synaptic reorganization due to an interaction between neuroplastic processes and aberrant environmental requirements, analogous to that following amputation, have thus been suggested as possible mechanisms (46,47).

Routine investigations of the central and peripheral nervous systems typically do not reveal any structural abnormalities in CRPS type I or posttraumatic dystonia. However, in patients with causalgia-dystonia abnormalities similar to those seen in primary dystonia, including impaired reciprocal inhibition of H-reflexes (48–50) and abnormal stretch reflexes (46,49), have been reported, and one group reported genetic susceptibilities related to the human leukocyte antigen (HLA) system (51,52). In addition, changes in contralateral thalamic perfusion on iodine-123-labelled SPECT imaging in cases of CRPS (53) have suggested that central adaptation mechanisms occur in CRPS. However, whether these central thalamic changes are primary or secondary to the clinical changes remains a matter of dispute.

Management in both posttraumatic dystonia and CRPS type I is conspicuously difficult. Treatments from pharmacologic pain management strategies to ganglion blockades and surgical sympathectomy have been inconsistent and disappointing (54), although spinal cord stimulation has been reported to provide pain relief for up to 2 years, and intrathecal baclofen (55) and botulinum toxin (56) have been reported in some studies to improve dystonia in these conditions.

Due to the lack of "hard" neurologic signs and structural abnormalities on routine investigations (excluding changes secondary to immobilization), and due to the overlap between the clinical features of PD and posttraumatic dystonia or CRPS, it has been suggested that at least a

---

TABLE 8.4
CRITERIA FOR COMPLEX REGIONAL PAIN SYNDROME (IASP/CRPS)

1. The presence of an initiating noxious event, or a cause of immobilization
2. Continuing pain, allodynia, or hyperalgesia where the pain is disproportionate to any inciting event
3. Evidence at some time of edema, changes in skin blood flow, or abnormal sudomotor activity in the region of pain
4. This diagnosis is excluded by the existence of conditions that would otherwise account for the degree of pain and dysfunction

Associated signs and symptoms of CRPS listed in IASP taxonomy but not used for diagnosis

1. Atrophy of the hair, nails, and other soft tissues
2. Alterations in hair growth
3. Loss of joint mobility
4. Impairment of motor function, including weakness, tremor, and dystonia
5. Sympathetically maintained pain may be present

From Merskey H, Bogduk N, eds. In: *Classification of chronic pain: descriptions of chronic pain syndromes and definitions of pain terms*, 2nd ed. Seattle: IASP Press, 1994:40–43, with permission.

proportion of patients with these disorders in fact suffer from a PD. Indeed, a patient with a diagnosis of CRPS type I who was shown by secret surveillance to be malingering for the purpose of insurance payments has been reported in the literature inclusive of a video-recording (57). In addition, many such patients show behavioral or personality abnormalities. Some have argued that causalgia-dystonia is purely a psychogenic condition. In one study none of the patients with this diagnosis had any structural abnormality upon investigations of the nervous system, all had other nonorganic signs, and in some cases, malingering was documented (58). However, others have reported conflicting results (53,59), have disputed an association between CRPS and psychological disorders (36), or have reported personality profiles in patients with CRPS similar to those in patients with other chronic pain syndromes (35).

Thus, considerable controversy remains on the nosology and pathogenesis of CRPS type I. It has also been argued that study of this condition is particularly complicated by the heterogeneous presentations of CRPS type I, and that the presentation of CRPS may represent a common end path of a variety of causes (37). One of the possible causes ultimately leading to CRPS could encompass PD.

REFERENCES

1. Oppenheim H. Über eine eigenartige krampfkrankheit des kindlichen und jugendlichen Alters (dysbasia lordotica progressiva, dystonia musculorum deformans). *Neurol Zentralblatt.* 1911;30:1090–1107.
2. Flatau E, Sterling W. Progressiver torsionsspasmus bei kindern. *Neurol Psychiatr.* 2004;7:586–612.
3. Fahn S, Eldridge R. Definition of dystonia and classification of the dystonic states. *Adv Neurol.* 1976;14:1–5.
4. Marsden CD. Dystonia: the spectrum of the disease. In: Yahr MD, ed. *The basal ganglia.* New York: Raven Press, 1976:351–367.
5. Miyasaki JM, Sa DS, Galvez-Jimenez N, et al. Psychogenic movement disorders. *Can J Neurol Sci.* 2003;30(Suppl. 1):S94–100.
6. Fahn S, Bressman SB, Marsden CD. Classification of dystonia. *Adv Neurol.* 1998;78:1–10.
7. Francis P, Baker GA. Non-epileptic attack disorder (NEAD): a comprehensive review. *Seizure.* 1999;8(1):53–61.
8. Wessely S, Nimnuan C, Sharpe M. Functional somatic syndromes: one or many? *Lancet.* 1999;354(9182):936–939.
9. Cohen ME, Robins E, Purtell JJ, et al. Excessive surgery in hysteria; study of surgical procedures in 50 women with hysteria and 190 controls. *J Am Med Assoc.* 1953;151(12):977–986.
10. Schrag A, Brown R, Trimble M. The reliability of self-reported diagnoses in patients with neurologically unexplained symptoms. *J Neurol Neurosurg Psychiatry.* 2004;75(4):608–611.
11. Ziv I, Djaldetti R, Zoldan Y, et al. Diagnosis of "non-organic" limb paresis by a novel objective motor assessment: the quantitative Hoover's test. *J Neurol.* 1998;245(12):797–802.
12. Stone J, Zeman A, Sharpe M. Functional weakness and sensory disturbance. *J Neurol Neurosurg Psychiatry.* 2002;73(3):241–245.
13. Goetz CG, Leurgans S, Raman R. Placebo-associated improvements in motor function: comparison of subjective and objective sections of the UPDRS in early Parkinson's disease. *Mov Disord.* 2002;17(2):283–288.
14. Williams DT, Ford B, Fahn S. Phenomenology and psychopathology related to psychogenic movement disorders. *Adv Neurol.* 1995;65:231–257.
15. Factor SA, Podskalny GD, Molho ES. Psychogenic movement disorders: frequency, clinical profile, and characteristics. *J Neurol Neurosurg Psychiatry.* 1995;59(4):406–412.
16. Feinstein A, Stergiopoulos V, Fine J, et al. Psychiatric outcome in patients with a psychogenic movement disorder: a prospective study. *Neuropsychiatry Neuropsychol Behav Neurol.* 2001;14(3):169–176.
17. Lang AE. Psychogenic dystonia: a review of 18 cases. *Can J Neurol Sci.* 1995;22(2):136–143.
18. Rief W, Hessel A, Braehler E. Somatization symptoms and hypochondriacal features in the general population. *Psychosom Med.* 2001;63(4):595–602.
19. Fahn S, Williams DT. Psychogenic dystonia. *Adv Neurol.* 1988;50:431–455.
20. Pringsheim T, Lang AE. Psychogenic dystonia. *Rev Neurol (Paris).* 2003;159(10 Pt 1):885–891.
21. Edwards MJ, Huang YZ, Wood NW, et al. Different patterns of electrophysiological deficits in manifesting and non-manifesting carriers of the DYT1 gene mutation. *Brain.* 2003;126(Pt 9):2074–2080.
22. Panizza M, Lelli S, Nilsson J, et al. H-reflex recovery curve and reciprocal inhibition of H-reflex in different kinds of dystonia. *Neurology.* 1990;40(5):824–828.
23. Farmer SF, Sheean GL, Mayston MJ, et al. Abnormal motor unit synchronization of antagonist muscles underlies pathological co-contraction in upper limb dystonia. *Brain.* 1998;121(Pt 5):801–814.
24. Tijssen MA, Marsden JF, Brown P. Frequency analysis of EMG activity in patients with idiopathic torticollis. *Brain.* 2000;123 (Pt 4):677–686.
25. Filipovic SR, Siebner HR, Rowe JB, et al. Modulation of cortical activity by repetitive transcranial magnetic stimulation (rTMS): a review of functional imaging studies and the potential use in dystonia. *Adv Neurol.* 2004;94:45–52.
26. Eidelberg D, Moeller JR, Antonini A, et al. Functional brain networks in DYT1 dystonia. *Ann Neurol.* 1998;44(3):303–312.
27. Jankovic J. Post-traumatic movement disorders: central and peripheral mechanisms. *Neurology.* 1994;44(11):2006–2014.
28. Jankovic J. Can peripheral trauma induce dystonia and other movement disorders? Yes! *Mov Disord.* 2001;16(1):7–12.
29. Weiner WJ. Can peripheral trauma induce dystonia? No! *Mov Disord.* 2001;16(1):13–22.
30. Truong DD, Dubinsky R, Hermanowicz N, et al. Posttraumatic torticollis. *Arch Neurol.* 1991;48(2):221–223.
31. Goldman S, Ahlskog JE. Posttraumatic cervical dystonia. *Mayo Clin Proc.* 1993;68(5):443–448.
32. Sa DS, Mailis-Gagnon A, Nicholson K, et al. Posttraumatic painful torticollis. *Mov Disord.* 2003;18(12):1482–1491.
33. O'Riordan S, Hutchinson M. Cervical dystonia following peripheral trauma—a case-control study. *J Neurol.* 2004;251(2):150–155.
34. Schrag A, Trimble M, Quinn N, et al. The syndrome of fixed dystonia: an evaluation of 103 patients. *Brain.* 2004;127:2360–2372.
35. Ciccone DS, Bandilla EB, Wu W. Psychological dysfunction in patients with reflex sympathetic dystrophy. *Pain.* 1997;71(3):323–333.
36. Lynch ME. Psychological aspects of reflex sympathetic dystrophy: a review of the adult and paediatric literature. *Pain.* 1992;49(3):337–347.
37. Schott GD. Reflex sympathetic dystrophy. *J Neurol Neurosurg Psychiatry.* 2001;71(3):291–295.
38. Schwartzman RJ, Kerrigan J. The movement disorder of reflex sympathetic dystrophy. *Neurology.* 1990;40(1):57–61.
39. Veldman PH, Reynen HM, Arntz IE, et al. Signs and symptoms of reflex sympathetic dystrophy: prospective study of 829 patients. *Lancet.* 1993;342(8878):1012–1016.
40. Bhatia KP, Bhatt MH, Marsden CD. The causalgia-dystonia syndrome. *Brain.* 1993;116:843–851.
41. Merskey H, Bogduk N. Complex regional pain syndromes: classification of chronic pain. *Descriptions of chronic pain syndromes and definitions of pain terms.* Seattle, WA: IASP Press, 1994:40–43.
42. Baron R, Levine JD, Fields HL. Causalgia and reflex sympathetic dystrophy: does the sympathetic nervous system contribute to the generation of pain? *Muscle Nerve.* 1999;22(6):678–695.

43. Birklein F, Schmelz M, Schifter S, et al. The important role of neuropeptides in complex regional pain syndrome. *Neurology.* 2001;57(12):2179–2184.

44. Schott GD. Mechanisms of causalgia and related clinical conditions. The role of the central and of the sympathetic nervous systems. *Brain.* 1986;109(Pt 4):717–738.

45. Schott GD. Induction of involuntary movements by peripheral trauma: an analogy with causalgia. *Lancet.* 1986;2(8509):712–716.

46. van Hilten JJ, van de Beek WJ, Vein AA, et al. Clinical aspects of multifocal or generalized tonic dystonia in reflex sympathetic dystrophy. *Neurology.* 2001;56(12):1762–1765.

47. Elbert T, Rockstroh B. Reorganization of human cerebral cortex: the range of changes following use and injury. *Neuroscientist.* 2004;10(2):129–141.

48. Koelman JH, Hilgevoord AA, Bour LJ, et al. Soleus H-reflex tests in causalgia-dystonia compared with dystonia and mimicked dystonic posture. *Neurology.* 1999;53(9):2196–2198.

49. van de Beek WJ, Vein A, Hilgevoord AA, et al. Neurophysiologic aspects of patients with generalized or multifocal tonic dystonia of reflex sympathetic dystrophy. *J Clin Neurophysiol.* 2002;19(1):77–83.

50. van de Beek WJ, Schwartzman RJ, van Nes SI, et al. Diagnostic criteria used in studies of reflex sympathetic dystrophy. *Neurology.* 2002;58(4):522–526.

51. van de Beek WJ, Roep BO, van der Slik AR, et al. Susceptibility loci for complex regional pain syndrome. *Pain.* 2003;103(1-2):93–97.

52. van Hilten JJ, van de Beek WJ, Roep BO. Multifocal or generalized tonic dystonia of complex regional pain syndrome: a distinct clinical entity associated with HLA-DR13. *Ann Neurol.* 2000;48(1):113–116.

53. Fukumoto M, Ushida T, Zinchuk VS, et al. Contralateral thalamic perfusion in patients with reflex sympathetic dystrophy syndrome. *Lancet.* 1999;354(9192):1790–1791.

54. Goldstein DS. Spinal cord stimulation for chronic reflex sympathetic dystrophy. *Ann Neurol.* 2004;55(1):5–6.

55. van Hilten BJ, van de Beek WJ, Hoff JI, et al. Intrathecal baclofen for the treatment of dystonia in patients with reflex sympathetic dystrophy. *N Engl J Med.* 2000;343(9):625–630.

56. Cordivari C, Misra VP, Catania S, et al. Treatment of dystonic clenched fist with botulinum toxin. *Mov Disord.* 2001;16(5):907–913.

57. Kurlan R, Brin MF, Fahn S. Movement disorder in reflex sympathetic dystrophy: a case proven to be psychogenic by surveillance video monitoring. *Mov Disord.* 1997;12(2):243–245.

58. Verdugo RJ, Ochoa JL. Abnormal movements in complex regional pain syndrome: assessment of their nature. *Muscle Nerve.* 2000;23(2):198–205.

59. Birklein F, Riedl B, Sieweke N, et al. Neurological findings in complex regional pain syndromes—analysis of 145 cases. *Acta Neurol Scand.* 2000;101(4):262–269.

Psychogenic Parkinsonism

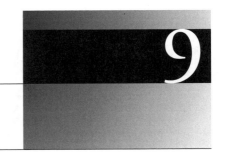

John C. Morgan   Kapil D. Sethi

ABSTRACT

Parkinson disease (PD) is characterized by bradykinesia, tremor, cogwheel rigidity, and, in later stages, postural instability. Bradykinesia is a requisite clinical feature for the diagnosis of PD by the United Kingdom Parkinson's Disease Society Brain Research Center (UKPDSBRC) criteria and correlates best with nigrostriatal degeneration. Slow movements, tremor, rigidity, and postural/gait disturbances can also occur in psychogenic parkinsonism (PP). In this chapter we will attempt to define the clinical features of PP. We will focus on how to differentiate PP from PD based upon a review of the literature and our own clinical experience.

Psychogenic movement disorders (PMDs) were estimated to constitute approximately 2% to 3% of all movement disorders seen in two large tertiary movement disorder centers (1,2). Tremor, dystonia, and myoclonus appear to be the most common PMDs in the tertiary setting, accounting for approximately 80% of PMDs (1–3). On the contrary, psychogenic parkinsonism is a rare PMD occurring in only 2% to 6% of all PMD patients (2–4). In the larger spectrum of parkinsonism, PP accounts for only 0.17% of all cases of parkinsonism in the movement disorders database of Columbia-Presbyterian Hospital (5), and only 0.5% of all the parkinsonism cases from 842 consecutive patients seen in 6 years of movement disorders practice (2).

PP appears to affect patients of ages ranging from 21 to 63 years with an approximately equal male-to-female ratio (2,5,6). The duration of symptoms before diagnosis is highly variable, ranging from 4 months up to 13 years (2,5). Onset is usually sudden, often with obvious precipitating factors such as work-related injuries, accidents, or psychological trauma. Patients usually reach maximum disability early and the dominant side may be most affected often (5). Prognosis of PP is highly variable, with some patients improving quickly and other patients suffering for 28 years or more without signs of improvement or progression (as in Case 1 below). In this chapter we will focus on differentiating PP from Parkinson disease based upon a review of the literature. We will also present three cases from our own practice that illustrate the varied clinical features of PP.

BRADYKINESIA/BRADYPHRENIA

Bradykinesia is a requirement to make the diagnosis of PD using the United Kingdom Parkinson Disease Society Brain Research Center (UKPDSBRC) criteria (7). Bradykinesia is best characterized as slowness of movement (8), and its presence is the best clinical correlate of nigrostriatal degeneration in PD (9). In Parkinson disease (PD), bradykinesia typically manifests as slowness in initiating movements with a progressive reduction in the speed and amplitude of the repetitive movements. Early fatiguing and arrests in movement are also components of the bradykinesia in PD (5). Psychogenic parkinsonism (PP) patients also have significant difficulty performing rapid repetitive movements. Unlike PD patients, PP patients typically demonstrate extreme effort, with sighing, grimacing, or using whole-body movements in order to perform a simple motor task (5). PP patients do not typically demonstrate fatigue or decrement in movement amplitude when performing rapid repetitive movements (5). A patient who manifests very slow, pained-appearing repetitive tasks for the examiner (such as finger taps) while easily performing other casual activities requiring similar finger dexterity and movements (easily opening and closing a purse) is demonstrating psychogenic bradykinesia, not the true bradykinesia of PD (5,10). In our experience, axial bradykinesia, hypomimia, and decreased blink rate are common in PD and rare in PP.

In addition to bradykinesia, PD patients also frequently suffer from slowed cognitive processing associated with impairment of concentration and apathy, or bradyphrenia (11–13). Patients with PP may also suffer from depression, which can cause psychomotor retardation (14), a condition which may be difficult to distinguish from the bradyphrenia of PD. In one study comparing PD patients and depressed patients, it appeared that both cognitive and motor slowing contributed to slowing of responses in both (13). The authors suggested that bradyphrenia in PD and psychomotor retardation in depression are closely related, and impairment of mesocorticolimbic dopaminergic systems may be involved in both conditions (13). Separating bradyphrenia from psychomotor retardation may even be difficult in a "pure" population of PD patients given that approximately half of them also suffer depressive symptoms (15).

TREMOR

PD tremor is classically a gradual-onset, 4 to 6 Hz rest tremor of consistent frequency, usually with transient dampening upon assuming a new posture (5,16,17). The amplitude may vary depending upon the activity and the emotional state of the patient. Tremor was present in 12 of 14 PP patients in the series by Lang et al. (5), with sudden onset in 10 of the 14 patients. Tremor of the arm or hand is most typical in PP and rest tremor of the chin or leg/foot would be highly unusual in PP. PP tremor is typical of other psychogenic tremors in that the amplitude and frequency of the tremor vary widely in an individual patient (5,18,19). Unlike what is typical of PD tremor, PP tremor is distractible in the affected limb by having the patient perform complex motor tasks in the contralateral limb or serial arithmetic (5). Patients with PP typically demonstrate entrainment, where the limb with psychogenic tremor will assume the frequency of a contralateral repetitive movement, unlike PD where the tremor itself often entrains the rate of repetitive movements (5). PP tremors also frequently persist with action or sustained postures, unlike PD tremors in most patients. When the examiner directs attention to the tremor of PP patients, the tremor usually worsens. The tremor may even spread from one contiguous body part to another, or even to contralateral limbs when the primarily affected joints are immobilized, especially with suggestion.

RIGIDITY

Cogwheel rigidity is a cardinal finding in PD and other forms of organic parkinsonism; however, this does not typically occur in PP (5). Rigidity in PP typically has a feature of voluntary resistance or difficulty relaxing and was only present in six of the 14 patients with PP in the series of Lang et al. (5). Performing synkinetic movements of a contralateral limb appears to help reduce the rigidity characteristically found in PP (presumably through distraction)—exactly the opposite of what occurs in PD (5). Visible cogwheeling during voluntary movement about a joint as an isolated symptom/sign is more typical of anxiety and not of PD.

GAIT/POSTURAL INSTABILITY

A shuffling gait with freezing and turning *en bloc* is typical in moderate to advanced PD; however, this is not typically seen in PP. Gait freezing in PD may have unusual relieving factors including improvement with visual/auditory cues leading to confusion with PP. Gait is frequently bizarre in PP, as is typical of PMDs. Only one patient in the Lang et al. (5) series was noted to have a shuffling gait, while four patients had unusual or bizarre gaits.

Postural stability is typically impaired in moderate to advanced PD, but not in early disease. Unlike PD patients, those with PP typically demonstrate postural instability regardless of the duration of symptoms. The PP patients in our practice typically have unusual or even bizarre gaits, and many have abnormal pull tests. PP patients with abnormal pull tests frequently demonstrate retropulsion or back arching and flailing of the arms without falling. Other PP patients will fall backwards into the examiner's arms "like a log," not attempting to take steps backward to avoid falling.

ASSOCIATED SYMPTOMS AND SIGNS IN PSYCHOGENIC PARKINSONISM

Patients may complain of a myriad of problems in addition to the motor features characteristic of PP. Impaired concentration and memory, alterations in speech or language function, functional or "give-way" weakness, nonanatomical sensory loss, and selective disabilities are typical. In our experience, some PP patients also demonstrate distractible, bizarre dysarthrias or stuttering. PP patients also commonly report pain in varied distributions (5), frequently chronic and unrelated to the development of PP, however, occasionally coincident with PP onset. Pain can also be a feature of the nonmotor fluctuations in PD (20,21), usually occurring in the "off" state and responding to levodopa or dopamine agonists. Pain, regardless of cause, does not usually respond to levodopa or dopamine agonists in patients with PP. Some PP patients complain of unusual, unexplained visual disturbances (such as bilateral tunnel vision) in addition to their PP motor symptoms.

CASE STUDIES

The following three cases from our own experience are illustrative of PP.

Case 1

A 73-year-old sinistral man recounted that he first developed symptoms of "Parkinson disease" manifested by tremor in his left hand at age 45. He is a Korean War veteran and has suffered posttraumatic stress disorder and depression related to his war experiences. He was never exposed to neuroleptic medications. He was treated with various medications including trihexyphenidyl, benztropine, and amantadine without benefit, complaining of various side effects. He also suffered a "stroke" 23 years prior to this evaluation with resultant chronic, mild left hemiparesis and dysarthria; however, his neuroimaging never substantiated his report. He has remained on a low dose of carbidopa/levodopa for at least 25 years, complaining of "extra movements" (as he shakes his head in a "no-no" fashion) when he was taking "too much." He was currently taking one to one and a half tablets of carbidopa/levodopa 25/100 four times per day. On a prior occasion he was admitted to the hospital and carbidopa/levodopa was withdrawn over 4 days with monitoring of his creatine kinase levels and clinical state. There was no change in his symptoms or signs and his creatine kinase levels were unchanged. He complained of "freezing" when he attempted to stand from a seated position during this clinic visit.

His examination was significant for no progression despite multiple evaluations by us over the past 18 years. He had a flat affect with normal cognition; however, he had a strange, stuttering speech not consistent with the tachyphemia of PD. He had a rest tremor of the left greater than the right upper extremity that appeared to vary in amplitude and frequency, especially with distraction. He had give-way weakness of the left hemibody with obvious poor effort. No cogwheeling was present in the upper extremities. He demonstrated slow finger taps and hand supination/pronation. His gait was bizarre with normal stride length, left leg circumduction, and intermittent left hand rest tremor. His pull test was normal.

Despite ongoing counseling, he remains convinced he suffers with PD. He and his son are active members in the local Parkinson support group.

Case 2

A 38-year-old dextral man presented for evaluation of right arm tremor and abnormal posturing of both feet. He had been in good health until 7 months prior to our evaluation, when he developed chest pain and was ruled out for myocardial infarction at an outside hospital. He was subsequently diagnosed with type 2 diabetes mellitus and hypertension, and treated for this. A month later he was treated with clarithromycin for a pulmonary infection and he suddenly became unconscious for 30 minutes without tonic-clonic movements, tongue biting, bladder incontinence, or evidence of arrhythmias. An extensive metabolic work-up and brain MRI/MRA and EEG at that time yielded normal results.

A week following this hospitalization, he developed a rather abrupt onset of right hand tremor within one day, followed a week later by the toes of his right foot curling under for a period of hours. His right hand tremor became worse at this time and his entire right foot became "dead numb." About two weeks later the toes of his left foot started curling under. Repeat MRI of the brain with contrast and EEG were normal. The right hand tremor was treated with nadolol without improvement. He was treated with pramipexole approximately one month after his right hand tremor began, given the suspicion that his condition may represent early-onset PD with dystonia. Pramipexole did not help his tremor or curled toes. Upon our initial evaluation, he was taking carbidopa/levodopa 25/100 (4.5 tablets per day) and nadolol 40 mg per day without benefit.

He had no prior psychiatric diagnoses. He had never taken neuroleptics or metoclopramide. He owned his own small engine repair shop and admitted to being under considerable stress secondary to financial problems. There was no family history of tremor, parkinsonism, or dystonia.

On examination, he had a depressed affect with rest and action tremor in the right arm. The tremor was regular and completely relented with distraction. He demonstrated deliberate slowing of his movements, not typical of PD bradykinesia. There was no cogwheel rigidity. His toes were flexed in an extreme position and this posture fluctuated with ambulation with his toes assuming normal positions at times. He did not exhibit a sensory trick and a vibrating tuning fork placed on his foot did not help relax his toes. His pull test was normal. We thought he had a diagnosis most consistent with PP and psychogenic dystonia, and advised him to discontinue use of the carbidopa/levodopa.

Three weeks after our evaluation he called and reported to his primary neurologist that both of his hands were balled into fists and he could not open them. He blamed his glyburide/metformin combination therapy for his movement disorder. He stopped this medication and immediately his right hand/arm tremor and the abnormal posturing of his hands and feet disappeared. He remained on glyburide alone for diabetic control with no return of symptoms.

Case 3

A 76-year-old man complained of bilateral tremors and slowing of his walking following a coronary artery bypass graft procedure at the age of 71. The gait difficulty progressed over the next 2 to 3 years with multiple falls resulting in his routine use of a wheelchair. He was noted to have a rest tremor in the right arm with bradykinesia bilaterally on exam at age 74 and was treated with amantadine and pramipexole, leading to hallucinations and nightmares. He was then started on carbidopa/levodopa, and the dose of levodopa was escalated to 1,200 mg per day without improvement in his tremors or bradykinesia, but with complaints of nausea. Concerned about vascular parkinsonism, doctors performed an MRI of the brain when the patient was age 74, and he demonstrated mild bilateral periventricular white matter disease, diffuse cortical atrophy, and per the neuroradiologist's interpretation, "decreased definition of the substantia nigra on T2-weighted images which might be consistent with a clinical diagnosis of Parkinson disease."

He suffered with depression and had anger management issues in his prior job in the military, leading to demotion. His tremors and disabilities were noted to improve when he was working in his woodshop. Otherwise, he was predominantly in his wheelchair due to gait difficulties.

On a recent examination he demonstrated a slightly blunted affect, with normal cognition and language. He had full appendicular strength with no evidence of cogwheel rigidity. He had a rest tremor of the right arm that was clearly distractible despite poor concentration on the distracting task. He displayed slow, rapidly alternating movements without arrests. He had no dyskinesias by history or on examination. His gait was slow and steady using a cane, with a floridly abnormal pull test, manifested by retropulsion/falling backward with the slightest of tugs or falling backward with a sudden loss of tone when lightly touched on the top of his head.

On recent follow-up, he had stopped his carbidopa/levodopa (1,200 mg of levodopa per day) suddenly without any adverse consequences, and he actually noted improvement in function while off the carbidopa/levodopa. He stopped the drug because he thought it was not doing him "any good." He was referred for psychiatric counseling and during that interview he complained that his tremors and other symptoms were worse while off the carbidopa/levodopa, and he felt the "neurology physicians were wrong" about his diagnosis of PP. The attending psychiatrist involved in his care indicated the patient appeared to have organic parkinsonism rather than PP. The patient did not feel that he needed further psychiatric follow-up.

DIAGNOSTIC EVALUATIONS

Usually, no diagnostic tests are needed to make the diagnosis of PP. A thorough clinical history and detailed examination are essential. The benefit of longitudinal follow-up to make or break the diagnosis of organic parkinsonism or PP is invaluable. Functional neuroimaging will also prove useful in cases of suspected psychogenic parkinsonism (see below). If the diagnosis remains in doubt, an additional opinion from another movement disorder neurologist may help. The categories of diagnostic certainty of Fahn and Williams (4) are useful for PP (and PMD in general) and are discussed elsewhere in this book.

Most of the PP patients in the series described by Lang et al. (5) had PD as their prior diagnosis; in one patient, thalamotomy had been suggested, and another patient was actually enrolled in a clinical trial for PD. Presumably, most cases of PP are diagnosed in tertiary movement disorder clinics given that many general neurologists appear uncomfortable making this diagnosis. Alternatively, other physicians misdiagnose patients as having PD, and refer them to our clinic for "difficult-to-manage" PD.

FUNCTIONAL NEUROIMAGING IN PSYCHOGENIC PARKINSONISM

The role of striatal dopamine transporter/dopamine uptake imaging in patients with parkinsonism is a subject of intense study. In organic parkinsonism, [^{123}I]β-CIT striatal dopamine transporter imaging and striatal [^{18}F]DOPA uptake are proving quite useful in a number of settings, particularly in helping to distinguish patients with drug-induced parkinsonism, Parkinson-plus disorders, and early PD (22). A recent [^{123}I]-FP-CIT striatal dopamine transporter imaging study by Benamer et al. (23) suggests that this technique may be useful for identifying early PD patients who do not meet strict clinical diagnostic criteria for PD.

The situation has become more complex of late. In the REAL-PET, CALM-PD, and ELLDOPA trials 11%, 4%, and 14% of early PD patients, respectively, had scans without evidence of dopaminergic deficit (SWEDD) (24) with [^{18}F]DOPA (25,26) or [^{123}I]β-CIT (24,27,28). Further longitudinal clinical history and repeated functional neuroimaging may identify some of these patients as misdiagnosed or alternatively could demonstrate clinical disease progression and imaging abnormalities typical of PD. [^{123}I]β-CIT striatal dopamine transporter and striatal [^{18}F]DOPA uptake imaging have been (26) and will be used as surrogate markers of disease progression in PD in the future.

[^{123}I]β-CIT striatal dopamine transporter imaging and striatal [^{18}F]DOPA uptake is also quite useful in cases of PP

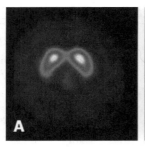 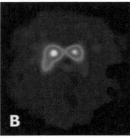 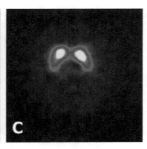

Figure 9.1 [^{123}I]β-CIT striatal dopamine transporter imaging in a (**A**) normal control patient, (**B**) a patient with Parkinson disease, and (**C**) a patient with psychogenic parkinsonism. (Courtesy of Kenneth L. Marek, MD, The Institute for Neurodegenerative Disorders, New Haven, Conn.)

(5,29–31). PP patients have normal [^{123}I]β-CIT striatal dopamine transporter imaging and striatal [^{18}F]DOPA uptake given intact nigrostriatal neuroanatomy. Figure 9.1 illustrates the potential utility of [^{123}I]β-CIT striatal dopamine transporter imaging in three patients: a normal control (Fig. 9.1A), a PD patient (Fig. 9.1B), and a patient with PP (Fig. 9.1C). The patient with PP (Fig. C) has similar [^{123}I]β-CIT striatal uptake as in a normal patient (Fig. 9.1A), providing significant corroboration of the clinical diagnosis of PP.

As mentioned above, it is essential to couple the longitudinal clinical history of the patient with the imaging results (and perhaps even repeat imaging). An excellent example of this comes from Booij et al. (29), who described 19 patients with inconclusive forms of parkinsonism and normal [^{123}I]-FP-CIT SPECT scans; four patients were eventually diagnosed with PP on further clinical follow-up.

[^{18}F]DOPA-PET or [^{123}I]β-CIT-SPECT imaging may not only help confirm the clinical diagnosis of PP in many patients, but these techniques may also help refute PP as the diagnosis in others. O'Sullivan et al. (32) reported three patients with suspected PP who were all found to have reduced [^{123}I]-FP-CIT uptake in the putamen and caudate, helping confirm the diagnosis of organic parkinsonism. Clouding the picture further is the fact that some patients with PD may embellish their symptoms/signs. In the 14 PP patients reported by Lang et al. (5), one of the patients actually had reduced [^{18}F]DOPA uptake in one striatum while exhibiting a placebo response to psychotherapy and haloperidol (5).

Treatment

There are no well-designed studies addressing treatment of PP given the rarity of this disorder. Treatment is aimed at improving the underlying psychiatric disorder, and many patients have evidence of multiple somatizations or previous conversion disorders. In two of the three PP patients we described above, and in the two PP patients described

TABLE 9.1

HISTORICAL FEATURES OF PARKINSON DISEASE AND PSYCHOGENIC PARKINSONISM

	Parkinson Disease	Psychogenic Parkinsonism
Onset	Gradual, typically in the 6th or 7th decade	Abrupt, varied age of onset
Presenting complaints	Unilateral tremor, bradykinesia, rigidity	Generalized weakness, tremor (bilateral in 50%), slowing of movements, abnormal postures, less common complaints of rigidity
Course	Slowly progressive	Usually static with maximum disability early, condition may abruptly or gradually remit
Precipitating factors	Usually none	Stressful life events and work injuries, ongoing litigation or disability proceedings
Psychiatric history	Depression may precede diagnosis	Previous conversion disorders, somatization, factitious disorder, anxiety, and depression
Impact of disease	Gradual loss of function with every attempt to maintain work, leisure activities, and to perform activities of daily living	Most unable to work very early, many unable to perform activities of daily living
Medication response	Responds well to dopamine agonists or levodopa	Usually unresponsive to multiple medical trials
Motor fluctuations	Dyskinesias in half of patients on levodopa after 5–7 years, "on"–"off" fluctuations	Very rare complaints of "extra movements" on levodopa, no dyskinesias after long-term levodopa treatment
Nonmotor problems	Dysautonomia, constipation, sexual dysfunction, sleep problems, hallucinations	Sexual dysfunction and sleep disturbances occur, hallucinations and dysautonomia very unlikely

TABLE 9.2

CLINICAL FEATURES OF PARKINSON DISEASE AND PSYCHOGENIC PARKINSONISM

	Parkinson Disease	Psychogenic Parkinsonism
Bradykinesia	Slowing of rapid repetitive movements without fatigue, arrests or decrement	Extremely slow movements without fatigue, arrests or decrement; grimacing, sighing, or whole-body movements when performing simple tasks; normal speed of movements when not being examined
Tremor	Typically unilateral at rest, gradual onset in either limb, 4–6 Hz, worsens with distraction, transiently dampens on assuming a new posture	Unilateral or bilateral; rest, postural, action; abrupt onset usually involving the dominant hand, varying frequency and amplitude, distractible, increases with attention, "spreads" when immobilizing the affected limb
Rigidity	Cogwheel rigidity	Cogwheeling absent, voluntary resistance which may decrease with distraction
Postural instability	Impaired in moderate to advanced disease, retropulsion on the pull test	Impaired early in the course of disease, may have exaggerated or bizarre responses to minimal displacement, falls "like a log" on a light pull backwards
Speech	Hypophonic, stuttering, tachyphemia	Stuttering, bizarre dysarthria, distractible
"False" signs	Unusual	"Give-way" weakness, nonanatomic sensory loss, memory deficits

by Factor et al. (2), there was evidence of previous conversion disorders. It should be emphasized that the existence of a PMD does not exclude the diagnosis of an underlying organic disorder, since up to 25% of patients with a PMD can have an organic movement disorder also (2,33). Anxiety and mood disorders are also common psychiatric comorbidities in PP, and they are frequently evident on initial evaluation of the patient presenting with PP, either historically or on examination. Factitious disorder, malingering, and personality disorders occur in PP patients as well.

Outcomes are highly variable and appear to correlate with the outcomes observed in other PMDs. Patients with a shorter duration of PP symptoms tend to do better than patients with chronic symptoms, especially if there are obvious triggers. Lempert et al. (34) found that 90% of patients admitted for neurologic conversion disorders experienced significant improvement or remission if symptoms were present for 2 weeks or less, while only 30% of patients had improvement or remission if symptoms were present for more than 6 months. If litigation is pending or a disability issue is unresolved, patients frequently improve after a legal settlement is reached. PP patients with chronic symptoms are frequently unable to work or are fully disabled in our experience and in published series (2,5).

Placebo treatment and suggestion are powerful medicines in many of these patients and may be a good adjunct to psychotherapy and pharmacotherapy in highly selected patients. Helping remove underlying stressors and triggers is important. Physical, occupational, and speech therapy are often helpful. Hypnosis can also help these patients, since many are quite susceptible to hypnosis (35). In medical climates where it is possible, long-term hospitalization

and multidisciplinary treatment with neurology, psychiatry, and paramedical therapies have proven effective over time in many patients with PMD (see chapter 33).

SUMMARY

Our three cases and the other cases in the literature (2,5,6) are illustrative of the varied presentations and factors surrounding the history, diagnosis, and treatment of PP. Table 9.1 summarizes the typical historical differences in patients with PD versus PP, and Table 9.2 summarizes the differences in clinical findings in PD versus PP patients.

REFERENCES

1. Fahn S. Psychogenic movement disorders. In: Marsden CD, Fahn S, eds. *Movement disorders 3*. Oxford: Butterworth-Heineman, 1994:359–372.
2. Factor SA, Podskalny GD, Molho ES. Psychogenic movement disorders: frequency, clinical profile, and characteristics. *J Neurol Neurosurg Psychiatry*. 1995;59:406–412.
3. Miyasaki JM, Sa DS, Galvez-Jimenez N, et al. Psychogenic movement disorders. *Can J Neurol Sci*. 2003;30(Suppl. 1):S94–S100.
4. Fahn S, Williams PJ. Psychogenic dystonia. *Adv Neurol*. 1988; 50:431–455.
5. Lang AE, Koller WC, Fahn S. Psychogenic parkinsonism. *Arch Neurol*. 1995;52:802–810.
6. Walters AS, Boudwin J, Wright D, et al. Three hysterical movement disorders. *Psychol Rep*. 1988;62:979–985.
7. Gibb WRG, Lees AJ. The relevance of the Lewy body to the pathogenesis of idiopathic Parkinson's disease. *J Neurol Neurosurg Psychiatry*. 1988;51:745–752.
8. Hallett M, Khoshbin S. A physiological mechanism of bradykinesia. *Brain*. 1980;103:301–314.

9. Vingerhoets FJG, Schulzer M, Calne DB, et al. Which clinical sign of Parkinson's disease best reflects the nigrostriatal lesion? *Ann Neurol.* 1997;41:58–64.

10. Sawle GV. Psychogenic movement disorders. In: Sawle GV, ed. *Movement disorders in clinical practice.* Oxford: Isis Medical Media Ltd, 1999:199–205.

11. Naville F. Études sur les complications et les séquelles mentales de l'encéphalite épidémique. La bradyphrénie. *Encéphale.* 1922; 17:369–375–423–436.

12. Rogers D. Bradyphrenia in parkinsonism: a historical review. *Psychol Med.* 1986;16:257–265.

13. Rogers D, Lees AJ, Smith E, et al. Bradyphrenia in Parkinson's disease and psychomotor retardation in depressive illness. An experimental study. *Brain.* 1987;110:761–776.

14. Sobin C, Sackeim A. Psychomotor symptoms of depression. *Am J Psychiatry.* 1997;154:4–17.

15. McDonald WM, Richard IH, DeLong MR. Prevalence, etiology, and treatment of depression in Parkinson's disease. *Biol Psychiatry.* 2003;54:363–375.

16. Sethi KD. Clinical aspects of Parkinson disease. *Curr Opin Neurol.* 2002;15:457–460.

17. Sethi KD. Tremor. *Curr Opin Neurol.* 2003;16:481–485.

18. O'Suilleabhain PE, Matsumoto JY. Time-frequency analysis of tremors. *Brain.* 1998;121:2127–2134.

19. Zuener KE, Shoge RO, Goldstein SR, et al. Accelerometry to distinguish psychogenic from essential or parkinsonian tremor. *Neurology.* 2003;61:548–550.

20. Quinn N, Koller WC, Lang AE, et al. Painful Parkinson's disease. *Lancet.* 1986;2:1366–1369.

21. Witjas T, Kaphan E, Azulay JP, et al. Nonmotor fluctuations in Parkinson's disease. *Neurology.* 2002;59:408–413.

22. Poewe W, Scherfler C. Role of dopamine transporter imaging in investigation of parkinsonian syndromes in routine clinical practice. *Mov Disord.* 2003;18(Suppl. 7):S16–S21.

23. Benamer HTS, Oertel WH, Patterson J, et al. Prospective study of presynaptic dopaminergic imaging in patients with mild parkinsonism and tremor disorders: part 1. Baseline and 3-month observations. *Mov Disord.* 2003;18:977–984.

24. Marek KL, Seibyl J. Parkinson study group. β-CIT scans without evidence of dopaminergic deficit (SWEDD) in the ELLDOPA-CIT and CALM-CIT study: long-term imaging assessment. *Neurology.* 2003;60(Suppl. 1):A293.

25. Whone AL, Remy P, Davis MR, et al. The REAL-PET study: slower progression in early Parkinson's disease treated with ropinirole compared with L-dopa. *Neurology.* 2002;58(Suppl. 3):A82–A83.

26. Whone AL, Watts RL, Stoessl AJ, et al. Slower progression of Parkinson's disease with ropinirole versus levodopa: the REAL-PET study. *Ann Neurol.* 2003;54:93–101.

27. Fahn S. Results of the ELLDOPA (Earlier vs. Later Levodopa) study. *Mov Disord.* 2002;17(Suppl. 5):S13–S14.

28. Parkinson study group. Dopamine transporter brain imaging to assess the effects of pramipexole vs. levodopa on parkinson disease progression. *JAMA.* 2002;287:1653–1661.

29. Booij J, Speelman JD, Norstink MW, et al. The clinical benefit of imaging striatal dopamine transporters with [123I]FP-CIT SPET in differentiating patients with presynaptic parkinsonism from those with other forms of parkinsonism. *Eur J Nucl Med.* 2001; 28:266–272.

30. Factor SA, Seibyl J, Innis R, et al. Psychogenic parkinsonism: confirmation of diagnosis with β-CIT SPECT scans. *Mov Disord.* 1998;13:860.

31. Tolosa E, Coelho M, Gallardo M. DAT imaging in drug-induced and psychogenic parkinsonism. *Mov Disord.* 2003;18 (Suppl. 7):S28–S33.

32. O'Sullivan JD, Costa DC, Lees AJ. Confirming Parkinson's disease with [123I]FP-CIT SPECT. *Eur J Neurol.* 1999;6(Suppl):131.

33. Ranawaya R, Riley D, Lang A. Psychogenic dyskinesias in patients with organic movement disorders. *Mov Disord.* 1990;5:127–133.

34. Lempert T, Dieterich M, Huppert D, et al. Psychogenic disorders in neurology: frequency and clinical spectrum. *Acta Neurol Scand.* 1990;82:335–340.

35. Anderson KE. Psychogenic movement disorders. *Curr Treat Options Neurol.* 2003;5:169–176.

Psychogenic Gait: An Example of Deceptive Signaling

10

3

John G. Morris   *Gregory Mark de Moore*   *Marie Herberstein*

ABSTRACT

Psychogenic gaits are characterized by a number of features (1): exaggerated effort or fatigue (often with sighing), extreme slowness, convulsive shaking (with "knee buckling"), fluctuations (with periods of normality), unusual postures, and bizarre movements. The onset may be abrupt; a sudden "cure," albeit short-lived, may also occur. Pain may be prominent, particularly where the problem follows an injury. There are usually no objective neurologic signs relevant to the disability, though a psychogenic gait may also complicate the presentation of a true physical disorder, with its associated signs. A psychiatric assessment often fails to identify a significant underlying psychiatric disorder such as major depression or psychosis. The current classification of psychogenicity lays much emphasis on the distinction between patients who knowingly seek to deceive and those in whom the behavior is unconscious. In practice it is often hard to make this distinction. There is a growing literature on behavioral deception in animals where the question of insight on the part of the deceiver does not arise. Behavioral deception in animals is discussed in terms of signaling and its effect on the receiver (2). Deceptive signals, by definition, benefit the deceiver and are costly to the receiver. That this behavior is so widespread affirms its value to those who practice it. Psychogenic behavior in humans equates most closely with injury-feigning, seen, for example, in chimpanzees, which induces nurturing behavior in receivers of the same species, or protects the signaler from stronger or more aggressive members of the group. The hallmark of the psychogenic gait is its emotive quality; it signals to the observer both disability and distress, and induces nurturing behavior. It is best conceived as an acquired behavioral response to stress in a predisposed individual.

INTRODUCTION

Neurologists training in the latter part of the 20th century were discouraged from applying the label of hysteria to patients with neurologic symptoms that could not be readily explained on the basis of any underlying physical disease. Interns who exposed "give-way" weakness, midline splitting of sensory loss, and distractible tremors were given dire warnings by their seniors that many such patients have, or go on to develop, major neurologic diseases. Eliot Slater's farewell address to his neurologic colleagues at the National Hospital, Queen Square, was often cited (3). In this scholarly essay, Slater quoted some of the great neurologists who have given this matter their attention ("Hysteria … the mocking bird of nosology"; "… as much a temperament as a disease …"; the diagnosis of "hysterical paralysis" is a "a negative verdict"; hysteria is "only half a diagnosis") before drawing, like Brain (4) before him, a distinction between adjectival and substantival views of hysteria. While it might be acceptable to label a symptom as hysterical, there was no justification for accepting hysteria as a syndrome: "Both on theoretical and practical grounds it is a term to be avoided." In 49 of 85 patients diagnosed as having hysteria in the years 1951, 1953, and 1955 at the National Hospital, Slater and Glithero (5) subsequently found an underlying organic illness. While this study has since been criticized on many grounds, it had a profound effect on neurologic practice for some decades to follow. Of even greater influence was David Marsden who, with Stanley Fahn, founded the subspecialty of movement disorders. One of Marsden's many achievements was to rescue organic disorders such as torticollis and writer's cramp from the "no man's land" of hysteria. While he wrote with his customary flair and authority on the subject of hysteria (6), Marsden himself was reluctant to make the diagnosis.

Faced with a patient who did not appear to have a neurologic disease yet was disabled by neurologic symptoms, neurologists turned to their colleagues in psychiatry, only to be told, in most cases, that there was no major psychiatric disease present. Often, there was anxiety and depression, but these, perhaps, were understandable in the circumstances. The term "hysterical," long contaminated by its everyday use, was replaced by "psychogenic," but the problem of how to think about these patients and, more important, manage them, remained. Psychogenic disorders account for a sizeable proportion of referrals to neurology clinics, and it is time that this important yet neglected aspect of neurologic practice receives the attention it is due.

In this chapter, we will discuss the key diagnostic features of the psychogenic gait by reviewing a number of specific cases. The hallmark of the psychogenic gait, namely, its emotive quality, will then be discussed in the light of the current classification of psychogenic disorders, and then from the perspective that this is an example of deceptive signaling, a common pattern of behavior throughout the animal kingdom.

CASES

A. Psychogenic Gait in Neurologic Disease

One of the most difficult and demanding roles of the neurologist is distinguishing psychogenic from "real" symptoms in a patient with proven neurologic disease. This is illustrated in the first two cases.

Case 1

A 67-year-old woman presented with a 10-year history of "collapses." These began after she discovered an indiscretion by her husband. There were bouts of tremor of the limbs. She had become disabled and dependent on her

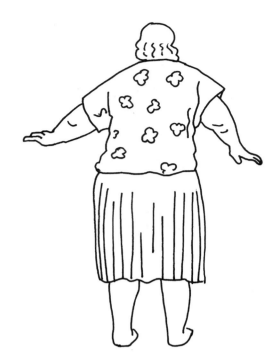

Figure 10.1   Tightrope walking in Case 1.

husband; by the time of her referral to our clinic, she was using a wheelchair outside the home. During the consultation, her manner was one of forced jollity. On standing, she developed a coarse tremor of her trunk and legs which settled after a minute or so. She then walked very slowly on a broad base with her arms extended in the manner of a tightrope walker (Fig. 10.1). While sitting in the chair, she developed a gross tremor of the right leg when it was extended, which was abolished by getting her to tap with the left foot at a varying rate set by the examiner. A diagnosis of psychogenic gait was made, but a tremor study confirmed the presence of a 16-Hz tremor in the legs. This patient had impairment of balance due to orthostatic tremor. She was a vulnerable person with marital problems and there was undoubtedly embellishment. With a program of rehabilitation, her confidence improved and with it, her gait.

Case 2

A teenage girl suddenly developed a generalized tremor and difficulty walking. She walked on a broad base with her feet inverted and her arms held out beside her. Her body bounced with a coarse tremor which increased in amplitude when she sat down, causing the couch to creak. As a child she had had a number of strokes, and an angiogram showed the typical features of Moya Moya disease with occlusion of the internal carotid arteries and the opening up of multiple co-lateral vessels. An MRI scan, performed after the onset of the tremor, showed a large area of infarction in the distribution of the right middle cerebral artery; this was unchanged from imaging studies she had had as a child. There were no signs on clinical examination, which could be related to the area of infarction. The problem continued and she had several admissions to the hospital. During one of these, she was seen to walk normally at a time that she thought she was unobserved. After 18 months she was cured by a faith healer. She then walked quite normally for several years until she gave birth to three children in three years. At this time of great emotional stress and physical exhaustion, her tremor and gait disturbance returned. She was treated as an inpatient with rehabilitation and made a rapid recovery. She was a girl of modest intelligence who had difficulty coping with the trials of adolescence and then motherhood, and expressed this through her physical symptoms; her many admissions to the hospital as a child may have influenced this process. While she had an undoubted underlying neurologic disease, which may have made her less able to cope with life's stresses, this had not caused her tremor and gait disturbance.

B. Gait in Major Psychiatric Disease

Gait disorders not uncommonly occur in the setting of major psychiatric disease and exposure to neuroleptic drugs.

Case 3

A young man with a 5-year history of schizophrenia, for which he had been treated with a number of neuroleptic drugs including fluphenazine and thioridazine, was referred because his father was concerned over the young man's gait. While sitting and conversing, he flapped his hands. Before attempting to walk, he wiggled his toes repeatedly and then walked in a curious creeping manner on his heels with his toes extended. In view of his long exposure to neuroleptic drugs, the posturing of his feet might have represented a form of tardive dystonia. When he put on his thongs, however, he walked quite normally, though before initiating gait he usually wiggled his toes. This patient had a stereotypy of his hands; his gait was ritualistic and related to his psychosis. It is probably better to distinguish this type of gait, which may be seen as another facet of psychotic behavior, from psychogenic gait, where the patient is signaling distress and disability (see below).

C. "Pure" Psychogenic Gait

The diagnosis of psychogenic gait is made with more confidence in younger patients, in whom the likelihood of an underlying physical cause is lower than in the elderly. It is also reassuring if there are no objective physical signs.

Case 4

A 9-year-old boy developed tremor of his hands and a gait disturbance. The tremor, which appeared when the arms

were raised, was distractible and the gait disturbance only occurred during the examination when he was asked to walk heel-to-toe. He then threw himself into a series of wild gyrations, flinging his arms about and leaping from one foot to another, while somehow staying upright, thereby revealing, if nothing else, that there was no problem with his balance. There were no other physical signs. He was of below average intelligence. His mother had multiple sclerosis. With firm encouragement and reassurance, he made a full recovery.

Case 5

A young woman who was a champion athlete came to the clinic with her coach, having suddenly lost her balance and her ability to open her left eye. She walked slowly and gingerly with her arms held out and fell repeatedly into the arms of her coach, who shadowed her for fear that she would fall and injure herself (Fig. 10.2). There were no objective signs. Her left eye was closed. That this was a "pseudoptosis," due to sustained contraction of orbicularis oculi rather than weakness of levator palpebrae superioris, was demonstrated by the fact that the eyebrow was lower on the affected side (not higher as usually occurs in patients with true ptosis where an attempt is made to overcome the ptosis using frontalis). The presence of this "false" sign was helpful in confirming the diagnosis of psychogenic gait. Extensive investigations, including imaging of the brain and spinal cord, had proven negative.

Case 6

A man of middle age miraculously escaped injury when a tree fell onto the hood of his car in a high wind. He was

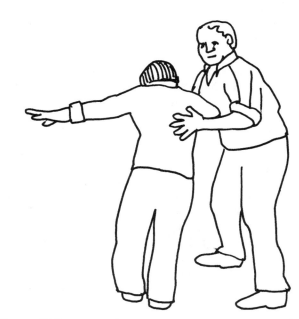

Figure 10.2 Astasia-abasia in Case 5.

severely shaken, and over the next few weeks began to have increasing difficulty in walking. He consulted a lawyer and, at the time of assessment, was bringing an action against the local council to whom the tree belonged. He walked with extraordinary slowness, pausing repeatedly and panting as though he were climbing a mountain. After a few steps, his knees buckled and he sank to the floor. There were no objective physical signs and all investigations were negative.

Case 7

A 41-year-old woman presented with a 10-year history of gait disturbance, poor vision, and difficulty in swallowing and speech. At times, her jaw would lock. On examination, she had a hobbling gait. She appeared to be in pain and leaned heavily on her walking stick. After a few steps, she leaned back heavily on the wall as though exhausted. She had a curious stammer, repeating whole syllables, rather than consonants (a feature of psychogenic stutter noted by Henry Head) (7), and enunciating words in an infantile fashion. Her face radiated misery and anguish. She professed to be completely blind, though she found her way around the room without bumping into the walls or furniture. Her hearing was normal but she incorrectly localized, by pointing, the direction from where the examiner's voice emanated. There were no objective neurologic signs. While the gait had no features particularly suggestive of a psychogenic disorder apart from the effort involved, the presence of psychogenic stutter and blindness were helpful in confirming the presence of a psychogenic gait.

Case 8

A young woman became numb from the neck down the day after a minor car accident. Subsequently, she developed a stammer, gait disturbance, and a tendency to strike herself with her right arm. She had had an abusive and unhappy childhood. After the break-up of her marriage, she had been admitted to a psychiatric unit with "nervous exhaustion." All investigations had been negative. Litigation was pending. On examination, she stammered as described in Case 7. She had a curious creeping gait punctuated by sudden bouts in which she clasped her back in apparent pain (Fig. 10.3).

Case 9

A 73-year-old doctor presented with a 50-year history of multiple symptoms including shin pain, malaise, foot drop, neck pain, and gait and speech disturbance. She trailed her right arm behind her and led with her left leg as though wading through water. Raising her left arm, but not her right, caused the gait to revert to normal. She was able to run normally. While these may have represented an unusual dystonia, she had another sign that made a psychogenic disorder more likely. When she turned her head to the left, she developed a foreign accent.

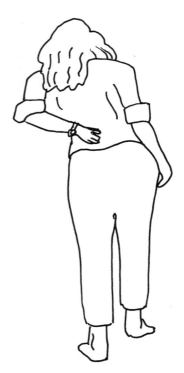

Figure 10.3 Signaling back in Case 8.

KEY FEATURES OF THE PSYCHOGENIC GAIT

These cases illustrate some of the key features which lead to a diagnosis of psychogenic gait (1). These include:

- Exaggerated effort or fatigue with groans and sighs.
- Extreme slowness of movement without evidence of diseases that might cause this such as parkinsonism or hypothyroidism.
- Appearance of pain suggested by grimaces or an antalgic gait where the time spent bearing weight on the painful side is minimized by hurrying the stride on the unaffected side.
- Convulsive tremor where the whole body succumbs to bouts of violent shaking, with the patient remaining conscious and maintaining balance.
- Knee-buckling.
- Unusual postures such as camptocormia or extreme flexion of the trunk, which requires considerable effort and physical strength to maintain. Camptocormia was a common feature of hysteria in soldiers in the First World War (8).
- Associated features such as psychogenic blindness and psychogenic speech disturbance.
- Periods of normality (often when observed covertly).
- Lack of relevant physical signs.

Psychogenic gaits take many forms: hemiparetic (dragging the leg rather than circumducting it, as in a true hemiparesis), paraparetic, ataxic, dystonic, stiff-legged, and slapping (8). In astasia-abasia, the patient experiences apparent difficulty standing or walking, yet has normal leg function on the bed. Midline cerebellar lesions, vestibular dysfunction, and apraxia of gait need to be considered in such patients. Holding the arms out like a tightrope walker (as in Case 1) is something which is not seen in physical diseases which impair balance.

While psychogenic gaits vary markedly in their manifestation, the key feature which alerts the physician to their true nature is most commonly their *emotive* quality. It eloquently signals that the patient is not only disabled but suffering. This is achieved by an exaggeration of the effort required to walk and by the posture, facial expression, and sounds that accompany the gait.

Most of these patients had no major underlying psychiatric illness. Some were receiving treatment for depression. Most were a little anxious. In two cases, litigation was pending. The most striking impression in most of these patients was that they were, for one reason or another, not coping well with life's vicissitudes.

AN APPROACH TO THE PSYCHOGENIC PATIENT

The diagnosis of a psychogenic neurologic disorder is one of the most challenging in clinical medicine (1,8–10), and one that is best dealt with by close collaboration among the neurology, psychiatry, and rehabilitation teams. The role of the neurologist is to determine whether there is an underlying neurologic disorder and whether it could explain the clinical features. The psychiatrist formally assesses the patient for disorders, such as depression, and for psychological factors in the patient and family which could have predisposed the patient to this form of behavior. A history of abuse in childhood, of similar unexplained illnesses in the past, and the presence of multiple unrelated symptoms may be helpful factors in considering this diagnosis. Often, this information is only gained after many consultations with the patients, caregivers, and family over many weeks. Uncovering past emotional traumas does not, in itself, usually improve the symptoms, but encouraging patients to accept that emotion can express itself in physical symptoms can be beneficial. Many patients, however, take exception to this approach, particularly if there is an implication that they are feigning symptoms. Treatment is often most acceptable and effective within the framework of conventional physical rehabilitation (11).

Our experience of using the classical psychoanalytic formulations (12), whereby unresolved psychological conflicts related to sexuality or aggression are channelled into symbolic physical expression, has been unrewarding. The process of linking specific symptoms to particular stresses in the patient's life is open to contrivance and overinterpretation. Certainly patients, even after full recovery, are rarely able to confirm such a link. Conversely, some patients with genuine physical disorders raise the question with their medical practitioners of whether their problem could be related to a particular stress in their lives.

The current classification of psychogenic disorders divides patients into two broad groups: factitious disorders, which are feigned or intentionally produced, and somatoform disorders, which are thought to reflect processes beyond the patient's consciousness or awareness (13). It might be assumed that this could readily be determined by a psychiatrist trained and experienced in this field. In fact, this is a very difficult task even for detectives whose job it is to detect lies (14). Very few patients, in our experience, are willing to admit, even after they have lost all their symptoms, that they had been intentionally producing them. While individual patients can sometimes be confidently labeled as having factitious or somatoform disorders, most patients fall somewhere on a continuum between complete awareness and lack of awareness of the true nature of their symptoms (15–18). The schema offered by Fahn and Williams (19), whereby psychogenic disorders are graded from "possible" to "clearly proven," goes some way to overcoming this impractical dichotomous approach toward classification.

There is further disadvantage to a classification based on whether the patient is deemed to be feigning symptoms. Patients with a label of factitious disorder or malingering are often given short shrift by their doctors. This assumed particular importance in the First World War where, it has been estimated, up to 10% of British officers developed psychogenic symptoms while exposed to the horrors of the trenches (20). Psychiatrists and neurologists were given the unenviable task of resolving whether the soldiers' symptoms reflected "shell shock"(unconscious) or cowardice (feigned). Some, as a result of this assessment, faced the firing squad.

An alternative approach is to view this form of behavior as deceptive signaling. Communication by signaling is one of the key areas of research in behavioral ecology, a relatively new discipline which combines evolution, ecology, and behavior. It aims to analyze decision-making in animals by comparing different communication systems and using economic models that consider costs and benefits of behavior (21). Animals communicate using signals, such as color, pheromones, or behavior, to manipulate a receiver in a way that is beneficial to the individual sending the signal (signaler) and to the individual responding to the signal (receiver) (21). In most systems, the signal mutually benefits signaler and receiver. However, signal deception, whereby the signaler manipulates the receiver and gains benefits at the cost of the receiver, is common.

Deceptive signals are seen in predator-prey interactions, when predators lure prey by deception, or prey use deceptive signals to confuse or deter predators. The bolas spider produces a chemical that is similar to the pheromone of female moths. Male moths are attracted to this chemical

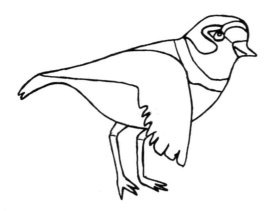

Figure 10.4   Piping plover.

and are subsequently captured by a sticky silk ball that the spider swings (22,23). The mimic octopus changes its shape and color when under attack (24) to mimic the appearance of the highly toxic banded sea snake. The piping plover (Fig. 10.4) lures predators away from its eggs by dragging its wings as if to signal that it is injured and is easy prey (25).

Among social groups, the close interaction of individuals provides ample opportunities for deception, but at the cost of being recognized, ignored, or even punished (2). Examples of deception include withholding information on the location of food by primates (26) and birds (27). By definition, this type of behavior is only considered deceptive if it carries a cost to the receiver and a benefit for the signaler (28). There are a number of accounts of deceptive behavior in nonhuman primates (2). A female baboon was seen to approach a male that had caught an antelope. She started to groom him, and while he was distracted, she snatched the antelope from him (29,30). Seyfarth and Cheney (31) observed a young vervet monkey give a false "leopard alarm" call as a new male and potential competitor attempted to join the social group. A chimpanzee which had been attacked and injured by another male subsequently limped, but only in his presence (32). Compared to other behaviors, deception seems to be rare in nonhuman primates. It may be that they are able to learn from experience which individuals send deceptive signals and ignore or punish them (27).

Deceptive behavior in most animal systems is shaped by natural selection. Signalers benefiting from the change in behavior induced in the receiver are more likely to survive and reproduce (31). Behavior which has evolved in this way is often constantly expressed (28). Deceptive behavior in nonhuman primates, by contrast, is probably acquired through learning and mimicry, and is more adaptive, changing according to the response that is elicited. While imitation and mimicry are highly developed in humans, the evidence for this in nonhuman primates is sparse

(30,33). However, for the purpose of this discussion we do not require a full understanding of the mechanism of non-human primate deception. It is our aim to apply approaches successfully used in behavioral ecology to gain a better understanding of the behavior observed in patients with psychogenic gait.

The approach used in the behavioral ecology of deceptive signals can be applied to humans and may help not only to better define this behavior, but also to gain a better understanding of why this behavior is expressed. Ultimately, this may lead to new approaches that may help patients. Rather than considering the patient a liar or a fraud, we may regard him or her as a *signaler* who is communicating to a *receiver*. The first question concerns the content of the signal. In our cases, the signal conveys a physical ailment. Importantly, our approach does not distinguish whether the patient knowingly or unknowingly displays the signal. Furthermore, this approach does not assume that the patient is healthy. All we assume is that the signal displayed by the patient does not reflect an actual physical state. Patients may or may not have a medical disorder; nevertheless they display signals that suggest a condition that is not present.

As important as the signaler is the person or people to whom the signal is directed: family members, caregivers, friends, employers, or the physician. The posture of the coach depicted in Case 5, poised as he was to catch the young woman, reveals how effective her signaling was in communicating to him her loss of balance. There is little point in trying to rehabilitate the signaler if, on returning to the home environment, the receiver encourages a resumption of this behavior. The family and caregivers have to be heavily involved in the rehabilitation process. There is probably a period in the establishment of this behavior pattern between signaler and receiver after which it is difficult to intervene successfully. Certainly, there was little prospect of altering the behavior of the patient in Case 9 after 50 years.

In assessing patients with psychogenic disorders from the perspective of deceptive signaling behavior, it is useful to weigh up the relative costs and benefits of this behavior. In most cases, the cost is a loss of independence and an inability to lead a full and normal life. The gain is removal from an unwanted activity and increased support and nurture from their family. In cases involving litigation, there is a clear financial incentive.

In naturally selected signals, once the costs outweigh the benefits, the signal will be selected against. In the human context, the loss of face associated with recovery may prolong this behavior even if the costs are very high. The aim of rehabilitation is to create an emotional environment where the patient feels safe to resume normal activities.

According to this approach, one might expect psychogenic gaits only to be exhibited when there is someone to receive the signal. Indeed, the resumption of a normal gait when the patient is observed covertly and worsening of gait in company are key findings in making the diagnosis. It was noteworthy that the patient in Case 8 had her arms at her side when she walked towards the camera and clutched her back (Fig. 10.3) as she walked away from it. Nevertheless, it is conceivable that such a behavior can become so entrenched, the patient so taken up with the role after many years, that it persists even when the patient is alone.

In conclusion, the hallmark of the psychogenic gait is its emotive quality reflecting its function of signaling pain, disability, or distress to the onlooker. It may be viewed as a biologic response to stress and an inability to cope. The current classification based on whether or not the patient consciously deceives is not useful.

REFERENCES

1. Hayes MW, Graham S, Heldorf P, et al. A video review of the diagnosis of psychogenic gait: appendix and commentary. *Mov Disord.* 1999;14:914–921.
2. Semple S, McComb K. Behavioural deception. *Trends Ecol Evol.* 1996;11:434–437.
3. Slater E. Diagnosis of "Hysteria." *BMJ.* 1965;1:1395–1399.
4. Brain WR. The concept of hysteria in the time of William Harvey. *Proc R Soc Med.* 1963;56:317–324.
5. Slater E, Glithero E. A follow-up of patients diagnosed as suffering from hysteria. *J Psychosom Res.* 1965;9:9–13.
6. Marsden CD Hysteria—a neurologist's view. *Psychol Med.* 1986; 16:277–288.
7. Head H. The diagnosis of hysteria. *BMJ.* 1922;i:827–829.
8. Keane JR. Hysterical gait disorders. *Neurology.* 1989;39:586–589.
9. Thomson APJ, Sills JA. Diagnosis of functional illness presenting with gait disorder. *Arch Dis Child.* 1988;63:148–153.
10. Lempert T, Brandt T, Dieterich M, et al. How to identify psychogenic disorders of stance and gait. A video study in 37 patients. *J Neurol.* 1991;238:140–146.
11. Speed J. Behavioural management of conversion disorder: retrospective study. *Arch Phys Med Rehabil.* 1996;77:147–154.
12. Meares R, Gordon E. Whose hysteria: Briquet's, Janet's or Freud's? *Aust N Z J Psychiatry.* 1985;19:256–263.
13. American Psychiatric Association. *Diagnostic and statistical manual of mental disorders.* Washington, DC: American Psychiatric Association, 2000.
14. Vrij A. Credibility judgments of detectives: the impact of nonverbal behaviour, social skills and physical characteristics on impression formation. *J Soc Psychol.* 1993;133:601–610.
15. Cunnien AJ. Psychiatric and medical syndromes associated with deception. In: Rogers R. ed. *Clinical assessment of malingering and deception.* New York, London: The Guildford Press, 1988:14–15.
16. Spivak H, Rodin G, Sutherland A. The psychology of factitious disorders. A reconsideration. *Psychosomatics.* 1994;35:25–34.
17. Jonas JM, Pope HG. The dissimulating disorders: a single diagnostic entity? *Compr Psychiatr.* 1985;26:58–62.
18. Hyler SE, Pitzer RL. Hysteria split asunder. *Am J Psychiatry.* 1978; 135:1500–1504.
19. Fahn S, Williams DT. Psychogenic dystonia. In: Fahn S. ed. *Advances in neurology: dystonia 2.* New York: Raven Press, 1988: 431–455.
20. Shephard B. *A war of nerves. Soldiers and psychiatrists.* London: Jonathan Cape, 2000:1914–1994.
21. Johnstone RA. The evolution of animal signals. In: Krebs J, Ra DNB, eds. *Behavioral Ecology.* Oxford: Blackwell Science, 1997: 155–178.
22. Stowe MK, Tumlinson JH, Heath RR. Chemical mimicry: bolas spiders emit components of moth prey species sex pheromones. *Science.* 1987;236:964–967.
23. Yeargan KV. Biology of bolas spiders. *Ann Rev Entomol.* 1994;39: 81–99.
24. Norman MD, Finn J, Tregenza T. Dynamic mimicry in an Indo-Malayan octopus. *Proc R Soc Lond B.* 2001;268:1755–1758.
25. Ristau C. Aspects of the cognitive ethology of an injury-feigning bird, the piping plover. In: Ristau C. ed. *Cognitive ethology: the minds of other animals.* Hillsdale, NJ: Lawrence Erlbaum Associates, 1991:91–126.
26. Gouzoules H, Gouzoules S. Primate communication: by nature honest, or by experience wise? *Int J Primatol.* 2002;23:821–848.
27. Bugnyar T, Kotrschal K. Observational learning and the raiding of food caches in ravens, corvus corax: is it "tactical" deception? *Anim Behav.* 2002;64:185–195.
28. Whiten A, Bryne RW. Tactical deception in primates. *Behav Brain Sci.* 1988;11:233–273.
29. Jolly A. *The evolution of primate behaviour.* New York: Macmillan, 1972.
30. Heyes CM. Theory of mind in nonhuman primates. *Behav Brain Sci.* 1998;21:101–148.
31. Seyfarth RM, Cheney DL. Signallers and receivers in animal communication. *Annu Rev Psychol.* 2003;54:145–173.
32. De Waal. *Chimpanzee politics: power and sex among the apes.* Baltimore: John Hopkins University Press, 1982.
33. Bryne RW. Imitation as behaviour parsing. *Philos Trans R Soc Lond B.* 2003;358:529–536.

Paroxysmal Psychogenic Movement Disorders

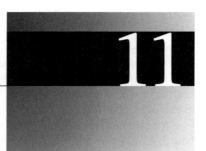

Marie Vidailhet   *Frédéric Bourdain*   *Philippe Nuss*   *Jean-Marc Trocello*

ABSTRACT

Paroxysmal psychogenic movement disorders are rare, but may be underdiagnosed because of two major limitations: the definition of "paroxysmal" and the positive diagnosis of "psychogenic" disorder. Several subtypes are identified (in order of frequency), such as paroxysmal dystonia and dyskinesia, stereotypies, myoclonus, and tics, and are illustrated by clinical "vignettes." The features that are the most useful clues to distinguish psychogenic from "organic" paroxysmal manifestations are discussed. Paroxysmal psychogenic movement disorders are rarely isolated (either intricate with other movement disorders or associated with other somatic symptoms over time). Nevertheless, paroxysmal psychogenic movement disorders share with the other psychogenic movement disorders common mechanisms, therapeutic strategies, and prognosis.

Psychogenic movement disorders may represent up to 20% of patients in a movement disorders clinic. Although the proportion of the different types of movement disorders varies from one tertiary referral center to another, the most frequent psychogenic movement disorders are, in descending order, tremor, dystonia, myoclonus, parkinsonism, gait disorders, and tics (1–6). Paroxysmal movement disorders are not mentioned in most of the series. The most likely reason is that even though many psychogenic movement disorders occur paroxysmally, they are not selected out and labeled separately as paroxysmal psychogenic movement disorders. Furthermore, paroxysmal movement disorders are often categorized as pseudoseizures and are, therefore, excluded from the series of psychogenic movement disorders.

The diagnosis of paroxysmal psychogenic movement disorder (as against an organic disorder) is very difficult and suffers two major limitations: the definition of "paroxysmal," and the positive diagnosis of "psychogenic" disorder applied to this particular category, as the field of "organic" paroxysmal disorders is still expanding with some difficulties in the classifications of the various subtypes.

DEFINITION: PAROXYSMAL

It is not easy to set the limits of the label "paroxysmal" because it refers, in some definitions, both to duration and to triggering factors (7,8). It can also be defined as abrupt onset, recurrence, or intensification of symptoms. The symptoms occur suddenly out of a background of normal motor behavior. Important characteristics such as the frequency, severity, type of movements, and duration are not included in some definitions, and features may vary from one attack to another, as well. The triggering factors can be similar to those incriminated in organic paroxysmal disorders (9–11) (e.g., kinesigenic, continuous exertion, startle, coffee, tea, alcohol, fasting, lack of sleep, fatigue, anxiety, stress, excitement, emotion), but can also include suggestion, distraction maneuvers, or emotional reactions (to the examiner, the family, or the environment).

It would be artificial to restrain the diagnosis of psychogenic paroxysmal disorders to the movements that "look like" paroxysmal dyskinesias (9–11). Paroxysmal psychogenic movement disorders do not only overlap with the clinical features of organic paroxysmal dyskinesias, but may be phenomenologically similar to tremor, myoclonus, tics, stereotypies, and other movement disorders. In a subgroup of sporadic paroxysmal dyskinesias, mainly representing nonfamilial, nonkinesigenic dyskinesias, the prevalence rate of psychogenic origin was 61% (5).

We use the term "paroxysmal" to describe a hyperkinetic movement disorder that occurs abruptly and unpredictably out of a background of normal motor activity and that generally lasts less than 24 hours [i.e., arbitrary definition by analogy with transient ischemic attacks (TIA) and paroxysmal movement disorders related to TIA, and by analogy with secondary paroxysmal dyskinesias]. In most cases, psychogenic paroxysmal movement disorders usually last only for a few seconds or minutes, often less than 1 hour.

POSITIVE DIAGNOSIS OF PSYCHOGENIC PAROXYSMAL MOVEMENT DISORDERS

The usual diagnostic criteria for psychogenic movement disorders (2,9) are partially inoperative in the situation of paroxysmal phenomena. One cannot rely on the clues such as "abrupt onset," "paroxysmal" or "paroxysmal worsening," "spontaneous remission," or "over-time variability," as they also can be observed in organic disorders. Moreover, organic movement disorders can be temporarily and voluntarily suppressed (tics) or restrained (chorea, akathisia) or may appear with voluntary movements (dystonia).

As a consequence, the important clues are restricted to a few items: incongruity with known organic movement disorders, selective disability (excessive slowness or clumsiness in voluntary movements), multiple somatizations, associated "odd" neurologic signs (e.g., weakness, false sensory loss), litigation, and secondary gain (2,3,6). Response to placebo or suggestion is to be considered with caution (up to 20% of organic disorders improve with placebo) (4).

Despite all these caveats, the diagnosis of paroxysmal psychogenic disorder should be a *positive* diagnosis, based on a set of clinical "clues," possibly supplemented by further diagnostic testing. Furthermore, a diagnostic workup for possible organic disorders should be performed. It also implies multiple observations under various conditions (patient alone, with family, with the staff, at home) at different times by experienced movement disorder specialists with a background in neuropsychiatric strategies (2,3,6).

CLINICAL PRESENTATION

Paroxysmal Dystonia and Paroxysmal Dyskinesias

Illustrative Cases

Case 1

A 17-year-old girl (right-handed) without prior medical history is the youngest of eight children. When her family

moved to another town, she had to adapt to a new school that she did not like, and she was rather lonely and distressed. She abruptly presented paroxysmal "dystonic" movements of the left hand, without any triggering factor. She clenched her fist, and flexed her elbow for 10 to 20 seconds, and meanwhile she could answer questions, smile, and behave normally. At the end of the episode, she could normally open her hand, without any sensory or motor abnormality. Then she said, "it is all over," sighed, and smiled. She was a childish, dependent girl, and she tried not to answer questions. Several episodes were triggered by suggestion. None occurred when secretly observed by the examiner and the family, but the episodes were markedly increased when the mother was present and especially when the girl had to go to school. Clinical examination and MRI were normal. The episodes completely disappeared when the girl was taken from school during the holidays and never reappeared thereafter (with a follow-up of 1 year). She was diagnosed as having psychogenic paroxysmal dystonia.

This observation illustrates several clues in favor of the psychogenic origin: an abrupt onset and end, the influence of suggestion, the fact that the episodes only occurred when somebody was around and concerned, the identification of a triggering factor and of its influence on the movement disorder (disappearance of dystonia when the triggering factor was removed), and predisposing factors (passive–dependent, immature personality). Favorable prognostic factors included young age, abrupt onset and short duration of evolution, identified triggering factor, and no underlying severe psychiatric disorder.

Case 2

A 38-year-old woman complained of the abrupt onset of twitching movements of the left upper lip, immediately after dental anesthesia 8 years earlier. She complained of transient paresthesias in the area of the movement disorder.

These movements mimicked those of a rabbit's mouth for less than 1 minute, increased with suggestion and during physical examination, and appeared mainly in stressful situations. She sometimes complained of pain in the precise location where anesthesia had been performed a few years earlier. Local injection of lidocaine led to resolution of the movement disorder for a few hours. She was then told that a local injection would "cure" the problem. This placebo test consisted of the injection of 0.1 mL of saline solution 1 centimeter over the lip. The paroxysmal movement immediately disappeared and did not recur for 3 weeks. She came back and asked for another "therapeutic" injection.

Neurologic examination was normal. Cranial and brain MRI were normal and extensive blood tests were normal.

She had a histrionic personality, and was deeply depressed. She described difficulties in her marriage (with conjugal violence and ongoing divorce procedure), and was the mother of an 8-year-old autistic child with little help at home. She described herself as "trapped between fate and duty." She recognized that she would recover from her symptoms when her family (at least marital) problems would be solved. Her brother testified that the movement disorder could disappear for several weeks during vacations or when she was less anxious.

She was diagnosed with paroxysmal facial dystonia.

This observation illustrates the role of rationalization (as she makes a connection between the dental anesthesia and the onset of the movement disorder), the utility of the placebo test, the recurrence of the movement disorder in a difficult personal and familial context, and a partial insight into the phenomenon (as the patient knows that the disappearance of the symptoms depends on the improvement of her personal life).

Comments

By definition, paroxysmal dystonia and paroxysmal dyskinesias consist of intermittent dystonia, chorea, athetosis, ballism, or any combination of these hyperkinetic disorders. Initially, paroxysmal dyskinesias were classified according to the duration of the attack and the precipitant factor [paroxysmal kinesigenic choreoathetosis or PKC (12), paroxysmal dystonic choreoathetosis or PDC (13,14), paroxysmal exercise-induced dystonia or PED] (15). A revised classification (8) is mainly based on precipitating factors, phenomenology, duration of attacks, and etiology: paroxysmal kinesigenic dyskinesias (PKD) induced by sudden movement; paroxysmal, nonkinesigenic dyskinesia (PNKD); and PED induced after prolonged exercise (8).

However, even in these apparently well-defined entities, several observations do not "fit" with the usual clinical features. For example, in PKD, paroxysmal attacks are triggered by sudden movement and last for a few seconds (less than 5 minutes), but in some cases, attacks may be also be triggered by hyperventilation, stress, startle, menses, heat, and cold (7,10,11). Moreover, incomplete atonic attacks (weakness of the legs) have been described; prolonged (longer than 5 minutes up to hours) (16), more dystonic episodes may also be observed in the same patient or within the same family; and benign infantile convulsions are sometimes present (17).

The variability in duration, provoking factor, and clinical pattern may be part of the disease and cannot be relied upon for the diagnosis of psychogenic movement disorder.

In PNKD, some patients report muscle tension or paresthesia in the limb prior to the onset of the attacks. This premonitory phenomenon is important because sensory symptoms can also be recorded in psychogenic disorders, but the duration and/or localization and the timing are incongruous. By definition, PNKDs are influenced by various endogenous and environmental factors, thus overlapping with organic and psychogenic disorders (e.g., stress, startle, passive movement of a limb) (18).

Family history (19) and a prolonged evolution with an early age at onset are strong elements in favor of genetic,

TABLE 11.1	
DIAGNOSIS	
Historical clues	**Clinical clues**
Abrupt onset	*Incongruous with organic movement disorders*
Static course	*Inconsistent* (mixed bizarre movement disorders)
Minor	Over-time variability
Trauma (compensation)	*Selective disabilities*
Purely paroxysmal	Role of distraction/attention
Spontaneous remissions	Response to placebo
Multiple somatizations	Suggestible
Other psychiatric illness	—
Clear secondary gain	—

organic paroxysmal disorders. In contrast, in sporadic, abrupt adult-onset cases, a psychogenic origin may be suspected after a complete workup for secondary causes, especially if multiple sensorimotor symptoms and behavioral disorders are also present (1,5,20,21).

Both in the literature and in our illustrative cases, suggestibility and response to placebo were observed. The most useful clues for differential diagnosis are summarized in Table 11.1 (6) and italicized. However, most of the accepted "reliable clues" refer to "abrupt onset" or variability in time (e.g., paroxysmal, remission, variability) and do not apply to paroxysmal psychogenic movement disorders.

Paroxysmal Stereotypies

Illustrative Case

A 17-year-old girl, without medical history complained of pain and paresthesias in her left arm. A few days later, she developed stereotyped movements of the left arm with rhythmic pounding of the chest. Despite the force of the blows, she did not have any self-inflicted injury on the chest. On examination, she performed repetitive voluntary movements of the right hand with difficulty and slowness, and the copying of the examiner's hand postures were very clumsy. In the meantime, the pounding of the chest was disorganized. An attempt to immobilize the left arm was followed by the girl's frantic movements of the hand and forearm. During the time of observation, paroxysmal reinforcements of the movements were detected. The patient was very indifferent to her trouble (la belle indifférence) and explained that she was not worried or tired and that she "could not help" as her arm had "its own life." Neurologic examination and extensive workup for an etiology were normal. She received placebo (saline) infusion and electrical stimulation. Subsequently, she explained that she had the feeling that she "will recover" and described tingling of the arm, heralding the future improvement. She "recovered" with a complete cessation of the paroxysmal movement, but she displayed (with equal indifference) a paralysis of her left arm.

She was very guarded on her history but explained that a few days before the onset of the trouble, she had a fight at school with a friend. The friend was injured and was admitted to the hospital. She was concerned, but did not want to tell more about it. It was thought that there were some relationships between this episode and the paroxysmal movement disorder.

This observation illustrates several features of the psychogenic disorder. The patient was fully indifferent to the trouble (la belle indifférence). There was marked variability, an inability to perform complex movements, and an influence of distraction (decrease in the amplitude and frequency of the movement). The most remarkable part is the replacement of the psychogenic movement disorder by hysterical sensorimotor loss (considered to be an "improvement" by the patient). This illustrates that positive (movement disorder) and negative (paralysis, blindness, sensory loss) symptoms are a common result of psychogenic disorders and can be observed either simultaneously or at different periods of time of the disease.

Comments

The characteristics of the movement disorders could correspond to the definition of stereotypies. Stereotypies are repetitive, patterned, rhythmic, purposeless, seemingly ritualistic movements or postures, sometimes associated with mannerism. These behaviors are interpreted as a self-generating sensory stimulus or a motor expression of underlying tension and anxiety. Most of the time, the subjects are not fully aware of the movements and do not complain about them. They can suppress them. They do not feel any increase of inner tension or urge to move (as opposed to tics). Recognition of stereotypies is often in a context of psychiatric (e.g., autism, mental retardation, schizophrenia, psychosis, Angelman syndrome, Rett syndrome) or neurologic disorders (neuroacanthocytosis, Lesch-Nyhan syndrome with self-inflicted mutilations, severe Gilles de la Tourette syndrome, obsessive–compulsive disorders). The fact that psychogenic paroxysmal stereotypies were not mentioned in the series of psychogenic movement disorders is not surprising, as most of the movements corresponding to the description were included either in abnormal movements associated with paroxysmal dystonia (e.g., dancing, throwing, lurching gait) or in psychogenic tics (5).

Paroxysmal Psychogenic Tics and Myoclonus

Illustrative Case

A 53-year-old woman had an onset over a few days of jerks in her neck, left shoulder, trunk, and right hand. The shoulder's jerk could mimic a shrug, and the trunk movements a startle. The jerks were repetitive but were variable in frequency, amplitude, and distribution, and appeared on a normal motor behavior. They were present at rest, without a triggering factor, but were also triggered or increased by stress, startle, or the presence of the examiner. On examination, she was not always aware of them, but could suppress them voluntarily (over 1 minute). There was no urge to move and no rebound after 1 minute of voluntary control of the movements.

She first developed these movements at work. She worked as a secretary and recently had to endure moral harassment from her hierarchy. She became very depressed and anxious, and had the feeling of being in a "mouse trap" and "victimized." She became very withdrawn both at work and in her social and personal life. She was successfully treated for depression, had to change her job, and fully recovered with a follow-up of 6 months.

This observation illustrates the difficulties in the differential diagnosis of some paroxysmal psychogenic disorders. The clinical features could be compatible with those of "organic" tics, myoclonus, and startle. On one hand, the movement shares most of the clinical characteristics of tics (i.e., brief, pseudopurposeful, upper body distributions, and voluntary control over 1 minute), but the "urge to move" and rebound phenomenon were not observed. On the other hand, it could be interpreted as myoclonus (i.e., sudden, brief, shocklike, involuntary movements, axial distribution–startle). However, the lack of consistency, the continuous changing pattern in anatomic distributions, latency from external stimuli (as opposed to startle), and amplitude are incongruous with the description of organic myoclonus. The adult abrupt onset and the resolution after removal of the identified triggering factor are in favor of psychogenic origin.

Comments

In contrast to this observation, in a series of psychogenic myoclonus (22), most of the patients had additional psychogenic disorders (tremor, gait abnormalities, etc.). Psychiatric comorbidity was often present prior to the onset of the movement disorders (e.g., depression, panic attacks, anxiety disorders, and personality disorders). However, similar psychiatric comorbidity is frequent in organic tic disorders and cannot be taken as a reliable clue in favor of psychogenic origin of the trouble and a long-term follow-up. Moreover, the adult onset, the spontaneous remission, and the occurrence on a background of pre-existence troubles emphasize the importance of vigilance in order to detect and differentiate an underlying organic or psychiatric disorder.

In such cases, extensive neurophysiologic explorations (23) could also detect characteristic patterns of startle, spinal or propriospinal myoclonus, or cortical myoclonus.

PITFALLS AND DIFFERENTIAL DIAGNOSIS

Why Paroxysmal Psychogenic Movement Disorders Are Rare. In psychogenic movement disorders, the symptoms are meant to attract attention and care (although for most patients there is no evidence that these symptoms are intentionally produced). The difficulties presented must be clinically significant with marked disability and impairment in social or personal functioning, and must require medical attention and evaluation. This implies a substantial duration of the dysfunction, and this is the case for most types of psychogenic movement disorders. In contrast, paroxysmal disorders are by definition brief and reversible, superimposed on normal motor behavior, and not distressing enough to fall into the category of a severe medical condition. Therefore, they are among the less frequent psychogenic disorders (with the exception of psychogenic seizures).

The Usual Diagnostic Clues Are Lacking or May Be Misleading. The classical behavioral features associated with conversion such as la belle indifférence, histrionic personality, and passive–dependant personality with extreme suggestibility may be lacking as reported by Factor (4) and Fahn (2). The initiation or exacerbation of the symptoms may be preceded by psychological conflicts or other stresses, as over 60% of the patients have a clear history of a precipitating event and 50% have a psychiatric diagnosis (depression). Moreover, psychogenic disorders and organic or psychiatric disorders can be intermingled. Several studies have suggested that one-fourth of individuals with psychogenic disorders have a current coexisting neurologic condition (4,24,25). On the other hand, up to 50% of patients with somatization disorders have associated psychiatric troubles (depression, anxiety, personality disorders) (26).

Special attention should be paid to patients with psychogenic disorders who have a current coexisting neurologic condition (4,25,26). In some cases, the classical characteristics of an organic disease are completely modified by superimposed "odd" incongruous symptoms that are labeled "psychogenic." In some cases, the patient is more or less consciously "overdoing" the organic symptoms in order to attract medical attention. Such behavior is more common in low socioeconomic and low-educated backgrounds. In brief, one can imitate well what one already has got as a disease (unrecognized or recognized). In such cases, special attention and care to the organic disease might help in the recovery of the superimposed psychogenic movement disorder.

Differential Diagnosis

Factitious Disorder and Malingering. In both conditions, the symptoms are produced under voluntary control. They are intentionally produced, due to psychological need (in factitious disorder) or in pursuit of a goal (e.g., economic gain) in malingering. By definition, factitious disorders are due to a mental disorder, whereas malingering is not. However, in clinical practice, it is sometimes difficult to know whether the abnormal behavior is under voluntary control or not, especially when secondary gains are present. In part for this reason, factitious disorder and malingering are usually included in the rubric of psychogenic movement disorder.

Psychogenic Nonepileptic Seizures. Pseudoseizures are paroxysmal episodes that resemble and are often misdiagnosed as epileptic seizures. They often occur in patients with epilepsy. Pseudoseizures can present in various forms, for example, convulsive-type pseudoseizures, "arc de cercle" opisthotonic posture, loss of tone, loss of awareness, and unresponsiveness accompanied by complicated behavior (where the risk of confusion with complex partial seizures is greatest). Movement disorders, particularly myoclonus, but also polymyoclonus, startle response, or dystonia, can be observed, but they are rarely the main features. They are part of a well-identified clinical pattern during known seizure disorders and are mixed with incongruent phenomena in the case of pseudoseizures. Electrophysiologic explorations (video-EEG) (27) combined with clinical workup (28) help in the differential diagnosis in most of the cases. Moreover, the red flags that raise the suspicion that seizures may be psychogenic rather than epileptic are often similar to those observed in paroxysmal psychogenic movement disorders (e.g., emotional triggers such as "stress," presence of an "audience," past medical history of somatic disorders), and these subjects have a greater degree of personality abnormalities (mainly maladaptative personality) (29).

TREATMENT

The treatment of paroxysmal psychogenic disorder is not different from that applied to other psychogenic movement disorders. As the symptom is supposed to be "less severe," the main discussion will be the indications, and inconvenience and expense of hospitalization. As the symptom is paroxysmal, more difficult to observe and to analyze, hospitalization may be a useful time to ascertain the clinical diagnosis and to detect the underlying organic or psychiatric disorders. Depression and anxiety are associated with psychogenic movement disorders in up to 50% of the cases (4) and must be treated independently from the psychogenic disorder. Nevertheless, hospitalization may also have an ambiguous effect: either protection as the patient "runs away" from an "aggressive environment" with which he or she cannot cope anymore, or a narcissistic withdrawal with increasing dependence (and hopeless therapeutic escalation) upon the medical environment. In any case, the hospitalization will be a temporary relief for the family circle and will help to find a new and more normal interaction among the protagonists. For the doctor and caregivers, the hospitalization will be a "break" in a one-to-one relationship, and will help to wind down the spiral of increasing unrealistic demand on the patient's side and the helplessness on the doctor's side.

CONCLUSION

Paroxysmal psychogenic movement disorders are rare, and rarely isolated (either intricate with other movement disorders or associated with other somatic symptoms over time). It is still unclear why patients express either movement disorders or sensorimotor deficiency in response to apparently similar underlying mechanisms.

Nevertheless, paroxysmal psychogenic movement disorders share with the other psychogenic movement disorders common mechanisms, therapeutic strategies, and prognosis. Overall, prognostic factors are poor in psychogenic sensorimotor loss (30) or psychogenic movement disorders with a prolonged course. In contrast, as mentioned by Fahn's and Lang's groups, the best prognostic factors are young age, recent and abrupt onset, identifiable underlying cause, and no serious psychiatric comorbidity (31,32). In keeping with the abrupt onset and the variability of the trouble, one could expect that paroxysmal psychogenic movement disorders would have a rather good prognosis, and, therefore, are underreported in tertiary referral centers, where more persistent movement disorders are more likely to be referred. In all cases, a reliable positive diagnosis and efficient treatment require a close interaction among experienced movement disorder specialists and psychiatrists trained in movement disorders (30).

ACKNOWLEDGMENTS

We thank Veronique Leteur for her helpful and efficient editorial assistance.

REFERENCES

1. Fahn S, Williams D. Psychogenic dystonia. *Adv Neurol.* 1988;50: 431–455.
2. Fahn S. Psychogenic movement disorders. In: Marsden CD, Fahn S, eds. *Movement disorders.* 3rd ed. Oxford: Butterworth-Heineman, 1994:359–372.
3. Williams DT, Ford B, Fahn S. Phenomenology and psychopathology related to psychogenic movement disorders. In: Lang AE, Weiner WJ, eds. *Advances in neurology.* Vol 65. New York: Raven Press, 1995:231–257.
4. Factor SA, Podskalny GD, Molho ES. Psychogenic movement disorders: frequency, clinical profile and characteristics. *J Neurol Neurosurg Psychiatry.* 1995;59:406–412.
5. Bressman SB, Fahn S, Burke RE. Paroxysmal non-kinesigenic dystonia. *Adv Neurol.* 1988;50:403–414.
6. Pringsheim P, Lang AE. Psychogenic dystonia. *Rev Neurol (Paris).* 2003;159:885–891.
7. Demirkiran M, Jankovic J. Paroxysmal dyskinesias: clinical features and classification. *Ann Neurol.* 1995;38:571–579.
8. Jankovic J, Demirkiran M. Classification of paroxysmal dyskinesias and ataxias. In: Fahn S, Frucht SJ, Hallet M et al., eds. *Advances in neurology.* Vol 89. Philadelphia, PA: Lippincott Williams & Wilkins, 2002:387–400.
9. Fahn S. The paroxysmal dyskinesias. In: Marsden CD, Fahn S, eds. *Movement disorders,* 3rd ed. Oxford: Butterworth-Heineman, 1994:310–345.
10. Bhatia KP. The paroxysmal dyskinesias. *J Neurol.* 1999;246: 149–155.
11. Vidailhet M. Paroxysmal dyskinesias as a paradigm of paroxysmal movement disorders. *Curr Opin Neurol.* 2000;13:457–462.
12. Sadamatsu M, Masui A, Sakai T, et al. Familial paroxysmal kinesigenic choreoathetosis: an electrophysiologic and genotypic analysis. *Epilepsia.* 1999;40:942–949.
13. Matsuo H, Kamakura K, Saito M, et al. Familial paroxysmal dystonic choreoathetosis: clinical findings in a large Japanese family and genetic linkage to 2q. *Arch Neurol.* 1999;56:721–726.
14. Fink JK, Hedera P, Mathay JG, et al. Paroxysmal dystonic choreoathetosis linked to chromosome 2q: clinical analysis and proposed pathophysiology. *Neurology.* 1997;49:177–183.
15. Barnett MH, Jarman PR, Heales SJ, et al. Further case of paroxysmal exercise-induced dystonia and some insights intopathogenesis. *Mov Disord.* 2002;17:1386–1387.
16. Fukuda M, Hashimoto O, Nagakubo S, et al. A family with an atonic variant of paroxysmal kinesigenic choreoathetosis and hypercalcitoninemia. *Mov Disord.* 1999;14:342–344.
17. Lee WL, Tay A, Ong HT, et al. Association of infantile convulsions with paroxysmal dyskinesias (ICCA syndrome): confirmation of linkage to human chromosome 16p12-q12 in a Chinese family. *Hum Genet.* 1998;103:608–612.
18. Nagamitsu S, Matsuishi T, Hashimoto K, et al. Multicenter study of paroxysmal dyskinesias in Japan—clinical and pedigree analysis. *Mov Disord.* 1999;14:658–663.
19. Bhatia KP. Familial (idiopathic) paroxysmal dyskinesias: an update. *Semin Neurol.* 2001;21:69–74.
20. Miyasaki JM, Sa DS, Galvez-Jimenez N, et al. Psychogenic movement disorders. *Can J Neurol Sci.* 2003;30(Suppl. 1):S94–100.
21. Blakeley J, Jankovic J. Secondary paroxysmal dyskinesias. *Mov Disord.* 2002;17:726–734.
22. Monday K, Jankovic J. Psychogenic myoclonus. *Neurology.* 1993; 43:349–352.
23. Brown PJ, Thompson PD. Electrophysiological aids to the diagnosis or psychogenic jerks, spasms and tremor. *Mov Disord.* 2001; 16:595–599.
24. Lang AE, Koller WC, Fahn S. Psychogenic parkinsonism. *Arch Neurol.* 1995;52:802–810.
25. Ranawaya R, Riley D, Lang A. Psychogenic dyskinesias in patients with organic movement disorders. *Mov Disord.* 1990;5:127–133.
26. Carson AJ, Best S, Postma K, et al. The outcome of neurology outpatients with medically unexplained symptoms: a prospective cohort study. *J Neurol Neurosurg Psychiatry.* 2003;74:897–900.
27. McGonigal A, Russell AJ, Mallik AK, et al. Use of short term video EEG in the diagnosis of attack disorders. *J Neurol Neurosurg Psychiatry.* 2004;75:771–772.
28. Leis M, Ross MA, Summers AK. Psychogenic seizures: ictal characteristics and diagnostic pitfalls. *Neurology.* 1992;42:95–99.
29. Reuber M, Pukrop R, Bauer J, et al. Multidismensional assessment of personality in patients with psychogenic non-epileptic seizures. *J Neurol Neurosurg Psychiatry.* 2004;75:667–668.
30. Marjama J, Troster AI, Koller WC. Psychogenic movement disorders. *Neurol Clin.* 1995;17:283–297.
31. Feinstein A, Stergiopoulos V, Fine J, et al. Psychiatric outcome in patients with a psychogenic movement disorder. *Neuropsychiatry Neuropsychol Behav Neurol.* 2001;14:169–176.
32. Stone J, Sharpe M, Rothwell PM, et al. The 12 year prognosis of unilateral functional weakness and sensory disturbance. *J Neurol Neurosurg Psychiatry.* 2003;74:591–596.

Treatment and Outcome of Psychogenic Nonepileptic Seizures

12

Ronald P. Lesser

ABSTRACT

Psychogenic nonepileptic seizures (PNES) are episodes that resemble epileptic seizures but are due purely to the emotions. Their clinical features vary considerably and it often is difficult to distinguish PNES from epileptic seizures without video-EEG monitoring. They can be due to a variety of underlying emotional difficulties, though some patients are found to be emotionally normal. Treatment varies, and depends upon the underlying etiology. Response to treatment also varies, and a substantial subset of patients continue to have episodes. We need to improve our abilities to determine etiologies underlying PNES in individual patients, in our abilities to treat these etiologies, and in the supply of personnel able to do this.

Psychogenic nonepileptic seizures (PNES) resemble epileptic seizures, and often are treated as such. Careful evaluation demonstrates that they are not due to epilepsy, but rather are caused purely by the emotions (1–12). A substantial proportion of patients referred for evaluation have PNES, with the incidence of PNES estimated to be about 3% to 9% that of epilepsy, 1.4 to 3.0 per 100,000 person years of observation (13,14). If these numbers are accurate, then there are about 50,000 to 100,000 people with this disorder in the United States, and similar numbers elsewhere (2,13,15,16). It is often difficult to differentiate PNES from epileptic seizures (12,17), and proper diagnosis can be delayed for decades (18). The literature indicates that 10% to 40% of PNES patients have both PNES and epilepsy (1,2,4–12,19). A corollary of these estimates is the conclusion that most patients have one diagnosis or the other. Perhaps because of the presence of psychological dysfunction, quality of life of patients with PNES is worse than that of patients with epilepsy (20).

Treatment of a disorder usually is based upon some understanding of the disorder and its etiology, so that the appropriate treatment can be directed at the appropriate cause. It is important to emphasize that PNES can have multiple causes. This is the case both for individual patients and for the total population of patients with PNES. Also, just as with movement disorders, there are patients who have epilepsy and do not have PNES, but whose epileptic seizures can be precipitated by their emotions.

CLINICAL MANIFESTATIONS

PNES can occur at any age; reported patients have ranged from 4 to 77 years (3). Three quarters are women (3).

The clinical manifestations of PNES can closely resemble those of epileptic seizures. Emergency room personnel, epilepsy monitoring unit staff, and even epilepsy experts have been fooled (12). Some motor manifestations such as pelvic thrusting or asynchronous movements have been reported to differentiate, but may not, because these can occur both with PNES and with epileptic, particularly frontal lobe seizures. Injury (21–23) and urine or fecal incontinence (21,23,24) can occur both with epileptic seizures and with PNES. Patients may be insensitive to pain testing, including standard clinical tests such as conjunctival stimulation (25). PNES patients may present in pseudoepileptic status and allow themselves to be intubated (16,26,27). PNES episodes may sometimes, but not always be longer than epileptic seizures (21,28–30). Some manifestations are more useful, however. Eyes and mouth are generally open during epileptic seizures, and often closed with PNES (31,32). Eyelids may flutter during PNES (25,30). Weeping can occur with PNES, and is unusual with epilepsy (33,34). PNES episodes do not occur during EEG-documented sleep (35,36).

The heart rate may not increase as much with PNES. A 30% increase has been suggested to differentiate between PNES and complex partial or generalized tonic-clonic seizures (37). Prolactin levels, if obtained within 15 to 30 minutes after the end of an episode, may increase severalfold with generalized tonic-clonic or complex partial seizures, and should not with PNES. However, both false-positive and false-negative results can occur (3). Episode induction during video-EEG monitoring can be very helpful, if a clinically typical episode is induced, but should be done carefully, and while maintaining respect for the dignity of the patient (24,38).

The most useful test is an ictal video-EEG. Careful video-EEG analysis usually can determine the etiology of the episode (3). Interictal EEGs are less useful; some individuals with no history of epilepsy have true interictal epileptiform discharges (3). Also, normal variant patterns are frequently mistaken to be epileptiform discharges, so the EEG needs to be evaluated carefully, and by an experienced reader (3).

ETIOLOGIES

It would be interesting to know if specific conversion symptoms would be more likely to have specific etiologies, but little is known about this in the case of PNES. Broadly, psychogenic nonepileptic seizures can present with prominent motor activity or with prominent changes in affect, or both (21,39). Presumably, a patient could have a psychogenic

nonepileptic seizure with purely sensory symptoms, but this is not the subject of comment in the PNES literature. Motor manifestations can vary: Shaking may be of greater amplitude in some patients, lesser amplitude in others, and still others may fall to the ground (40). One study found that patients with prominent motor components to their PNES were less likely to achieve seizure control (41). Similarly, a second study found that patients without rigidity or shaking, ictal incontinence, or tongue biting, no episodes of PNES status, and without admissions to intensive care units had better outcomes (42). However, another study reported that patients with prominent affectual components and less prominent motor components to their episodes might be more disturbed emotionally (43). Such a finding suggested that PNES episodes might be more likely to persist in these patients, although the study was not designed to assess that question. Therefore, the clinical manifestations of PNES may or may not help in determining prognosis. On the other hand, if patients who are more emotionally disturbed nonetheless subsequently are more likely to improve, interesting questions could be raised regarding the relationships among the underlying etiology of a patient's PNES, the clinical manifestations, and the capacity of the patient for emotional improvement.

The psychological causes for PNES vary; a great many have been described in the literature (Table 12.1) (3,44–46). It is likely that the etiologies underlying other "conversion reactions" similarly vary.

First, episodes can occur due to a disturbance in the patient's interactions with others, or in others' interactions with the patient. These include patients with inadequate personalities, adjustment reactions, family conflicts, or who have been victims of sexual or physical abuse. It also includes circumstances in which other people have reinforced a patient's PNES behaviors and in which patients have difficulties managing anger or hostility.

Second, episodes can be due to intrinsic emotional problems or to internalized conflicts. These etiologies include affective disorders, panic attacks, anxiety, obsessive–compulsive disorders, conversion/somatization disorders, dissociative/depersonalization disorders, and posttraumatic stress disorders. Patients may, for internal reasons, misinterpret, or overinterpret occurrences in the environment. These include patients in whom simple partial seizures may occur, but elaborate into PNES (53).

Third, patients may be psychotic or schizophrenic.

Fourth, they may have personality disorders. This group includes patients with borderline, histrionic, narcissistic, antisocial, passive–aggressive, avoidant, and passive–dependent personality. Etiologies such as malingering, factitious disorder, and substance abuse can be included in this group.

Fifth, cognitive difficulties may be present or there may be a history of head trauma (54,55). At least some studies

TABLE 12.1

CAUSES OF PSYCHOGENIC NONEPILEPTIC SEIZURES

Interactions with others
   Adjustment reaction
   Family conflicts
   Inadequate personality
   Reinforced behaviors
   Sexual or physical abuse

Intrinsic emotional problems
   Affective disorders, anxiety disorder, anger, hostility
   Conversion/dissociative/depersonalization/somatization disorders
   Highlighting or misinterpretation (including epileptic seizures)
   Obsessive–compulsive disorder, panic attacks
   Posttraumatic stress disorder

Psychoses, schizophrenia

Personality disorders
   Antisocial personality, avoidant personality, borderline personality,
   factitious disorder, histrionic personality, malingerer, narcissistic
   personality, passive–aggressive personality disorder,
   passive–dependent personality disorder, substance abuse

Structural, developmental, or genetic defects
   Cognitive difficulties, head trauma, EEG abnormalities,
   MRI abnormalities, genetic predispositon

Miscellaneous disorders
   Attention deficit disorder, tic

No psychiatric disease

Note: The table shows one possible way of grouping causes of psychogenic nonepileptic seizures (PNES). An individual patient could have more than one etiology for episodes. In addition, etiologies in one grouping could have a relationship to those in another. For example, a reaction to sexual abuse pertains to what someone did to the patient, but the emotional reaction to it in many ways could be considered a posttraumatic reaction. Some of the etiologies are taken from standard psychiatric nosology (47), others from articles in the literature, which consider etiologies for PNES *per se*, regardless of whether these are listed in the standard nomenclature (44,45,48). Finally, some patients have been found psychiatrically normal (27,49–52).

report an increased likelihood of MRI or EEG abnormalities in patients with PNES (49,50,56–59). It also is worth pointing out that there are data demonstrating that somatization disorder may have a genetic component. Patients with PNES do not necessarily fulfill the criteria for somatization disorder. However, these findings point out that behaviors of this type can have an "organic" basis.

Sixth, there are etiologies such as attention deficit disorder and tic that are mentioned in the literature, but are difficult to classify elsewhere.

Finally, there is a significant subgroup of patients in whom a psychiatric diagnosis cannot be made (27,49–52). These patients may be variants, even if extreme variants, of normal. Because they seem like us, it may be harder for us to understand why PNES is occurring. However, these patients may fare relatively well clinically, as will be discussed below.

More than one etiology can occur in a patient: Who you are and how you interact with others are closely intertwined.

Experience with psychometric testing instruments such as the Minnesota Multiphasic Personality Inventory (MMPI) similarly indicate that the etiologies underlying PNES can be complex, multiple, and variable (60–63).

TREATMENT AND OUTCOME

Once the diagnosis has been made, telling the patient the diagnosis is the first step in treatment (2,3,24,64–68). This should be done carefully and tactfully, and usually by the neurologist primarily responsible for evaluating or for following the patient (24,67,68). This can be complicated when patients are admitted for video-EEG monitoring. Many caregivers have access to the chart and to the patient, and some may discuss the diagnosis, or possible diagnosis, with the patient prematurely. However, the preliminary diagnosis of PNES, perhaps based on the initial outpatient assessment, may be wrong. Also, caregivers do not always treat patients with conversion symptoms well, and may not inform the patient of the diagnosis as tactfully as they should. Therefore, it is a good idea not to write in the chart that the patient may have PNES until one is sure that the patient does have it, and not to write this until after the patient has been informed properly.

The next step is to explore with the patient why the events are occurring. Some patients may know, and this should be discussed. These conversations alone are sufficient to allow control of PNES in some patients (11,21,69–71). Most patients will need additional evaluation and treatment. Patients often resist recommendations for emotional assessment. This makes it particularly important to present the diagnosis and recommend treatment in a manner that is sensitive to the patient's sense of personal dignity (68). It is also important to find a therapist who is comfortable assessing and treating patients with conversion symptoms; not all are. Keep in mind that some patients with emotional disorders are extremely difficult to treat either psychiatrically or neurologically (72). Be aware of such patients, and find professional colleagues who are experienced with managing them and who can help you to do so.

In general, one should tailor the treatment to the underlying emotional cause(s) of the PNES. Different treatments are available for different goals, and these are outlined in Table 12.2. Although the treatments listed are based upon clinical experience with a broad range of disorders, there are few systematic studies regarding the appropriate treatment for PNES. Broadly, conversion disorders can be considered to occur in patients who select a physical way to express a concern or desire. This predisposition can occur in some patients because of the organic "ground" in which the conversion symptom grows. The presence or absence of this "ground" can be important in selecting the most appropriate treatment for a patient.

Pakalnis et al. (27) reported on a group of patients with psychogenic status. They treated patients found to have

TABLE 12.2
TREATMENT OF PSYCHOGENIC NONEPILEPTIC SEIZURES

Goals	Means
Acceptance	Explanation
Motivation	Exploration
Understanding	Counseling
	Psychotherapy
Control	Biofeedback
	Counseling
	Meditation
	Medication
	Psychotherapy
	Relaxation therapy
Consolidation	Follow-up

The table outlines potential goals for patients with psychogenic nonepileptic seizures in the left column. The right column outlines potential therapeutic means to meet these goals.

conversion disorders as inpatients, with psychotherapy and discontinuation of anticonvulsants. Three became episode-free; episodes were reduced in five, and continued in three. Patients with mental retardation were treated as outpatients, with behavioral modification and neuroleptics. One improved; episodes decreased in three. Patients with personality disorders resisted the diagnosis and did not comply with treatment. In one, episodes decreased; in four there was no change.

Walczak et al. (52) reported that in 51 patients, PNES stopped in 18 and continued in 33. Psychotherapy had occurred for 13 of 18 and 28 of 33 patients in these two groups; the difference was not statistically significant. A psychiatric history was present in 8 of 18 and 24 of 33—a significant difference ($p = 0.008$). Ettinger et al. (73) reported that 30 of 56 patients with PNES were rehospitalized for PNES or other symptoms. In their population, 29 were found to be depressed; 22 had suicidal ideation, and 11 had made suicide attempts.

Kanner et al. (49) studied the outcome of patients treated with observation alone, medications, psychotherapy, or medications plus psychotherapy. They reported on the occurrence of spells 1 month and 2 to 6 months postdiagnosis. Four patients treated with observation alone were episode-free. Of patients treated with psychiatric medication, six were episode-free, while two had some episodes. Of ten patients treated with psychotherapy, seven had some episodes, and three had an unchanged number of episodes. Of patients treated with psychiatric medication and psychotherapy, three had no episodes, three had some, and 17 had an unchanged number of episodes. Of patients who refused psychotherapy, one had no episodes, eight some, and four had persistent episodes. These numbers do not suggest that psychotherapy or medication improved prognosis. It appears possible, however, that the underlying diagnosis determined the treatment: Those less sick were observed; sicker patients received psychotherapy and/or medication. When the authors grouped their patients by psychiatric diagnoses, none of the patients did well overall, but patients who had experienced one major depressive episode were most likely to be episode-free. Those with somatoform, dissociative, or personality disorders; recurrent depression; or who had experienced chronic abuse were more likely to have persistent episodes. Similarly, Reuber et al. found that patients with somatization or dissociative disorders were less likely to respond to therapy (42). In many cases, any emotional treatment probably was given by practitioners with only limited familiarity with epilepsy and with PNES; results are likely to be better when the treating personnel are experienced with these entities (27,70), but there are both staffing and health insurance barriers. The insurance barriers can be especially troublesome, and also are surprising, particularly from the economic point of view. For example, one study concluded that the per-capita health care expenditures were up to nine times greater for patients with somatization disorder (66). Expenditures declined by half among patients who received psychiatric consultation. Patients with somatization disorder accounted for 48% of sick-leave days among a cohort of adopted women studied in Sweden (74).

An important actor on this stage remains the primary neurologist or epileptologist who made the diagnosis or who is following the patient. That person should see the patient again, and find out whether treatment has been initiated and how effective it has been.

How many patients improve? Among six studies of a total of 317 patients, from 29% to 52% became seizure-free; 15% to 43% experienced seizure reduction (21,51, 52,75–77). Patients were more likely to improve if they were women or children (21,64), if their episodes began more recently (27,41,49,51), if they were normal on psychiatric examination (51), if they did not have personality disorders (27,49), and if there was no ongoing litigation linked to their PNES (77). As just discussed, not only the presence or absence of psychiatric diagnoses, but also the diagnoses made seem to help predict long-term outcome (3,27,49–52,68).

Some have concluded that likelihood of long-term seizure control depends more on the presence or absence of an underlying psychiatric diagnosis than it does on the treatment. Lempert and Schmidt (51) compared PNES patients with and without additional psychiatric diagnoses. Of those with psychiatric diagnoses, seven became episode-free, while 23 did not. Of those without psychiatric diagnoses, six became seizure-free, and two did not. The difference was significant ($p < 0.05$).

In summary, PNES vary in their clinical manifestations and in their etiologies. No single treatment can be prescribed for patients with PNES, any more than a single treatment can be prescribed for patients with epilepsy. Because of their underlying emotional makeup, some patients resist treatment and control of their episodes (72), while others are better able to control their episodes and their lives. Treatment is probably more successful for patients with specific kinds of etiologies, and when given by personnel with appropriate experience.

How does an understanding of PNES help in the evaluation and treatment of patients with movement disorders? Video, accelerometric, and electromyographic analyses can help differentiate "psychogenic" from "organic" disorders (78–81). More data are needed regarding the results of these kinds of testing. Information is becoming available regarding the underlying emotional etiologies for these psychogenic movement disorders (82–84) as well as the responses to treatment (82,85–87). Do etiologies vary between movement disorders and PNES? If so, what are the differences? If not, do certain psychopathologies result in certain kinds of clinical manifestations? A comparison of clinical findings, underlying etiologies, and treatment results may help us better understand the reasons for the occurrence of both PNES and psychogenic movement disorders.

REFERENCES

1. Benbadis SR. Provocative techniques should be used for the diagnosis of psychogenic nonepileptic seizures. *Arch Neurol.* 2001;58:2063–2065.
2. Gumnit RJ. Psychogenic seizures. In: Wyllie E, ed. *The treatment of epilepsy: principles and practice.* Philadelphia, PA: Lea & Febiger, 1993:692–695.
3. Lesser RP. Psychogenic seizures. *Neurology.* 1996;46:1499–1507.
4. Ramsay RE, Coen A, Brown MC. Coexisting epilepsy and non-epileptic patients. In: Rowan AJ, Gates JR, eds. *Nonepileptic seizures.* Boston, MA: Butterworth-Heineman, 1993:47–54.
5. Olafsson E, Hauser WA, Ludvigsson P, et al. Incidence of epilepsy in rural Iceland: a population-based study. *Epilepsia.* 1996;37: 951–955.
6. Hauser WA, Annegers JF, Kurland LT. Incidence of epilepsy and unprovoked seizures in Rochester, Minnesota: 1935–1984. *Epilepsia.* 1993;34:453–468.
7. Hauser WA, Olafsson E, Ludvigsson P, et al. Incidence of unprovoked seizures in Iceland. *Epilepsia.* 1997;38(Suppl. 18):136.
8. Fakhoury T, Abou-Khalil B, Newman K. Psychogenic seizures in old age: a case report. *Epilepsia.* 1993;34:1049–1051.
9. Gates JR, Luciano D, Devinsky O. Classification and treatment of nonepileptic events. In: Devinsky O, Theodore WH, eds. *Epilepsy and behavior.* New York: Wiley-Liss, 1991:251–263.
10. Desai BT, Porter RJ, Penry JK. Psychogenic seizures. A study of 42 attacks in six patients, with intensive monitoring. *Arch Neurol.* 1982;39:202–209.
11. Lesser RP, Lueders H, Dinner DS. Evidence for epilepsy is rare in patients with psychogenic seizures. *Neurology.* 1983;33:502–504.
12. King DW, Gallagher BB, Murvin AJ, et al. Pseudoseizures: diagnostic evaluation. *Neurology.* 1982;32:18–23.
13. Sigurdardottir KR, Olafsson E. Incidence of psychogenic seizures in adults: a population-based study in Iceland. *Epilepsia.* 1998; 39(7):749–752.
14. Szaflarski JP, Ficker DM, Cahill WT, et al. Four-year incidence of psychogenic nonepileptic seizures in adults in Hamilton County, OH. *Neurology.* 2000;55:1561–1563.
15. Hauser WA, Hesdorffer DC. *Epilepsy: frequency, causes and consequences.* New York: Demos Publications, 1990.
16. Howell SJ, Owen L, Chadwick DW. Pseudostatus epilepticus. *Q J Med.* 1989;71:507–519.
17. Smith D, Defalla BA, Chadwick DW. The misdiagnosis of epilepsy and the management of refractory epilepsy in a specialist clinic. *Q J Med.* 1999;92:15–23.
18. Reuber M, Fernandez G, Bauer J, et al. Diagnostic delay in psychogenic nonepileptic seizures. *Neurology.* 2002;58:493–495.
19. Lesser RP. Psychogenic seizures. *Psychosomatics.* 1986;27:823–829.
20. Szaflarski JP, Hughes C, Szaflarski M, et al. Quality of life in psychogenic nonepileptic seizures. *Epilepsia.* 2003;44:236–242.
21. Meierkord H, Will B, Fish D, et al. The clinical features and prognosis of pseudoseizures diagnosed using video-EEG telemetry. *Neurology.* 1991;41:1643–1646.
22. Luther JS, McNamara JO, Carwile S, et al. Pseudoepileptic seizures: methods and video analysis to aid diagnosis. *Ann Neurol.* 1982;12:458–462.
23. Peguero E, Abou-Khalil B, Fakhoury T, et al. Self-injury and incontinence in psychogenic seizures. *Epilepsia.* 1995;36:586–591.
24. Lesser RP. Psychogenic seizures. In: Pedley TA, Meldrum BS, eds. *Recent advances in epilepsy.* Edinburgh: Churchill Livingstone, 1985:273–296.
25. Gowers WR. *Epilepsy and other chronic convulsive diseases: their causes, symptoms, and treatment.* New York: Dover Publications, 1964.
26. Özkara C, Dreifuss FE. Differential diagnosis in pseudoepileptic seizures. *Epilepsia.* 1993;34:294–298.
27. Pakalnis A, Drake ME Jr, Phillips B. Neuropsychiatric aspects of psychogenic status epilepticus. *Neurology.* 1991;41:1104–1106.
28. Gates JR, Ramani V, Whalen SM. Ictal characteristics of pseudoseizures. *Epilepsia.* 1983;24:246–247.
29. Leis AA, Ross MA, Summers AK. Psychogenic seizures: ictal characteristics and diagnostic pitfalls [see comments]. *Neurology.* 1992;42:95–99.
30. Gates JR, Ramani V, Whalen S, et al. Ictal characteristics of pseudoseizures. *Arch Neurol.* 1985;42:1183–1187.
31. DeToledo JC, Ramsay RE. Patterns of involvement of facial muscles during epileptic and nonepileptic events: review of 654 events. *Neurology.* 1996;47:621–625.
32. Flügel D, Bauer J, Käseborn U, et al. Closed eyes during a seizure indicate psychogenic etiology: a study with suggestive seizure provocation. *J Epilepsy.* 1996;9:165–169.
33. Bergen D, Ristanovic R. Weeping as a common element of pseudoseizures. *Arch Neurol.* 1993;50:1059–1060.
34. Walczak TS, Bogolioubov A. Weeping during psychogenic nonepileptic seizures. *Epilepsia.* 1996;37(2):208–210.
35. Thacker K, Devinsky O, Perrine K, et al. Nonepileptic seizures during apparent sleep. *Ann Neurol.* 1993;33:414–418.
36. Herman ST, Walczak TS, Bazil CW. Distribution of partial seizures during the sleep—wake cycle: differences by seizure onset site. *Neurology.* 2001;56:1453–1459.
37. Opherk C, Hirsch LJ. Ictal heart rate differentiates epileptic from non-epileptic seizures. *Neurology.* 2002;58:636–638.
38. Devinsky O, Fisher R. Ethical use of placebos and provocative testing in diagnosing nonepileptic seizures. *Neurology.* 1996;47: 866–870.
39. Leis AA, Ross MA, Summers AK. Psychogenic seizures: ictal characteristics and diagnostic pitfalls. *Neurology.* 1992;42:95–99.
40. Groppel G, Kapitany T, Baumgartner C. Cluster analysis of clinical seizure semiology of psychogenic nonepileptic seizures. *Epilepsia.* 2000;41:610–614.
41. Selwa LM, Geyer J, Nikakhtar N, et al. Nonepileptic seizure outcome varies by type of spell and duration of illness. *Epilepsia.* 2000;41(10):1330–1334.
42. Reuber M, Pukrop R, Bauer J, et al. Outcome in psychogenic nonepileptic seizures: 1 to 10 year follow-up in 164 patients. *Ann Neurol.* 2003;53:305–311.
43. Holmes GL, Sackellares JC, McKiernan J, et al. Evaluation of childhood pseudoseizures using EEG telemetry and video tape monitoring. *J Pediatr.* 1980;97:554–558.
44. Gumnit RJ, Gates JR. Psychogenic seizures. *Epilepsia.* 1986; 27(Suppl. 2):S124–S129.
45. Gates JR, Erdahl P. Classification of non-epileptic events. In: Rowan AJ, Gates JR, eds. *Non-epileptic seizures.* Stoneham, Massachusetts, MA: Butterworth-Heineman, 1993:21–30.

46. Gates JR, Luciano D, Devinsky O. The classification and treatment of nonepileptic events. In: Devinsky O, Theodore WH, eds. *Epilepsy and behavior*. New York: Wiley-Liss, 1991:251–263.

47. Spitzer RL, Williams JB, Gibbon M, et al. *Structured clinical interview for DSM-III-R*. Patent edition-SCID-P, version 1.0. Washington, DC: American Psychiatric Press, 1990.

48. Gumnit RJ. Behavior disorders related to epilepsy. *Electroencephalogr Clin Neurophysiol Suppl*. 1985;37:313–323.

49. Kanner AM, Parra J, Frey M, et al. Psychiatric and neurologic predictors of psychogenic pseudoseizure outcome. *Neurology*. 1999;53:933–938.

50. Mokleby K, Blomhoff S, Malt UF, et al. Psychiatric comorbidity and hostility in patients with psychogenic nonepileptic seizures compared with somatoform disorders and healthy controls. *Epilepsia*. 2002;43:193–198.

51. Lempert T, Schmidt D. Natural history and outcome of psychogenic seizures: a clinical study in 50 patients. *J Neurol*. 1990;237:35–38.

52. Walczak TS, Papacostas S, Williams DT, et al. Outcome after diagnosis of psychogenic nonepileptic seizures. *Epilepsia*. 1995;1131:1137.

53. Kapur J, Pillai A, Henry TR. Psychogenic elaboration of simple partial seizures. *Epilepsia*. 1995;36(11):1126–1130.

54. Barry E, Krumholz A, Bergey GK, et al. Nonepileptic posttraumatic seizures. *Epilepsia*. 1998;39:427–431.

55. Conder RL, Zasler ND. Psychogenic seizures in brain injury: diagnosis, treatment and case study. *Brain Inj*. 1990;4:391–397.

56. Reuber M, Fernandez G, Bauer J, et al. Interictal EEG abnormalities in patients with psychogenic nonepileptic seizures. *Epilepsia*. 2002;43:1013–1020.

57. Wesbrook LE, Devinsky O, Geocadin R. Nonepileptic seizures after head injury. *Epilepsia*. 1998;39(9):978–982.

58. Kalogjera-Sackellares D, Sackellares JC. Impaired motor function in patients with psychogenic pseudoseizures. *Epilepsia*. 2002;42:1600–1606.

59. Kalogjera-Sackellares D, Sackellares JC. Intellectual and neuropsychological features of patients with psychogenic pseudoseizures. *Psychiatry Res*. 1999;86:73–84.

60. Wilkus RJ, Dodrill CB. Factors affecting the outcome of MMPI and neuropsychological assessments of psychogenic and epileptic seizure patients. *Epilepsia*. 1989;30:339–347.

61. Wilkus RJ, Dodrill CB, Thompson PM. Intensive EEG monitoring and psychological studies of patients with pseudoepileptic seizures. *Epilepsia*. 1984;25:100–107.

62. Storzbach D, Binder LM, Salinsky MC, et al. Improved prediction of nonepileptic seizures with combined MMPI and EEG measures. *Epilepsia*. 2000;41(3):332–337.

63. Kalogjera-Sackellares D, Sackellares JC. Analysis of MMPI patterns in patients with psychogenic pseudoseizures. *Seizure*. 1997;6:419–427.

64. Wyllie E, Friedman D, Lüders H, et al. Outcome of psychogenic seizures in children and adolescents compared with adults. *Neurology*. 1991;41:742–744.

65. Betts T. Pseudoseizures: seizures that are not epilepsy. *Lancet*. 1990;336:163–164.

66. Smith GR, Monson RA, Ray DC. Psychiatric consultation in somatization disorder: a randomized controlled study. *N Engl J Med*. 1986;314:1407–1413.

67. Shen W, Bowman ES, Markand ON. Presenting the diagnosis of pseudoseizure. *Neurology*. 1990;40:756–759.

68. Lesser RP. Treating psychogenic nonepileptic seizures: easier said than done. *Ann Neurol*. 2003;53:285–286.

69. Betts T, Boden S. Diagnosis, management and prognosis of a group of 128 patients with non-epileptic attack disorder. *Seizure*. 1992;1:19–32.

70. Aboukasm A, Mahr G, Gahry BR, et al. Retrospective analysis of the effects of psychotherapeutic interventions on outcomes of psychogenic nonepileptic seizures. *Epilepsia*. 1998;39:470–473.

71. Tergau F, Wischer S, Somal HS, et al. Relationship between lamotrigine oral dose, serum level and its inhibitory effect on CNS: insights from transcranial magnetic stimulation. *Epilepsy Res*. 2003;56:67–77.

72. Groves JE. Taking care of the hateful patient. *N Engl J Med*. 1978;298:883–887.

73. Ettinger AB, Devinsky O, Weisbrot DM, et al. A comprehensive profile of clinical, psychiatric, and psychosocial characteristics of patients with psychogenic nonepileptic seizures. *Epilepsia*. 1999;40(9):1292–1298.

74. Sigvardsson S, von Knorring AL, Bohman M, et al. An adoption study of somatoform disorders. I. The relationship of somatization to psychiatric disability. *Arch Gen Psychiatry*. 1984;41:853–859.

75. Krumholz A, Niedermeyer E. Psychogenic seizures: a clinical study with follow-up data. *Neurology*. 1983;33:498–502.

76. Kristensen O, Alving J. Pseudoseizures—risk factors and prognosis. A case-control study. *Acta Neurol Scand*. 1992;85:177–180.

77. Ettinger AB, Devinsky O, Weisbrot DM, et al. A comprehensive profile of clinical, psychiatric, and psychosocial characteristics of patients with psychogenic nonepileptic seizures. *Epilepsia*. 1999;40:1292–1298.

78. Lempert T, Brandt T, Dieterich M, et al. How to identify psychogenic disorders of stance and gait. A video study in 37 patients. *J Neurol*. 1991;238:140–146.

79. Milanov I. Electromyographic differentiation of tremors. *Clin Neurophysiol*. 2001;112:1626–1632.

80. Tijssen MA, Marsden JF, Brown P. Frequency analysis of EMG activity in patients with idiopathic torticollis. *Brain*. 2000;123 (Pt 4):677–686.

81. Rapoport A, Stein D, Shamir E, et al. Clinico-tremorgraphic features of neuroleptic-induced tremor. *Int Clin Psychopharmacol*. 1998;13:115–120.

82. Feinstein A, Stergiopoulos V, Fine J, et al. Psychiatric outcome in patients with a psychogenic movement disorder: a prospective study. *Neuropsychiatry Neuropsychol Behav Neurol*. 2001;14:169–176.

83. Marjama J, Troster AI, Koller WC. Psychogenic movement disorders. *Neurol Clin*. 1995;13:283–297.

84. Williams DT, Ford B, Fahn S. Phenomenology and psychopathology related to psychogenic movement disorders. *Adv Neurol*. 1995;65:231–257.

85. Lang AE. Psychogenic dystonia: a review of 18 cases. *Can J Neurol Sci*. 1995;22:136–143.

86. Dooley JM, Stokes A, Gordon KE. Pseudo-tics in tourette syndrome. *J Child Neurol*. 1994;9:50–51.

87. Monday K, Jankovic J. Psychogenic myoclonus. *Neurology*. 1993;43:349–352.

Functional Paralysis and Sensory Disturbance

13

Jon Stone   Michael Sharpe

ABSTRACT

Paralysis or sensory loss unexplained by disease and often described as functional or psychogenic is a common clinical presentation, especially in neurologic practice.

Despite their frequency, functional paralysis and sensory loss have received remarkably little research attention. In this chapter, we summarize the available epidemiologic and clinical research literature that specifically relates to functional paralysis and sensory symptoms. We also discuss hypotheses that try to answer the question of why patients develop paralysis rather than another symptom such as fatigue or pain. Lastly, we suggest how conceptualizing these symptoms as arising from reversible dysfunction of the nervous system, rather than as purely psychogenic, is both consistent with recent research findings and a way of achieving greater transparency of communication with the patient.

TERMINOLOGY

Doctors use a wide variety of terms to describe symptoms unexplained by disease. All have theoretic and practical shortcomings, however (1,2). Table 13.1 lists some of the commonly used words, together with their respective advantages and pitfalls.

In Edinburgh we have studied the perceptions of different diagnostic terms for paralysis by general neurology outpatients. We asked them to imagine that they had a weak leg, that their tests were normal, and that the doctor was giving them one of ten diagnoses (see Table 13.2) (4). The diagnoses "all in the mind," "hysterical," and "psychosomatic" were interpreted as meaning "mad," "imagining

symptoms," or "making up symptoms" by more than half of the subjects. The diagnosis of functional weakness was, however, no more offensive than that of stroke.

The diagnosis of functional nervous disorder was in common use as a description of "hysterical" symptoms from the late 19th century to the middle of the 20th century. Using it avoids having to make a meaningless distinction between symptoms that are arising from the mind rather than from the brain; it implies that the problem is one of nervous system functioning rather than structural damage. However, the term "functional" continues to have a pejorative meaning for some doctors. Whilst this is perhaps more of a problem for doctors than patients, it may also be argued that the term will inevitably acquire stigma with the general public if widely used. The term may also be criticized as being simply too broad in meaning, as other conditions such as epilepsy and migraine can also be described as functional. Despite these reservations, we will use the term "functional" because we consider it to be the best currently available, theoretically and practically.

HOW COMMON IS FUNCTIONAL PARALYSIS AND SENSORY LOSS?

Studies in Nonneurologic Populations

There have been few population-based studies of functional weakness. These have estimated the prevalence at 2% (5,6). One of these, a study of functional symptoms in over 2,000 people found this rate was maintained even in people aged less than 45 years (Rief, *personal communication*, 2000). By way of contrast, another study of 600 people did not find anyone with functional paralysis (7). A

TABLE 13.1

WORDS USED TO DESCRIBE PARALYSIS UNEXPLAINED BY DISEASE

Diagnosis

Psychogenic	Suggests a purely psychological etiology, when increasingly most workers in the field of somatic symptoms accept that a biopsychosocial model fits the data best.
Psychosomatic	In its true intended sense, it means an interaction between mind and body, but has become shorthand for "psychogenic" (3). Likely to offend (4).
Nonorganic	A "nondiagnosis" that indicates what the problem isn't rather than what it is.
Hysterical	Suggests uterine etiology. Likely to offend (4). It has the advantage that it cannot mean malingering.
Conversion disorder	Little clinical evidence to support the psychodynamic conversion hypothesis for most cases. Conversion symptoms typically have a high rate of comorbid distress.
Dissociative motor disorder	Although dissociation can be an important mechanism in some cases, there is no evidence that all patients develop paralysis or sensory loss because of dissociation.
Medically unexplained	More theoretically neutral but untrue since we do have some understanding of these symptoms and can recognize them clinically. Does not distinguish symptoms that present with a hallmark of inconsistency from symptoms which are consistent but with poorly understood pathology (e.g., cervical dystonia or unexplained spastic paraplegia). Also impractical when talking to patients (4).
Functional	Avoids psychological vs. physical debate in keeping with biopsychosocial model. Describes abnormal functioning of nervous system. Not offensive to patients. Can also mean malingering. Too broad a term for some.

TABLE 13.2

PERCEPTION OF DIAGNOSTIC LABELS FOR WEAKNESS "IF YOU HAD LEG WEAKNESS, YOUR TESTS WERE NORMAL, AND A DOCTOR SAID YOU HAD X, WOULD HE BE SUGGESTING THAT YOU WERE Y (OR HAD Y)"[a]

	Y Connotations (% response, n = 86)							
X Diagnoses	**Putting It On (Yes)**	**Mad (Yes)**	**Imagining Symptoms (Yes)**	**Can Control Symptoms (Yes)**	**Medical Condition (No)**	**Good Reason to be Off Sick from Work (No)**	**Offense Score (%)[b]**	**The Number Needed to Offend (95% CI)[c]**
Symptoms all in the mind	83	31	87	83	66	70	93	2 (2-2)
Hysterical weakness	45	24	45	48	33	42	50	2 (2-3)
Medically unexplained weakness	24	12	31	33	37	41	42	3 (2-4)
Psychosomatic weakness	24	12	40	28	21	28	35	3 (3-4)
Depression-associated weakness	21	7	20	28	15	28	31	4 (3-5)
Stress-related weakness	9	3	14	30	14	23	19	6 (4-9)
Chronic fatigue	9	1	10	23	19	14	14	8 (5-13)
Functional weakness	7	2	8	17	8	20	12	9 (5-16)
Stroke	2	5	5	7	6	12	12	9 (5-16)
Multiple sclerosis	0	1	3	2	3	8	2	43 (13-∞)

CI, confidence intervals.
[a]Percent responses among 86 new neurology outpatients, offense score, and number needed to offend (i.e., the number of patients to whom you would have to give this diagnostic label before one patient is offended).
[b]The proportion of subjects who responded "Yes" to one or more of: "putting it on," "mad," or "imagining symptoms."
[c]Calculated according to the offense score.
Adapted and reprinted from Stone J, Wojcik W, Durrance D, et al. What should we say to patients with symptoms unexplained by disease? The "number needed to offend." *BMJ.* 2002;325:1449–1450, with permission.

prospective consecutive study of neurologic inpatients with functional paralysis in Sweden found a minimum population incidence of functional paralysis of 5 per 100,000 (8). This incidence is similar to that of other neurologic disorders, for example, amyotrophic lateral sclerosis (2 per 100,000) and multiple sclerosis (3 per 100,000) (9).

In older studies from the St. Louis group, the lifetime reported prevalence of an episode of unexplained paralysis in psychiatric patients, postpartum women, and medically ill patients was much higher at 7%, 9%, and 12%, respectively (10–12).

Carrying out high-quality epidemiology on a symptom such as weakness is not easy, and there are significant limitations to all of the studies listed above. First, functional weakness can be a difficult clinical diagnosis, and basing figures on patient self-report or retrospective note review is likely to lead to errors in over- and underreporting, respectively. Second, doctors and patients are likely to have varying views on what "medically unexplained weakness" encompasses. For example, is sleep paralysis—a type of paralysis that many people have experienced at one time or other in their lives—unexplained by disease? Or is the temporary weakness felt in a limb that has been injured normal or abnormal? Consequently, a much more detailed survey than any carried out so far will be needed to obtain robust estimates of the nature, incidence, and prevalence of various forms of functional weakness in the general population.

Outpatients

There have been no studies that have specifically examined the prevalence of functional paralysis and sensory loss in neurologic outpatients. A number of studies in European practice have established that around one third of all outpatients seen by neurologists have symptoms that are only somewhat or not at all explained by disease (13,14). Unfortunately, it remains unclear how many of these patients have paralysis or sensory loss. The best estimate is from a case series reported by a neurologist in London who diagnosed conversion hysteria in 3.8% of 7,836 consecutive patients (15).

Inpatients

The reported frequency of functional paralysis in neurologic inpatients varies from 1% to 2% (8,16) and after back surgery, as high as 3% (17). Further information comes from studies of the prevalence of "hysteria" or conversion disorder in neurologic inpatients which varies between 1% to 18% (18–21). Between a third to a half of patients with conversion disorder have paralysis as their main symptom (22), which would suggest the true frequency may be even higher.

In conclusion, the limited epidemiologic evidence available suggests that the symptoms of functional paralysis and sensory disturbance are relatively common in neurologic practice and may also have a surprisingly high prevalence and incidence in the general population.

ETIOLOGY OF FUNCTIONAL PARALYSIS AND SENSORY LOSS:

General Factors

There is a large literature on the possible causes of conversion disorder/hysteria. It approaches the problem from a variety of perspectives: psychoanalytic, psychogenic, cultural, and biologic. However, the fundamental problem with these general approaches is that they make the assumption that all patients presenting with symptoms imitating neurologic disease have the same disorder (23,24). Until the validity of grouping together patients with different pseudoneurologic symptoms can be established, it seems more sensible to study patients defined by sharing specific symptoms.

There has been only one controlled study that has addressed the etiology of functional paralysis and none in patients with functional sensory symptoms. There have, however, been several studies of wider groups of patients that have contained high proportions of patients with paralysis or sensory loss (25–32).

Binzer et al. carried out a prospective case control study of 30 patients with functional paralysis and 30 patients with neurologic paralysis (8,33,34). They found a higher rate of so-called axis 1 psychiatric disorders (such as depression) as well as axis 2 disorders (personality disorders) in the functional paralysis group. They also found that functional paralysis patients tended to have received less education and to have experienced more negatively perceived life events prior to symptom onset. Contrary to many other studies of conversion disorder (26), they did not find a higher rate of childhood abuse in the cases, although the cases did report their upbringing to be more negative (34). A study of illness beliefs in the same cases and controls was remarkable for showing that patients with motor conversion symptoms were more likely to be convinced that they had a disease and to reject psychological explanations than were patients who actually had a neurologic disease.

Other studies have examined patients with conversion disorder, a high proportion of whom have paralysis. They have confirmed the importance of childhood factors, psychiatric comorbidity, personality variables, and the importance of organic disease as risk factors for functional symptoms.

The problem remains that all of these studies, although relatively specific to patients with functional paralysis, are still examining questions relating to the generality of why people might develop symptoms unexplained by disease. Childhood factors, psychiatric morbidity, disease, and personality factors are relevant to the development of many kinds of functional somatic symptoms, and for that matter, depression and anxiety (35). What researchers have found much harder to tackle is the specific question, "Why do people develop paralysis and not some other symptom?"

Why Do People Develop Paralysis?

The Psychodynamic Perspective

For the last century, the dominant view of the etiology of functional paralysis has been psychodynamic. Figure 13.1 shows a classic case of a soldier who has lost the ability to perform his duties because of paralysis of the right hand. He complained, "I cannot salute and I cannot handle a gun with this hand; it has to be treated." Figure 13.1A shows the patient at presentation and Figure 13.1B after psychotherapeutic treatment.

According to the psychodynamic model, the loss of function implicit in paralysis is said to arise as a result of mental conflict in a vulnerable individual—the mental conflict being partially or even completely resolved by the expression of physical symptoms—so-called primary gain. In addition to communicating distress that cannot be verbalized and "escaping" the conflict, the individual receives the status and advantage of being regarded as an invalid—so-called secondary gain. Some have regarded conversion hysteria purely as a form of communication. In the case of paralysis, the symptom may be regarded as communicating a conflict over action, for example, a pianist who cannot move his or her fingers. In the case shown in Figure 13.1, the potential symbolism of the loss of the saluting hand is obvious.

While the hypothesis that conversion results from a transformation of distress into physical symptoms is clinically plausible for some patients, it remains merely a hypothesis. The evidence is that most patients have obvious "unconverted," emotional distress as demonstrated by a number of studies which have found greater prevalence of emotional disorder in patients with functional symptoms compared to controls with an equivalently disabling symptom caused by disease (8). Further evidence against the conversion hypothesis is the poor sensitivity and specificity of la belle indifférence as a clinical sign (see below). When emotional distress is apparently hidden, it is often the case that the patient is not *unaware* of their emotional symptoms; rather, they simply *do not want to tell a doctor* about them for fear of being labeled as mentally ill. Wessely (36) has made a cogent plea for revision of the *Diagnostic and Statistical Manual of Mental Disorders*, Fourth Edition (DSM-IV) criteria to a more practical and theoretic symptom-based classification which would entail removing the name "Conversion Disorder." In our view, this would be a great step forward, although it would be wrong to abandon all of the things we have learned from psychodynamic theory in doing so.

The Psychogenic Perspective and Dissociation

Ross Reynolds (37), Charcot (38), and others observed more than a century ago that ideas and suggestion could play a central role in the formation of particular symptoms. Janet extended this notion further with the idées fixes and dissociation (39). Here is a famous example:

A man traveling by train had done an imprudent thing: While the train was running, he had got down on the step in order to pass from one door to the other, when he became aware that the train was about to enter a tunnel. It occurred to him that his left side, which projected, was going to be knocked slantwise and crushed against the arch of the tunnel. This thought caused him to swoon away but happily for him, he did not fall on the track, but was taken back inside the carriage, and his left side was not even grazed. In spite of this, he had a left hemiplegia (39).

Janet referred to the principle process in hysteria as a "retraction of the field of personal consciousness and a

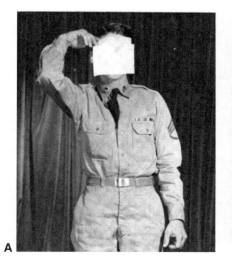 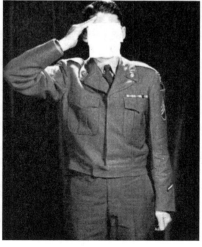

Figure 13.1 A soldier with functional paralysis before **(A)** and after **(B)** treatment. (Reprinted from Abse W. *Hysteria and Related Mental Disorders*. Bristol: Wright, 1966.)   A   B

tendency to the dissociation and emancipation of the system of ideas and functions that constitute personality." In the example above, the idea of paralysis, brought on by terror of an imminent injury, has become dissociated from the patient's consciousness and is acting independently. He was keen to point out, however, that it is not necessarily the idea itself that is the cause of the symptom, but the action of that idea on a biologically and psychologically vulnerable individual. His conception of the idées fixes was also more sophisticated than "I'm paralyzed" or "I'm numb." He thought in many cases the idées fixes could be something less immediately related to the symptom, for example, the fixed idea of a mother's death or the departure of a spouse.

Surprisingly, there has been little systematic work since the efforts of Janet (39) that has examined the phenomenon of dissociation in patients with functional paralysis, even though dissociation assumes the role of a principal etiologic factor in the *International Classification of Diseases* (ICD-10) classification. Two studies by Roelofs et al. found relationships between somatic and cognitive aspects of dissociation, hypnotisability, and child abuse in a cohort most of whom had functional motor symptoms (26,40). More work is needed in this area, specifically controlled data, and studies looking at dissociation as a transient trigger of symptoms rather than a general trait.

The Social Perspective

A social perspective on the generation and shaping of functional paralysis can also be advanced (41). It has been suggested that patients respond to social pressures and expectations by choosing, consciously or subconsciously, to present with certain symptoms. The symptoms of paralysis may be chosen because it is a more culturally accepted presentation of ill health than is depression. This idea is supported by studies finding greater disease conviction among patients with functional paralysis compared to neurologic controls (33). A strong belief in, or less often fear of a disease, is a recurring theme in this patient group. However, in our experience, the conviction that, whatever it is, it is "not a psychological problem" is even more prevalent and may reflect socially determined stigma about psychological problems. The social dimension of hysterical paralysis is explored further in Shorter's book *From Paralysis to Fatigue* (42), although his hypothesis that paralysis is "now a rare symptom and seen mostly in 'backward' working-class and rural patients" (43) requires revision in light of more recent studies.

The Biologic Perspective

For decades, researchers have been sporadically searching for biologic correlates of functional paralysis or sensory loss. Only with the advent of functional neuroimaging is this avenue proving fruitful, although studies thus far remain preliminary.

Transcranial Magnetic Stimulation

Eleven studies and case reports (17,44–53) with a total of 73 patients have used transcranial magnetic stimulation (TMS) to test motor function in patients with functional paralysis. Almost without exception they have reported normal findings. This suggests that TMS may be a useful adjunct in distinguishing neurologic from functional weakness. Two papers have described therapeutic benefit from diagnostic (50) and repetitive TMS (54), although one suspects the mechanism here is primarily persuasion that recovery is possible rather than anything specific to TMS itself.

Evoked Responses and the P300 Response

An early study of functional hemianesthesia suggested that patients may have impaired standard evoked sensory responses in their affected limbs (55), but this was refuted by several even earlier (56) and later studies (57–62) including a recent study using magnetoencephalography (63). Most recently transiently absent scalp somatosensory evoked responses have been seen in two patients with conversion disorder that subsequently recovered (64).

Of greater interest are the nature of the P300 and other late components of the evoked response in patients with functional sensory loss. One study found that it was diminished in one case of unilateral functional sensory loss but not in a subject feigning sensory loss (65), and another found reduction in P300 components in patients with hypnotically induced sensory loss (66).

Cognitive Neuropsychology

Two older studies (both with around ten patients each) found that patients with conversion symptoms had reduced habituation compared to ten controls with anxiety, suggesting an impairment in attention (67,68). These studies found different degrees of physiologic arousal detectable in patients with conversion symptoms compared to controls. Another study suggested that arousal was high even when la belle indifférence was present (69). A series of studies in this area by Roelofs et al. have suggested deficits in higher level central initiation of movement with relative preservation of lower level motor execution (as measured, e.g., by reaction times) in patients with functional paralysis (70,71). Detailed studies of attention in this patient group have been consistent with a high-level voluntary attentional deficit (72). Spence has argued that functional paralysis is a disorder of action, drawing analogies with other disorders, including depression and schizophrenia (73).

Functional Imaging

Charcot spent many years later in his career applying the clinicoanatomic method to hysteria. He believed that there must be a dynamic lesion in the brain to explain the symptoms he was observing. The small body of work on the functional neuroimaging of hysteria that is now able to look for such a dynamic lesion is presented elsewhere in this symposium. The studies published in relation to the symptom of paralysis and sensory loss are summarized in Table 13.3 below.

The data so far published is conflicting. This is perhaps not surprising and was acquired from different experimental paradigms. It is discussed further in Chapter 26.

At their best, newer studies based in cognitive neuroscience are leading the way to a more integrated cognitive neuropsychiatric approach to the problem of functional paralysis with a focus on mechanism rather than cause. But although these studies challenge conventional psychogenic models of causation, a purely biologic interpretation of this data is just as unsatisfactory as a purely psychogenic theory of hysterical paralysis.

TABLE 13.3
STUDIES OF FUNCTIONAL BRAIN IMAGING IN FUNCTIONAL, FEIGNED AND HYPNOTIC PARALYSIS AND SENSORY LOSS

First Author/year		Subjects	Paradigm	Activations and Deactivations Seen
Conversion Disorder				
Tiihonen, 1995 (74)	1	Weak + sensory (L)	SPECT during electrical stimulation of left median nerve, before and after symptoms	Increased perfusion of right frontal lobe and hypoperfusion in right parietal lobe during symptomatic state compared to recovery
Marshall, 1997 (75)	1	Paralysis (L)	PET, attempted movement of leg against resistance	Activation of right anterior cingulate and orbitofrontal cortex
Yazici, 1998 (76)	5	Gait (L + R)	SPECT	Predominantly left-sided temporal (4/5) and parietal (2/5) hypoactivation
Spence, 2000 (77)	3	Paralysis (L + R)	PET, a hand joystick task of affected limb	Hysterical paralysis associated with deactivations in left dorsolateral prefrontal cortex during movements but not at rest; feigners showed deactivation in right anterior frontal cortex regardless of laterality of weakness
Vuilleumier, 2001 (78)	8	Weak + sensory (L + R)	SPECT, buzzers applied to all four limbs. Four patients had before and after scans	Reduced cerebral blood flow in the contralateral thalamus and basal ganglia; less severe hypoactivation predicted recovery
Mailis-Gagnon, 2003 (79)	4	Pain + sensory (L + R)	fMRI, sensory stimulation	When stimulus not perceived—anterior cingulate activation; deactivation in somatosensory, prefrontal, inferior frontal and parietal cortex; failure to activate thalamus and posterior cingulate
Werring, 2004 (80)	5	Visual loss controls	fMRI, 8 Hz visual stimulation	Reduced activation of visual cortices, with increased activation of left inferior frontal cortex, left insula-claustrum, bilateral striatum and thalami, left limbic structures, left posterior cingulate cortex
	7			
Hypnotically (Hyp) induced paralysis				
Halligan, 2000 (81)	1	Hyp paralyzed (L)	PET, attempted movement of paralyzed leg	Right anterior cingulate and right medial orbitofrontal cortex activation similar to that seen in the single patient described by Marshall et al.
Ward, 2003 (82)	12	Hyp paralyzed (L)	PET, attempted movement of paralyzed leg	*Hypnotic paralysis vs rest*: activation of putamen bilaterally, left thalamus, right orbitofrontal cortex, left cerebellum, left supplementary motor area
	12	Feigned paralysis (L)		*Hypnotic compared to feigned paralysis*: right orbitofrontal cortex, right cerebellum, left thalamus and left putamen

fMRI, functional magnetic resonance imaging; PET, positron emission tomography; SPECT, single photon emission computed tomography.

The Importance of Panic, Dissociation, Physical Injury, or Pain at Onset

Little attention has been paid to the circumstances and symptoms surrounding the onset of functional paralysis. In our experience, the circumstances around onset reported by individual patients provide intriguing clues to the possible mechanisms behind functional paralysis. We tend to think of paralysis, unlike abdominal bloating, as a symptom outside everyday experience and normal physiology. Yet paralysis occurs in all of us during REM sleep, when we are terrified, when we are tired and our limbs feel like lead, or as a very transient protective response when we experience acute pain in a limb. Is it possible that some of these more "everyday" causes of transient paralysis are acting as triggers to more long-lasting symptoms?

Panic and Dissociation

When given in-depth interviews, many patients reluctantly report symptoms of panic just before the onset of functional paralysis. Specifically, they may report that they became dizzy, (by which they often mean the dissociative symptoms of depersonalization or derealization), and autonomic symptoms such as sweating, nausea, and breathing difficulties. Sometimes the patient either refuses to volunteer or genuinely didn't experience fear in association with other autonomic symptoms—so called "panic without fear" (83). This idea is not new. Savill comments on it in his 1909 book (84) extending the range of attack types at onset to include nonepileptic seizures, something we have also seen:

> If the patient is under careful observation at the time of onset, it will generally be found that cases of cerebral paresis, rigidity or tremor are actually initiated, about the time of onset, by a more or less transient hysterical cerebral attack....
>
> Affirmative evidence on this point is not always forthcoming unless the patient was at the time under observation, or is himself an intelligent observer. I found affirmative evidence of this point in 47/50 cases of hysterical motor disorder which I investigated particularly. Sometimes there was only a "swimming" in the head, or a slight syncopal or vertiginous attack, slight confusion of the mind, or transient loss of speech, but in quite a number there was generalized trepidation or convulsions (84).

Hyperventilation

Hyperventilation may also occur at the onset of symptoms, either alone or in combination with panic and dissociation. The link between hyperventilation and unilateral sensory symptoms is well-established clinically (85,86) and experimentally (87), but the mechanism for this remains in doubt as both central and peripheral factors may be responsible (88).

Physical Injury

Careful reading of the numerous case reports of functional paralysis indicates a large number of cases arising after a physical injury rather than a primarily emotional or psychological shock (although, clearly, physical injury is itself an emotional trauma). The relevance of physical trauma, and its psychological correlates, in precipitating hysteria in vulnerable individuals was well-understood by clinicians, such as Charcot (89), Page (90), Fox (91), and Janet (39), in the late 19th and early 20th century. Subsequently, trauma and shock acquired a much more psychological flavour, and the possibility that simple physical injury, even of a trivial nature, could be enough in itself to produce hysterical symptoms has been lost (although interestingly, similar debate continues with respect to whiplash injury and reflex sympathetic dystrophy).

Pain

A trivial injury could trigger functional paralysis because of panic, dissociation, or hyperventilation as described above. But pain does not have to cause a shock to cause symptoms. It is well-established that pain in itself causes a degree of weakness, which can be overcome only with effort (92). Motor symptoms (predominantly weakness) are prominent in case series of reflex sympathetic dystrophy and complex regional pain. In one case series, 79% of 145 patients described weakness, mostly of the give-way variety, and 88% sensory disturbance (93). When sensory signs and symptoms are sought they seem to be remarkably common in patients with chronic pain (94). Ochoa and Verdugo (95,96) have produced convincing evidence that much of the sensory disturbance and movement disorder seen in complex regional pain is clinically identical to that seen in functional or psychogenic disorders. In one study of 27 patients with complex regional pain syndrome type 1 and sensory symptoms, 50% of the patients had complete reversal of their hypoaesthesia with placebo compared to none out of 13 patients with a nerve injury (95).

Other Pathways

There are many other pathways to the development of functional paralysis. We have seen patients who develop functional paralysis after surgery (who simultaneously experienced intense depersonalization as they came out of the anesthetic), and several whose first experience of paralysis was an episode of undiagnosed sleep paralysis precipitated by depression and insomnia that later snowballed into more permanent nonsleep-related symptoms. Perhaps one of the commonest routes to functional paralysis is that of a patient with mild chronic fatigue or pain who then becomes aware of an asymmetry of symptoms. Either for biologic reasons or for attentional reasons (but probably because of both), this asymmetry escalates over weeks and months until it appears more dramatically unilateral.

These are hypotheses regarding onset and they require testing. They could, however, open a window on the proximal mechanisms of functional paralysis.

Etiology—Conclusions

Functional paralysis is a symptom, like headache or fatigue, which almost certainly has multiple causes. Some predisposing factors, like childhood neglect, are nonspecific and apply to many illnesses; others such as dissociation are perhaps more specific to pseudoneurologic symptoms. Similarly, stress and emotional disorder may be nonspecific precipitating factors, whereas pain or sleep paralysis and the asymmetry of the brain's functioning in emotional disorder and panic may be more specific triggers. Illness beliefs, such as a belief or fear of stroke, are probably just one of many factors that can play a role in perpetuating the specific symptom of paralysis. Neuroimaging and other biologic approaches may prove helpful in increasing our understanding of the neural mechanisms of functional paralysis. It seems likely that there are a variety of different factors that lead to the development of an apparently identical symptom and that these may differ among patients.

CLINICAL ASSESSMENT

The clinical diagnosis of functional paralysis presents one of the most fascinating and challenging problems in clinical neurology. The neurologist must be able to take a careful and probing history, paying attention to psychologic and social aspects whilst not alienating the patient by appearing too "psychiatric". The examination remains a crucial element in distinguishing functional paralysis from disease, its importance being to find positive signs of a functional disorder as well as to establish the absence of disease. Finally, the explanation of the diagnosis, perhaps using the examination to do so, is a chance to change the trajectory of a patient's illness, for good or for bad. In this section, we outline an approach that we find helpful, paying attention specifically to the symptoms of paralysis and sensory loss.

History

Age of Onset and Sex

Functional paralysis can occur in a wide range of ages from children aged 5 up the mid-seventies (97). The average age of onset seems to be in the mid-thirties (8,98–100), in contrast to patients with pseudoseizures, who characteristically develop attacks in their mid-twenties (only two papers out of 22 in the possession of the author reported a mean age higher than 30 years).

Surprisingly, the literature does not show any gender predominance. An analysis of seven studies of 167 patients with paralysis produced a mean proportion of 48% women (8,44,101–104). In one further study, 57% of 1,316 patients seen at a Chinese hysterical paralysis treatment center were women (97). A review of the 46 studies of pseudoseizures of which we are aware, with a total of 2,103

patients, indicated that the majority (74%) were women (references available from authors).

Mode of Onset

We have discussed above the value of closely questioning patients with functional paralysis and sensory loss about the circumstances at onset. However, this questioning has to proceed with caution if it is to avoid verbal landmines (a negative patient response to direct inquiry into psychological factors) that may prevent the true story being given. For example, many patients will deny having a panic attack, but if asked "Did you get lots of symptoms just before the paralysis?" and "Was it frightening?" will answer positively. If patients reported dizziness, did they mean derealization/depersonalization? Was there a physical injury, a history of pain in the limb, or a story of snowballing fatigue?

Other Functional Symptoms

There is now good evidence that the more symptoms a patient has, the more likely the primary symptom is to be unexplained by disease (35). In Crimlisk's study of patients with motor symptoms, additional unexplained symptoms such as paraesthesia (65%), pseudoseizures (23%), and dysphonia (5%) were common (25). In Binzer's study of unexplained motor symptoms (8), 20% had a prior history of conversion symptoms compared to none of the controls with neurologic disease. A history of repeated surgical procedures without clear evidence of pathology should ring alarm bells that the current symptom may be functional.

Patients with functional paralysis may be exceptionally forthcoming about the presence of other somatic symptoms, even bringing a long and exhaustive list with them to the clinic. Many, however, will just focus on the paralysis and sensory loss, and omit to mention fatigue, sleep disturbance, memory and concentration problems, headache, dizziness, chronic pain, and other functional symptoms such as irritable bowel symptoms, unless specifically questioned about these. These patients may be aware that the more symptoms they present with, the less seriously their presenting symptom will be viewed. The same applies to a past history of functional symptoms; in some cases this is obvious by the size of the file, but in others it will have to be teased out of the notes or obtained from other sources such as the primary care physician. Patients may also inaccurately recall (or be misinformed about) their past medical histories, for example, reporting previous disease diagnoses such as asthma and cervical cancer when in fact these were not proven (105).

Neurologic Disease

A large number of studies have reported that functional neurologic symptoms often occur in patients who also have established neurologic disease. In Crimlisk's study

(25), 42% of patients with unexplained motor symptoms had a comorbid neurologic disease and, interestingly, half of these had a peripheral origin. In other studies of mixed functional symptoms, the range of disease comorbidity ranges from around 20% to 60%, although the method of case ascertainment has a large effect on these estimates (16,18,28,29,31,106–114). The relationship between disease and a coexisting functional paralysis is likely to be complex. Diseases of the nervous system can lead (by biologic and psychological mechanisms) to emotional and personality changes, which in turn render some individuals susceptible to more disability or paralysis than they would otherwise have had. However, some patients with mild organic paralysis may appear to have functional overlay when examined merely because they are keen to convince the doctor that they have a problem.

Modeling

Although it is often suggested that patients copy symptoms or model the symptoms of friends and family (115), there is little actual evidence for this in patients with paralysis or sensory disturbance. Whilst 22% of the patients in Crimlisk's study (25) had worked in medical or paramedical professions, which may have increased the scope for symptom modeling, the specificity of this association has not been examined in a controlled study.

Illness Beliefs

A number of studies have suggested that patients with functional somatic symptoms tend to have similar illness beliefs to those of patients with comparable organic diagnoses. For example, one study (116) found that people with chronic fatigue syndrome had similar illness beliefs to patients with multiple sclerosis. Their belief in an organic cause may, however, be even stronger (33).

The patient with functional weakness may have specific anxieties about a certain diagnosis (health anxiety) or simply be convinced about a certain diagnosis, such as multiple sclerosis, without apparently being worried about it. The beliefs of family and friends may also be important: Do they believe, or have they been told, that they have nerve damage or a stroke? Do they think using the limb could make that damage worse? Will the patient be hostile or offended by a psychological diagnosis—even a comorbid one? Whilst these questions are not helpful diagnostically, they are crucial in orientating the explanation of the problem that will be given to the patient at the end of the consultation. They may also be important in estimating prognosis, because a strong belief in the physicality of the illness is associated with a poor prognosis (117). We believe that rather than focus on whether the diagnosis is medical or psychiatric, it is more helpful to focus discussion on whether the illness is considered to be permanent or reversible.

Laterality of the Symptoms

For many years it has been accepted that functional motor and sensory symptoms are more common on the left. Briquet himself had said so (118), and a number of studies tailored to this question had appeared to confirm it (119–121). This data seemed to tie in nicely with a number of theories, including those suggesting a relationship with the "emotional right hemisphere," a relationship to "neglect" (seen particularly in right hemisphere lesions), or perhaps simply an asymmetry determined by the inconvenience of having a weak dominant hand.

We have carried out a systematic review of the relevant literature published since 1965 (122). While studies that specifically set out to examine this issue (headline studies) often reported a positive answer, studies that reported laterality incidentally (nonheadline studies) did not find an asymmetry (see Fig. 13.2) (122). The net result from all studies combined suggested that while there may be a slight preponderance of left-sided symptoms over right (about 55% left-sided for paralysis and 60% for sensory symptoms), a form of publication bias may account for most of this apparent asymmetry. The results of this study are backed up by a similar systematic analysis carried out by Ernest Jones in 1908 (123), who found no lateralizing

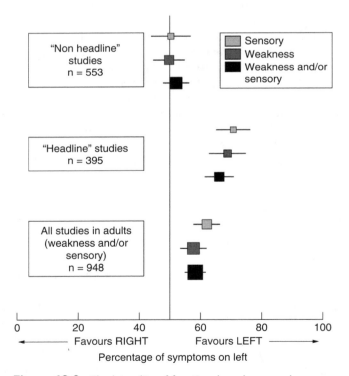

Figure 13.2 The laterality of functional weakness and sensory disturbance—a systematic review of all studies from 1965–2000. Demonstrating that studies in which laterality is specifically studied find a preponderance on the left, whereas those which report the data incidentally do not. (Reprinted from Stone J, Sharpe M, Carson A, et al. Are functional motor and sensory symptoms really more common on the left? *JNNP.* 2002;73:578–581, with permission.)

effect in 277 cases drawn from 164 articles. The diagnosis of functional weakness should therefore certainly not be made based on the side of the symptoms.

Other aspects of history-taking such as the eliciting of symptoms of psychiatric disorder, childhood factors, life events, and difficulties, the complications of chronic illness such as financial benefits, legal involvement, and iatrogenesis are necessary but will not be described here.

Examination

Functional Weakness

The diagnosis of patients with functional weakness and sensory disturbance depends on finding positive features on examination as well as the absence of signs of organic disease. This simple idea has been somewhat lost in neurologic practice over the last century. Fifty years ago, textbooks such as those of Purves-Stewart contained a large section on the positive physical manifestations of hysteria (124). Although some can still be found, a lot of this information has been marginalized or lost in most modern textbooks.

When considering any sign of functional weakness, it is important to remember the following caveats:

- Any sign that depends on inconsistency does not distinguish hysterical from malingered weakness.
- The presence of a positive sign of functional weakness does not exclude the possibility that the patient also has an organic disease.
- All physical signs have limited sensitivity, specificity, and interrater reliability (125).

Preliminary Observation

The assessment of patients with functional weakness should begin as the patients get up from their chairs in the waiting room and not end until they are leaving the consulting room (or the hospital). The primary objective is to look for evidence of *inconsistency*. It may be particularly helpful to watch patients:

- taking their clothes on or off.
- removing and replacing something from a bag (for example, a list of medications).
- walking into the room as compared to walking out of the room or out of the outpatient building.

La Belle Indifférence

La belle indifférence, or an apparent lack of concern about the nature or implications of conversion symptoms, is a clinical feature that continues to receive prominence in standard descriptions. However, the evidence, such as it is, suggests that it is a highly unreliable clinical sign. Its survival may owe more to the persistence of the concept of conversion than to clinical reality. The high rates of depression and anxiety found in studies of these patients are incompatible

with a high proportion manifesting indifference. As Lewis and Berman observed (113), "in marked contrast to their alleged indifference many hysterical patients manifest a deep interest...in describing their ailments."

Combining the results of studies published since 1966, most of which are of poor quality and uncontrolled, we have found that la belle indifférence is reported in roughly the same proportion of patients with hysteria (around 20%) (29,110–113,126–130) as it is in patients with organic disease (29,110,126,128,130). However, none of these studies have operationalized the concept of la belle indifférence. This is important because la belle indifférence could be easily misdiagnosed in (i) patients who are making an effort to appear cheerful in a conscious attempt to not be labeled as depressed; (ii) patients with sensory signs of which they were unaware (something Janet and Charcot emphasized but which is not the same as indifference to disability); (iii) patients who are concerned about a limb symptom when asked about it but appear absent-minded, apathetic, or distracted the rest of the time; and (iv) patients whose symptoms are factitious (they may not be concerned since they know from where the symptoms are arising) (131).

The Hoover Sign

The Hoover sign is probably the most useful test for functional weakness and the only one that has been subjected to scientific study with a neurologic control group (99, 132). It is a simple, repeatable test which does not require skilled surreptitious observation. The test relies on the principle that virtually all people, whether they have a disease or not, extend their hip when flexing their contralateral hip against resistance. This finding is thought to be a result of the crossed extensor reflex, described by Sherrington (133), which enables normal walking, and is present even in decorticate animals. The test as described by Hoover in 1908 (134) can be performed in two ways:

A. *Hip extension.* In patients with functional weakness, a discrepancy can be observed between their voluntary hip extension (which is often weak) and their involuntary hip extension when the opposite hip is being flexed against resistance (which is normal). This test is illustrated in Figure 13.3. It is important when testing involuntary hip extension to ask patients to concentrate hard on their good leg.

B. *Hip flexion.* The opposite test, where hip flexion in the weak leg is tested while the examiner's hand is held under the good heel is also described, although it has not been adequately evaluated. In this test, the absence of downward pressure in the good leg indicates a lack of effort transmitted to either leg.

Head (135) described an additional variant in which patients lie on their front and are asked to extend their good hip while hip flexion is tested in the weak leg. Raimiste (136) has described a similar phenomenon of

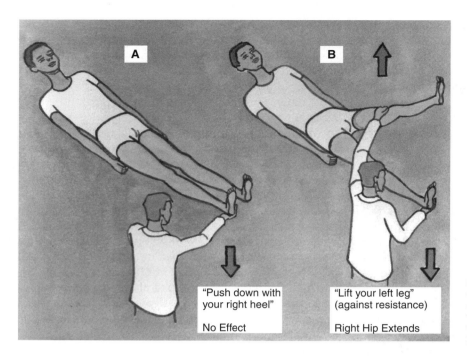

Figure 13.3 The Hoover sign. **A:** Hip extension is weak when tested directly. **B:** Hip extension is normal when the patient is asked to flex the opposite hip. (Reprinted from Stone J, Zeman A, Sharpe M. Functional weakness and sensory disturbance. *JNNP.* 2002;73:241–245, with permission.)

simultaneous leg adduction and abduction which has recently been tested and elaborated by Sonoo (137) with promising results.

False positives may occur if:

- pain in the affected hip may produce greater weakness on direct, compared with indirect, testing as a result of attentional phenomena (related to pain rather than weakness).
- patients with organic disease may be trying to "help" you or "convince" you that they are ill.
- there are insufficient data to rule out the possibility that a similar phenomenon may sometimes occur as a direct result of organic brain disease, for example, multiple sclerosis.
- it could be predicted that Hoover sign may be positive in patients with neglect.
- it is not clear whether some normal subjects have a slightly stronger involuntary hip extension than voluntary hip extension, and "mildly positive" Hoover signs should be interpreted with caution.

False negatives may occur if patients are not concentrating sufficiently on flexing their good hip when you are testing involuntary extension of the weak hip. If so, you should find that flexion in the good leg is stronger when you remove your hand from under the weak leg.

The Hoover sign has been evaluated in two controlled studies. In the first, computer myometry demonstrated a significant difference in the "involuntary:voluntary hip extension ratio" in seven patients with nonorganic weakness compared to ten controls with organic weakness (Fig. 13.4) (99). An equivalent study using simple weighing scales

comparing nine subjects having functional weakness with control groups having organic weakness, back pain, and no weakness produced similar results (132). These studies were not blinded and did not measure the reliability of the test as used in the real world. They do, however, provide preliminary support for its use.

The Hoover Sign in the Arms?

Hoover described a similar phenomenon of "complementary opposition" in the arms. In this test, elevation against resistance of an arm stretched out in front of the patient can produce downward pressure of the other arm. Analyzing this phenomenon, Ziv et al. (99) obtained results comparable to those in the legs. A related test of shoulder adduction has also been described based on the principle that often when shoulder adduction is tested on one side, the contralateral side will also adduct (138).

Collapsing Weakness

A common finding in functional weakness is that of collapsing weakness. This is the phenomenon in which a limb collapses from a normal position with a light touch (or occasionally, even before your hand has touched the limb). Normal power can often be achieved transiently with encouragement. The instruction, "At the count of three, stop me from pushing down" is often helpful in this respect. Another method to obtain normal power is to gradually increase the force applied to the limb starting extremely gently and building imperceptibly up to normal force. The intuitive explanation of collapsing weakness is that the patient simply isn't trying. Whilst this is sometimes undoubtedly the case, in our experience the performance of

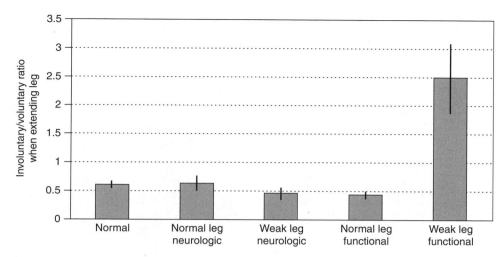

Figure 13.4 The validity of the Hoover sign (the ratio of involuntary hip extension compared to voluntary hip extension) in the lower limbs of seven patients with functional paralysis compared to ten with disease. A unique pattern is observed in the affected weak limbs of patients with psychogenic weakness, in contrast to their unaffected limb, normal controls, and patients with neurologic weakness. [Redrawn from Ziv I, Djaldetti R, Zoldan Y, et al. Diagnosis of "non-organic" limb paresis by a novel objective motor assessment: the quantitative Hoover's test. *J Neurol.* 1998;245(12):797–802.]

most patients with functional weakness seems to get worse, the more effort and attention they expend on the limb.

The problem with collapsing weakness is that, like the Hoover sign, it may also occur for a number of reasons unrelated to the diagnosis. These include an inability to understand the instruction, pain in the relevant joint, being generally unwell, and a misguided eagerness of some patients to help the doctor or convince the doctor even though they actually have organic disease.

Collapsing or give-way weakness has been investigated neurophysiologically (139–141). These studies have suggested the following abnormalities in patients with functional weakness: (i) the force generated by a limb at the point the examiner overcomes the muscle force can be unusually *high* when compared to the force generated by normal resistance (140); (ii) there may be significantly variable amounts of force in their limbs compared to controls (139–141); and (iii) they produce less force the slower the movement is (141).

Collapsing weakness has only been put to test in one real life controlled clinical study and was found in 20% of patients with conversion disorder compared to 5% of patients with disease (126). Gould et al. (130) found that of 30 patients with acute neurologic pathology (mostly stroke), 10 had collapsing weakness, emphasizing the need for caution with this sign.

The Monoplegic and Hemiplegic Gait

Unilateral functional weakness of a leg, if severe, tends to produce a characteristic gait in which the leg is dragged behind the body as a single unit, like a sack of potatoes (Fig. 13.5). The hip is either held in external or internal rotation so that the foot points inwards or outwards. We have also seen a number of patients who have a tendency to flex their affected arm while walking even if they don't at other times.

Functional Weakness of the Face, Pseudoptosis and "Wrong Way Tongue Deviation"

Pseudoptosis or functional ptosis is occasionally encountered, often in association with photophobia. At the end of the 19th century, there was considerable debate about whether functional weakness could develop in the face. Charcot, amongst others, pointed out that functional limb weakness is usually accompanied by "the absence of any participation of the face" and does not seem to have reported a case (38). Janet, however, wrote that he had seen "many cases of hysterical facial paralysis" that were "typical" (39). Given the rarity of pseudoptosis, it's always worth considering whether an underlying or coexistent problem such as blepharospasm and myasthenia gravis is present. Organic unilateral ptosis is usually associated with frontalis overactivity, whereas in pseudoptosis a *persistently* depressed eyebrow with a variable inability to elevate frontalis and overactivity of orbicularis oculis is characteristic (Fig. 13.6).

Functional weakness of the lower half of the face is not described in recent literature, but we have seen striking cases in which the apparent weakness is caused by a similar overcontraction, this time of orbicularis oris.

In neurologic hemiplegia, the tongue may sometimes deviate towards the paretic side. Keane (142) has described four patients with functional paralysis whose tongues deviated towards the normal rather than the paretic side, again suggesting overactivity of the affected side rather than underactivity.

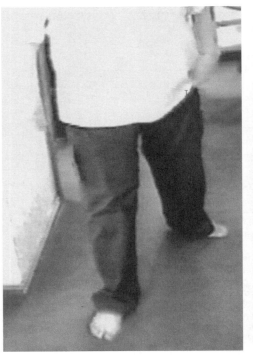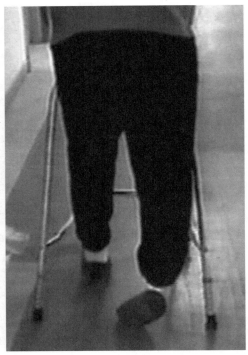

A   B

Figure 13.5 Functional monoplegic gait. In both cases the leg is dragged at the hip. External or internal rotation of the hip or ankle inversion/eversion is common. (Reprinted from Stone J, Zeman A, Sharpe M. Functional weakness and sensory disturbance. *JNNP.* 2002;73:241–245, with permission.)

Monoparesis

There is a suggestion that monoparesis may be overrepresented among cases of unexplained motor weakness. In Binzer's controlled study (8), 30% of cases had a monoparesis against none of 30 controls with organic paralysis. In Lempert's large consecutive series (16), there were 31 cases of monoparesis against 20 of hemiparesis, 18 of tetraparesis, ten of paraparesis and two cases of bibrachial weakness.

Other Signs of Functional Weakness

- *Co-contraction.* It may be possible to feel the contraction of an antagonist muscle, for example, triceps, when the agonist muscle, biceps, is being tested. Knutsson et al. (141) showed in 12 patients with functional weakness that knee flexion was weaker than it would have been if they had just let the weight of the lower leg carry out the movement, indicating antagonist activation.

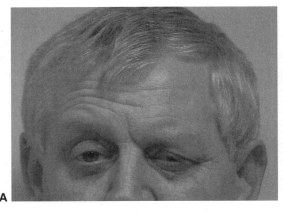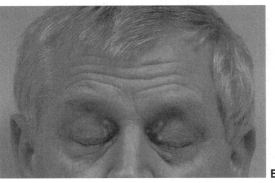

A   B

Figure 13.6 Pseudoptosis. This man presented with photophobia and difficulty elevating the right side of his forehead. The photograph shows his normal resting state **(A)** and normal movement of his forehead with his eyes shut **(B)**. The problem was overactivity of his left orbicularis oculis with functional weakness of his left frontalis, which had been incorrectly interpreted as ptosis. It improved with gradual exposure to light. (Reprinted from Stone J. Pseudoptosis. *Practical Neurology.* 2002;2:364–365, with permission.)

- *The "arm-drop."* This describes dropping a supposedly paralyzed arm over patients' faces to see if they will protect themselves from its fall. This has also been described as a test on the unconscious patient. However, the arm must be so weak for this test to be interpretable that we suggest it rarely adds information. A less aggressive variation is to watch the speed and smoothness with which arms fall down from an outstretched position onto the lap. In functional weakness, this may be slower and jerkier. This has not been validated.
- *Pseudowaxy flexibility.* Occasionally, patients complaining of weakness may find that if their limbs are put into a certain position, for example, with the arms outstretched, they will inexplicably maintain their position even to the point of not being able to get them down again. This phenomenon is similar to that seen in people undergoing stage hypnosis.
- *Sternocleidomastoid (SCM) test.* Recently Diukova et al. (143) have reported that 80% of 30 patients with functional hemiparesis had SCM weakness, usually ipsilateral, whereas only 11% of 27 patients with a vascular hemiparesis had weakness of SCM (which is bilaterally innervated and so is rarely weak in upper motor neuron lesions).

Important Absent Signs in Functional Weakness

We have emphasized the importance of looking for positive signs of functional weakness and sensory disturbance. The absence of certain specific signs is also important. Tone and reflexes should be normal, although pain may increase tone and there may be mild asymmetry, particularly if there is attentional interference from the patient (91,144). Clonus is not necessarily an organic sign. Pseudoclonus was well-described at the turn of the 20th century as a clonus with irregular and variable amplitude (91,145). The plantar response may be mute on the affected side particularly if there is marked sensory disturbance but should not be upgoing.

Sensory Disturbance

The clinical detection and localization of sensory dysfunction is probably one of the least reliable areas of the neurologic examination (146). What evidence exists suggests that these signs are just as untrustworthy in the detection of functional symptoms.

Functional sensory disturbance may be noticed by the patient, or as is often the case, be detected by the examiner and come as a surprise to the patient. It typically affects all sensory modalities either in a hemisensory distribution ("I feel as if I'm cut in half") or affects a whole limb. In the latter, sharply demarcated boundaries at the shoulder and at the groin are common (39,147). If the trunk is involved, the front is more commonly involved than the back. If patients have functional weakness, they usually have functional sensory disturbance as well, perhaps suggesting a

shared pathophysiology. Whilst a number of functional sensory signs have been described, none appear to be specific and should not, therefore, be used to make a diagnosis.

Midline Splitting and the Hemisensory Syndrome

The hemisensory syndrome has been described for over a century and continues to be a well-known but rarely studied clinical problem in neurology (Fig. 13.7). The intensity of the sensory disturbance often varies, and while it may be complete, it is usually rather patchy but with a distinct complaint from the patient that something is "not right" down one side.

Patients with hemisensory disturbance frequently complain of intermittent blurring of vision in the ipsilateral eye (asthenopia) and sometimes ipsilateral hearing problems, as well. Hemisensory symptoms are increasingly recognized in patients with chronic pain (79,94) and in patients diagnosed as having reflex sympathetic dystrophy (95).

Recently, Toth (148) has published a study of 34 outpatients with the hemisensory syndrome finding that the majority of patients improved at follow-up.

It has been commonly assumed that exact splitting of sensation in the midline cannot occur in organic disease. The reason usually given is that cutaneous branches of the intercostal nerves overlap from the contralateral side, so sensory loss should be paramedian, that is 1 or 2 centimeters from the midline. But midline splitting can occur in thalamic stroke when a profound loss of several modalities in a manner similar to functional sensory loss can occur. Similar hemisensory disturbance can be provoked by hyperventilation (88) or hypnotic suggestion (87). The

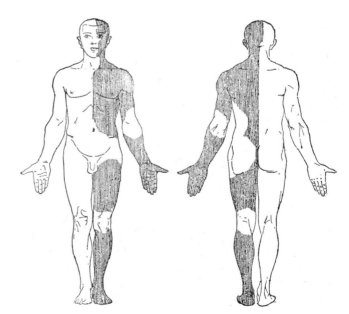

Figure 13.7 Hemisensory disturbance. (Reprinted from Charcot JM. *Clinical lectures on diseases of the nervous system.* London: New Sydenham Society, 1889.)

finding of contralateral thalamic and basal ganglia hypoactivation in patients with this symptom using SPECT is also intriguing in this respect (78). Rolak (149) reported midline splitting in six out of 80 patients with organic disease. Chabrol et al. found midline splitting in 26% of 15 conversion disorder patients compared to 15% of 40 neurologic controls.

Splitting of Vibration Sense

Common sense decrees that there should be little difference in the sensation of a tuning fork placed over the left and right side of the sternum or frontal bone as the bone is a single unit and must vibrate as one. Toth found this sign in 68% of his sample (148). However, in Gould's study mentioned earlier, 21 out of 30 patients with organic disease exhibited this sign (130). Similarly, Rolak found that 69 out of 80 patients with organic disease had this sign versus 19 out of 20 patients with functional sensory loss (149). Again, perhaps our model of the sensory system and its thalamocortical representation has been too simplistic when devising these tests.

Tests Involving Doctor Trickery

These include, "Say 'yes' when you feel me touch you and 'no' when you don't," (originally described by Janet) and sensory examination of the hands while they are either crossed behind the back or interlocked and rotated on the chest (the Bowlus maneuver) (138). Forced choice procedures have also been described in which testing is made sufficiently complicated that a performance worse than chance can be achieved (150,151), suggesting systematic underperformance. However, this finding does not discriminate conscious from unconscious intentions and is unlikely to add to the diagnosis or management. These tests are rarely necessary, although they may have a role in medicolegal assessment.

Speech, Visual and Other Functional Motor and Sensory Symptoms

A number of other functional motor and sensory symptoms may coexist in patients with paralysis or occur in isolation. A brief summary of other symptoms (excluding cognition, pain, and fatigue) is given here to direct the interested reader to relevant literature.

Speech and Swallowing Symptoms

Dysarthria can sometimes accompany paralysis, and although very little has been written on this in recent times (152) there are good descriptions in the older literature (124,153). Typically, the speech is slow and may resemble a stutter or be extremely slow with long hesitations. Despite long gaps in the speech, it may be noticeable that these occur in the middle but not the ends of sentences, and the patient will often still be difficult to interrupt. The emotional content of the speech may have a noticeable influence on its fluency with anger, often producing more fluency and discussion of emotional state, leading to greater hesitation. Sometimes the speech will become telegrammatic and become reduced to the main verbs and nouns in a sentence. In its extreme form the patient may become mute. Just as the act of physical examination can make functional paralysis appear much worse, so patients with functional dysarthria tend to be at their very worst when asked to repeat particular phrases.

Word-finding difficulty is a common symptom in anyone with significant fatigue or concentration problems, and may compound a functional dysarthria. True dysphasia as a more severe functional symptom, however, is rare.

Dysphonia is a much more common functional speech complaint, and there is now quite a large literature outlining approaches to diagnosis and management (154). Often the clinical presentation is of whispering or hoarse speech that is initially thought to be laryngitis by the patient but then persists for months or years. The possibility of spasmodic adductor or abductor dysphonia must always be considered. A recent randomized trial of voice therapy suggests that this can be an effective treatment (155).

Globus pharyngis or functional dysphagia also has a sizable literature. The patient normally complains of a sensation of a "ball in the throat" and investigations do not reveal a cause. There remains controversy regarding how extensively patients with globus should be investigated before this diagnosis is made (156,157), but there is no doubt this most ancient of functional symptoms remains common (158).

Visual Symptoms

Blurred vision, or asthenopia, is commonly described by patients with functional weakness and sensory symptoms. Meaning literally "tired eyes," the patient with this symptom usually describes intermittent blurring of vision that returns to normal if they screw up their eyes tight, then relax them again. Some of these patients have convergence or accommodative spasm, the tendency for the convergence reflex to be transiently overactive, either unilaterally or bilaterally (159). In this situation, lateral gaze restriction can sometimes appear to be present, but the presence of miosis may help to confirm that the problem is convergence spasm (160). Voluntary nystagmus is described and appears to be a "talent" possessed by around 10% of the population (161).

There is a large literature of functional visual acuity problems and the tests available to diagnose them. These are reviewed elsewhere (162–164). Spiral or tubular fields are commonly seen clinically, are often asymptomatic, and can be elicited at the bedside. Keane (165) has described functional hemianopia as the "missing half defect." Patients with functional hemianopia are typically found to have homonymous hemianopia with both eyes open and then, inconsistent with this, have a monocular hemianopia in the affected eye with full fields in the normal eye—one of the clearest examples of ideogenic symptoms in this area of neurology.

Auditory Symptoms

The literature on functional deafness is somewhat smaller than that for visual symptoms. Basic tests for complete deafness relying on a startle response have been described, such as making a loud unexpected clap out of sight of the patient or seeing if the patient wakes to an alarm clock in the middle of the night (166). In addition to audiometry, which relies on good cooperation from the patient, additional tests such as auditory brainstem evoked responses or evoked otoacoustic emissions may be necessary to fully investigate a patient with this symptom (167).

Pseudocyesis

According to Evans writing in 1984 (168), only three men and 100 women had been reported in the previous 45 years with the symptom of abdominal swelling imitating pregnancy. Pseudocyesis is the extreme end of what the French have labeled *couvade* (to hatch). *Couvade* simply refers to general symptoms of pregnancy such as nausea and weight gain. Estimates of its frequency range widely in studies that are largely uncontrolled for the general rate of these symptoms in the population. Psychotic delusion of pregnancy is also well-reported in men and women. The mechanism of pseudocyesis must be something to do with exaggerated lordosis and persistent relaxation of abdominal muscles, but its well-studied presence in animals and rarity in humans mean that judgment must be reserved about its true nature.

Investigations

Laboratory Investigation

It should be remembered that positive evidence of functional weakness does not exclude the presence of coexisting disease. In many patients with disabling symptoms, a focused set of investigations may be unavoidable. Preferably these should be performed as quickly as possible, as protracted testing or minor abnormalities on these tests can maintain a focus on looking for disease rather than rehabilitation. It may also be necessary to make two diagnoses: one of an organic disease such as multiple sclerosis and another of additional functional weakness or disability.

Examination Under Sedation or Hypnosis

The use of interview after administration of intravenous sodium amytal was initially promoted as a method of uncovering the hidden psychic conflict causing the patient's symptom. More recently, *examination* under sedation, including the use of benzodiazepines (169), has been used therapeutically to demonstrate to the neurologist, and by means of video to the patient, that the apparently paralyzed limb can move. White et al. (170) report positively on this technique in 11 patients with functional locomotor disorders, who had been disabled for several years. Ideally, this kind of procedure should be filmed and played back to the patient as a method of persuasion in treatment and ongoing transparency about the diagnosis. These methods merit more systematic study.

Explaining the Diagnosis and Management

Explaining the Diagnosis

We have already outlined our own reasons, both pragmatic and scientific, for preferring the use of the diagnosis of functional weakness or functional sensory disturbance. It is a diagnosis that sidesteps physical versus psychological debates with the patient, avoids offense, and although broad, is consistent with our current understanding of the mechanism of these symptoms.

It is at the first point of contact that diagnostic label of functional weakness becomes particularly helpful, as it allows for a transparent discussion with the patient. At a first encounter, we would generally explain the diagnosis to the patient using the following key points:

- We describe the symptoms as due to a common problem in the function of the nervous system which is not damaged and has the potential to recover. Analogies are often helpful here and include:
  - "It's like a piano/car that's out of tune and isn't working properly. All the parts are there, they just aren't working right together."
  - "The hardware is fine but there is a problem with the software."
  - "Its like the opposite of phantom limb; they feel a limb that is not there, you cannot feel a limb that is."
- We pay particular attention to overcoming the patient's fear that you don't believe them or think they are mad, imagining or putting on their symptoms. Sometimes simply saying, "I don't think you're mad, imagining or putting on your symptoms" can be very effective.
- We avoid verbal landmines, initially at least, for example, using the phrase "not sinister" instead of "not serious"; or "not structural" instead of "not physical." In a patient hostile to psychological explanations, we use the word "functional" instead of "psychological."
- We may show patients their positive physical signs, in particular, their Hoover sign, in order to demonstrate how the diagnosis is being made and why we do not think they have another disorder. This is one reason why we find tests involving a high degree of deception on the part of the doctor or placebos unacceptable in hospital practice.
- We don't expect a patient to be glad they haven't got a disease unless they are given a coherent alternative explanation. Reassurance does not seem as important as explanation.

- We copy the letter to the patient and give them other written information.
- We try to explain the diagnosis to important family and friends so that they can reinforce it.

An example of an explanation to a patient with functional weakness and sensory disturbance:

> You have functional weakness. This is a common problem which hundreds of people in this area also suffer from. Your nervous system is not damaged but it is not working properly. This is why when you try to send the messages to your limbs, they do not move properly. Similarly, this is why the sensations from your body are also not being felt properly (or in the case of pain, amplified). The most important thing about this condition is that because your nervous system is not damaged, the problem is potentially reversible.

In apparently overmedicalizing the diagnosis of functional weakness, we run the risk of leaving patients with the impression that they have a neurologic disorder over which they have no control. We acknowledge this risk, but our experience is that although these initial explanations are deliberately nonpsychiatric, they allow the rapid development of a therapeutic relationship that permits the subsequent emergence and discussion of psychological factors that might otherwise never have taken place.

Further Management

In some patients with mild symptoms, explanation and reassurance with encouragement to resume normal activity may be sufficient. In those with more resistant symptoms, the following treatment modalities may be helpful:

- *Cognitive–behavioral therapy (CBT).* Evidence exists at systematic review levels that CBT is effective for a wide range of functional somatic symptoms (171). Chalder (172) has described specific CBT-based treatment for this group of patients. In our own practice, we build on the implications of the functional model in longer-term treatment. This is in many ways simply a variant of the "rational persuasion" that Dubois and others used at the beginning of the 20th century to help patients with these disorders get better (173).
- *Physical rehabilitation.* Patients with physical problems often need physical treatments to get better. Some of our best treatment successes have been accomplished by our experienced neurophysiotherapists who are able to combine hands-on, "no-nonsense" physical treatments with suggestion and encouragement. Wade has reviewed the rehabilitation literature of functional paralysis and gait disorder (174). Many studies report encouraging results but none of these are randomized. Shapiro and Teasell describe a behavioral technique in which the patient is placed in a "double bind"; they are told that if their disease is organic, it should respond to physiotherapy (175). This is an interesting technique

but appears contrary to the desire for an honest therapeutic relationship.

- *Antidepressants.* There is evidence from a systematic review that antidepressants are of benefit in patients with functional symptoms (176). The main problem in using them is one of stigma and a perception that they are addictive or harmful (177). One solution is to explain their purpose as medications which improve general nervous system functioning and which are not specific to depression.
- *Hypnosis and intravenous sedation.* There is only one group which has performed randomized controlled trials of any type of treatment in these patients. Moene et al. (178,179) have studied both inpatients and outpatients with functional motor symptoms using multidisciplinary rehabilitative techniques and hypnosis as an additional treatment modality in randomized patients. In 22 outpatients, 10 weeks of additional hypnosis produced a significant improvement in cases, compared to 22 waiting-list controls. In the inpatient trial, both cases and controls improved equally and no extra effect from hypnosis was found. Thus, it appears that hypnosis is better than doing nothing, but it is unclear whether it is superior to other interventions of a similar intensity and duration. In our practice, where we do not have hypnosis skills, we have found the use of IV sedatives, particularly propofol, helpful in persuading some patients with whom we already have a good relationship that they can eventually make a recovery. We would be cautious, however, in applying a potentially invasive procedure to all patients.
- *Other forms of psychotherapy.* For some patients, where possible, a more in-depth psychotherapy that looks back at antecedents of symptoms as well as forward will be of value, but has not been specifically evaluated in randomized trials.

PROGNOSIS

Misdiagnosis

We have already discussed how functional paralysis and sensory disturbance can be often accompanied by both comorbid psychiatric disorders and by neurologic disease. But how often is the diagnosis of functional symptoms simply wrong and the original symptoms actually those of organic disease? This has been an important question over the last 35 years after an influential paper by Slater in 1965 (180). Slater claimed that 61% of his cohort of patients with "hysteria" developed neurologic disease. His analysis, however, is flawed, and his conclusion that hysteria is a "delusion and a snare" highly misleading (181). Although contemporaries, including Francis Walshe (182), protested, the paper is frequently quoted in textbooks, perhaps because it is consistent with doctors' fears about misdiagnosing symptoms as functional. (And dare we say it gave psychiatrists an excuse not to take on a difficult patient group?)

Slater's views have now been refuted by several recent studies reporting rates of misdiagnosis of under 10% in regional and tertiary neurologic centers (Table 13.4). A study of patients referred to a specialist psychiatric service (183) is a notable outlier with a rate of misdiagnosis of 13% (although there was a prior "suspicion of neurologic disorder" in 80% of these "misdiagnosed" cases). Pooling the results of the five studies in which the neurologic

TABLE 13.4

COMPARISON OF OUTCOMES AND PROGNOSTIC FACTORS IN PATIENTS WITH FUNCTIONAL MOTOR AND SENSORY SYMPTOMS[a]

	Year	Size	Population Sampled	Mean Years of Follow-up	Neurologic Disorder Missed (Clinical Features)	Disability at Follow-up	Prognostic Factors
Couprie et al. (184)	1995	56	Neurologic Inpatients 73% weakness 12% gait 5% sensory only Retrospective	4.5	2 cases (1 bizarre transient paralysis due to cerebral ischaemia; 1 ataxia with posturing due to multiple sclerosis)	41% with Rankin scores worse than 2 ("I have symptoms which have caused some changes in my life, but I am still able to look after myself")	*Positive*: Recent onset and recovery by the time of discharge
Crimlisk et al. (25)	1998	64	Neurologic Inpatients 50% weakness 50% movement disorder Retrospective	6	3 cases [all gait disorder due to (i) myotonic dystrophy, (ii) spinocerebellar degeneration, and (iii) paroxysmal hemidystonia]	50% had either retired on grounds of ill health or were on sick leave; 36% had a psychiatric disorder	*Positive*: symptoms present for less than one year; the presence of an axis 1 psychiatric disorder *Negative*: receipt of benefits, and litigation
Binzer and Kullgren (185)	2000	30	Neurologic Inpatients 100% weakness Prospective	1[b]	None	43% not working at 1 year	*Negative*: the presence of a personality disorder, hopelessness, and a concurrent somatic diagnosis
Moene (183)	2000	76[c]	Psychiatric In- and outpatients 58% weakness or movement disorder 37% motor and sensory 5% sensory Prospective	2.4	10 cases (1 weakness due to ALS; 5 movement disorders proven to be organic; 3 gait disorders due to MS, MSA, and dementia; 1 leg pain due to radicular disease)	Not stated	Higher age at onset, longer duration of symptoms, and "suspicion of neurologic disorder" predicted misdiagnosis
Stone (186)	2002	47	Neurologic Inpatients 55% weakness 45% sensory only Retrospective	12.5	1 case (intermittent paresis due to multiple sclerosis)	30% had taken medical retirement; 38% limited in moderate activities; 43% with severe or very severe pain;	*Positive*: sensory symptoms and signs alone rather than weakness and/or sensory symptoms
Toth (148)	2003	34	Neurologic Outpatients 100% hemisensory	1.4	1 case (lacunar infarct)	20% had persisting symptoms	Not mentioned

[a] Excluding studies with high proportions of other functional neurologic symptoms, for example, nonepileptic attacks, pain, nonorganic visual symptoms.
[b] Length of time after assessment (mean 3.75 years after symptom onset).
[c] Two patients with visual symptoms and seven with pseudoepileptic attacks also reported.
Note: Three studies report limited data on motor symptoms alone: Carter (1946) (187), 22% unchanged or worse at 5 years; Ljungberg (1957) (101), 32% unchanged or worse at 5 years; Mace and Trimble (1996) (24), 34% not improved at 10 years.

misdiagnoses of patients with functional motor and sensory symptoms are described in detail shows that there were 16 cases in 273 patients (6%). Other studies looking at the prognosis of conversion disorder have included significant numbers of patients with other functional neurologic symptoms such as nonepileptic attacks and blindness. These are reviewed elsewhere (181) and we do not elaborate on them here.

Misdiagnosis is common in medicine. For example, reported rates of misdiagnosis in epilepsy vary from 26% (188) to 42% (189). In a population-based study of 387 subjects diagnosed with multiple sclerosis, 17% subsequently turned out to be wrongly diagnosed, half because they had another neurologic disorder and half because the symptoms were functional or psychological in origin (190). Similar misdiagnosis rates have been reported in motor neuron disease (8%) (191) and schizophrenia (6%) (192). The process by which neurologists decide that weakness or sensory disturbance is functional or medically unexplained has come under remarkably little scrutiny (193). The data suggest that this process is as least as accurate as the diagnosis of other neurologic disorders.

Symptomatic Recovery and Other Measures of Outcome

This aspect of prognosis has received less attention than that of misdiagnosis. Studies examining outcomes in patients with functional weakness and sensory disturbance are shown in Tables 13.4 and 13.5. Around one third to half of all patients appear to remain symptomatic in the long term depending on the nature of the initial sample. In longer studies, many patients accumulate other symptoms suggestive of a diagnosis of somatization disorder (24, 186,194). Toth's study of sensory symptoms and a subgroup analysis from our study in Edinburgh suggest that sensory symptoms have a more benign prognosis (148, 186). The only consistent predictor of poor recovery is symptom duration (25,184), although personality disorder is likely to indicate poor prognosis. Interestingly, one study found the presence of an axis 1 disorder and a change in marital status were both positive prognostic factors (25). Patients in that particular study were also found to frequently change their primary care physician and gain repeat referrals both to neurology and other specialties, even after a firm diagnosis had been made (195).

MALINGERING/FACTITIOUS DISORDER IN RELATION TO PARALYSIS AND SENSORY LOSS

Neurologists, are generally good at telling whether illnesses are associated with organic disease or not, in that their diagnoses usually remain stable over time (25,184,185). However, discriminating between consciously produced and

TABLE 13.5

ADDITIONAL STUDIES REPORTING OUTCOME BUT NOT PROGNOSTIC FACTORS IN PATIENTS WITH FUNCTIONAL PARALYSIS

	Year	Sample Size	Population Sampled	Mean Years of Follow-up	Disability at Follow-up
Knutsson (141)	1985	25	Neurology outpatients and inpatients, Stockholm	6 mo–6 y	44% (11/25) improvement seen within 1–7 wk 56% (14/25) sustained paresis over 1–9 y
Apple (103)	1989	17	Spinal unit Paralysis (mostly traumatic onset)	3–112 d	At discharge (avg. 3–112 d) 13 were normal, 3 had weakness in one leg and 1 sent to psychiatric ward
Baker (102)	1987	20	Spinal unit	18 d	All had recovered at 18 d, 13 within first 48 h
			Paralysis (with injuries)		2 developed seizures, 1 seen rowing, other illness behavior
Heruti (196)	2002	34	Spinal unit Paralysis	Discharge	9 had complete recovery, 10 partial recovery, and 15 unchanged
Zhang (97)	1987	1,316	Hysterical paralysis treatment center	Immediate and after >20 y	1,287/1,316 cured after acupuncture (97.8%), 16 improved, 13 no change 900 received only 1 treatment
			Paralysis		Postfollow-up: 125 followed up; 78% (108) recovered and could work; 3% still had symptoms; 18% relapsed but paralysis milder than before

unconsciously produced functional symptoms is altogether more difficult, if not impossible. Patients' awareness of control over symptoms is probably not an all-or-nothing phenomenon but rather on a continuum. It may also vary over time so that a patient may begin an illness with little awareness about what is happening, but gradually gain a degree of conscious control with time (or vice versa).

Doctors are almost certainly worse at detecting deception by a patient than we would like to think (82,197). Covert surveillance demonstrating a *major discrepancy* in function or a direct confession are probably the only reliable methods available in patients with functional paralysis, but are rarely obtained other than as part of the lawyers' investigation in medical legal disputes (198).

Among those patients who are consciously generating symptoms and signs, it is important to distinguish between those whose aim is to obtain medical care and those in pursuit of material gain. Behavior of the first kind comes under the diagnosis of factitious disorder and is a medical diagnosis analogous to that of deliberate self-harm, another "conscious" act. Those who simulate for financial or other material gain are malingerers and are not considered to have a medical condition. The difficulty is in not allowing them to cloud our view of other patients who are genuinely suffering with similar complaints.

After a bad experience of discovering that you have been deceived by a patient, it can be tempting to believe that a large proportion of patients with apparently functional symptoms are in fact factitious. At times like this it is useful to pose the following questions to oneself: Why do so many patients present such similar stories of bafflement and fear about their symptoms? Why do follow-up studies show persistence of symptoms in the majority in the long term? Why are patients with these symptoms so keen to have investigations to hunt down an organic cause for their symptoms? If they knew they were malingerers, they would know that this could weaken their case. Is it really a doctor's job to detect malingering, anyway? Finally, when you see a patient clearly exaggerating a symptom or groaning heavily during an examination, is this exaggeration to deceive or exaggeration to convince?

CONCLUSION

Functional paralysis and sensory disturbance is common in neurologic practice. The causes are often complex, although patients may share common psychophysiologic mechanisms for their symptoms. The diagnosis of functional weakness and sensory disturbance is not easy. Positive signs are just as important as looking for the absence of signs of disease. Motor signs, particularly the Hoover sign, are more reliable than sensory signs, but none should be used in isolation and all must be interpreted in the overall context of the presentation. Always bear in mind the possibility that your patient may have both a functional *and*

an organic disorder. Using the functional model allows a transparent explanation and interaction with the patients that can facilitate later physical and psychological treatments. If made by a neurologist, a diagnosis of functional as opposed to organic disorder is usually correct.

ACKNOWLEDGMENTS

We would like to thank our colleagues in Edinburgh, especially Dr. Adam Zeman, Dr. Alan Carson, and Professor Charles Warlow, for their valuable collaboration and support of this work.

REFERENCES

1. Mace CJ, Trimble MR. "Hysteria", "functional" or "psychogenic"? A survey of British neurologists' preferences. *J R Soc Med.* 1991; 84:471–475.
2. Wessely S. To tell or not to tell? The problem of medically unexplained symptoms. In: Zeman A, Emmanuel L, eds. *Ethical dilemmas in neurology.* London: WB Saunders, 2000:41–53.
3. Stone J, Colyer M, Feltbower S, et al. "Psychosomatic": a systematic review of its meaning in newspaper articles. *Psychosomatics.* 2004;45:287–290.
4. Stone J, Wojcik W, Durrance D, et al. What should we say to patients with symptoms unexplained by disease? The "number needed to offend". *BMJ.* 2002;325:1449–1450.
5. Rief W, Hessel A, Braehler E. Somatization symptoms and hypochondriacal features in the general population. *Psychosom Med.* 2001;63:595–602.
6. Spalt L. Hysteria and antisocial personality. A single disorder? *J Nerv Ment Dis.* 1980;168(8):456–464.
7. Franz M, Schepank H, Schellberg D. Unspecific neurologic symptoms as possible psychogenic complaints. *Eur Arch Psychiatry Clin Neurosci.* 1993;243:1–6.
8. Binzer M, Andersen PM, Kullgren G. Clinical characteristics of patients with motor disability due to conversion disorder: a prospective control group study. *J Neurol Neurosurg Psychiatry.* 1997;63:83–88.
9. Kurtzke J. The current neurologic burden of illness and injury in the United States. *Neurology.* 1982;32:1207–1214.
10. Farley J, Woodruff RA Jr, Guze SB. The prevalence of hysteria and conversion symptoms. *Br J Psychiatry.* 1968;114:1121–1125.
11. Woodruff RA Jr. Hysteria: an evaluation of objective diagnostic criteria by the study of women with chronic medical illnesses. *Br J Psychiatry.* 1968;114:1115–1119.
12. Woodruff RA Jr, Clayton PJ, Guze SB. Hysteria: an evaluation of specific diagnostic criteria by the study of randomly selected psychiatric clinic patients. *Br J Psychiatry.* 1969;115:1243–1248.
13. Carson AJ, Ringbauer B, Stone J, et al. Do medically unexplained symptoms matter? A prospective cohort study of 300 new referrals to neurology outpatient clinics. *J Neurol Neurosurg Psychiatry.* 2000;68:207–210.
14. Nimnuan C, Hotopf M, Wessely S. Medically unexplained symptoms: an epidemiological study in seven specialties. *J Psychosom Res.* 2001;51:361–367.
15. Perkin GD. An analysis of 7836 successive new outpatient referrals. *J Neurol Neurosurg Psychiatry.* 1989;52:447–448.
16. Lempert T, Dieterich M, Huppert D, et al. Psychogenic disorders in neurology: frequency and clinical spectrum. *Acta Neurol Scand.* 1990;82:335–340.
17. Janssen BA, Theiler R, Grob D, et al. The role of motor evoked potentials in psychogenic paralysis. *Spine.* 1995;20:608–611.
18. Marsden CD. Hysteria—a neurologist's view. *Psychol Med.* 1986; 16:277–288.
19. Schiffer RB. Psychiatric aspects of clinical neurology. *Am J Psychiatry.* 1983;140:205–207.

20. Ewald H, Rogne T, Ewald K, et al. Somatization in patients newly admitted to a neurological department. *Acta Psychiatr Scand.* 1994;89:174–179.
21. Metcalfe R, Firth D, Pollock S, et al. Psychiatric morbidity and illness behavior in female neurological in-patients. *J Neurol Neurosurg Psychiatry.* 1988;51:1387–1390.
22. Stone J, Zeman A. Hysterical conversion—the view from clinical neurology. In: Halligan PW, Bass C, Marshall JC, eds. *Contemporary approaches to the study of hysteria.* Oxford: Oxford University Press, 2001:102–125.
23. Birket-Smith M, Mortensen EL. Pain in somatoform disorders: is somatoform pain disorder a valid diagnosis? *Acta Psychiatr Scand.* 2002;106:103–108.
24. Mace CJ, Trimble MR. Ten-year prognosis of conversion disorder. *Br J Psychiatry.* 1996;169:282–288.
25. Crimlisk HL, Bhatia K, Cope H, et al. Slater revisited: 6-year follow up study of patients with medically unexplained motor symptoms. *BMJ.* 1998;316:582–586.
26. Roelofs K, Keijsers GP, Hoogduin KA, et al. Childhood abuse in patients with conversion disorder. *Am J Psychiatry.* 2002;159:1908–1913.
27. Wilson-Barnett J, Trimble MR. An investigation of hysteria using the illness behaviour questionnaire. *Br J Psychiatry.* 1985;146:601–608.
28. Kapfhammer HP, Dobmeier P, Mayer C, et al. Konversions-syndrome in der neurologie: eine psyhopathologische und psychodynamische differenzierung in Konversionsstörung, Somatisierungsstörung und artifizielle Störung. *Psychother Psychosom Med Psychol.* 1998;48:463–474.
29. Raskin M, Talbott JA, Meyerson AT. Diagnosis of conversion reactions. Predictive value of psychiatric criteria. *JAMA.* 1966;197:530–534.
30. Okasha A, Seif ED, Asaad T. Presentation of hysteria in a sample of Egyptian patients—an update. *Neurol Psychiatry Brain Res.* 1993;1:155–159.
31. Lecompte D. Organic disease and associated psychopathology in a patient group with conversion symptoms. *Acta Psychiatr Belg.* 1987;87:662–669.
32. Krull F, Schifferdecker M. Inpatient treatment of conversion disorder: a clinical investigation of outcome. *Psychother Psychosom.* 1990;53:161–165.
33. Binzer M, Eisemann M, Kullgren G. Illness behavior in the acute phase of motor disability in neurological disease and in conversion disorder: a comparative study. *J Psychosom Res.* 1998;44:657–666.
34. Binzer M, Eisemann M. Childhood experiences and personality traits in patients with motor conversion symptoms. *Acta Psychiatr Scand.* 1998;98:288–295.
35. Wessely S, Nimnuan C, Sharpe M. Functional somatic syndromes: one or many? *Lancet.* 1999;354:936–939.
36. Wessely S. Discrepancies between diagnostic criteria and clinical practice. In: Halligan P, Bass C, Marshall JC, eds. *Contemporary approaches to the science of hysteria.* Oxford: Oxford University Press, 2001:63–72.
37. Reynolds JR. Paralysis and other disorders of motion and sensation dependent on idea. *BMJ.* 1869;2:483–485.
38. Charcot J-M. *Clinical lectures on diseases of the nervous system.* London: New Sydenham Society, 1889:220–259.
39. Janet P. *The major symptoms of hysteria.* London: Macmillan, 1907.
40. Roelofs K, Hoogduin KA, Keijsers GP, et al. Hypnotic susceptibility in patients with conversion disorder. *J Abnorm Psychol.* 2002;111:390–395.
41. Showalter E. *Hystories.* London: Picador, 1997.
42. Shorter E. *From paralysis to fatigue.* New York: The Free Press, 1992.
43. Shorter E. Paralysis: the rise and fall of a "hysterical" symptom. *J Soc Hist* 1986;19:549–582.
44. Cantello R, Boccagni C, Comi C, et al. Diagnosis of psychogenic paralysis: the role of motor evoked potentials. *J Neurol.* 2001;248:889–897.
45. Meyer BU, Britton TC, Benecke R, et al. Motor responses evoked by magnetic brain stimulation in psychogenic limb weakness: diagnostic value and limitations. *J Neurol.* 1992;239:251–255.
46. Mullges W, Ferbert A, Buchner H. Transkranielle magnetstimulation bei psychogenen paresen. *Nervenarzt.* 1991;62:349–353.
47. Schriefer TN, Mills KR, Murray NME, et al. Magnetic brain stimulation in functional weakness. *Muscle Nerve.* 1987;10:643.
48. Hageman G, Eertman-Meyer CJ, Tel-Hampsink J. The clinical diagnostic value of studies using magnetic stimulation (see comments) [Dutch]. *Ned Tijdschr Geneeskd.* 1993;137:2323–2328.
49. Foong J, Ridding M, Cope H, et al. Corticospinal function in conversion disorder. *J Neuropsychiatry Clin Neurosci.* 1997;9:302–303.
50. Jellinek DA, Bradford R, Bailey I, et al. The role of motor evoked potentials in the management of hysterical paraplegia: case report. *Paraplegia.* 1992;30:300–302.
51. Pillai JJ, Markind S, Streletz LJ, et al. Motor evoked potentials in psychogenic paralysis. *Neurology.* 1992;42:935–936.
52. Morota N, Deletis V, Kiprovski K, et al. The use of motor evoked potentials in the diagnosis of psychogenic quadriparesis. A case study. *Pediatr Neurosurg.* 1994;20:203–206.
53. Gomez L, Fernandez A, Mustelier R, et al. Evoked motor potentials in the diagnosis of conversion hysteria [letter]. *Rev Neurol.* 1998;26:839–840.
54. Schonfeldt-Lecuona C, Connemann BJ, Spitzer M, et al. Transcranial magnetic stimulation in the reversal of motor conversion disorder. *Psychother Psychosom.* 2003;72:286–288.
55. Hernández-Peón R, Chávez-Ibarra G, Aguilar E. Somatic evoked potentials in one case of hysterical anaesthesia. *Electroencephalogr Clin Neurophysiol.* 1963;15:889–892.
56. Alajouanine T, Scherrer J, Barbizet J, et al. Potentiels évoqués corticaux chez de sujets atteints de troubles somesthesiques. *Rev Neurol.* 1958;98:757–792.
57. Levy R, Behrman J. Cortical evoked responses in hysterical hemianaesthesia. *Electroencephalogr Clin Neurophysiol.* 1970;29:400–402.
58. Levy R, Mushin J. The somatosensory evoked response in patients with hysterical anaesthesia. *J Psychosom Res.* 1973;17:81–84.
59. Halliday AM. Computing techniques in neurological diagnosis. *Br Med Bull.* 1968;24:253–259.
60. Moldofsky H, England RS. Facilitation of somatosensory average-evoked potentials in hysterical anesthesia and pain. *Arch Gen Psychiatry.* 1975;32:193–197.
61. Howard JE, Dorfman LJ. Evoked potentials in hysteria and malingering. *J Clin Neurophysiol.* 1986;3:39–49.
62. Kaplan BJ, Friedman WA, Gravenstein D. Somatosensory evoked potentials in hysterical paraplegia. *Surg Neurol.* 1985;23:502–506.
63. Hoechstetter K, Meinck HM, Henningsen P, et al. Psychogenic sensory loss: magnetic source imaging reveals normal tactile evoked activity of the human primary and secondary somatosensory cortex. *Neurosci Lett.* 2002;323:137–140.
64. Yazici KM, Demirci M, Demir B, et al. Abnormal somatosensory evoked potentials in two patients with conversion disorder. *Psychiatry Clin Neurosci.* 2004;58:222–225.
65. Lorenz J, Kunze K, Bromm B. Differentiation of conversive sensory loss and malingering by P300 in a modified oddball task. *Neuroreport.* 1998;9:187–191.
66. Spiegel D, Chase RA. The treatment of contractures of the hand using self-hypnosis. *J Hand Surg (Am).* 1980;5:428–432.
67. Horvath T, Friedman J, Meares R. Attention in hysteria: a study of Janet's hypothesis by means of habituation and arousal measures. *Am J Psychiatry.* 1980;137:217–220.
68. Lader M, Sartorius N. Anxiety in patients with hysterical conversion symptoms. *J Neurol Neurosurg Psychiatry.* 1968;31:490–495.
69. Rice DG, Greenfield NS. Psychophysiological correlates of la belle indifference. *Arch Gen Psychiatry.* 1969;20:239–245.
70. Roelofs K, Naring GW, Keijsers GP, et al. Motor imagery in conversion paralysis. *Cognit Neuropsych.* 2001;6:21–40.
71. Roelofs K, van Galen GP, Keijsers GP, et al. Motor initiation and execution in patients with conversion paralysis. *Acta Psychol (Amst).* 2002;110:21–34.
72. Roelofs K, van Galen GP, Eling P, et al. Endogenous and exogenous attention in patients with conversion disorders. *Cognit Neuropsychol.* 2003;20:733–745.
73. Spence SA. Hysterical paralyses as disorders of action. *Cognit Neuropsych.* 1999;4:203–226.

74. Tiihonen J, Kuikka J, Viinamaki H, et al. Altered cerebral blood flow during hysterical paresthesia. *Biol Psychiatry.* 1995;37:134–135.

75. Marshall JC, Halligan PW, Fink GR, et al. The functional anatomy of a hysterical paralysis. *Cognition.* 1997;64:B1–B8.

76. Yazici KM, Kostakoglu L. Cerebral blood flow changes in patients with conversion disorder. *Psychiatry Res.* 1998;83:163–168.

77. Spence SA, Crimlisk HL, Cope H, et al. Discrete neurophysiological correlates in prefrontal cortex during hysterical and feigned disorder of movement. *Lancet.* 2000;355:1243–1244.

78. Vuilleumier P, Chicherio C, Assal F, et al. Functional neuroanatomical correlates of hysterical sensorimotor loss. *Brain.* 2001;124:1077–1090.

79. Mailis-Gagnon A, Giannoylis I, Downar J, et al. Altered central somatosensory processing in chronic pain patients with "hysterical" anesthesia. *Neurology.* 2003;60:1501–1507.

80. Werring DJ, Weston L, Bullmore ET, et al. Functional magnetic resonance imaging of the cerebral response to visual stimulation in medically unexplained visual loss. *Psychol Med.* 2004;34:583–589.

81. Halligan PW, Athwal BS, Oakley DA, et al. Imaging hypnotic paralysis: implications for conversion hysteria. *Lancet.* 2000;355: 986–987.

82. Ward NS, Oakley DA, Frackowiak RS, et al. Differential brain activations during intentionally simulated and subjectively experienced paralysis. *Cognit Neuropsych.* 2003;8:295–312.

83. Kushner MG, Beitman BD. Panic attacks without fear: an overview. *Behav Res Ther.* 1990;28:469–479.

84. Savill TD. *Lectures on hysteria and allied vasomotor conditions.* London: Glaisher, 1909.

85. Perkin GD, Joseph R. Neurological manifestations of the hyperventilation syndrome. *J R Soc Med.* 1986;79:448–450.

86. Blau JN, Wiles CM, Solomon FS. Unilateral somatic symptoms due to hyperventilation. *BMJ.* 1983;286:1108.

87. Fleminger JJ, McClure GM, Dalton R. Lateral response to suggestion in relation to handedness and the side of psychogenic symptoms. *Br J Psychiatry.* 1980;136:562–566.

88. O'Sullivan G, Harvey I, Bass C, et al. Psychophysiological investigations of patients with unilateral symptoms in the hyperventilation syndrome. *Br J Psychiatry.* 1992;160:664–667.

89. Micale MS. Charcot and Les nevroses traumatiques: scientific and historical reflections. *J Hist Neurosci.* 1995;4:101–119.

90. Page HW. *Injuries of the spine and spinal cord without apparent mechanical lesions.* London: J & A Churchill, 1883.

91. Fox CD. *The psychopathology of hysteria.* Boston, MA: The Gorham Press, 1913.

92. Le Pera D, Graven-Nielsen T, Valeriani M, et al. Inhibition of motor system excitability at cortical and spinal level by tonic muscle pain. *Clin Neurophysiol.* 2001;112:1633–1641.

93. Birklein F, Riedl B, Sieweke N, et al. Neurological findings in complex regional pain syndromes—analysis of 145 cases. *Acta Neurol Scand.* 2000;101:262–269.

94. Rommel O, Gehling M, Dertwinkel R, et al. Hemisensory impairment in patients with complex regional pain syndrome. *Pain.* 1999;80:95–101.

95. Verdugo RJ, Ochoa JL. Reversal of hypoaesthesia by nerve block, or placebo: a psychologically mediated sign in chronic pseudoneuropathic pain patients. *J Neurol Neurosurg Psychiatry.* 1998;65: 196–203.

96. Verdugo RJ, Ochoa JL. Abnormal movements in complex regional pain syndrome: assessment of their nature. *Muscle Nerve.* 2000;23: 198–205.

97. Zhang ZY, Yuan YM, Yan BW, et al. An observation of 1316 cases of hysterical paralysis treated by acupuncture. *J Tradit Chin Med.* 1987;7:113–115.

98. Ehrbar R, Waespe W. Funktionelle Gangstörungen. *Schweiz Med Wochenschr.* 1992;122:833–841.

99. Ziv I, Djaldetti R, Zoldan Y, et al. Diagnosis of "non-organic" limb paresis by a novel objective motor assessment: the quantitative Hoover's test. *J Neurol.* 1998;245(12):797–802.

100. Teasell RW, Shapiro AP. Diagnosis of conversion disorders in a rehabilitation setting. *NeuroRehabilitation.* 1997;8:163–174.

101. Ljungberg L. Hysteria: a clinical, prognostic and genetic study. *Acta Psychiatr Neurol Scand.* 1957;32(Suppl. 112):1–162.

102. Baker JH, Silver JR. Hysterical paraplegia. *J Neurol Neurosurg Psychiatry.* 1987;50:375–382.

103. Apple DF Jr. Hysterical spinal paralysis. *Paraplegia.* 1989;27: 428–431.

104. Heruti RJ, Reznik J, Adunski A, et al. Conversion motor paralysis disorder: analysis of 34 consecutive referrals. *Spinal Cord.* 2002; 40:335–340.

105. Schrag A, Brown RJ, Trimble MR. Reliability of self-reported diagnoses in patients with neurologically unexplained symptoms. *J Neurol Neurosurg Psychiatry.* 2004;75:608–611.

106. Merskey H, Buhrich NA. Hysteria and organic brain disease. *Br J Med Psychol.* 1975;48:359–366.

107. Whitlock FA. The aetiology of hysteria. *Acta Psychiatr Scand.* 1967;43:144–162.

108. McKegney FP. The incidence and characteristics of patients with conversion reactions, I: a general hospital consultation service sample. *Am J Psychiatry.* 1967;124:542–545.

109. Kligerman MJ, McKegney FP. Patterns of psychiatric consultation in two general hospitals. *Psychiatry Med.* 1971;2:126–132.

110. Barnert C. Conversion reactions and psychophysiologic disorders: a comparative study. *Psychiatry Med.* 1971;2:205–220.

111. Roy A. Cerebral disease and hysteria. *Compr Psychiatry.* 1977;18: 607–609.

112. Ebel H, Lohmann T. Clinical criteria for diagnosing conversion disorders. *Neurol Psychiatry Brain Res.* 1995;3:193–200.

113. Lewis WC, Berman M. Studies of conversion hysteria. *Arch Gen Psychiatry.* 1965;13:275–282.

114. Folks DG, Ford CV, Regan WM. Conversion symptoms in a general hospital. *Psychosomatics.* 1984;25:285.

115. Lazare A. Current concepts in psychiatry. Conversion symptoms. *N Engl J Med.* 1981;305:745–748.

116. Trigwell P, Hatcher S, Johnson M, et al. "Abnormal" illness behaviour in chronic fatigue syndrome and multiple sclerosis. *BMJ.* 1995;311:15–18.

117. Sharpe M, Hawton K, Seagroatt V, et al. Follow up of patients presenting with fatigue to an infectious diseases clinic. *BMJ.* 1992;305:147–152.

118. Briquet P. *Traité clinique et thérapeutique de l'Hysterie.* Paris: J.B. Ballière, 1859.

119. Stern DB. Handedness and the lateral distribution of conversion reactions. *J Nerv Ment Dis.* 1977;164:122–128.

120. Galin D, Diamond R, Braff D. Lateralization of conversion symptoms: more frequent on the left. *Am J Psychiatry.* 1977;134: 578–580.

121. Pascuzzi RM. Nonphysiological (functional) unilateral motor and sensory syndromes involve the left more often than the right body. *J Nerv Ment Dis.* 1994;182:118–120.

122. Stone J, Sharpe M, Carson A, et al. Are functional motor and sensory symptoms really more frequent on the left? A systematic review. *J Neurol Neurosurg Psychiatry.* 2002;73:578–581.

123. Jones E. Le côté affecté par l'hémiplégie hystérique. *Rev Neurol.* 1908;16:193–196.

124. Purves-Stewart J, Worster-Drought C. The psychoneuroses and psychoses. *Diagnosis of nervous diseases.* Baltimore, MD: Williams & Wilkins, 1952:661–758.

125. Hansen M, Sindrup SH, Christensen PB, et al. Interobserver variation in the evaluation of neurological signs: observer dependent factors. *Acta Neurol Scand.* 1994;90:145–149.

126. Chabrol H, Peresson G, Clanet M. Lack of specificity of the traditional criteria of conversion disorders. *Eur Psychiatry.* 1995;10: 317–319.

127. Kapfhammer HP, Buchheim P, Bove D, et al. Konverssionssymptome bei patienten im psychiatrischen konsiliardienst. *Nervenarzt.* 1992;63:527–538.

128. Weinstein EA, Lyerly OG. Conversion hysteria following brain injury. *Arch Neurol.* 1966;15:545–548.

129. Sharma P, Chaturvedi SK. Conversion disorder revisited. *Acta Psychiatr Scand.* 1995;92:301–304.

130. Gould R, Miller BL, Goldberg MA, et al. The validity of hysterical signs and symptoms. *J Nerv Ment Dis.* 1986;174:593–597.

131. Stone J, Smyth R, Carson A, et al. La belle indifference in conversion disorder and hysteria—a systematic review. *Br J Psychiatry* 2005 *(in press).*

132. Diukova G, Liachovitskaia NI, Begliarova AM, et al. Simple measurement of Hoover's test in patients with psychogenic and with organic pareses. *Nevrol Zhurnal.* 2001;5:19–21.

133. Sherrington CS. Flexion-reflex of the limb, crossed extension reflex, and reflex stepping and standing. *J Physiol (Lond).* 1910; 40:28–121.

134. Hoover CF. A new sign for the detection of malingering and functional paresis of the lower extremities. *JAMA.* 1908;51:746–747.

135. Head H. The diagnosis of hysteria. *BMJ.* 1922;27:827–829.

136. Raimiste J. Deux signes d'hèmiplegie organique du membre inférieur. *Rev Neurol.* 1909;17:125–129.

137. Sonoo M. Abductor sign: a reliable new sign to detect unilateral non-organic paresis of the lower limb. *J Neurol Neurosurg Psychiatry.* 2004;73:121–125.

138. DeJong R. Examination in cases of suspected hysteria and malingering. *The neurologic examination.* New York: Harper & Row, 1967:989–1015.

139. McComas AJ, Kereshi S, Quinlan J. A method for detecting functional weakness. *J Neurol Neurosurg Psychiatry.* 1983;46:280–282.

140. van der Ploeg RJ, Oosterhuis HJ. The "make/break test" as a diagnostic tool in functional weakness. *J Neurol Neurosurg Psychiatry.* 1991;54:248–251.

141. Knutsson E, Martensson A. Isokinetic measurements of muscle strength in hysterical paresis. *Electroencephalogr Clin Neurophysiol.* 1985;61:370–374.

142. Keane JR. Wrong-way deviation of the tongue with hysterical hemiparesis. *Neurology.* 1986;36:1406–1407.

143. Diukova GM, Stolajrova AV, Vein AM. Sternocleidomastoid (SCM) muscle test in patients with hysterical and organic paresis. *J Neurol Sci.* 2001;187(Suppl. 1):S108.

144. Stam J, Speelman HD, van Crevel H. Tendon reflex asymmetry by voluntary mental effort in healthy subjects. *Arch Neurol.* 1989;46:70–73.

145. Gowers WR. Hysteria. *A Manual of diseases of the Nervous System.* London: Churchill Livingstone, 1892:903–960.

146. Lindley RI, Warlow CP, Wardlaw JM, et al. Interobserver reliability of a clinical classification of acute cerebral infarction. *Stroke.* 1993;24:1801–1804.

147. Freud S. Quelques considerations pour une étude comparative des paralysies motrices organiques et hystériques. *Arch Neurologie.* 1893;26:29–43.

148. Toth C. Hemisensory syndrome is associated with a low diagnostic yield and a nearly uniform benign prognosis. *J Neurol Neurosurg Psychiatry.* 2003;74:1113–1116.

149. Rolak LA. Psychogenic sensory loss. *J Nerv Ment Dis.* 1988; 176:686–687.

150. Tegner R. A technique to detect psychogenic sensory loss. *J Neurol Neurosurg Psychiatry.* 1988;51:1455–1456.

151. Miller E. Detecting hysterical sensory symptoms: an elaboration of the forced choice technique. *Br J Clin Psychol.* 1986;25(Pt 3):231–232.

152. Matas M. Psychogenic voice disorders: literature review and case report. *Can J Psychiatry.* 1991;36:363–365.

153. Janet P. The troubles of speech. *The major symptoms of hysteria.* New York: The Macmillan Company, 1907:208–226.

154. Roy N. Functional dysphonia. *Curr Opin Otolaryngol Head Neck Surg.* 2003;11:144–148.

155. MacKenzie K, Millar A, Wilson JA, et al. Is voice therapy an effective treatment for dysphonia? A randomised controlled trial. *BMJ.* 2001;323:658–661.

156. Back GW, Leong P, Kumar R, et al. Value of barium swallow in investigation of globus pharyngeus. *J Laryngol Otol.* 2000;114: 951–954.

157. Farkkila MA, Ertama L, Katila H, et al. Globus pharyngis, commonly associated with esophageal motility disorders. *Am J Gastroenterol.* 1994;89:503–508.

158. Deary IJ, Wilson JA, Kelly SW. Globus pharyngis, personality, and psychological distress in the general population. *Psychosomatics.* 1995;36:570–577.

159. Rutstein RP, Daum KM, Amos JF. Accommodative spasm: a study of 17 cases. *J Am Optom Assoc.* 1988;59:527–538.

160. Troost BT, Troost EG. Functional paralysis of horizontal gaze. *Neurology.* 1979;29:82–85.

161. Zahn JR. Incidence and characteristics of voluntary nystagmus. *J Neurol Neurosurg Psychiatry.* 1978;41:617–623.

162. Beatty S. Non-organic visual loss. *Postgrad Med J.* 1999;75: 201–207.

163. Keane JR. Neuro-ophthalmic signs and symptoms of hysteria. *Neurology.* 1982;32:757–762.

164. Bose S, Kupersmith MJ. Neuro-ophthalmologic presentations of functional visual disorders. *Neurol Clin.* 1995;13:321–339.

165. Keane JR. Hysterical hemianopia. The 'missing half' field defect. *Arch Ophthalmol.* 1979;97:865–866.

166. Weintraub MI. Hysteria. A clinical guide to diagnosis. *Clin Symp.* 1977;29:1–31.

167. Qiu WW, Yin SS, Stucker FJ, et al. Current evaluation of pseudohypacusis: strategies and classification. *Ann Otol Rhinol Laryngol.* 1998;107:638–647.

168. Evans DL, Seely TJ. Pseudocyesis in the male. *J Nerv Ment Dis.* 1984;172:37–40.

169. Ellis SJ. Diazepam as a truth drug. *Lancet.* 1990;336:752–753.

170. White A, Corbin DO, Coope B. The use of thiopentone in the treatment of non-organic locomotor disorders. *J Psychosom Res.* 1988;32:249–253.

171. Kroenke K, Swindle R. Cognitive-behavioral therapy for somatization and symptom syndromes: a critical review of controlled clinical trials. *Psychother Psychosom.* 2000;69:205–215.

172. Chalder T. Cognitive behavioral therapy as a treatment for conversion disorders. In: Halligan P, Bass C, Marshall JC, eds. *Contemporary approaches to the study of hysteria: clinical and theoretical perspectives.* Oxford: Oxford University Press, 2001:298–311.

173. Dubois P. *The psychic treatment of nervous disorders.* New York: Funk & Wagnalls, 1909.

174. Wade D. Rehabilitation for conversion symptoms. In: Halligan P, Bass C, Marshall JC, eds. *Contemporary approaches to the study of hysteria.* Oxford: Oxford University Press, 2001:330–346.

175. Shapiro AP, Teasell RW. Strategic-behavioral intervention in the in-patient rehabilitation of non-organic (factitious/conversion) motor disorders. *Neurorehabilitation.* 1997;8:183–192.

176. O'Malley PG, Jackson JL, Santoro J, et al. Antidepressant therapy for unexplained symptoms and symptom syndromes. *J Fam Pract.* 1999;48:980–990.

177. Stone J, Durrance D, Wojcik W, et al. What do medical outpatients attending a neurology clinic think about antidepressants? *J Psychosom Res.* 2003;56:293–295.

178. Moene FC, Spinhoven P, Hoogduin KA, et al. A randomised controlled clinical trial on the additional effect of hypnosis in a comprehensive treatment programme for in-patients with conversion disorder of the motor type. *Psychother Psychosom.* 2002; 71:66–76.

179. Moene FC, Spinhoven P, Hoogduin CA, et al. A randomized controlled clinical trial of a hypnosis-based treatment for patients with conversion disorder, motor type. *Int J Clin Exp Hypn.* 2003;51:29–50.

180. Slater ET. Diagnosis of 'hysteria'. *BMJ.* 1965;i:1395–1399.

181. Ron M. The prognosis of hysteria/somatisation disorder. In: Halligan P, Bass C, Marshall JC, eds. *Contemporary approaches to the study of hysteria.* Oxford: Oxford University Press, 2001:271–281.

182. Walshe F. Diagnosis of hysteria. *BMJ.* 1965;2:1451–1454.

183. Moene FC, Landberg EH, Hoogduin KA, et al. Organic syndromes diagnosed as conversion disorder. Identification and frequency in a study of 85 patients. *J Psychosom Res.* 2000;49:7–12.

184. Couprie W, Wijdicks E-FM, Rooijmans H-GM, et al. Outcome in conversion disorder: a follow-up study. *J Neurol Neurosurg Psychiatry.* 1995;58:750–752.

185. Binzer M, Kullgren G. Motor conversion disorder. A prospective 2-to 5-year follow-up study. *Psychosomatics.* 1998;39:519–527.

186. Stone J, Sharpe M, Rothwell PM, et al. The 12-year prognosis of unilateral functional weakness and sensory disturbance. *J Neurol Neurosurg Psychiatry.* 2003;74:591–596.

187. Carter AB. The prognosis of certain hysterical symptoms. *BMJ.* 1949;1:1076–1079.

188. Smith D, Defalla BA, Chadwick DW. The misdiagnosis of epilepsy and the management of refractory epilepsy in a specialist clinic. *QJM.* 1999;92:15–23.

189. Zaidi A, Crampton S, Clough P, et al. Head-up tilting is a useful provocative test for psychogenic non-epileptic seizures. *Seizure.* 1999;8:353–355.

190. Hankey GJ, Stewart-Wynne EG. Pseudo-multiple sclerosis: a clinico-epidemiological study. *Clin Exp Neurol.* 1987;24:11–19.

191. Davenport RJ, Swingler RJ, Chancellor AM, et al. Avoiding false positive diagnoses of motor neuron disease: lessons from the scottish motor neuron disease register. *J Neurol Neurosurg Psychiatry.* 1996;60:147–151.

192. Johnstone EC, Macmillan JF, Crow TJ. The occurrence of organic disease of possible or probable aetiological significance in a population of 268 cases of first episode schizophrenia. *Psychol Med.* 1987;17:371–379.

193. Stone J, Zeman A, Sharpe M. Functional weakness and sensory disturbance. *J Neurol Neurosurg Psychiatry.* 2002;73:241–245.

194. Kent DA, Tomasson K, Coryell W. Course and outcome of conversion and somatization disorders. A four-year follow-up. *Psychosomatics.* 1995;36:138–144.

195. Crimlisk HL, Bhatia KP, Cope H, et al. Patterns of referral in patients with medically unexplained motor symptoms. *J Psychosom Res.* 2000;49:217–219.

196. Heruti RJ, Reznik J, Adunski A, et al. Conversion motor paralysis disorder: analysis of 34 consecutive referrals. *Spinal Cord.* 2002; 40:335–340.

197. Lempert T, Brandt T, Dieterich M, et al. How to identify psychogenic disorders of stance and gait. A video study in 37 patients. *J Neurol.* 1991;238:140–146.

198. Sharpe M. Malingering and psychiatric disorder. In: Halligan P, Bass C, Oakley DA, eds. *Malingering.* Oxford: Oxford University Press, 2002.

Phenomenology:
Psychiatry

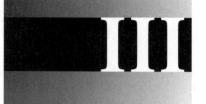

An Overview of the Psychiatric Approach to Conversion Disorder

Fred Ovsiew

ABSTRACT

This overview of the psychiatry of conversion disorder
addresses the reliability of the diagnosis and the psychiatric features concurrent with the pseudoneurologic
symptom. In particular, the issues of traumatic experience
in childhood and dissociative symptoms are explored.
An attempt is made to formulate the nature of the
psychological defect that underlies the still-mysterious
use of bodily symptoms as an expression of distress. To
this end, the relevance of attachment theory is proposed.

Let's start with a case from the medical literature. This case
of "malingering associated with hysterical ataxia, scissor
gait, and aggressive outbursts" was recorded by the late
Richard Asher, a physician specializing in psychological
medicine (and coiner of the term Münchausen syndrome,
among other contributions) (1):

> One Sunday, when my daughter was two years old, I prom-
> ised my wife that, if it was not taken as a precedent, I would
> myself get her up from her afternoon rest, dress her, and
> take her for a walk. I performed these duties without diffi-
> culty or loss of dignity, until the walk started. Then there
> was trouble. The child kept falling to the left; she walked
> with a ridiculous scissor gait, and she frequently fell to the
> ground. She cried and said she had a pain. She behaved
> abominably, and I spent a wretched afternoon in Park
> Square West attempting to coax her into good behaviour. I

knew this was sheer devilment, a malignant aggressive
demonstration against the father figure; I would not submit.

> At last my wife returned and undressed her for her
> evening bath. There was a sudden cry: "Do you realise
> you've put both her legs through the same hole in her
> knickers?" I can still remember, after those tortured limbs
> had been freed from the crippling garments, how that gay,
> naked figure raced unrestrictedly to the bathroom without
> a trace of malingering.

Asher's account raises several points of immediate clinical relevance. Asher notes both the motor phenomena and
the poor girl's nonorganic somatic complaints ("she had a
pain"), and emotional and behavioral aberrations—he
even has a psychodynamic explanation for them. We will
take up the theme of psychiatric disorder in patients with
conversion symptoms shortly. Asher makes little distinction between hysteria and malingering—she must have
known what she was doing, he implies. We will address
this question at the end of the chapter. But prior to both of
these issues is a concern central to Asher's account: when
we make the psychiatric diagnosis of conversion disorder,
are we missing organic disease? Here is the lesson that
Asher took from his experience:

> That incident taught me to be cautious about diagnosing
> malingering or hysteria. These diagnoses must not be made
> for the sole reason that the clinical picture is not yet hung
> in the clinical picture gallery of the doctor in charge. It may

be something he hasn't heard of. There are too many examples of apparent malingering turning out to be cases of organic disease, and jokes about the high mortality of malingering or hysteria are commonplace.

At around the same time as Asher made this point, so did Eliot Slater, writing from the National Hospital, Queen Square, London. Hysteria, he said, is "a disguise for ignorance, and a fertile source of clinical error. It is in fact not only a delusion but a snare (2)." His argument was based on follow-up data (3). Eighty-five patients (of 99 consecutive patients) diagnosed with hysteria were followed up at 7 to 11 years after the diagnosis. Seventy of these were seen for assessment, the remainder rediagnosed from notes or information from relatives. Twelve of the 85 had died, four by suicide. Twenty-two of the remaining 73 (and presumably of the 85) had gone on to receive a diagnosis of organic disease in lieu of hysteria, an alarming 30% (or 26%) of the series. The authors noted that for the most part, this rediagnosis represented a reinterpretation of unchanged medical facts, rather than the result of new information. On these data, one cannot but quaver in announcing a diagnosis of hysteria.

We now know that this concern is exaggerated. To be sure, at times patients with psychiatric symptoms can be disregarded by doctors, their somatic complaints not evaluated with due care. However, when proper evaluations are performed and a diagnosis of conversion disorder made, that diagnosis usually proves to be correct on follow-up; organic disease explanatory of the original symptoms is infrequently found. By way of parallel to Slater's series, Crimlisk et al. reported the outcome of six years on 73 consecutive patients diagnosed at the National Hospital with "medically unexplained" motor symptoms from 1989 to 1991 (4). Adequate data were available for 64, of whom only three had developed neurologic disorders that "fully or partly explained" their undiagnosed symptoms, in all cases including disordered gait. One was a woman with a learning disability who at follow-up clearly had myotonic dystrophy. A second was a man with whom communication was said to be difficult because English was not his first language, and who proved to have a spinocerebellar degeneration. (Was he interviewed in his native language? The authors do not say.) A final misdiagnosed patient had paroxysmal hemidystonia, a condition not well-recognized at the time of misdiagnosis. In an earlier series from the same institution, Mace and Trimble found that 11 of 73 patients had a neurologic rediagnosis at 10-year follow-up (5). A similar study from Edinburgh was able to ascertain the outcome in 66 of 90 patients with medically unexplained symptoms from a neurology clinic (6). None had acquired a neurologic diagnosis eight months on. In a separate study from the same group, information as to diagnostic outcome was available in 48 of 60 patients with purportedly pseudoneurologic symptoms after a lapse of a mean of

12.5 years (7). In only one had an apparently explanatory diagnosis been made.

All these studies are open to methodological question, for example, as to the representativeness of the patient population at these tertiary care hospitals, or as to how typical the evaluations they underwent might be in ordinary clinical practice. On the other hand, diagnostic tools surely have improved since the time of the cohort studied by Slater more than 4 decades ago. The lesson seems to be that clinicians who take due care in evaluation, especially with regard to adequate communication with patients who may at times be difficult, are justified in a high level of confidence in a diagnosis of conversion disorder. Perfect accuracy, no; importance of keeping an open mind, certainly; but the disorder being a delusion and a snare, hardly.

What of the remaining 51 of the 73 patients in the Slater and Glithero series, those in whom the diagnosis of hysteria was not judged to be in error? Of those, 19 had known organic disease along with a "hysterical overlay," which was regarded as "temporary" and not influential on the course of the basic disease. Nonetheless, the recognition of this group requires explanation of a mental mechanism productive of the "overlay." Indeed, Slater fully recognized the existence of hysterical symptoms; "... the dissociative mechanisms of hysteria are known of old, and can lead to symptoms which deserve no other name," he wrote (8). His allegation was that the presence of the hysterical symptoms and the poor relationship between doctor and patient that resulted from an interaction between the patient's abnormal personality and the doctor's impatience to make a diagnosis might lead the doctor to ignore important diagnostic considerations. Further, Slater and Glithero (really Slater, who slipped into the first person singular late in the essay) believed that the personality disorder might itself be due to a fundamental organic brain disease, which "may bring about a general disturbance involving the personality. This personality change may then be a basis for hysterical conversion reactions, or by causing affective lability, hypochondriasis, attention-seeking, self-concern, suggestibility, variability of symptoms, and so forth, lead directly to an unfavorable reaction on the part of the clinician (3)."

The same concern animated his stressing that of the final 32 patients who had no evidence of organic disease on follow-up, in ten a psychiatric diagnosis came to light: Two developed schizophrenia, eight, cyclothymia. The authors speculated that the original diagnosis of hysteria was made during an unrecognized episode of depression.

The concern for missed psychiatric disorder in the Slater and Glithero paper is unfortunate, because subsequent studies clearly demonstrate that other psychiatric disorders are common in patients with conversion disorder. Brown and Ron summarized the literature as suggesting that perhaps three quarters of patients with conversion disorder merit another psychiatric diagnosis (9). A mood disorder is present in 40% to 80%, an anxiety disorder in a similar proportion, and personality disorder in the majority. These aspects will be taken up in detail in other chapters in this volume. Moreover, the prognosis of conversion disorder itself is poor, if outcome assessment includes psychosocial functioning beyond the presence or resolution of the presenting symptom (10). Having signaled the theme of concurrent psychiatric disorder, I want to focus in this chapter on a particular set of psychiatric symptoms, namely, dissociative symptoms.

A link has been drawn between dissociation and hysteria since the late 19th century, beginning with the work of Janet (11). Dissociation refers to "a disruption in the usually integrated functions of consciousness, memory, identity, or perception of the environment (12)." Perhaps the exact meaning of the term cannot be gleaned from this definition, but fortunately, reliable scales for the ascertainment of dissociative symptoms have been constructed. The most commonly used, the Dissociative Experiences Scale (DES), has factors related to memory symptoms, capacity for absorption in experience, and derealization (Table 14.1).

Applying the DES to an inpatient population of conversion disorder patients, in comparison with a mixed group of psychiatric inpatients, Spitzer and coworkers found that the conversion disorder patients had more dissociative symptoms, despite the lack of a significant difference in a broad range of other symptoms (although there was a consistent trend for the comparison group to have more symptoms in other domains) (15). This finding has not always been replicated, and not all studies have as carefully controlled for the effects of psychopathology in general. However, Nijenhuis et al. argued that the DES does not fully account for the dissociative process in regard to somatic experience (as opposed to perceptions and ideas experienced in the mental realm) (13). They devised a supplementary scale, the Somatoform Dissociation Questionnaire-20 (SDQ-20), and applied this to a group of patients with conversion disorder as well as a number of other psychiatric conditions (Table 14.1). They found that the patients with somatoform disorders had elevated scores on the SDQ-20, in comparison with mood disorder or eating disorder patients, even after covarying out the effect of general psychopathology. In contrast, the DES did not allow this distinction.

The postulated connection between dissociation and conversion disorder has been sufficiently convincing that the *International Classification of Diseases* (ICD-10) devised an alternative to the *Diagnostic and Statistical Manual of Mental Disorders* (DSM) categorization of the so-called somatoform disorders. In ICD-10, "dissociative (conversion) disorders" are defined to include pseudoneurologic syndromes, such as pseudoseizures, as well as dissociative fugue or amnesia. This highlights a presumed commonality of underlying mental mechanisms.

Since Janet, and certainly in contemporary psychiatry, dissociative symptoms and dissociation as a mechanism are taken to point to a role for trauma in pathogenesis. In particular, sexual abuse and physical abuse in early life are taken to be key factors in the creation of vulnerability to nonorganic somatic symptoms. Many studies have found an elevated rate of abuse in childhood in patients with pseudoseizures (16) and with other nonorganic somatic symptoms (17). In accord with this conclusion, in the first study of a group of patients with more various sensory and motor conversion symptoms, Roelofs et al. found an association with early abuse (18).

Several difficulties with this evidence require attention toward the goal of a more precise delineation of the

---

TABLE 14.1

SAMPLE ITEMS FROM THE DISSOCIATIVE EXPERIENCES SCALE AND THE SOMATOFORM DISSOCIATION QUESTIONNAIRE-20[a]

Dissociative Experiences Scale

> Finding themselves in a place and having no idea how they got there.
> Finding themselves dressed in clothes that they don't remember putting on.
> Having no memory of some important event in their lives (e.g., a wedding or graduation).
> Sometimes remembering an event so vividly they feel as if they were reliving that event.
> Sometimes having the ability to ignore pain.

Somatoform Dissociation Questionnaire-20

> My body, or a part of it, feels numb.
> I dislike smells that I usually like.
> I cannot swallow, or can swallow only with great effort.
> I am paralyzed for a while.

[a]For each item in each scale, subjects are asked to estimate how often the experience applies to themselves. From Nijenhuis ER, van Dyck R, Spinhoven P, et al. Somatoform dissociation discriminates among diagnostic categories over and above general psychopathology. *Aust N Z J Psychiatry.* 1999;33:511–520; and Wright DB, Loftus EF. Measuring dissociation: comparison of alternative forms of the dissociative experiences scale. *Am J Psychol.* 1999;112:497–519.

background of patients with conversion symptoms. One concern is the retrospective nature of the reports of abuse. For obvious reasons, prospective data are much harder to obtain. In a potentially relevant study—there are no prospective studies of the issue directly focused on conversion disorder—Raphael et al. could not confirm a link between documented abuse in childhood and medically unexplained pain complaints in adulthood (19).

This is not to say that abuse in childhood is unrelated to psychopathology. In fact, several longitudinal studies demonstrate the strength of such an association. For example, Fergusson et al. in New Zealand found elevated risks of mood, anxiety, and substance abuse disorders in subjects with abuse in childhood, with an odds ratio for conduct disorder in those experiencing intercourse in childhood of 11:9 (20). Unfortunately, major reviews of the risk of psychiatric illness after childhood trauma do not mention conversion disorder; studies did not seek this outcome (21,22).

To raise questions about the evidence relating early abuse to conversion disorder is also not to deny that early experience determines later psychopathology. In a striking demonstration of the relevance of early experience, Van Ommeren et al. studied a group of Bhutanese refugees—forced to leave their homes by political persecution—in a camp for displaced persons in Nepal (23). During an epidemic of medically unexplained dizziness, fainting, and other symptoms, the authors were able to construct a case-control series of carefully interviewed subjects. Cases showed more childhood trauma, including early loss of parents by death or separation, even under these enormously stressful present circumstances.

To raise these questions is certainly not to disbelieve that horrible things happen to children or to dismiss patients' reports of abuse. However, whether sexual abuse is itself the culpable factor in conversion disorder or whether it serves as a proxy for other features of an adverse environment of development remains uncertain. Findings as to the relationship between nonorganic symptoms and childhood experiences have been inconsistent, with some suggesting a link to sexual abuse, others to physical or emotional abuse. In respect to dissociation, Mulder et al. employed the DES in a general population sample (24). In the logistic regression analysis, early physical abuse and current psychiatric disorder were associated with dissociative symptoms, but early sexual abuse dropped out of the equation. Salmon et al. suggested that the very inconsistency of findings across studies suggests that these markers are proxies for other pathogenic influences in the family (25,26).

In sum, abuse in childhood may be associated with conversion disorder later in life, as it is with many other adverse psychiatric outcomes. The nonspecific nature of the connection between abuse and conversion disorder—abuse has various outcomes, including good functioning (27), and risk of conversion disorder may be raised by various childhood experiences—is not surprising in psychiatry,

where nonlinear developmental processes are the rule, not the exception. Nonetheless, we are left, from the available data, without a compelling explanation of the somatic form of the symptoms resulting from deviant development (28). We can see, however, that the psychiatric inquiry in the patient with conversion disorder must be comprehensive.

The last theme to be explored here—the question raised by Asher's vignette as to the relation between hysteria and malingering—is complex. Conversion disorder? Is this anything more than psychiatric obfuscation? Don't these people know what they're doing? Isn't this, in other words, nothing other than malingering? How, one might ask, could it be otherwise—how could someone *not* know? And how could we hope to know what is truly in the minds of the sufferers—if indeed they are sufferers?

The British neurologist Sir Charles Symonds addressed this point forcefully with regard to hysterical fugue, which he considered always to be malingered (29). He advocated saying to the patient, "I know from experience that your pretended loss of memory is the result of some intolerable emotional situation. If you will tell me the whole story I promise absolutely to respect your confidence, will give you all the help I can and will say to your doctor and relatives that I have cured you by hypnotism." He asserted that his method "has never failed." His approach, I have been told, was that taken in World War II in the British Forces, when conversion disorder had the appellation LMF—lack of moral fiber—and could be treated by a sympathetic but firm physician who told the patient, essentially, "I'm a doctor; you can trust me." Physicians expected that the pretense of not knowing could under these circumstances be given up and the truth would out.

But this is not fair to Symonds. Actually, he made this claim only about hysterical fugue. With regard to conversion symptoms generally, he held a subtler point of view. He believed that, in many instances, hysterics showed a peculiar mixture of knowing and not knowing. He quoted the neurologist James Birley as saying that "the capacity for self-deception in the hysteric might be regarded as a specific kind of mental deficiency." (Symonds alludes to the provenance of this remark in imprecise terms, as set down "in a paper on the hysterical personality, I think in the *St. Thomas's Hospital Gazette*." Unfortunately, despite the best efforts of the St. Thomas's and National Hospital librarians on my behalf, such an article has not come to light.) I consider Birley's remark to be astute beyond its times. In the remainder of this chapter, I will examine what light the developmental evidence throws on the nature of this "specific kind of mental deficiency."

From a Jacksonian perspective, the delineation of a mental "deficiency"—a negative symptom—is the counterpart of understanding the production of novel, or "positive," symptoms. This point stands in regard to conversion disorder even if the "positive" nonorganic symptoms are "negative" in a neurologic sense, for example, weakness or sensory loss. To put the point in more contemporary or psychodynamic terms, the development of conversion symptoms can be seen as compensatory for a deficit in managing emotion, or memories, or interpersonal transactions in a more effective fashion, and the symptoms cannot be understood without accounting for the deficit. This perspective owes more to Janet than to the early Freud, for whom hysterical symptoms resulted from processes of symbolization and repression, with no implication that the processes themselves were malfunctioning. Tracing the way in which the recognition of "ego defects" entered psychoanalytic conceptualization is far beyond the scope of this chapter, but it is fair to say that no one should now put forth a simple view of hysterical symptoms as symbolic transformations of repressed ideas (30).

Rather, something has gone decidedly wrong with the very representation of ideas or emotions, such that patients find themselves "thinking with the body." Attachment theory provides a scientific framework for conceptualizing how representation of emotion can go awry, and it is to this framework that I now turn.

Attachment theory derives from the work of John Bowlby and others in applying concepts from evolutionary theory and ethology to psychiatric problems (31). The creation of a standardized, quasi-naturalistic structured setting for observation of separations and reunions of a child with a parent—the Ainsworth Strange Situation—allowed the description of categories of observable attachment behavior. With *secure* attachment, the child is able to explore actively, show distress upon separation, and re-engage actively with the parent upon reunion. Two categories of *insecure* attachment were recognized. In *avoidant* attachment, signs of distress upon separation are muted, and re-engagement upon reunion is actively avoided. The child's focus is on the environment rather than the relationship. In *resistant* (or *ambivalent*) attachment, the child is preoccupied with the parent rather than the toys in the environment, showing distress even before the separation and failing to be comforted upon reunion. Later, in trying to understand observations that remained unclassifiable in the existing scheme, Mary Main et al. described *disorganized* attachment behavior (32). These children display contradictory or undirected movement and behavior patterns, such as stereotypies, freezing, or anomalous postures. They may show apprehension about the parent, as if the parent were a source of fear rather than comfort.

Observations within the Strange Situation paradigm are behavioral, but few observers can watch children for long without wondering, imagining, or assuming what the children are thinking and feeling. Often in psychiatry, understanding meaningful connections between ideas, emotions, and symptoms is taken to be antithetical, or at least orthogonal, to scientific explanation of etiology and pathogenesis (33). To be sure, abuse of hermeneutic thinking is easy

(34)—of making many meanings for symptoms, there is no end, so to say. However, attachment theory provides a scientific framework for studying the process of meaning attribution in narratives and allows the integration of a perspective from child development with a description of a patient's representational capacities (35,36).

Bowlby himself (37), who was particularly interested in the "internal working models" developed on the basis of early experience and in the ways those models determined the deployment of attention in the interpersonal world, prefigured the "move to the level of representation." In his theory, "[d]efensive exclusion [of information] is regarded as being at the heart of psychopathology … cognitive disconnection of a response from the interpersonal situation that elicited it I believe to play an enormous role in psychopathology." In this way, the attachment paradigm is open to integration with theories in the cognitive neurosciences, including those proposed to explain dissociative psychopathology (38).

The decisive step in approaching the "level of representation" was the development, by Main et al., of the Adult Attachment Interview (AAI) (39). This instrument allows the clinical observer to make judgments on the form (as opposed to the content) of the adult subject's narrative account of early attachment experiences. The subject is asked to describe the relationship with the parents, the ways in which emotions were handled, experiences of loss and violence, and the understanding of the parents' personalities and motivations. The resulting protocol is assessed for the "state of mind in respect to attachment," with such categories as coherence and lapses or contradictions in the narrative, realistic appraisal or idealization of attachment figures, and tolerance of attachment-related emotions as against their dismissal or derogation. The outcome is a set of classification categories corresponding to those of the Strange Situation. Secure/autonomous subjects provide a coherent narrative with objective appraisal of relationships. Dismissing subjects show less coherent and briefer accounts, with devaluing of relationships and vague, generalized descriptors inconsistent with reported events. Preoccupied subjects produce less coherent and often long accounts, and are preoccupied by the past experiences with associated anger and fear. Unresolved/disorganized subjects show lapses of reasoning and discourse, such as logical contradictions or bizarre ideas, sometimes with prolonged silences.

Evidence gathered using these methods demonstrates that disorganized attachment in childhood is associated with childhood trauma and with abnormal narratives in later childhood and adulthood, characterized by lapses in reasoning and discourse, plausibly understood as representing poorly modulated shifts in self-state (32). Further, disorganized attachment appears to have a striking relationship with dissociative psychopathology. Observationally, disorganization in infants in the Strange Situation bears a resemblance to dissociative symptoms in adolescents and adults. Dissociative symptoms correlated with "unresolved" status on the AAI in a clinical sample of adolescents (40). Most compelling, longitudinal data show disorganized infants to have an excess of dissociative symptoms when studied in adolescence (41–43). More specifically, Lyons-Ruth reported that both disorganized attachment and measures of disrupted mother–infant communication contributed to dissociative symptoms in adolescents, though documented maltreatment in early childhood did not. She epitomized the communication failure by saying that "the mother's seeing and not knowing in infancy may constitute one contribution to the child's knowing and not knowing in late adolescence (42)."

In summary, strong connections, based on systematic empirical data, can be drawn between trauma and attachment disorganization, between attachment disorganization and dissociation, and among trauma, dissociation, and conversion disorder. Data are lacking, because the relevant studies are lacking, to delineate a connection directly between disorganized attachment and a psychiatric diagnosis of conversion disorder. A plausible interpretation is that these connections depend on a disorder of the representation of experience such that coherent narrative and effective thought are impaired. This, I propose, is the "specific defect" to which Birley and Symonds referred.

From this perspective, in reply to Asher's point of view, patients "don't know" not because they forget or dissemble. They exhibit the peculiar mixture of knowing and not knowing because they are unable to mentalize distress, the result of an inhibition or failure of thinking about distress in the context of disorganized attachment and its aberrant internal working models. *Faute de mieux*, an inadequate form of representation and communication using the body, is undertaken. Even under normal circumstances, much of one's way of relating to others is unformulated or unsymbolized; this recognition has led to conceptualizations of "implicit relational knowing" (44) and the "unthought known" (45). However, under normal circumstances, a person is able to make use of representational capacities to keep unpleasant or conflicting affects in mind when doing so is necessary for problem solving. In patients with conversion disorder, this capacity is deficient. From the viewpoint of cognitive neuroscience, this indicates a defect in attention or working memory (46). Specifically why certain people adopt "thinking with the body" as an outcome of this developmental process is not known. Most likely, multiple factors may contribute to the pathway to conversion disorder, perhaps including parental illness in the patient's childhood, early childhood illness, concurrent somatic illness in adolescence or adulthood, and organic cerebral disease. The disorder of symbolic thought emphasized here serves, in this interpretation, as a permissive factor in many or most such patients.

By way of historical footnote, linking conversion symptoms to impairment of narrative processes would not have surprised Freud. To the contrary, in his early essay on hysteria, the so-called Dora case, he wrote:

> I cannot help wondering how it is that the authorities can produce such smooth and precise histories in cases of hysteria. As a matter of fact the patients are incapable of giving such reports about themselves….The connections—even the ostensible ones—are for the most part incoherent…. The patients' inability to give an ordered history of their life in so far as it coincides with the history of the illness is … characteristic of the neurosis (47).

Several caveats are in order. First, to say that experiential factors, such as abuse in childhood, are influential in the development of conversion disorder is not to deny the relevance of genetic or organic factors. Untangling the roles and interactions of genetic, organic, and experiential factors in psychiatric illness is complex, but it is fair to say that a person's genetic endowment is likely to play a role in the development of any illness in which personality is significant. Moreover, psychiatric symptoms, including conversion symptoms, are reflective of the integrity of the function of the brain. Considerable evidence indicates that the presence of concomitant neurologic disease is a risk factor for pseudoneurologic complaints. This may occur because of the psychosocial stress produced by illness, and the organic symptoms may provide a behavioral model for the development of the nonorganic ones, notably in the case of the patient with both epilepsy and pseudoseizures. However, organic alteration of personality, of the sort emphasized by Slater, may well be a factor, at least in certain cases. Deterioration of the capacity for coherent thought about complex and emotionally powerful matters may be the mechanism by which personality regression due to organic disease leads to conversion symptoms.

As an additional caveat, psychiatric symptoms always can occur in a range of severity, and conversion symptoms are no exception. Patients with conversion disorder may have a chronic, severe, and polysymptomatic illness, or they may have a relatively isolated outcropping of nonorganic symptoms. Correlatively, the underlying deficit may be more or less pervasive in the personality, across a broader or narrower range of emotional domains and narrative demands. The generally poor psychosocial outcome of conversion disorder implies that the patients are more impaired than the sometimes-good outcome of the presenting symptoms has suggested to some. The proposal made here is that even the apparently milder forms of conversion disorder are more like the severe forms of psychosomatic illness than is often recognized in contemporary psychiatry or neurology. Further study of these patients with sophistication as to the nature of the relevant processes in the personality should confirm or refute these proposals.

REFERENCES

1. Asher R. Malingering. In: Avery Jones F, ed. *Richard Asher talking sense.* London: Pitman, 1972:145–155.
2. Slater E. Diagnosis of "Hysteria." *Br Med J.* 1965;5447:1395–1399.
3. Slater ET, Glithero E. A follow-up of patients diagnosed as suffering from "hysteria." *J Psychosom Res.* 1965;9:9–13.
4. Crimlisk HL, Bhatia K, Cope H, et al. Slater revisited: 6-year follow up study of patients with medically unexplained motor symptoms. *Br Med J.* 1998;316:582–586.
5. Mace CJ, Trimble MR. Ten-year prognosis of conversion disorder. *Br J Psychiatry.* 1996;169:282–288.
6. Carson AJ, Best S, Postma K, et al. The outcome of neurology outpatients with medically unexplained symptoms: a prospective cohort study. *J Neurol Neurosurg Psychiatry.* 2003;74:897–900.
7. Stone J, Sharpe M, Rothwell PM, et al. The 12-year prognosis of unilateral functional weakness and sensory disturbance. *J Neurol Neurosurg Psychiatry.* 2003;74:591–596.
8. Slater E. Hysteria 311. *J Ment Sci.* 1961;107:359–371.
9. Brown RJ, Ron MA. Conversion disorders and somatoform disorders. In: Ramachandran VS, ed. *Encyclopedia of the human brain,* Vol 2. Amsterdam: Academic Press, 2002:37–49.
10. Reuber M, Pukrop R, Bauer J, et al. Outcome in psychogenic nonepileptic seizures: 1- to 10-year follow-up in 164 patients. *Ann Neurol.* 2003;53:305–311.
11. Brown P, Macmillan MB, Meares R, et al. Janet and Freud: revealing the roots of dynamic psychiatry. *Aust N Z J Psychiatry.* 1996;30:480–489; discussion:489–491.
12. American Psychiatric Association. *Diagnostic and statistical manual of mental disorders,* 4th ed. Washington, DC: American Psychiatric Association, 1994.
13. Nijenhuis ER, van Dyck R, Spinhoven P, et al. Somatoform dissociation discriminates among diagnostic categories over and above general psychopathology. *Aust N Z J Psychiatry.* 1999;33:511–520.
14. Wright DB, Loftus EF. Measuring dissociation: comparison of alternative forms of the dissociative experiences scale. *Am J Psychol.* 1999;112:497–519.
15. Spitzer C, Spelsberg B, Grabe HJ, et al. Dissociative experiences and psychopathology in conversion disorders. *J Psychosom Res.* 1999;46:291–294.
16. Alper K, Devinsky O, Perrine K, et al. Nonepileptic seizures and childhood sexual and physical abuse. *Neurology.* 1993;43:1950–1953.
17. Leserman J, Li Z, Drossman DA, et al. Selected symptoms associated with sexual and physical abuse history among female patients with gastrointestinal disorders: the impact on subsequent health care visits. *Psychol Med.* 1998;28:417–425.
18. Roelofs K, Keijsers GP, Hoogduin KA, et al. Childhood abuse in patients with conversion disorder. *Am J Psychiatry.* 2002;159:1908–1913.
19. Raphael KG, Widom CS, Lange G. Childhood victimization and pain in adulthood: a prospective investigation. *Pain.* 2001;92:283–293.
20. Fergusson DM, Horwood LJ, Lynskey MT. Childhood sexual abuse and psychiatric disorder in young adulthood: II. Psychiatric outcomes of childhood sexual abuse. *J Am Acad Child Adolesc Psychiatry.* 1996;35:1365–1374.
21. Molnar BE, Buka SL, Kessler RC. Child sexual abuse and subsequent psychopathology: results from the National Comorbidity Survey. *Am J Public Health.* 2001;91:753–760.
22. Cohen P, Brown J, Smaile E. Child abuse and neglect and the development of mental disorders in the general population. *Dev Psychopathol.* 2001;13:981–999.
23. Van Ommeren M, Sharma B, Komproe I, et al. Trauma and loss as determinants of medically unexplained epidemic illness in a Bhutanese refugee camp. *Psychol Med.* 2001;31:1259–1267.
24. Mulder RT, Beautrais AL, Joyce PR, et al. Relationship between dissociation, childhood sexual abuse, childhood physical abuse, and mental illness in a general population sample. *Am J Psychiatry.* 1998;155:806–811.
25. Salmon P, Al-Marzooqi SM, Baker G, et al. Childhood family dysfunction and associated abuse in patients with nonepileptic seizures: towards a causal model. *Psychosom Med.* 2003;65:695–700.
26. Salmon P, Skaife K, Rhodes J. Abuse, dissociation, and somatization in irritable bowel syndrome: towards an explanatory model. *J Behav Med.* 2003;26:1–18.
27. McGloin JM, Widom CS. Resilience among abused and neglected children grown up. *Dev Psychopathol.* 2001;13:1021–1038.
28. Bulik CM, Prescott CA, Kendler KS. Features of childhood sexual abuse and the development of psychiatric and substance use disorders. *Br J Psychiatry.* 2001;179:444–449.
29. Symonds C. Hysteria. In: Merskey H, ed. *The analysis of hysteria.* London: Balliere Tindall, 1979:258–265.
30. Gottlieb RM. Psychosomatic medicine: the divergent legacies of Freud and Janet. *J Am Psychoanal Assoc.* 2003;51:857–881.
31. Goldberg S, Muir R, Kerr J. *Attachment theory: social, developmental, and clinical perspectives.* Hillsdale, NJ: Analytic Press, 1995.
32. Hesse E, Main M. Disorganized infant, child, and adult attachment: collapse in behavioral and attentional strategies. *J Am Psychoanal Assoc.* 2000;48:1097–1127; discussion 1175–1087.
33. Jaspers K. Causal and meaningful connexions between life history and psychosis. In: Hirsch SR, Shepherd M, eds. *Themes and variations in european psychiatry.* Bristol: John Wright & Sons, 1974:81–93.
34. Slavney PR. Pseudoseizures, sexual abuse, and hermeneutic reasoning. *Compr Psychiatry.* 1994;35:471–477.
35. Holmes J. Borderline personality disorder and the search for meaning: an attachment perspective. *Aust N Z J Psychiatry.* 2003;37:524–531.
36. Main M, Kaplan N, Cassidy J. Security in infancy, childhood, and adulthood: a move to the level of representation. In: Bretherton I, Waters E, eds. *Growing points of attachment theory and research.* Chicago: University of Chicago Press, 1985:66–104.
37. Bowlby J. *Loss: sadness and depression.* New York: Basic Books, 1980.
38. Brown RJ. The cognitive psychology of dissociative states. *Cognit Neuropsych.* 2002;7:221–235.
39. Hesse E. The adult attachment interview: historical and current perspectives. In: Cassidy J, Shaver PR, eds. *Handbook of attachment: theory, research, and clinical applications.* New York: Guildford Press, 1999:395–433.
40. West M, Adam K, Spreng S, et al. Attachment disorganization and dissociative symptoms in clinically treated adolescents. *Can J Psychiatry.* 2001;46:627–631.
41. Ogawa JR, Sroufe LA, Weinfield NS, et al. Development and the fragmented self: longitudinal study of dissociative symptomatology in a nonclinical sample. *Dev Psychopathol.* 1997;9:855–879.
42. Lyons-Ruth K. Dissociation and the parent-infant dialogue: a longitudinal perspective from attachment research. *J Am Psychoanal Assoc.* 2003;51:883–911.
43. Carlson EA. A prospective longitudinal study of attachment disorganization/disorientation. *Child Dev.* 1998;69:1107–1128.
44. Stern DN, Sander LW, Nahum JP, et al. Non-interpretive mechanisms in psychoanalytic therapy. The 'something more' than interpretation. The process of change study group. *Int J Psychoanal.* 1998;79:903–921.
45. Bollas C. *The shadow of the object: psychoanalysis of the unthought known.* New York: Columbia University Press, 1987.
46. Meares R, Stevenson J, Gordon E. A Jacksonian and biopsychosocial hypothesis concerning borderline and related phenomena. *Aust N Z J Psychiatry.* 1999;33:831–840.
47. Freud S. Fragment of an analysis of a case of hysteria. In: Strachey J, ed. *Standard edition of the complete psychological works of Sigmund Freud.* Vol VII. London: Hogarth Press, 1905:7–122.

The Role of Personality in Psychogenic Movement Disorders

15

C. Robert Cloninger

ABSTRACT

The quantitative measurement of personality provides a rigorous quantitative approach to understanding the psychobiology of movement disorders. Individual differences in temperament and character distinguish patients with psychogenic movement disorders from others and identify quantitative variables that can be reliably measured and investigated in clinical practice. In addition, research through brain imaging, neurophysiology, and molecular genetics are rapidly clarifying the role of personality in information processing in general and in susceptibility to psychogenic movement disorders in particular. The activity of brain networks that regulate attention, affect, and motor activity are well-measured by Temperament and Character Inventory (TCI) character dimensions that are heritable but also influenced by variables unique to each individual, which can be voluntarily developed regardless of antecedent or initial conditions. The measurement of character allows reliable assessment of individual differences in levels of specific components of self-aware consciousness that regulate voluntary motor behavior. Patients with inadequate self-awareness can be treated with specific mental exercises to increase their awareness and decrease any psychogenic contribution to their disability.

PSYCHIATRIC DESCRIPTION

Psychogenic movement disorders refer to functional abnormalities in the modulation of voluntary movement. In this chapter, I will describe evidence that the fundamental abnormalities involve specific deficits in self-aware consciousness, which can be reliably quantified by specific measures of personality in my Temperament and Character Inventory (TCI) (1,2). Much is now known about the modulation of self-aware consciousness (3,4), and further work on movement disorders should extend and clarify this growing body of knowledge in ways that will be clinically and theoretically valuable.

Psychogenic movement disorders are classified as conversion disorders in the American Psychiatric Association's *Diagnostic and Statistical Manual of Mental Disorders*, Fourth Edition (DSM-IV) (5). A conversion disorder refers to a symptom or deficit "affecting voluntary motor or sensory function that suggests a neurologic or other general medical condition." The official criteria further stipulate that the symptoms or deficits cannot be explained by a neurologic or general medication condition and are not intentionally produced or feigned. On the other hand, psychological factors may be judged to be associated with the symptom or deficit "because the initiation or exacerbation of the symptom or deficit is preceded by conflicts or other stressors." However, all these criteria require judgments that are difficult and sometimes unreliable because patients with involuntary neurologic deficits also experience conflict and distress, which may lead to a functional overlay to an involuntary neurologic disorder.

The unreliability of diagnosis of individual conversion disorders led Eli Robins, Samuel Guze, and me to develop criteria for what is now called somatization disorder in DSM-IV (6). Somatization disorder requires the presence of four pain symptoms, two gastrointestinal symptoms, and one sexual symptom in addition to a pseudoneurologic symptom. These criteria identify a group of patients with chronic unexplained somatic and neurologic complaints. The disorder has a chronic fluctuating course with many complaints, and unnecessary medical treatment and surgeries, often highly disabling and expensive. The disorder is heritable, as shown by adoption studies I carried out in Sweden through access to national registers of all medical treatment and sick-leave disability (7,8). The vulnerability factors for somatization disorder can also be measured reliably as personality traits, and much is now known about the brain imaging, neurobiology, and molecular genetics of personality traits underlying somatization and conversion disorders (4,9–11). The heritability of vulnerability to psychogenic movement disorders suggests that there are real psychobiologic processes underlying these complex phenomena, as described later.

Most patients with unexplained somatic and neurologic complaints do not satisfy the stringent criteria for somatization disorder. As a result, physicians are usually still in great need of a valid and reliable way to evaluate the psychobiologic processes that modulate voluntary choice and movement in patients who do not satisfy criteria for somatization disorder. Much can be learned from careful observation and interpretation of the mental status examination of patients with unexplained somatic complaints or conversion disorders.

At the time when conversion symptoms occur, a person is lacking in awareness of their voluntary control of what they are doing. This lack of self-aware consciousness is characterized by little or no ability to recollect the spatiotemporal and psychosocial context in which the symptoms are occurring. As a result, clinicians describe such patients as "vague and inconsistent historians" when trying to elicit the history and doing mental status examination. They may be unable to provide an account of relevant stressors that collateral informants can readily describe or that can be observed directly. They may be able to report the occurrence of events as separate facts, but still are unaware of interdependent relationships that define the context in which their sensations and movements occur.

The patient may be excessively dramatic or excessively emotionally detached because they do not have much awareness or understanding of their psychosocial context. Often doctors are frustrated by the inconsistent, vague, and overdramatic history, failing to realize that this style of presentation actually characterizes the fundamental deficit in self-awareness and episodic memory underlying the disorder. If a person has a chronic deficit in self-awareness (i.e., their usual thoughts are childlike, immature, or lacking in self-awareness), then they are described as having a chronic personality disorder. Most often the patients have impulsive ("Cluster B") personality disorders, such as antisocial, histrionic, or borderline personality disorder. However, individuals without a chronic personality disorder may regress to an immature state of consciousness that is brief or sustained while they are under unusual stress. The mental status at the time that the patient's conversion symptoms are active is what is most important to observe.

PSYCHOBIOLOGY OF PERSONALITY AND MOVEMENT

I developed a comprehensive model of human personality over the past 15 years to understand the psychobiologic factors underlying vulnerability to psychopathology, such as somatization and conversion disorders (9,12–15). Most previous models of personality describe traits that differ among individuals, but do not explain the psychobiological processes within an individual that lead to these differences. For example, DSM-IV is a purely descriptive system that distinguishes several categories of personality disorder, such as antisocial, avoidant, and schizoid personality disorders. DSM-IV provides behavioral criteria for identifying these disorders, but provides no explanation whatsoever of the brain processes that cause these disorders. Fortunately, I have been able to develop a model of personality that explains the observable differences among individuals (as described in DSM-IV) and provides a testable model of the psychobiologic processes that cause these variations in personality and susceptibility to mental disorders, including psychogenic movement disorders (4).

Human personality can be described in terms of three systems of learning and memory: (i) procedural learning of habits and skills, which involves four dimensions of temperament; (ii) declarative or semantic learning of facts, which involves three dimensions of character; and (iii) self-aware consciousness or episodic memory, which involves autobiographic recollection of personal continuity, subjective time, and the spatiotemporal context in which facts about events occur in experience (4,11). The four temperament dimensions are measured as individual differences in associative conditioning of responses to simple emotional stimuli, eliciting fear (Harm Avoidance, anxiety-prone vs. risk-taking); anger (Novelty Seeking, impulsive vs. rigid); disgust (Reward Dependence, sociable vs. aloof); and ambition (Persistence, overachieving vs. underachieving). The three character dimensions are measured as individual differences in supervisory cognitive processes, including executive functions (Self-directedness, or the sense of personal agency); legislative functions (Cooperativeness, or the sense of flexible voluntary choice based on making rules to govern social interactions); and judicial functions (Self-transcendence, or the intuitive understanding of when rules apply and should be executed). The self-report of usual patterns of emotional response and mental self-government are reliably reported facts or semantic knowledge that is abstracted from self-aware consciousness in episodic memory. In addition, the dynamic movement of thought in time can be quantified in terms of a nonlinear matrix of subplanes of thought through which human beings move from moment to moment in self-aware consciousness. This movement in autobiographic memory has multiple steps and stages that can be reliably rated and quantified with interrater reliability around 0.88 using methods I have recently developed and described (4), as described in the next section.

Each of the four dimensions of temperament and three dimensions of character have heritabilities of about 50% estimated from large-scale twin studies in the United States and Australia. Each of the seven dimensions has unique genetic determinants (16). Each dimension has specific brain circuitry and carries out specific information-processing tasks, as has been demonstrated by functional brain imaging and evoked potential studies (11,17–21). A detailed description is provided elsewhere (4).

Each dimension measures variability in a complex adaptive system involving the nonlinear interaction of multiple genetic and environmental variables. In fact, there is a hierarchy of such complex coupled networks at increasing levels of information or self-aware consciousness. The hierarchy extends from the level of the matter to the cell, then the physiology of individual organisms, the psychology of individuals in social groups, and so on. Human beings are unique in their capacity for self-aware consciousness, so that a self-aware human being can be described as development and evolution conscious of itself. Great apes have intellectual reasoning and mirror recognition, but not self-aware consciousness in which there is autobiographical recollection of events in a spatiotemporal context (22). Other primates can learn facts, but only human beings can recollect when or where they learned those facts.

The succession of human thoughts in consciousness involves abrupt transitions between thoughts that are synchronous with transitions in spatiotemporal connections between changing sets of brain networks. Discrete thoughts are linked with distinct brain microstates that can be measured by segmentation of abrupt transitions in EEGs (23–25). Different thoughts are associated with distinct brain microstates. These discrete mind–brain states recur in a nonlinear fashion. In other words, different thoughts occur in complex sequences that are not fully predictable in terms of initial conditions or antecedent events.

The content of human thought can be defined in terms of the variability encompassed by individual differences in the seven dimensions of personality measured by the TCI. It is also possible to rank order the range of thought in terms of level of coherence or integration, which I have done by studies of disorganization of thought by induction of fears and increasing coherence of thought by induction of relaxation and meditative states. Then the movement of thought through the hierarchy of varying levels of coherence can be quantified. The modulation of movement of thought is measured by the TCI character dimensions, which correspond to individual differences in higher cognitive processes instantiated as supervisory brain networks regulating attention, affect, and motor activity (4,26). For example, individual differences in TCI Self-directedness are strongly correlated ($r = 0.75$) with individual differences in efficiency of activation of the medial prefrontal cortex (Brodmann areas 9/10) during tasks of executive function (19).

Individual differences in the content and movement of thought are about equally influenced by genetic factors and by variables unique to each individual. Judicial functions, as measured by TCI Self-transcendence, are correlated -0.7 with individual differences in 5HT1a receptor density in the neocortex, hippocampus, and raphe nuclei (27). Presynaptic 5HT1a receptors inhibit neuronal firing in the raphe and all projection areas, providing a means of modulating the activity of a widespread distributed network. The expression of the dopamine D4 (DRD4) receptor is also correlated with this same character trait (28). DRD4 is one of the most variable human genes known, and most of its diversity is the result of variation in a 48-base pair tandem repeat in exon 3 that encodes the third intracellular loop of the DRD4 dopamine receptor (29). Different allelic forms of DRD4 influence the sensitivity of the receptor to dopamine, so that individuals with the seven-repeat allele have much greater neuronal excitability than those with the ancestral four-repeat allele. As a result, the levels of TCI Novelty Seeking and Self-transcendence vary substantially as a result of gene–gene interactions among the DRD4 polymorphism and other genes that regulate the catabolism and transport of dopamine, such as catechol-O-methyltransferase and the dopamine transporter (4,30,31). Also gene–environment interactions influence the development of personality, so that childhood experience of a hostile environment and adult experience of stressful life events modify gene expression and personality development (32,33). In this way, each individual can adapt to his unique experiences in a flexible manner in ways that are partly heritable and partly creative (i.e., free of initial conditions and antecedent influences).

STEPWISE NATURE OF SELF-AWARE CONSCIOUSNESS

Much discussion of consciousness has been confused because of a failure to recognize that the movement of thought in self-aware consciousness is a quasi-continuous process with multiple stages. All human thinking has five steps that are modulated by three processes, as summarized in Table 1. The five steps in thought are: (i) the initial perspective in which there is intuitive recognition of what is given in experience; (ii) labeling the intuition and reasoning about intentions; (iii) emotional responses to those labels and intentions; (iv) intellectual judgments to execute the intention; and (v) the action itself, which with repetition leads to habits. The degree of coherence of a person's thought (that is, their level of character development) passes through stages that differ qualitatively as a person becomes consciously self-aware of these processes underlying their thinking. Individuals with conversion and personality disorders usually operate in the intuitive step without self-aware consciousness of the later steps in thought. Ordinary adults operate with self-awareness of the first two or three steps in thought, which is called

reflection or ordinary adult cognition ("first stage of self-aware consciousness") (4). Self-awareness of the fourth step in thought involves metacognition, which is "thinking about thinking" or meditation in which we become aware of thoughts that were previously subconscious. Self-awareness of all the stages of thought involve spontaneous flow states in which there is simultaneous coherence of intuition, intention, and action without effort or conflict, which is called contemplation ("third stage of self-aware consciousness") (4).

The first four steps are each regulated by one of the temperaments: intuition by Harm Avoidance, reasoning by Novelty Seeking, emotion by Reward Dependence, and intellectual judgments and intentions by Persistence. The emotional aspects of these steps are also supervised by the three processes indicated in Table 1: Agency or the executive initiation of responses, as measured by TCI self-directedness; Flexibility or the legislative selection of voluntary responses, as measured by TCI Cooperativeness; and Understanding or the judicial monitoring of responses, as measured by TCI Self-transcendence. The fifth step is the result of the character processes.

Each of the three character processes has five subscales corresponding to the five steps in thought, as summarized in Table 1. For example, the intuitive step is regulated by the first subscales of the three character dimensions: SD1, responsible versus controlled and victimized; CO1, tolerant

TABLE 15.1

FIVE STAGES OF HUMAN THOUGHT AND UNDERLYING DYNAMIC PROCESSES MEASURED BY TCI CHARACTER SUBSCALES OF SELF-DIRECTEDNESS, COOPERATIVENESS, AND SELF-TRANSCENDENCE

Step in Self-aware Consciousness	TCI Measures of Functional Processes		
	Agency (SD)	**Flexibility (CO)**	**Understanding (ST)**
Step 1: Intuition	Responsible vs. controlled	Tolerant vs. prejudiced	Sensible vs. repressive
Step 2: Reasoning	Purposeful vs. aimless	Forgiving vs. revengeful	Idealistic vs. practical
Step 3: Emotion	Accepting vs. approval-seeking	Empathic vs. inconsiderate	Transpersonal vs. individual
Step 4: Intention	Resourceful vs. inept	Helpful vs. unhelpful	Faithful vs. skeptical
Step 5: Action	Hopeful sublimation vs. compromising deliberation	Charitable principles vs. self-serving opportunism	Spiritual awareness vs. local realism

TCI, Temperament and Character Inventory; SC, Self-directedness; CO, Cooperativeness; ST, Self-transcendence.

versus prejudiced and hateful; ST1, sensible versus hysterical and repressive. The first step corresponds to the onset of preparatory activity in the brain as measured by the cortical "readiness potential" in experiments of Libet and others. The degree of preparatory activity is also measured by the P300 evoked potential in oddball experimental paradigms, which is moderately correlated with TCI Self-directedness (18). The time course of cortical event-related potentials allows the dissociation of the early intuitive recognition of stimuli from later decision making (34). Intuitions are only immediately conscious in the third stage of self-aware consciousness.

The second step of thought involves labeling and reasoning, which vary from purposeful planning to capricious wants and aversions. The longer the objective deliberation in the second stage, the slower will be the reaction time of subjects because of reduced spontaneity of agency. The second step defines our wants when our actions are purposeful, as in Libet's experiments in which subjects were asked to plan their movements thoughtfully.

The labels and plans of the second stage elicit emotional responses in the third step, which are modulated by the emotion-related aspects of the character dimensions (accepting, empathic, transpersonal vs. striving, inconsiderate, individualistic). The third step defines our wants when our actions are capricious, as in Libet's experiments in which subjects were asked to act "spontaneously" and "capriciously." The fourth step involves the actual intention to act, which corresponds to Libet's subjects awareness of movement beginning before it is actually measurable by the EMG. The final step is the overt action, measured by Libet as physical movement in the EMG.

The stepwise movement of thought has the same hierarchical structure whether observed as the movement of thought from moment to movement, or as the development of character or ego states over years across the lifespan (4,35,36). As thought increases in coherence, there is an expansion of the social radius and depth of understanding. Hence, the development of self-aware consciousness can be visualized as a spiral path of increasing radius with each rotation corresponding to expanded awareness of the next step in thought (4). Thought and its development do not proceed along a linear staircase, but make sudden, discrete jumps in content and level of coherence from moment to moment.

BRAIN REGULATION OF ATTENTION, AFFECT, AND MOVEMENT

The conflict between biases for unpleasant and pleasant stimuli is resolved by the elevation of thought to allow impartial purposeful actions, which require reality-testing and a sense of following a meaningful direction in one's life regardless of the hedonic valence of one's context, as measured by increasing TCI Self-directedness (37). The coherence

of such self-directed behavior requires prospective autobiographic memories that depend on the medial and rostral prefrontal cortex (Brodmann areas 9 and 10) (38–40), which are highly correlated with TCI Self-directedness (19,41,42).

Likewise, the alertness (arousal) brain network is another well-known distributed brain network that involves primarily the right frontal and right parietal cortex, as well as noradrenergic projections from the locus coeruleus in the brainstem (26,43,44). Drugs like clonidine, which block the activity of norepinephrine, reduce or eliminate the normal effect of warning signals on reaction time, but have no effect on orienting to the target location. The alertness brain network seems to continue to mature well into adulthood according to Posner's developmental studies (26). The development of the ability to modulate arousal is impaired in individuals with neuropsychiatric disorders involving the right inferior parietal cortex and anterior insula (45,46). The posterior superior temporal sulcus region nearby the insula is also consistently activated during both implicit and explicit mentalizing tasks, and has been proposed as the site for the detection of agency (i.e., the qualia of voluntariness or free will) (47). Being aware of wanting or voluntarily intending to cause an action is associated with activation of the anterior insula, whereas being aware of external control of an action is associated with activation of the inferior parietal cortex (45,46). These two regions are thought to be involved in the perception of complex representations of an individual and interactions with the external world. The anterior insula integrates all the concordant multimodal sensory signals associated with voluntary movements, thereby representing an egocentric representation of space. The inferior parietal, in contrast, represents voluntary actions in an allocentric coding system that can be applied to the actions of others as well as the self. Such an allocentric representation is necessary for cooperative behavior, which requires flexibility of choice in representations of self–other relationships as measured by TCI cooperativeness.

The three brain networks modulating character development are partially overlapping, so they are dissociable but may also function coherently. For example, the inferior parietal cortex is a prominent part of the networks proposed here to be associated with Cooperativeness and Self-transcendence. The inferior parietal cortex is hyperactive in individuals who feel they are being externally controlled, such as schizophrenics with delusions of passivity or alien control, or normal individuals under constrained experimental conditions (48–52). The representations of the current and predicted state of the motor system are encoded in the parietal cortex, whereas the representations of intended actions are found in the prefrontal and premotor cortex (49). The awareness of internal control of when an action is initiated is associated with the activation of the anterior cingulate and dorsolateral prefrontal cortex, whereas actions that are externally triggered do not activate these brain regions (53–55).

The control aspect of agency (i.e., awareness of the judicial control of motor responses), as measured by TCI Self-Transcendence, is associated with the activation of the anterior cingulate and dorsolateral prefrontal cortex, and is involved in the selective sculpting of motor responses (46,51). Likewise, the inhibitory control network of attention described by Posner depends on the same brain regions and is involved in the suppression or inhibition of conflicts, such as the inhibition of conditioned responses that are no longer adaptive. For example, a typical conflict test is measured by the Stroop task, which requires the subject to learn to respond to the color of ink (e.g., red) when the target is a competing color word (e.g., blue). Conflict is present when the cues are incongruent rather than when they are congruent. Such conflict tasks activate a distributed brain network, including the basal ganglia, the lateral prefrontal cortex, and the anterior cingulate gyrus (26,48, 51,56), just as does awareness of the judicial control of internally initiated movements. The lateral prefrontal cortex is particularly involved in working memory. The anterior cingulate is a place of convergence for motor control, homeostatic drive, emotion, and cognition (48,54,57). The judicial control network matures in late childhood along with self-aware consciousness, increasing substantially from ages 4 to 7 years and then stabilizing (26). Other work shows that flexibility and efficiency in carrying out multiple tasks develops around 4 years of age, along with the emergence of self-aware consciousness (58,59).

Hence, distributed brain networks regulating the three processes of agency, flexibility, and understanding can be experimentally activated, demonstrating predictably their role in the modulation of sensory, motor, emotional, cognitive, and integrative functions, which can be reliably measured by the three character dimensions of the TCI and their subscales. The convergence of the psychological results and the brain imaging results suggests that self-aware consciousness is truly three-dimensional and modulated by the character traits of TCI Self-directedness, Cooperativeness, and Self-transcendence.

PSYCHOGENIC PROCESSES IN MOVEMENT DISORDERS

The extent to which consciousness has real effects on physical movement has been experimentally examined in ground-breaking neurophysiologic studies by Benjamin Libet (60–64). Libet observed that there was a consistent sequence of observable phenomena prior to voluntary physical movements (62), as described by Mark Hallett elsewhere in this volume. Libet concluded that "cerebral initiation of a spontaneous, freely voluntary act can begin unconsciously, that is, before there is any (at least recallable) subjective awareness that a decision to act has already been initiated cerebrally." In other experiments, Libet concluded that it takes about 500 milliseconds for

the sensation evoked by any given external stimulus to reach conscious awareness, but that the time of the sensation is subjectively "back-referred" to the time of the stimulus, so that there does not seem subjectively to be a half-second lag in our awareness of the world (64,65). Both the studies of sensory stimulation of brain and brain activity prior to motor activity suggest that conscious awareness of sensorimotor events occurs after preparatory brain activity has already begun. Such data have been used to support the belief that consciousness is an inconsequential epiphenomenon of complex sequences of unconscious brain activity (66). We become consciously aware of wanting to move *after* the brain has already initiated its preparations for action, so how could consciousness represent anything but an illusion of agency and voluntary choice? This question has been called the "deep problem" in the concept of will, which is defined as voluntary agency or the capacity to choose what action to perform or withhold (67,68).

Libet's findings describe replicable phenomena that must be explained by any adequate theory of consciousness and mind–body relationships, but the interpretation of the results has been highly controversial, as evidenced by the acrimonious debates in an entire issue of the journal *Consciousness and Cognition* in June 2002 (65). In my opinion, the controversy over interpretation of Libet's replicable results has occurred because both Libet and other interpreters have assumed that self-aware consciousness is a dichotomous variable that is either fully present or totally absent. In fact, the movement of self-aware consciousness has multiple stages that are modulated by multiple quantitative variables, as described in the prior section, so treating consciousness as a dichotomous variable is inadequate, as evidenced by the controversy about the interpretation of the results. The interpretation of the findings becomes clarified once it is realized that the subject's self-reports indicate variably incomplete degrees of self-aware consciousness. Measures of individual differences in self-aware consciousness are needed in order to describe and interpret the timing of the five steps of development of self-aware consciousness in human thought. The onset of the readiness potential was usually substantially earlier than the awareness of wanting to move, but the difference varied from 1,010 milliseconds to only 15 milliseconds (62). Libet himself has begun to recognize the need to take personality into account in understanding such individual differences. For example, individual differences in self-transcendence (measured as tendency toward repression rather than sensory responsivity) are correlated moderately with length of sensory stimulation needed to elicit awareness of sensation (69). Less transcendent (i.e., more hysterical and repressive) subjects take longer to become aware of sensory stimulation.

The impression that self-aware consciousness occurs after the initiation of preparatory activity in the brain is, in my opinion, a misleading artifact of treating consciousness as a dichotomous variable that is either fully present or totally absent. TCI Self-directedness is moderately correlated with the P300, which may measure initial brain preparatory activity for action (70,71). For example, the amplitude of the P300 is positively correlated with TCI Self-directedness in parietal leads about 0.4 (18). In addition, TCI Self-directedness is positively correlated ($r = 0.6$) with total reaction times in tests of executive function requiring a simple motor response like a finger movement (19,42). When actions are capricious, the readiness potential consists mainly of the negative slope component. Similarly, contingent negative variation (CNV) in parietal leads is correlated with TCI Cooperativeness and Self-transcendence, but not Self-directedness (10). The parietal cortex is the region in which allocentric mapping of relationships occurs, which is necessary for cooperative behavior, as previously described.

Available data show that individual differences in TCI character scales will help us understand the stages of self-aware consciousness more rigorously than has been possible when consciousness is treated as a dichotomous variable. Much more work is needed about the higher stages of consciousness in which agency becomes increasingly spontaneous and free of emotional conflicts and intellectual deliberations. Little can be gained by assuming that consciousness is dichotomous and that everyone is equally aware.

In fact, there is substantial evidence that there are significant differences among individuals in their self-efficacy, and that self-efficacy can be enhanced voluntarily regardless of prior conditioning and biologic predisposition. Self-efficacy is the confidence that one can change and that one wants to change, which is a combination of basic confidence and awareness of flexibility in choice of what one wants. Self-efficacy corresponds to what is also called initiative, which is the beginning of the first stage of self-aware consciousness. Self-efficacy requires awareness of both personal agency (i.e., the will to be responsible and purposefully self-directed, rather than controlled by external circumstances) plus awareness of flexibility (i.e., the freedom to forgive oneself and change bad habits rather than continuing self-defeating behavior) in the intuitive and reasoning steps of thought (Table 15.1). In other words, individuals with self-efficacy should score average or higher on the TCI character subscales that modulate harm avoidance and novelty seeking (i.e., steps 1 and 2 in Table 12.1). Substantial evidence shows that individuals with substance dependence can give up the dependence without treatment if they have awareness of their self-efficacy. Success in quitting substance abuse can be predicted from a person's level of self-efficacy, not his or her degree of physiologic dependence on a substance of abuse, such as heroin (72) or tobacco (72–76).

Some people lack awareness of their self-efficacy because they lack the sense of responsibility (measured by the SD1 subscale) and sensibility (measured by the ST1

subscale). Such patients are usually described as having conversion disorders or as being hysterical and repressive (69). Patients with conversion disorders, such as nonepileptic seizures or "psychogenic" tremors, exhibit behaviors that appear to be voluntary but do not have explicit self-awareness of voluntary agency or motivation for their actions. They do have an intuitive awareness of what they are doing, which they can recall and describe vaguely as stated in the first section of this chapter (12). Their recall and descriptions lack contextual understanding as in children without full self-object differentiation, so they are often inconsistent historians. In the absence of explicit self-awareness, individuals with conversion disorders regard their actions as involuntary. The interpretation of their motivation is highly vulnerable to suggestions from others. EEG studies of individuals with conversion disorders have observed movement-related cortical readiness potentials that appear normal (77,78). Such readiness potentials do not indicate awareness of agency because patients with tics regard their movements as voluntary but frequently have a cortical readiness potential that is absent or brief (79). Differences between individuals in their awareness of agency are correlated with individual differences in the activation of the prefrontal cortex and parietal cortex (47,80), which are also highly correlated with TCI Self-directedness (19,41). Hysterical features are also correlated with sensory numbing and slower awareness of sensory stimulation (69).

A person can also voluntarily increase his or her awareness of self-efficacy. Most people can do this without treatment once they recognize that they have developed a maladaptive habit. For example 95% of cigarette smokers who quit do so on their own without any treatment (81). Among bulimics seeking treatment, the pretreatment level of TCI Self-directedness is the best predictor of success with cognitive–behavioral therapy (CBT) (82). Regardless of the initial level of character development, antidepressant medications and/or CBT increase the posttreatment levels of self-directedness, thereby establishing an upward spiral of increasing character development in ongoing therapy (82–84).

A BIOPSYCHOSOCIAL PARADIGM OF MOVEMENT DISORDERS

The quantitative measurement of personality provides a rigorous quantitative approach to understanding the psychobiology of psychogenic movement disorders. Individual differences in temperament and character distinguish patients with psychogenic movement disorders from others and identify quantitative variables that can be investigated in clinical practice. A fuller account of the biopsychosocial paradigm in neuropsychiatry is presented in detail elsewhere (4). Further information about the temperament and character inventory and how to order it can be obtained from the TCI website (85).

A major advantage of the perspective described in this chapter is its holistic biopsychosocial foundation. Dualistic distinctions between functional versus organic, imagined versus real, and psychogenic or neurologic are too reductionistic and are inevitably offensive to the sensibility of patients and counterproductive in their treatment. The brain networks that regulate attention, affect, and motor activity are well-measured by TCI character dimensions that are heritable but also influenced by each individual's unique variables, which can be voluntarily developed regardless of antecedent or initial conditions. The measurement of character allows recognition of contributions of character development to susceptibility to movement disorders, while also recognizing the important roles of free will and therapeutic guidance in character development. Patients with inadequate self-awareness can be encouraged to enter treatment to increase their awareness and decrease any psychogenic contribution to their disability. Many practical and theoretical lessons can be learned from the ongoing study of psychogenic movement disorders using a quantitative approach to personality measurement.

REFERENCES

1. Cloninger CR, Svrakic DM, Przybeck TR. A psychobiological model of temperament and character. *Arch Gen Psychiatry*. 1993; 50:975–990.
2. Cloninger CR, Przybeck TR, Svrakic DM, et al. *The temperament and character inventory: a guide to its development and use.* St. Louis, MO: Washington University Center for Psychobiology of Personality, 1994.
3. Tulving E. Episodic memory: from mind to brain. *Annu Rev Psychol*. 2002;53:1–25.
4. Cloninger CR. *Feeling good: the science of well being.* New York: Oxford University Press, 2004.
5. American Psychiatric Association. *Diagnostic and statistical manual of mental disorders.* Washington, DC: American Psychiatric Association, 1994.
6. Cloninger CR. The origins of DSM and ICD criteria for conversion and somatization disorders. In: Halligan PW, Bass C, Marshall JC, eds. *Contemporary approaches to the study of hysteria.* Oxford: Oxford University Press, 2001:49–62.
7. Cloninger CR, Sigvardsson S, von Knorring AL, et al. An adoption study of somatoform disorders: II. Identification of two discrete somatoform disorders. *Arch Gen Psychiatry*. 1984;41:863–871.
8. Cloninger CR, von Knorring AL, Sigvardsson S, et al. Symptom patterns and causes of somatization in men. II. Genetic and environmental independence from somatization in women. *Genet Epidemiol*. 1986;3:171–185.
9. Cloninger CR. The genetics and psychobiology of the seven factor model of personality. In: Silk KR, ed. *The biology of personality disorders.* Washington, DC: American Psychiatric Press, 1998:63–84.
10. Cloninger CR. Biology of personality dimensions. *Curr Opin Psychiatry*. 2000;13:611–616.
11. Cloninger CR. Functional neuroanatomy and brain imaging of personality and its disorders. In: D'haenen H, den Boer JA, Willner P, eds. *Biological psychiatry.* Chichester: John Wiley and Sons, 2002:1377–1385.
12. Cloninger CR. A unified biosocial theory of personality and its role in the development of anxiety states. *Psychiatr Dev*. 1986;3: 167–226.
13. Cloninger CR. A systematic method for clinical description and classification of personality variants: a proposal. *Arch Gen Psychiatry*. 1987;44:573–587.
14. Cloninger CR. Temperament and personality. *Curr Opin Neurobiol*. 1994;4:266–273.
15. Cloninger CR, ed. *Personality and psychopathology.* Washington, DC: American Psychiatric Press, 1999.
16. Gillespie NA, Cloninger CR, Heath AC, et al. The genetic and environmental relationship between Cloninger's dimensions of temperament and character. *Pers Individ Dif*. 2003;35:1931–1946.
17. Hansenne M. The P300 cognitive event-related potential. I. Theoretical and psychobiologic perspective. *Biol Psychol*. 1999; 50:143–155.
18. Vedeniapin AB, Anokhin AA, Sirevaag E, et al. Visual P300 and the self-directedness scale of the temperament-character inventory. *Psychiatry Res*. 2001;101:145–156.
19. Gusnard DA, Ollinger JM, Shulman GL, et al. Persistence and brain circuitry. *Proc Natl Acad Sci U S A*. 2003;100(6):3479–3484.
20. Hansenne M, Pinto E, Scantamburlo G, et al. Harm avoidance is related to mismatch negativity (MMN) amplitude in healthy subjects. *Pers Individ Dif*. 2003;34:1039–1048.
21. Turner RM, Hudson IL, Butler PH, et al. Brain function and personality in normal males: a SPECT study using statistical parametric mapping. *Neuroimage*. 2003;19:1145–1162.
22. Povinelli DJ. *Folk physics for apes: the chimpanzee's theory of how the world works.* New York: Oxford University Press, 2000.
23. Lehmann D, Grass P, Meier B. Spontaneous conscious covert cognition states and brain electric spectral states in canonical correlations. *Int J Psychophysiol*. 1995;19:41–52.
24. Lehmann D, Koenig T. Spatio-temporal dynamics of alpha brain electric fields and cognitive modes. *Int J Psychophysiol*. 1997; 26:99–112.
25. Lehmann D. Deviant microstates (atoms of thought) in brain electric field sequences of acute schizophrenics. *Eur Psychiatry*. 1998;13(Suppl. 4):197s–198s.
26. Posner MI, Fan J. Attention as an organ system. In: Pomerantz J, ed. *Neurobiology of perception and communication: from synapse to society.* Cambridge, MA: Cambridge University Press, 2003.
27. Borg J, Andree B, Soderstrom H, et al. The serotonin system and spiritual experiences. *Am J Psychiatry*. 2003;160(11):1965–1969.
28. Comings DE, Gonzales N, Saucier G, et al. The DRD4 gene and the spiritual transcendence scale of the character temperament index. *Psychiatr Genet*. 2000;10:185–189.
29. Ding YC, Chi HC, Grady DL, et al. Evidence for positive selection acting at the human dopamine receptor D4 gene locus. *Proc Natl Acad Sci U S A*. 2002;99:309–314.
30. Benjamin J, Osher Y, Kotler M, et al. Association of tridimensional personality questionnaire (TPQ) traits and three functional polymorphisms: dopamine receptor D4 (DRD4), serotonin transporter promoter region (5-HTTLPR) and catechol O-methyltransferase (COMT). *Mol Psychiatry*. 2000;5: 96–100.
31. Benjamin J, Ebstein EP, Belmaker RH et al., eds. *Molecular genetics and the human personality.* Washington, DC: American Psychiatric Publishing, 2002.
32. Caspi A, Sugden K, Moffitt TE, et al. Influence of life stress on depression: moderation by a polymorphism in the 5-HTT gene. *Science*. 2003;301:386–389.
33. Keltikangas-Jaervinen L, Raeikkoenen K, Ekelund J, et al. Nature and nurture in novelty seeking. *Mol Psychiatry*. 2004;9(3):308–311.
34. VanRullen R, Thorpe SJ. The time course of visual processing: from early perception to decision-making. *J Cogn Neurosci*. 2001; 13(4):454–461.
35. Vaillant GE, Milofsky E. Natural history of male psychological health: IX. Empirical evidence for Erikson's model of the life cycle. *Am J Psychiatry*. 1980;137:1348–1359.
36. Vaillant GE. *The wisdom of the ego.* Cambridge, MA: Harvard University Press, 1993.
37. Guillem F, Bicu M, Semkovska M, et al. The dimensional structure of schizophrenia and its association with temperament and character. *Schizophr Res*. 2002;56:137–147.
38. Burgess PW, Quayle A, Frith CD. Brain regions involved in prospective memory as determined by positron emission tomography. *Neuropsychologia*. 2001;39:545–555.

39. Maguire EA, Henson RN, Mummery CJ, et al. Activity in prefrontal cortex, not hippocampus, varies parametrically with the increasing remoteness of memories. *Neuroreport.* 2001;12(3):441–444.

40. Burgess PW, Scott SK, Frith CD. The role of the rostral frontal cortex (area 10) in prospective memory: a lateral versus medial dissociation. *Neuropsychologia.* 2003;41(8):906–918.

41. Gusnard DA, Akbudak E, Shulman GL, et al. Medial prefrontal cortex and self-referential mental activity: relation to a default mode of brain function. *Proc Natl Acad Sci USA.* 2001;98(7): 4259–4265.

42. Gusnard DA, Ollinger JM, Shulman GL, et al. Personality differences in functional brain imaging. *Soc Neurosc Abstr.* 2001; 27(80):11.

43. Marrocco RT, Davidson RJ. Neurochemistry of attention. In: Parasuraman R, ed. *The attention brain.* Cambridge, MA: MIT Press, 1998:35–50.

44. Davidson RJ, Marrocco RT. Local infusion of scopolamine into intraparietal cortex slows covert orienting in rhesus monkeys. *J Neurophysiol.* 2000;83:1536–1549.

45. Bottini G, Karnath HO, Vallar G, et al. Cerebral representations of egocentric space: functional-anatomical evidence from caloric vestibular stimulation and neck vibration. *Brain.* 2001;124(Pt 6): 1182–1196.

46. Farrer C, Frith CD. Experiencing oneself vs another person as being the cause of an action: the neural correlates of the experience of agency. *Neuroimage.* 2002;15(3):596–603.

47. Frith U, Frith CD. Development and neurophysiology of mentalizing. *Philos Trans R Soc Lond B.* 2003;358(1431):459–473.

48. Spence SA, Brooks DJ, Hirsch SR, et al. A PET study of voluntary movement in schizophrenic patients experiencing passivity phenomena (delusions of alien control). *Brain.* 1997;120(Pt 11): 1997–2011.

49. Frith CD, Blakemore S, Wolpert DM. Explaining the symptoms of schizophrenia: abnormalities in the awareness of action. *Brain Res Rev.* 2000;31(2–3):357–363.

50. Frith CD, Blakemore SJ, Wolpert DM. Abnormalities in the awareness and control of action. *Philos Trans R Soc Lond B.* 2000; 355(1404):1771–1788.

51. Nathaniel-James DA, Frith CD. The role of the dorsolateral prefrontal cortex: evidence from the effects of contextual constraint in a sentence completion task. *Neuroimage.* 2002;16(4):1094–1102.

52. Blakemore SJ, Oakley DA, Frith CD. Delusions of alien control in the normal brain. *Neuropsychologia.* 2003;41(8):1058–1067.

53. Jahanshahi M, Jenkins IH, Brown RG, et al. Self-initiated versus externally triggered movements. I: An investigation using measurement of regional cerebral blood flow with PET and movement-related potentials in normal and Parkinson's disease subjects. *Brain.* 1995;118:913–933.

54. Paus T. Primate anterior cingulate cortex: where motor control, drive and cognition interface. *Nat Rev Neurosci.* 2001;2:417–424.

55. Stephan V, Schall JD. Neuronal control and monitoring of initiation of movements. *Muscle Nerve.* 2002;26:326–339.

56. Fan J, Fossella J, Sommer T, et al. Mapping the genetic variation of executive attention onto brain activity. *Proc Natl Acad Sci U S A.* 2003;100:7406–7411.

57. MacLean PD. Brain evolution relating to family, play, and the separation call. *Arch Gen Psychiatry.* 1985;42:405–417.

58. Povinelli DJ, Simon BB. Young children's understanding of briefly versus extremely delayed images of the self: emergence of the autobiographical stance. *Dev Psychol.* 1998;34:188-194.

59. Povinelli DJ, Giambrone S. Reasoning about beliefs: a human specialization? *Child Dev.* 2001;72:691–695.

60. Libet B. Brain stimulation in the study of neuronal functions for conscious sensory experiences. *Hum Neurobiol.* 1982;1(4): 235–242.

61. Libet B, Wright EW Jr, Gleason CA. Readiness-potentials preceding unrestricted "spontaneous" vs. pre-planned voluntary acts. *Electroencephalogr Clin Neurophysiol.* 1982;54(3):322–335.

62. Libet B, Gleason CA, Wright EW, et al. Time of conscious intention to act in relation to onset of cerebral activity (readiness-potential): the unconscious initiation of a freely voluntary act. *Brain.* 1983;106(3):623–642.

63. Libet B, Wright EW Jr, Gleason CA. Preparation- or intention-to-act, in relation to pre-event potentials recorded at the vertex. *Electroencephalogr Clin Neurophysiol.* 1983;56(4):367–372.

64. Libet B. *Neurophysiology of consciousness: selected papers and new essays by benjamin Libet.* Boston, MA: Birkhauser, 1993.

65. Pockett S. On subjective back-referral and how long it takes to become conscious of a stimulus: a reinterpretation of Libet's data. *Conscious Cogn.* 2002;11:144–161.

66. Wegner DM. *The illusion of conscious will.* Cambridge, MA: The MIT Press, 2002.

67. Spence SA, Hunter MD, Harpin G. Neuroscience and the will. *Curr Opin Psychiatry.* 2002;15:519–526.

68. Hunter MD, Farrow TF, Papadakis NG, et al. Approaching an ecologically valid functional anatomy of spontaneous "willed" action. *Neuroimage.* 2003;20:1264–1269.

69. Shevrin H, Ghannam JH, Libet B. A neural correlate of consciousness related to repression. *Conscious Cogn.* 2002;11(2):334–341.

70. Fuster JM. Behavioral electrophysiology of the prefrontal cortex. *Trends Neurosci.* 1984;7:408–414.

71. Fuster JM. *The prefrontal cortex: anatomy, physiology, and neuropsychology of the frontal lobes.* New York: Lippincott–Raven Publishers, 1997.

72. Robins LN, Helzer JE, Davis DH. et al. Narcotic use in southeast Asia and afterward. An interview study of 898 Vietnam returnees. *Arch Gen Psychiatry.* 1995;32:955–961.

73. DiClemente CC, Prochasta JO, Gibertini M. Self-efficacy and the stages of self-change of smoking. *Cogn Ther Res.* 1985;9:181–200.

74. Kavanagh DJ, Pierce J, LO SK, et al. Self-efficacy and social support as predictors of smoking after a quit attempt. *Psychiatry Health.* 1993;8:231–242.

75. Hill HA, Schoenbach VJ, Kleinbaum DG, et al. A longitudinal analysis of predictors of quitting smoking among participants in a self-help intervention trial. *Addict Behav.* 1994;19:159–173.

76. Kenford SL, Fiore MC, Jorenby DE, et al. Predicting smoking cessation: who will quit with and without the nicotine patch. *J Am Med Assoc.* 1994;271:589–594.

77. Toro C, Torres F. Electrophysiological correlates of a paroxysmal movement disorder. *Ann Neurol.* 1986;20:731–734.

78. Terada K, Ikeda A, Van Ness PC, et al. Presence of bereitschafts potential preceding psychogenic myoclonus: clinical application of jerk-locked back averaging. *J Neurol Neurosurg Psychiatry.* 1995;58:745–747.

79. Karp BI, Porter S, Toro C, et al. Simple motor tics may be preceded by a premotor potential. *J Neurol Neurosurg Psychiatry.* 1996;61:103–106.

80. Spence SA, Crimlisk HL, Cope H, et al. Discrete neurophysiological correlates in prefrontal cortex during hysterical and feigned disorder of movement. *Lancet.* 2000;355:1243–1244.

81. Surgeon-General US. *Reducing the health consequences of smoking: 25 years of progress.* Washington, DC: US Department of Health and Human Services, 1989.

82. Bulik CM, Sullivan PF, Joyce PR, et al. Predictors of 1-year treatment outcome in bulimia nervosa. *Compr Psychiatry.* 1998;39: 206–214.

83. Tome MB, Cloninger CR, Watson JP, et al. Serotonergic autoreceptor blockade in the reduction of antidepressant latency: personality and response to paroxetine and pindolol. *J Affect Disord.* 1997;44:101–109.

84. Anderson CB, Joyce PR, Carter FA, et al. The effect of cognitive-behavioral therapy for bulimia nervosa on temperament and character as measured by the temperament and character inventory. *Compr Psychiatry.* 2002;43(3):182–188.

85. TCI Web site: www.psychobiology.wustl.edu.

Dissociation and Conversion in Psychogenic Illness

16

Richard J. Brown

ABSTRACT

The concepts of dissociation and conversion have been central to theories of unexplained illness since the late19th century. In this chapter, research and theory concerning the role of dissociation and conversion in unexplained illness is critically evaluated. Evidence for different aspects of the conversion model, including the role of la belle indifférence, psychological precipitation, conflict resolution, secondary gain, and childhood abuse in unexplained illness is reviewed. Although most of the empirical evidence for conversion theory is anecdotal, inconclusive, or contradictory, there is good evidence that childhood abuse is often reported by patients with unexplained symptoms. However, it is unclear what etiologic role childhood trauma plays in the development of these conditions. Studies investigating the occurrence of dissociative phenomena in patients with unexplained symptoms are then summarized and the conceptual and methodologic limitations of this research are explored. Problems with existing definitions of dissociation are identified and a recent attempt to provide a more precise definition of dissociation is described. By this view, depersonalization and derealization ("detachment" phenomena) are qualitatively different from dissociative symptoms characterized by an abnormal separation of material from conscious awareness ("compartmentalization" phenomena), and that only the latter are relevant to unexplained illness. Theory and research pertaining to this account of dissociation and psychogenic illness are then reviewed. This research provides good support for the idea that some, but not all, forms of "dissociation" are involved in the pathogenesis of unexplained symptoms.

INTRODUCTION

Although a psychological basis for medically unexplained illness has been recognized since the 17th century (1), a systematic psychological account of this phenomenon was lacking until the late 19th century and the work of Janet, Breuer, and Freud. According to Janet (2,3), unexplained symptoms are generated when traumatic events cause a fragmentation in the memory structures that constitute the patient's personality. By this view, trauma causes a spontaneous narrowing of attention (or "retraction in the field of consciousness") that prevents new information from being integrated with existing memories in the system. As a result, traumatic knowledge structures that are separated (or *dissociated*) from the rest of memory are created, with unexplained symptoms arising from the activation of these dissociated structures by internal or external events. According to Janet, a similar process of dissociation is responsible for comparable symptoms produced by hypnosis, which he regarded as a pathologic phenomenon possible only in "hysterical" individuals (the popularity of the terms "hysteria" and "hysterical," widely used at that time to refer to the phenomena and sufferers of psychogenic illness, have declined in recent years, for obvious reasons) (4,5).

Janet's model was later developed by Breuer and Freud (6), who argued that dissociation reflects the operation of a psychological defense mechanism rather than the disorganizing effects of trauma per se. According to this approach, dissociation protects the individual from the negative affect associated with memories of trauma by *converting* it into somatic symptoms; this process allows traumatic affect to be expressed without its origin being consciously acknowledged. The reduction of negative affect produced by this process represents the "primary gain" from developing symptoms; this is expressed as an apparent lack of concern about being symptomatic (so-called "la belle indifférence"). Symptoms may also reduce negative affect by resolving the emotional conflict giving rise to it. Thus, a wife who fears estrangement may develop symptoms that prevent her husband's departure, or employees who doubt their ability to meet important deadlines may develop symptoms that make it impossible for them to complete their work on time. According to conversion theory, the nature of the unexpressed emotion or conflict can often be inferred from the nature of the symptom, which is thought to be a symbolic representation of the underlying psychodynamics. Unexplained aphonia, for example, may be regarded as symbolic of an "unspeakable" past trauma, while a fixed dystonic fist could be viewed as an expression of unconscious anger. Once symptoms have developed, they may confer further benefits to the patient (e.g., social interaction, avoidance of unwanted activities, etc.) or "secondary gains." Importantly, conversion theory assumes that primary and secondary gains contribute to the development and maintenance of unexplained symptoms through *unconscious* psychological mechanisms.

Although over a century old, the concepts of dissociation and conversion continue to influence our understanding of psychogenic symptoms, and the way in which these conditions are classified and treated. Both the *Diagnostic and Statistical Manual of Mental Disorders*, Fourth Edition (DSM-IV), and the *International Classification of Diseases* (ICD-10) (7,8) include dissociative and conversion disorder categories that encompass some of the most common unexplained symptoms, for example, and both systems imply that a disruption of previously integrated mental functions (i.e., dissociation) or the transformation of traumatic affect (i.e., conversion) may be important etiological factors in these conditions. Despite this ongoing influence, it is unclear whether the concepts of dissociation and conversion provide an accurate and comprehensive account of these conditions. With this in mind, the current chapter reviews empirical evidence concerning the role of conversion and dissociation in psychogenic illness and considers whether these concepts provide a useful way of

understanding this phenomenon. As relatively few studies have addressed psychogenic movement disorders in isolation, research concerning the whole spectrum of medically unexplained syndromes will be considered.

EVIDENCE FOR CONVERSION THEORY

Several predictions from the conversion model have been investigated empirically, pertaining to the presence of la belle indifférence in patients with unexplained symptoms and the role of psychosocial stress, conflict resolution, secondary gain, and childhood abuse in the development of these conditions.

La Belle Indifférence

Studies indicate that between 6% and 41% of patients with psychogenic symptoms display an apparent lack of concern about their symptoms (9–12), suggesting that it is far from universal in these conditions. This wide variation in prevalence estimates probably reflects the different criteria used to select patients in these studies, and the use of subjective physician ratings of la belle indifférence without a clear operational definition of this phenomenon. Indeed, psychophysiologic research shows that physicians are actually quite poor at judging patients' attitude to their symptoms. Lader and Sartorius (13), for example, found that conversion disorder patients who were identified by their physicians as indifferent to their symptoms showed more physiologic symptoms of anxiety than did organic controls, in line with patients' own self-reports; a similar pattern of findings was obtained by Meares and Horvath (14) in patients with chronic conversion symptoms. Rice and Greenfield (15) also found that patients who were rated as indifferent to their symptoms showed more physiologic reactivity to emotional and illness stimuli than did organic controls, and there were few psychophysiologic differences between the two groups at rest. Thus, it may be that physician ratings of la belle indifférence reflect a confirmational bias resulting from a traditional psychiatric training in the features of psychogenic illness, rather than an accurate appraisal of patient behavior.

Other studies have shown that an apparent lack of concern about symptoms is also observed in patients with general medical conditions (16) and may be just as common in organic controls as in psychogenic illness (9,11). This clearly undermines the use of la belle indifférence as a diagnostic indicator in unexplained illness (17) and casts doubt on the theoretical significance of the phenomenon for these conditions.

Symptoms as Conflict Resolution

With the exception of case reports, only two published studies could be found that have empirically assessed whether unexplained symptoms solve an emotional conflict being faced by the sufferer (9,18). In a blinded, prospective study of this issue (9), it was found that conversion symptoms were significantly more likely to be rated as offering a solution to an ongoing conflict than organic symptoms; in addition, patients with conversion symptoms were more likely to report a history of previous unexplained symptoms occurring in response to psychosocial stressors than were organic controls. Although these findings seem encouraging, no information about how these ratings were made was included in the published report, making it difficult to confirm the validity of this study or to replicate its findings. A similar criticism can also be leveled at the only other study in this area (18), which apparently found evidence of symptoms serving a "defensive and expressive function" in patients with psychogenic illness. This study was also limited by its retrospective case-note design, an approach that would be particularly sensitive to physician biases in record-keeping and which might explain any recorded differences between the groups. The conflict resolution hypothesis is clearly difficult to assess, however, as demonstrated by the paucity of studies in this area.

Psychosocial Precipitation

Other studies have attempted to investigate whether unexplained symptoms are precipitated by psychosocial stressors. Evidence suggests that many unexplained symptoms develop at times of stress (9,11,12,18–20), although clinically it is often difficult to establish a clear etiologic link between such stressors and symptom onset (21,22). This is particularly problematic given that psychosocial stress is reported by a similar proportion of patients with established organic conditions (11,19,23). Although case-control studies of this sort do not rule out the possibility that psychosocial stress is an important factor in the development of unexplained symptoms, they clearly invalidate its role as a differential indicator in the diagnosis of these conditions. It remains a challenge for future researchers to develop meaningful but ethical methods for assessing the causal role of stress in the development of psychogenic illness.

Secondary Gain

The idea that unexplained symptoms are maintained by external benefits or secondary gains has been addressed in a number of studies. Although most studies have concluded that such gains are important in many cases of unexplained illness, the same appears to be true for general medical conditions (9,12,16,18,24,25). This pattern of findings appears to be more consistent with a learning theory account of illness behavior *per se* rather than a psychodynamic model of unexplained illness.

On the face of it, the available empirical evidence concerning la belle indifférence, conflict resolution, psychosocial precipitation, and secondary gain in psychogenic illness

is limited and raises important questions about the validity of conversion theory. Most clinicians working in this area have, however, encountered cases of unexplained illness where the role of psychodynamic and psychosocial factors seems unquestionable, and it remains an important task to address these factors in the assessment and treatment of these patients. Nevertheless, future researchers should aim to establish how, and to what extent, these factors are specific to psychogenic illness as opposed to emotional disturbance more generally.

Childhood Abuse

A substantial number of studies have investigated the occurrence of childhood abuse in patients with unexplained symptoms, providing probably the strongest support for the conversion concept. Table 16.1 summarizes cross-sectional studies that have directly compared the retrospective abuse histories of patients with psychogenic symptoms and those without unexplained complaints. All of the studies in this area have addressed the early Freudian hypothesis that childhood sexual abuse is an important etiologic factor in the development of psychogenic illness; a proportion of these studies have also addressed early physical and emotional abuse. Abuse in a range of unexplained syndromes has been considered, with the majority of studies addressing patients with chronic pelvic pain, functional gastrointestinal complaints, or nonepileptic attacks. With very few exceptions, these studies have shown that a history of childhood sexual abuse is reported significantly more often by patients with unexplained symptoms than by organic controls. A smaller proportion of studies have found that physical abuse histories are also more common in patients with psychogenic conditions, although the smaller number of studies in this area makes it more difficult to confirm the reliability of this difference. Other studies have reported a relationship between abuse history and the occurrence of unexplained symptoms, without reporting a direct comparison of patients with and without unexplained symptoms (50–58).

As most studies in this area have included an organic illness rather than a psychiatric control group, it is unclear whether the occurrence of childhood victimization is more common in psychogenic illness than in other emotional disorders. Moreover, many of these studies have measured abuse using unstandardized and poorly described clinical interviews, which are of questionable reliability and validity, or questionnaires that tend to underestimate the occurrence of abuse (59). Also problematic is the dichotomous coding of abuse as either present or absent, which is employed in most studies in this area. Such a practice precludes analyses concerning the role of abuse severity, frequency, and chronicity in the development of unexplained symptoms (60). Furthermore, although sexual and physical victimization are commonly reported by patients with unexplained symptoms, much less is known about exposure to

TABLE 16.1
SUMMARY OF CHILDHOOD ABUSE STUDIES[a]

Study	Psychogenic Condition	Group Difference in Sexual Abuse?	Group Difference in Physical Abuse?	Group Difference in Emotional Abuse?
Brown et al. (2005) (26)	Somatization disorder	✗	✓	✓
Pribor et al. (1993) (27)	Somatization disorder	✓	✓	✓
Morrison (1989a) (28)	Somatization disorder	✓	—	—
Drossman et al. (1996) (29)	Functional GI disorder	✓	✓	—
Talley et al. (1995) (30)	Functional GI disorder	✗	✗	✗
Drossman et al. (1990) (31)	Functional GI disorder	✓	—	—
Roelofs et al. (2002a) (32)	Motor conversion disorder	✓	✓	—
Binzer and Eisemann (1998) (33)	Motor conversion disorder	✗	✗	✓
Binzer et al. (2004) (34)	Nonepileptic attacks	—	—	✓
Kuyk et al. (1999) (35)	Nonepileptic attacks	✓	—	—
Reilly et al. (1999) (36)	Nonepileptic attacks	✓	✓	✓
Alper et al. (1993) (37)	Nonepileptic attacks	✓	✓	—
Betts and Boden (1992) (38)	Nonepileptic attacks	✓	—	—
Bodden-Heidrich et al. (1999) (39)	Chronic pelvic pain	✓	—	—
Ehlert et al. (1999) (40)	Chronic pelvic pain	✓	✗	—
Walker et al. (1995) (41)	Chronic pelvic pain	✓	✗	✗
Walker et al. (1992) (42)	Chronic pelvic pain	✓	—	—
Rapkin et al. (1990) (43)	Chronic pelvic pain	✗	✓	—
Walker et al. (1988) (44)	Chronic pelvic pain	✓	—	—
Harrop-Griffiths et al. (1988) (45)	Chronic pelvic pain	✓	—	—
Reiter et al. (1991) (46)	Nonorganic pelvic pain	✓	—	—
Total number of studies (proportion in parentheses)		16 (80%)	7 (64%)	5 (71%)

GI, gastrointestinal.
[a] Studies addressing the occurrence of childhood trauma in patients with DSM-IV-defined dissociative disorders (e.g., 47–49) are not included.

early emotional abuse in these patients. One study in this area used a single question to assess psychological abuse ("When you were a child did an older person insult, humiliate, or try to make you feel guilty?") (36), which is unlikely to provide an adequate measure of this phenomenon. Exposure to insults or criticism from an older sibling is unlikely to be as damaging as similar treatment from a parent, for example, a difference that is obscured by the single-question approach. More meaningful information has been obtained in two studies that have used questionnaire measures of perceived parental care (33,34), both finding that emotionally rejecting parents may contribute to the later development of unexplained symptoms. Nevertheless, further information about the role of emotional abuse in childhood is clearly required to assess which aspects of early victimization are most relevant to unexplained illness. It is possible, for example, that the relatively high prevalence of childhood sexual trauma reflects a pathogenic early environment more generally for patients with unexplained illness rather than the etiologic importance of sexual abuse per se (61). Other dimensions of childhood experience may also be important in unexplained illness, including early losses and parental neglect.

In order to address some of these issues, we (26) have recently conducted a study investigating the occurrence of child abuse in patients with somatization disorder using the Childhood Trauma Interview (CTI) (60). The CTI is a validated, semistructured interview measure that assesses six domains of early interpersonal trauma: separations/ losses, neglect, emotional abuse, physical abuse, witnessing violence, and sexual abuse. Participants are asked a series of probe questions within each trauma domain, followed by a set of follow-up questions depending on participant responses; questions are repeated until information about all perpetrators within each domain has been obtained. All responses are coded using a detailed manual. In this way, information about trauma frequency, severity, chronicity, and number of perpetrators within each domain can be obtained; these pieces of information can also be used to calculate composite exposure scores for each form of trauma. Using this approach, it was found that patients with somatization disorder reported significantly more severe forms of childhood physical abuse than did organic controls, but had not experienced more severe forms of emotional or sexual abuse. When composite trauma scores were compared, there was no significant difference between the two groups in overall exposure to early sexual or physical abuse. In contrast, the somatization group had significantly higher emotional abuse exposure scores than the controls did, suggesting that they had been exposed to this form of abuse far more often and over a much longer period. There were no differences among the groups in terms of exposure to early separations/losses or violence committed against others. Taken together, these findings seem to suggest that exposure to a distant and critical early environment characterized by frequent rejection, humiliation, and physical punishment may be more important in the development of unexplained illness than sexual abuse itself. Future research adopting a similar approach with less severe cases of unexplained illness is clearly warranted. Importantly, the use of dimensional measures such as the CTI allow for comparisons among conditions and assessment of the obvious hypothesis that more severe forms of unexplained illness will be associated with a greater degree of early trauma.

One of the limitations of this study, as with all of the abuse studies described so far, is the use of retrospective and subjective trauma reports. The reliability of such reports has been the subject of fierce debate over the years (59,62–64), encompassing the possibility of distortions and biases in recall due to psychological state, personality, the type of recall cues available, and the way in which questions are asked, in addition to the simple degradation of memory over time. One way around this problem is to conduct prospective studies addressing the occurrence of unexplained symptoms following independently corroborated episodes of trauma. This approach was adopted by Rimsza et al. (51), who found that sexually abused children and adolescents were more likely to develop somatic complaints than were matched controls who had not experienced abuse. In contrast, a much larger, prospective cohort study conducted by Raphael et al. (65) failed to find evidence for a link between early victimization and the subsequent development of unexplained pain symptoms. (The author is grateful to Fred Ovsiew for bringing this study to his attention.)

In this study, a large group (n = 676) of individuals with a history of early sexual abuse, physical abuse, or neglect that was documented in criminal justice system records was interviewed 20 years postvictimization using the revised version of the diagnostic interview schedule (DIS-III-R) (66) and validated, retrospective self-report measures of childhood trauma. This group was compared to a matched control group (n = 520) which did not have a documented history of abuse or neglect but which was broadly comparable in other respects. No significant differences were found in the number of unexplained pain symptoms reported by control participants and those who had a documented history of abuse or neglect. There was a trend for physically abused participants to report more problematic pain symptoms (either explained or unexplained) than were reported by control participants, but this was not significant after controlling for multiple comparisons. In contrast, participants who self-reported early abuse or neglect on the retrospective measures had significantly more unexplained pain symptoms than did those who did not report early victimization.

These findings appear to cast doubt on the hypothesized relationship between unexplained illness (at least in the form of psychogenic pain) and early victimization, as well as the reliability of the retrospective trauma reports made by patients with these conditions. One obvious problem with this interpretation is the fact that group allocation was based on court-recorded instances of childhood abuse or neglect, an approach that will inevitably identify only a small proportion of patients who have been exposed to early victimization. As a result, it is likely that many of the control participants had also experienced significant abuse, which would have contaminated any comparison of symptom reports based only on documented abuse history. In fact, 49% of the control participants in this study reported early abuse on the retrospective measures, compared to only 73% of the participants with a documented history of victimization. Not only does this suggest that many of the control participants had been abused, but it also shows that many of the abused group failed to report their early experiences of victimization. This is consistent with research showing that retrospective reports tend to underestimate rather than overestimate the occurrence of early trauma (59). Indeed, this may be particularly likely in patients with unexplained symptoms due to psychogenic amnesia or defense mechanisms such as repression. If this is the case, the difference between patients with unexplained illness and controls in terms of exposure to early abuse may be even more marked than the available studies suggest.

Ultimately, we have no reason to doubt the available evidence concerning the occurrence of abuse in patients with unexplained symptoms unless we assume that these individuals are more likely to fabricate episodes of abuse than are other psychiatric patients. As there is no evidence to suggest that this is the case, we must take the abuse reports of patients with unexplained symptoms at face value. Equally, however, the available evidence demonstrates that many patients with unexplained symptoms have not experienced significant childhood victimization. Thus, when patients deny such experiences, we must not assume that they are necessarily repressing early memories of abuse simply because of a theoretical tradition that propounds this view. Evidently, there is more to the development of unexplained illness than difficult experiences in childhood.

Efficacy of Dynamic Psychotherapy

A common argument cited in favor of the conversion model is that some cases of unexplained illness respond well to psychodynamic therapies that focus on helping the patient identify, explore, and work through the emotional conflicts underlying their symptoms. There are many case reports attesting to the apparent efficacy of psychodynamic therapy with this group of conditions, apparently supporting the conversion model. There is also evidence from clinical trials to suggest that dynamic psychotherapy can be effective in treating conditions such as irritable bowel syndrome (67), which may be part of the somatoform spectrum. Randomized controlled trials investigating the efficacy of dynamic psychotherapy in patients with more clear-cut medically unexplained symptoms are sadly lacking, however. Until such studies are conducted, the efficacy of this therapeutic approach in psychogenic illness remains to be demonstrated.

EVIDENCE FOR DISSOCIATION THEORY

Questionnaire Studies

The fact that many patients with unexplained symptoms report childhood victimization is consistent with both conversion theory and its conceptual precursor, dissociation theory. Other studies have attempted to validate dissociation theory by demonstrating that patients with psychogenic illness have a tendency to experience "dissociative" states more generally. The majority of studies in this area have used the Dissociative Experiences Scale (DES) (68), a 28-item self-report measure encompassing different types of dissociative phenomena. Each item describes a specific dissociative experience, and participants are asked to rate the proportion of time that they encounter that experience in everyday life on a scale ranging from 0% to 100%. The DES is premised on the concept of the "dissociative continuum," the idea that the various dissociative phenomena included in the DES are qualitatively similar, differing only in terms of severity and associated disability (Fig. 16.1).

At one end of the continuum are dissociative experiences such as daydreaming and absorption that are experienced by most people and are therefore considered "normal" phenomena. At the other end of the continuum are highly pathologic states of dissociation, including extensive periods of amnesia and major alterations in identity, which are only experienced by individuals with relatively rare conditions such as dissociative identity disorder (DID). Other dissociative phenomena, such as relatively brief episodes of amnesia and states of depersonalization/derealization, fall between these two extremes. According to this approach,

total DES scores provide a measure of an individual's capacity to experience dissociation in general, with higher scores indicating a tendency to experience more profound and clinically disabling dissociative phenomena. A large number of studies have been conducted using the DES, apparently validating this approach to measuring dissociative capacity. Scores on the DES reliably differentiate between patients with dissociative disorders and psychiatric controls, for example, while more severe forms of dissociative psychopathology (e.g., DID) are associated with higher DES scores than are less severe forms such as posttraumatic stress disorder (PTSD) and dissociative disorder not otherwise specified (DD NOS; Fig. 16.2) (69).

A list of studies that have used the DES to measure dissociation in patients with unexplained symptoms is provided in Table 16.2. Also included are two studies (35,72) that measured dissociative capacity using the Dissociation Questionnaire (DIS-Q) (80), a self-report measure of dissociation similar to the DES and correlating at 0.85 with that scale. In general, this research does not provide strong support for the hypothesis that patients with unexplained symptoms have greater levels of dissociativity than do comparable organic illness populations. Indeed, only one third of studies found a significant group difference. Moreover, according to these studies, the average DES score for patients with medically unexplained symptoms is within the normal range and even slightly lower than that found in many other psychiatric conditions. In the main, patients with nonepileptic attack disorder (NEAD) have a higher DES score than other somatoform patients, although only slightly higher than the average seen in patients with depression or schizophrenia. In addition, NEAD patients did not score significantly higher than epilepsy controls in two out of the three studies that compared these groups.

These findings based on DES and DIS-Q scores appear to cast doubts on the idea that dissociation is a basic feature of medically unexplained illness. Research investigating the occurrence of unexplained symptoms in patients with dissociative disorders suggests a rather different story, however. Evidence indicates, for example, that patients with dissociative disorders can be reliably differentiated from psychiatric controls using the Somatoform Dissociation Questionnaire (SDQ-20) (81–83), a measure of unexplained neurologic symptomatology. Other studies have shown that patients with multiple personality disorder

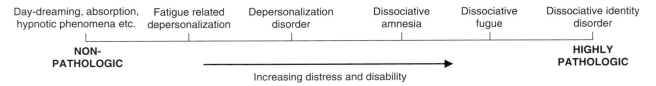

Figure 16.1 The Hypothetical Dissociative Continuum (not to scale).

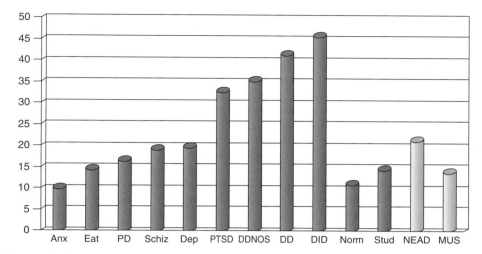

Figure 16.2 Graph Showing Average DES Scores across Conditions. Somatoform conditions shown in white. Anx, anxiety disorders; Eat, eating disorders; PD, personality disorders; Schiz, schizophrenia; Dep, depression; PTSD, posttraumatic stress disorder; DDNOS, dissociative disorder, not otherwise specified; DD, dissociative disorder; DID, dissociative identity disorder; Norm, normals; Stud, normal students; NEAD, nonepileptic attack disorder; MUS, medically unexplained symptoms (excluding NEAD). [Adapted from van Ijzendoorn MH, Schuengel C. The measurement of dissociation in normal and clinical populations: Meta-analytic validation of the Dissociative Experiences Scale (DES). *Clin Psychol Rev.* 1996;16:365–382.]

TABLE 16.2

QUESTIONNAIRE STUDIES OF DISSOCIATION IN PATIENTS WITH DIFFERENT PSYCHOGENIC CONDITIONS

Study	Condition	Dissociation Scale	Mean DES Score	Significant Group Difference?
Salmon et al. (2003) (70)	Irritable bowel syndrome	DES	13–15[a]	✓
Roelofs et al. (2002b) (71)	Motor conversion disorder	DES	11.7	✗
Moene et al. (2001) (72)	Motor conversion disorder	DIS-Q	—	✗
Goldstein et al. (2000) (73)	Nonepileptic attack disorder	DES	22.6	✓
Spitzer et al. (1999) (74)	Motor conversion disorder	DES	16.5	✓
Kuyk et al. (1999) (35)	Nonepileptic attack disorder	DIS-Q	—	✗
Alper et al. (1997) (75)	Nonepileptic attack disorder	DES	15.1	✗
Bowman and Markand (1996) (76)	Nonepileptic attack disorder	DES	20.2	No comparison group
Walker et al. (1995) (77)	Irritable bowel syndrome	DES	10.5	✗
Pribor et al. (1993) (27)	Somatization disorder	DES	Not recorded	✗
Bowman (1993) (78)	Nonepileptic attack disorder	DES	26.7	No comparison group
Walker et al. (1992) (42)	Chronic pelvic pain	DES	19	✓
Brown et al. (unpub)[b]	Somatization disorder	DES-VQ	10.4	✗
	average across all conditions	DES	16.7	Proportion significant = 36%[c]
	average in NEAD studies	DES	21.1	—
	average in non-NEAD studies	DES	13.7	—

DES, Dissociative Experiences Scale; DIS-Q, Dissociation Questionnaire; DES-VQ, Dissociative Experiences Scale with verbal qualifiers (79); NEAD, Nonepileptic attack disorder.
[a]Mean score not given (range represents estimate taken from graph.)
[b]Brown RJ, Schrag A, Trimble MR. Unpublished data from the National Hospital of Neurology and Neurosurgery, London, 2001.
[c]Not including studies without comparison groups.

(dissociative identity disorder in DSM-IV) have an average of 15 unexplained symptoms (84), while up to 64% of dissociative disorders patients meet criteria for somatization disorder (85). How are these apparently contradictory findings to be reconciled?

One possible explanation is the relatively limited range of dissociative experiences encompassed by the DES. Out of all of the unexplained neurologic symptoms, only unexplained amnesia is included in the scale, which was one of the primary motivations behind the development of the SDQ-20 (81). There is also an issue about the wording of DES items. All of the items on the scale consist of a statement describing a dissociative experience (e.g., "Some people have the experience of feeling that their body does not seem to belong to them"), followed by a prompt asking them to indicate how often they have that experience on a day-to-day basis ("Place a cross to show how much of the time this happens to you"). As such, the wording of the DES clearly implies that participants are to rate how often they have had particular dissociative experiences in the recent past, rather than in their life more generally. Although patients with a history of medically unexplained symptoms may have had many of the experiences included in the DES in the past, if they had not experienced them recently, their score on the measure would be low. This may obscure any differences between groups in terms of their tendency to experience dissociative events in general. Such an explanation could account for the elevated DES scores of patients presenting with nonepileptic attacks and/or dissociative amnesia when compared to patients with other somatoform symptoms, who may have a history of unexplained seizures or memory loss but no ongoing problems in these areas.

Detachment and Compartmentalization

This cannot be the whole story, however. Like the DES, the SDQ-20 implies that participants should consider recent symptoms only, and unexplained neurologic symptom scores on this scale are consistently elevated in patients with conditions such as dissociative amnesia and dissociative identity disorder. According to one recent account (86), the contradictory findings in this area could be attributed to the way in which the DES conflates different kinds of phenomena within the same unitary measure of "dissociation." By this view, the DES contains items pertaining to at least two qualitatively distinct forms of dissociation, known as "detachment" and "compartmentalization" (87–91). Detachment phenomena are characterized by an altered state of consciousness associated with a sense of separation from the self, the body, or the world. Depersonalization, derealization, and out-of-body experiences constitute archetypal examples of detachment in this account. Evidence suggests that these phenomena are generated by a common pathophysiologic mechanism involving the top-down

inhibition of limbic emotional processing by frontal brain systems (92). This mechanism serves to dampen down potentially disorganizing emotion in circumstances of extreme threat, allowing for more adaptive behavioral control. In benign circumstances, however, this process serves to strip normal stimuli of their emotional significance, creating a potentially pathologic state of detachment. Compartmentalization phenomena, in contrast, are characterized by an impairment in the ability to control processes or actions that would usually be amenable to such control and which are otherwise functioning normally. This category encompasses unexplained neurologic symptoms (including dissociative amnesia) and benign phenomena such as those produced by hypnotic suggestion, all of which involve a common psychological mechanism that is fundamentally different from that responsible for detachment. By this view, therefore, the traditional dissociative continuum misrepresents the nature of dissociation by incorporating qualitatively distinct phenomena within the same scale. According to these authors, a more appropriate approach is to conceive of two separate continua, one each for detachment and compartmentalization phenomena of varying degrees of severity and disability.

Evidence suggests that these two forms of "dissociation" are separable empirically as well as conceptually (86). Several factor analytic studies of the DES, for example, have found two statistically separable factors corresponding to detachment (i.e., depersonalization/derealization) and compartmentalization (i.e., amnesia) symptoms, and a third factor encompassing various experiences associated with the normal phenomenon of absorption (e.g., 93–96). Other studies have shown that clinically significant compartmentalization phenomena often occur in the absence of detachment symptoms. Brown et al. (26), for example, administered the Structured Clinical Interview for DSM-IV Dissociative Disorders (SCID-D) (97) to a group of patients with somatization disorder presenting with unexplained neurologic symptoms and a matched group of organic controls. In this study, almost 50% of somatization disorder participants reported a history of moderate to severe dissociative amnesia, which was significantly more common than in the control group. In comparison, moderate to severe depersonalization and derealization were relatively rare in the somatization disorder participants, and were equally common in the controls. Thus, the somatization disorder participants had a history of other compartmentalization symptoms (in addition to their presenting complaints), but showed no evidence of having experienced abnormal levels of detachment.

Viewed from this perspective, the fact that patients with unexplained symptoms rarely have significantly greater total DES scores than do controls is easily understood. By this view, the total DES score does not provide a useful measure of the kind of dissociation that is involved in psychogenic illness. Although the score is partly determined by amnesia experiences—a phenomenon involving a similar process of "dissociation" to other unexplained neurologic symptoms (i.e., compartmentalization)—it is also contaminated by items pertaining to detachment and absorption phenomena, neither of which involves this process. Even amnesia factor scores derived from the DES cannot provide an adequate measure of an individual's propensity to compartmentalization, as they encompass only a very limited part of this phenomenon. A more valid measure of the tendency to experience compartmentalization would be the SDQ-20, which almost entirely comprises items pertaining to this process. This is reflected in the consistently elevated SDQ-20 score of patients with dissociative disorders.

The Nature of Compartmentalization

Ultimately, even the SDQ-20 can only provide a measure of the tendency to experience certain kinds of symptoms; despite its name, it says nothing about the mechanisms responsible for those symptoms. What is known about the processes involved in compartmentalization? Our current understanding of this phenomenon owes much to Hilgard's neodissociation theory (98) and its conceptual derivative dissociated control theory (99–101), both of which provide an explicit reworking of Janet's original approach in contemporary cognitive psychological terms. According to neodissociation theory, the cognitive system comprises a large set of control modules ("schemas") organized beneath an executive system associated with attention, consciousness, and volition. The processing modules are organized in a nested hierarchy, with high-level schemas consisting of organized information about the processing involved in executing global acts (e.g., driving a car) and intermediate schemas detailing the processing involved in specific components of those acts (e.g., changing gears, reversing, etc.). Although the executive ego selects the most appropriate schemas to deal with current processing concerns, once

those schemas have been selected, they can function with a large degree of autonomy from the executive. This "dissociation" between the executive ego and control schemas preserves cognitive resources by allowing well-learned acts to be performed effortlessly, concurrently, and without awareness. In this model, therefore, dissociation is a fundamental aspect of cognitive processing in general, rather than a pathologic product of traumatic events or maneuvers designed to protect the individual from emotionally unacceptable material. Although Hilgard's model was originally developed to account for the alterations in mental activity often encountered in the hypnotic context, this approach can also be applied to unexplained symptoms. By this view, unexplained symptoms reflect an abnormal dissociation between the executive ego and the control systems responsible for processing certain kinds of information. In conversion blindness, for example, the visual system continues to process information as normal, but the executive ego is unable to receive that information due to an inhibitory process that prevents the systems from communicating with each other (Fig. 16.3); as consciousness is associated with the receipt of information by the executive, the individual experiences a subjective sense of blindness.

However, the visual system remains intact and is able to influence behavior through its effect on other processing modules in the system; in this sense, visual processing has become "compartmentalized." A similar explanation can easily be applied to other forms of unexplained sensory loss and phenomena such as dissociative amnesia, paralysis, certain seizures, and so on (101,102).

There is good evidence in support of this approach to psychogenic illness. A number of case studies, for example, have shown that patients with unexplained sensory loss display intact processing in the apparently damaged perceptual modality, a phenomenon known as "implicit processing" (102). Patients with conversion blindness, for example, will often display below-chance responding

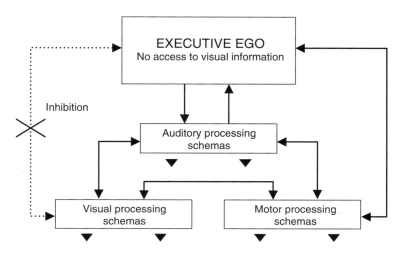

Figure 16.3 Neodissociation Account of Unexplained Blindness. (Adapted from Hilgard ER. *Divided Consciousness: multiple controls in human thought and action.* New York: John Wiley and Sons, 1977.)

in a forced-choice recognition paradigm, demonstrating an implicit sensitivity to complex visual information. Importantly, the preserved processing in these patients tends to be much more sophisticated than that observed in cases of blindsight associated with striate lesions (103). A similar effect has also been found in patients with unexplained deafness. An even more compelling demonstration of compartmentalization has been reported by Kuyk et al. (104), who compared patients with amnesia following nonepileptic attacks to a matched group of patients with amnesia following generalized epileptic seizures. Subjects in both groups were hypnotized and given suggestions designed to facilitate the recovery of information about events occurring during a recent seizure. While none of the epilepsy patients were able to recall ictal information under hypnosis, 85% of the nonepileptic attack group recovered significant amounts of previously unavailable material during the procedure; this material was corroborated by independent observers who had witnessed the seizure in question. This study clearly demonstrates that the amnesia associated with nonepileptic attacks is due to a retrieval deficit that prevents stored information from being accessed by the individual; until that information is accessed (e.g., by hypnotic suggestion), it remains "compartmentalized" within the cognitive system and unavailable to deliberate recall. In contrast, the amnesia resulting from a generalized epileptic event reflects a disruption in encoding during the seizure; as a result, no ictal information is available for later recall during hypnosis. This study is particularly important, as it also demonstrates that hypnotic suggestion can be used to access compartmentalized information, which has obvious clinical implications. However, as the role of hypnosis and hypnotizability in the etiology and treatment of psychogenic illness will be discussed elsewhere in this volume, they will not be considered further here.

Support for the compartmentalization model also comes from psychophysiologic research showing that only the later (300 ms or more), postconscious components of the auditory event-related potential are abnormal in patients with unexplained hearing loss (105). This is clearly consistent with the idea that unexplained symptoms are associated with a deficit in high-level cognition (i.e., at the level of the executive ego), despite preserved low-level processing (i.e., at the level of schema control). Put another way, it suggests that psychogenic illness is associated with a deficit in attentional, conscious processing and the preservation of preattentive, preconscious processes (91,106,107). This is in line with other studies showing that patients with unexplained symptoms often show a deficit on cognitive tasks involving an executive/explicit processing component or selective attention (108–110).

Although the compartmentalization concept is able to explain most "negative" unexplained symptoms (i.e., those involving an abnormal loss of certain functions, e.g., sensory loss, paralysis, amnesia, etc.), it is less obvious how this approach can account for symptoms where there is the abnormal *presence* of something that should be absent (i.e., "positive" symptoms, e.g., pseudohallucinations, tremor, dystonia, abnormal gait, etc.). How could such symptoms be generated by the abnormal separation (i.e., compartmentalization) of processing within the cognitive system? According to Brown (91,107), there is very little difference between these two forms of unexplained symptoms in terms of basic underlying mechanisms. By this view, all symptoms result from a loss of normal high-level attentional control over low-level processing systems; in this sense, all symptoms can be thought of as involving a form of compartmentalization. In each case, this "dissociation" between high- and low-level control results from the repetitive reallocation of high-level attention onto "rogue representations" in memory, causing low-level attention to misinterpret this stored information as an account of current rather than past processing activity. This misinterpretation is experienced as a distortion in consciousness (e.g., in the body image) or a loss of high-level control over any process that has been mistakenly identified as damaged by low-level systems. In this account, the only difference between positive and negative unexplained symptoms is in the rogue representation responsible for the symptom in question. Thus, a negative motor symptom may result from the chronic activation of a representation specifying movement inhibition, whereas the chronic activation of a representation specifying movement initiation might be implicated in a positive motor symptom. In both cases, however, there is a loss of high-level control over processing systems that are essentially undamaged and which can therefore be regarded as compartmentalized.

SUMMARY AND CONCLUSIONS

In this chapter, evidence pertaining to the conversion and dissociation models of unexplained illness has been described and evaluated. The available evidence does not provide strong support for conversion theory. Contrary to this approach, la belle indifférence is no more common in patients with medically unexplained symptoms than in those with general medical conditions; moreover, many patients who display apparent indifference to their symptoms are actually experiencing considerable anxiety. In contrast, there is some evidence to suggest that unexplained symptoms are often preceded by stressful psychosocial events and/or are associated with possible intrinsic and extrinsic gains. The available research demonstrates, however, that many cases of organic illness also develop at times of stress and have the potential to be maintained by the advantages associated with the sick role. As such, it is impossible to determine whether these factors play a central etiological role in the development of unexplained symptoms or relate to illness behavior more generally. That notwithstanding, there is good evidence to suggest that many patients with unexplained symptoms have experienced sexual, physical, and/or psychological abuse in childhood, which may be important in the pathogenesis of these conditions. More research addressing the impact of psychological abuse in unexplained illness is required, as is work concerning the role of abuse severity, frequency, and chronicity. At present, it is unclear what role early trauma plays in the development of psychogenic illness. According to conversion theory, unexplained symptoms reflect the operation of a primitive defense mechanism that facilitates the avoidance of traumatic affect. Dissociation theory, in contrast, suggests that trauma has a more general disorganizing effect on the cognitive system that is associated with the development of unexplained symptoms. At our current level of knowledge, it is impossible to determine whether either of these explanations is an appropriate account of the relationship between early trauma and psychogenic illness. Similarly, without further research into the efficacy of psychodynamic therapy, it is impossible to evaluate the available case material concerning the resolution of unexplained symptoms in response to this therapeutic approach.

Several studies have attempted to assess whether patients with unexplained symptoms experience more "dissociative" phenomena than do patients with general medical conditions. In the main, studies using the Dissociative Experiences Scale have not found a higher rate of dissociativity in patients with unexplained symptoms, in apparent contradiction of dissociation theory. However, studies using the Somatoform Dissociation Questionnaire or other unexplained symptom counts to investigate the occurrence of psychogenic illness in patients with dissociative disorders demonstrate that these conditions often co-occur and are probably part of the same spectrum of complaints. One recent classification suggests that the indifferent findings using the DES can be partly attributed to the scale conflating two qualitatively distinct forms of dissociation—detachment and compartmentalization—with only the latter being relevant to unexplained illness. By this view, definitions of dissociation need to be much more precise than those adopted in current psychiatric taxonomies. A number of theoretical, clinical, cognitive, and psychophysiologic studies indicate that the concept of compartmentalization provides a useful description of the mechanisms underlying psychogenic illness. One important component of the compartmentalization process appears to be a disturbance in high-level, explicit cognition alongside the preservation of low-level implicit processing.

According to the approach outlined here, the unqualified use of the term "dissociation" can only lead to further confusion about the nature and mechanisms of the different phenomena that have been associated with the label over the years. In contrast, the terms "dissociative detachment" and "dissociative compartmentalization" provide a language that would allow for unambiguous communication among researchers, clinicians, and patients in this area.

REFERENCES

1. Merskey H. *The analysis of hysteria*. London: Balliere, Tindall & Cassell, 1979.
2. Janet P. *L'automatisme psychologique*. Paris, NE: Felix Alcan, 1889.
3. Janet P. *The major symptoms of hysteria*. New York: Macmillan, 1907.
4. Brown RJ, Ron MA. Conversion and Somatoform Disorders. In: Ramachandran VS, ed. *Encyclopedia of the human brain*, Vol. 2. San Diego, CA: Academic Press, 2002:37–49.
5. Stone J, Wojcik W, Durrance D, et al. What should we say to patients with symptoms unexplained by disease? The "number needed to offend." *Br Med J*. 2002;325:1449–1550.
6. Breuer J, Freud S. Studies on hysteria. In: Strachey J, Strachey A, eds. *The standard edition of the complete psychological works of Sigmund Freud*, (Vol. 2). London: Hogarth Press & the Institute of Psycho-Analysis, 1893–1895/1955.
7. American Psychiatric Association. *Diagnostic and statistical manual of mental disorders*, 4th ed. Washington, DC: American Psychiatric Association, 1994.
8. World Health Organisation. *The ICD-10 classification of mental and behavioural disorders: clinical descriptions and diagnostic guidelines*. Geneva: World Health Organisation, 1992.
9. Raskin M, Talbott JA, Meyerson AT. Diagnosis of conversion reactions. Predictive value of psychiatric criteria. *J Am Med Assoc.* 1966;197:530–534.
10. Lewis WC, Berman M. Studies of conversion hysteria: I. Operational study of diagnosis. *Arch Gen Psychiatry.* 1965;13:275–282.
11. Chabrol H, Peresson G, Clanet M. Lack of specificity of the traditional criteria for conversion disorders. *Eur Psychiatry.* 1995;10: 317–319.
12. Sharma P, Chaturvedi SK. Conversion disorder revisited. *Acta Psychiatr Scand.* 1995;92:301–304.
13. Lader M, Sartorius N. Anxiety in patients with hysterical conversion symptoms. *J Neurol, Neurosurg & Psychiatry.* 1968;31:490–495
14. Meares R, Horvath T. "Acute" and "chronic" hysteria. *Br J Psychiatry.* 1972;121:653.
15. Rice DG, Greenfield NS. Psychophysiological correlates of la belle indifférence. *Arch Gen Psychiatry.* 1969;20:239–245.
16. Gould R, Miller BM, Goldberg MA, et al. The validity of hysterical signs and symptoms. *J Nerv Ment Dis.* 1986;174:593–597.
17. Lazare A. Conversion symptoms. *N Engl J Med.* 1981;305: 745–748.
18. Bishop ER, Torch EM. Dividing "hysteria": a preliminary investigation of conversion disorder and psychalgia. *J Nerv Ment Dis.* 1979;167:348–356.
19. Watson CG, Buranen C. The frequency and identification of false positive conversion reactions. *J Nerv Ment Dis.* 1979;167: 243–247.
20. Factor SA, Podskalny GD, Molho ES. Psychogenic movement disorders: frequency, clinical profile, and characteristics. *J Neurol Neurosurg Psychiatry.* 1995;59:406–412.
21. Ron MA. Somatisation in neurological practice. *J Neurol Neurosurg Psychiatry.* 1994;57:1161–1164.
22. Wessely SM. Discrepancies between diagnostic criteria and clinical practice. In: Halligan PW, Bass C, Marshall J, eds. *Contemporary approaches to the study of hysteria: clinical and theoretical perspectives.* Oxford, UK: Oxford University Press, 2001:63–72.
23. Slater E. Diagnosis of hysteria. *Br Med J.* 1965;1:1395–1399.
24. Eisendrath SJ, Valan MN. Psychiatric predictors of pseudoepileptic seizures in patients with refractory seizures. *J Neuropsychiatry Clin Neurosci.* 1994;6:257–260.
25. Craig TKJ, Drake H, Mills K, et al. The South London somatisation study: II. The influence of stressful life events, and secondary gain. *Br J Psychiatry.* 1994;165:248–258.
26. Brown RJ, Schrag A, Trimble MR. Dissociation, childhood interpersonal trauma and family functioning in somatization disorder. *Am J Psychiatry* 2005;162:899–905.
27. Pribor EF, Yutzy SH, Dean JT, et al. Briquet's syndrome, dissociation, and abuse. *Am J Psychiatry.* 1993;150(10):1507–1511.
28. Morrison J. Childhood sexual histories of women with somatization disorder. *Am J Psychiatry.* 1989;146:239–241.

29. Drossman DA, Li Z, Leserman J, et al. Health status by gastrointestinal diagnosis and abuse history. *Gastroenterology.* 1996;110:1301–1304.
30. Talley NJ, Fett SL, Zinsmeister AR. Self-reported abuse and gastrointestinal disease in outpatients: association with irritable bowel-type symptoms. *Am J Gastroenterol.* 1995;90:366–371.
31. Drossman DA, Leserman J, Nachman G, et al. Sexual and physical abuse in women with functional or organic gastrointestinal disorders. *Ann Intern Med.* 1990;113:828–833.
32. Roelofs K, Keijsers GPJ, Hoogduin KAL, et al. Childhood abuse in patients with conversion disorder. *Am J Psychiatry.* 2002;159:1908–1913.
33. Binzer M, Eisemann M. Childhood experiences and personality traits in patients with motor conversion symptoms. *Acta Psychiatr Scand.* 1998;98:288–295.
34. Binzer M, Stone J, Sharpe M. Recent onset pseudoseizures—clues to aetiology. *Seizure.* 2004;13:146–155.
35. Kuyk J, Spinhoven P, van Emde Boas W, et al. Dissociation in temporal lobe epilepsy and pseudo-epileptic seizure patients. *J Nerv Ment Dis.* 1999;187:713–720.
36. Reilly J, Baker GA, Rhodes J, et al. The association of sexual and physical abuse with somatization: characteristics of patients presenting with irritable bowel syndrome and non-epileptic attack disorder. *Psychol Med.* 1999;29:399–406.
37. Alper K, Devinsky O, Perrine K, et al. Nonepileptic seizures and childhood sexual and physical abuse. *Neurology.* 1993;43:1950–1953.
38. Betts T, Boden S. Diagnosis, management and prognosis of a group of 128 patients with non-epileptic attack disorder. Part II. Previous childhood sexual abuse in the aetiology of these disorders. *Seizure.* 1992;1:27–32.
39. Bodden-Heidrich R, Kuppers V, Beckmann MW, et al. Chronic pelvic pain syndrome (CPPS) and chronic vulvar pain syndrome (CVPS): evaluation of psychosomatic aspects. *J Psychosom Obstet Gynaecol.* 1999;20:145–151.
40. Ehlert U, Heim C, Hellhammer DH. Chronic pelvic pain as a somatoform disorder. *Psychother Psychosom.* 1999;68:87–94.
41. Walker EA, Gelfand AN, Gelfand MD,et al. Psychiatric diagnoses, sexual and physical victimization, and disability in patients with irritable bowel syndrome or inflammatory bowel disease. *Psychol Med.* 1995;25:1259–1267.
42. Walker EA, Katon WJ, Neraas K, et al. Dissociation in women with chronic pelvic pain. *Am J Psychiatry.* 1992;149:534–537.
43. Rapkin AJ, Kames LD, Darke LL, et al. History of physical and sexual abuse in women with chronic pelvic pain. *Obstet Gynecol.* 1990;76:92–96.
44. Walker EA, Katon WJ, Harrop-Griffiths J, et al. Relationship of chronic pelvic pain to psychiatric diagnoses and childhood sexual abuse. *Am J Psychiatry.* 1988;145:75–80.
45. Harrop-Griffiths J, Katon WJ, Walker EA, et al. The association between chronic pelvic pain, psychiatric diagnoses, and childhood sexual abuse. *Obstet Gynecol.* 1988;71:589–594.
46. Reiter RC, Shakerin LR, Gambone JC, et al. Correlation between sexual abuse and somatization in women with somatic and non-somatic chronic pelvic pain. *Am J Obstet Gynecol.* 1991;165:104–109.
47. Chu JA, Dill DL. Dissociative symptoms in relation to childhood physical and sexual abuse. *Am J Psychiatry.* 1990;147:887–892.
48. Coons PM. Confirmation of childhood abuse in child and adolescent cases of multiple personality disorder and dissociative disorder not otherwise specified. *J Nerv Ment Dis.* 1994;182:461–464.
49. Irwin HJ. Proneness to dissociation and traumatic childhood events. *J Nerv Ment Dis.* 1994;182:456–460.
50. Gross RJ, Doerr H, Caldirola D, et al. Borderline syndrome and incest in chronic pelvic pain patients. *Int J Psychiatry Med.* 1980–81;10:79–96.
51. Rimsza ME, Berg RA, Locke C. Sexual abuse: Somatic and emotional reactions. *Child Abuse Negl.* 1988;12:201–208.
52. Schofferman J, Anderson D, Hines R, et al. Childhood psychological trauma correlates with unsuccessful lumbar spine surgery. *Spine.* 1992;17:S138–S144.
53. Schofferman J, Anderson D, Hines R, et al. Childhood psychological trauma and chronic refractory low-back pain. *Clin J Pain.* 1993;9:260–265.
54. Talley NJ, Fett SL, Zinsmeister AR, et al. Gastrointestinal tract symptoms and self-reported abuse: A population-based study. *Gastroenterology.* 1994;107:1040–1049.
55. Atlas JA, Hiott J. Dissociative experience in a group of adolescents with history of abuse. *Percept Mot Skills.* 1994;78:121–122.
56. Leserman J, Drossman DA, Li Z, et al. Sexual and physical abuse history in gastroenterology practice: How types of abuse impact health status. *Psychosom Med.* 1996;58:4–15.
57. Farley M, Keaney JC. Physical symptoms, somatization, and dissociation in women survivors of childhood sexual assault. *Women Health.* 1997;25:33–45.
58. Morrison J. Childhood molestation reported by women with somatization disorder. *Ann Clin Psychiatry.* 1989;1:25–32.
59. Brewin CR, Andrews B, Gotlib IH. Psychopathology and early experience: a reappraisal of retrospective reports. *Psychol Bull.* 1993;113:82–98.
60. Fink LA, Bernstein D, Handelsman L, et al. Initial reliability and validity of the Childhood Trauma Interview: a new multidimensional measure of childhood interpersonal trauma. *Am J Psychiatry.* 1995;152:1329–1335.
61. Nash MR, Hulsey TL, Sexton MC, et al. Long-term sequelae of childhood sexual abuse: Perceived family environment, psychopathology, and dissociation. *J Consult Clin Psychol.* 1993;61:276–283.
62. Briere J, Conte J. Self-reported amnesia for abuse in adults molested as children. *J Trauma Stress.* 1993;6:21–31.
63. Berliner L, Williams LM. Memories of child sexual abuse: response to Lindsay and Read. *Appl Cognit Psychol.* 1994;8:379–387.
64. Lindsay SD, Read JD. Psychotherapy and memories of childhood sexual abuse: A cognitive perspective. *Appl Cognit Psychol.* 1994;8:281–338.
65. Raphael KG, Widom CS, Lange G. Childhood victimization and pain in adulthood: a prospective investigation. *Pain.* 2001;92:283–293.
66. Robins LN, Helzer JE, Cottler L, et al. *National Institute of Mental Health diagnostic interview schedule, version III revised (DIS-III-R).* St Louis, MO: Washington University; 1989.
67. Blanchard EB, Scharff L. Psychosocial aspects of assessment and treatment of irritable bowel syndrome in adults and recurrent abdominal pain in children. *J Consult Clin Psychol.* 2002;70:725–738.
68. Bernstein EM, Putnam FW. Development, reliability and validity of a dissociation scale. *J Nerv Ment Dis.* 1986;174:727–735.
69. van Ijzendoorn MH, Schuengel C. The measurement of dissociation in normal and clinical populations: Meta-analytic validation of the Dissociative Experiences Scale (DES). *Clin Psychol Rev.* 1996;16:365–382.
70. Salmon P, Skaife K, Rhodes J. Abuse, dissociation, and somatization in irritable bowel syndrome: towards an explanatory model. *J Behav Med.* 2003;26:1–18.
71. Roelofs K, Hoogduin KAL, Keijsers GPJ, et al. Hypnotic susceptibility in patients with conversion disorder. *J Abnorm Psychol.* 2002;111:390–395.
72. Moene F, Spinhoven P, Hoogduin KAL, et al. Hypnotizability, dissociation and trauma in patients with a conversion disorder: an exploratory study. *Clin Psychol Psychother.* 2001;8:400–410.
73. Goldstein LH, Drew C, Mellers J, et al. Dissociation, hypnotizability, coping styles and health locus of control: characteristics of pseudoseizure patients. *Seizure.* 2000;9:314–322.
74. Spitzer C, Spelsberg B, Grabe HJ, et al. Dissociative experiences and psychopathology in conversion disorders. *J Psychosom Res.* 1999;46:291–294.
75. Alper K, Devinsky O, Perrine K, et al. Dissociation in epilepsy and conversion nonepileptic seizures. *Epilepsia.* 1997;38:991–997.
76. Bowman ES, Markand ON. Psychodynamics and psychiatric diagnoses of pseudoseizure subjects. *Am J Psychiatry.* 1996;153:57–63.
77. Walker EA, Gelfand AN, Gelfand MD, et al. Psychiatric diagnoses, sexual and physical victimization, and disability in patients with irritable bowel syndrome or inflammatory bowel disease. *Psychol Med.* 1995;25:1259–1267.
78. Bowman ES. Etiology and clinical course of pseudoseizures: relationship to trauma, depression, and dissociation. *Psychosomatics.* 1993;34:333–342.

79. Wright DB, Loftus EF. Measuring dissociation: comparison of alternative forms of the Dissociative Experiences Scale. *Aust J Clin Exp Hypn*. 2000;28:103–126.

80. Vanderlinden J, Dyck RV, Vandereyken H, et al. The dissociation questionnaire: development and characteristics of a new self-reporting questionnaire. *Clin Psychol Psychother*. 1993;1:21–27.

81. Nijenhuis ERS, Spinhoven P, Van Dyck R, et al. The development and psychometric characteristics of the Somatoform Dissociation Questionnaire (SDQ-20). *J Nerv Ment Dis*. 1996;184:688–694.

82. Nijenhuis ERS, Spinhoven P, van Dyck R, et al. The development of the Somatoform Dissociation Questionnaire (SDQ-5) as a screening instrument for dissociative disorders. *Acta Psychiatr Scand*. 1997;96:311–318.

83. Nijenhuis ERS, van Dyck R, Spinhoven P, et al. Somatoform dissociation discriminates among diagnostic categories over and above general psychopathology. *Aust N Z J Psychiatry*. 1999;33:511–520.

84. Ross CA, Miller SD, Reagor P, et al. Structured interview data on 102 cases of multiple personality disorder from four centres. *Am J Psychiatry*. 1990;147:596–601.

85. Saxe GN, Chinman G, Berkowitz R, et al. Somatization in patients with dissociative disorders. *Am J Psychiatry*. 1994;151:1329–1334.

86. Holmes EA, Mansell W, Brown RJ, et al. Are there two qualitatively distinct forms of dissociation? A review and some clinical implications. Clin Psychol Rev 2005;25:1-23.

87. Cardena E. The domain of dissociation. In: Lynn SJ, Rhue JW, eds. *Dissociation: clinical and theoretical perspectives*. New York: Guilford Press, 1994: 15–31.

88. van der Kolk BA, Fisler R. Dissociation and the fragmentary nature of traumatic memories: overview and exploratory study. *J Trauma Stress*. 1995;8:505–525.

89. Putnam FW. *Dissociation in children and adolescents: a developmental perspective*. New York: Guilford Press, 1997.

90. Allen JG. *Traumatic relationships and serious mental disorders*. New York: John Wiley and Sons, 2001.

91. Brown RJ. The cognitive psychology of dissociative states. *Cogn Neuropsychiatry*. 2002;7:221–235.

92. Sierra M, Berrios GE. Depersonalization: neurobiological perspectives. *Biol Psychiatry*. 1998;44:898–908.

93. Carlson EB, Putnam FW, Ross CA, et al. Factor analysis of the dissociative experiences scale: a multi-center study. In: Braun BG, Carlson EB, eds. *Proceedings of the eight international conference on multiple personality and dissociative states*. Chicago, IL: Rush Presbyterian, 1991:16.

94. Darves Bornoz JM, Degiovanni A, Gaillard P. Validation of a French version of the Dissociative Experiences Scale in a rape-victim population. *Can J Psychiatry*. 1999;44:271–275.

95. Ross CA, Ellason JW, Anderson G. A factor analysis of the Dissociative Experiences Scale (DES) in dissociative identity disorder. *Dissociation*. 1995;8:229–235.

96. Stockdale GD, Gridley BE, Balogh DW, et al. Confirmatory factor analysis of single- and multiple-factor competing models of the Dissociative Experiences Scale in a nonclinical sample. *Assessment*. 2002;9:94–106.

97. Steinberg M. *Structured clinical interview for DSM-IV Dissociative Disorders (SCID-D)*. Washington, DC: American Psychiatric Association, 1993.

98. Hilgard ER. *Divided consciousness: multiple controls in human thought and action*. New York: John Wiley and Sons, 1977.

99. Woody EZ, Bowers KS. A frontal assault on dissociated control. In: Lynn SJ, Rhue JW, eds. *Dissociation: clinical and theoretical perspectives*. New York: Guilford Press, 1994:52–79.

100. Kirsch I, Lynn SJ. The altered state of hypnosis. *Am Psychol*. 1995;50:846–858.

101. Brown RJ. Epilepsy, dissociation and nonepileptic seizures. In: Trimble MR, Schmitz B, eds. *The neuropsychiatry of epilepsy*. Cambridge: Cambridge University Press, 2002:189–209.

102. Kihlstrom JF. Dissociative and conversion disorders. In: Stein DJ, ed. *Cognitive science and clinical disorders*. San Diego, CA: Academic Press , 1992:247–270.

103. Weiskrantz L, Warrington EK, Sanders MD, et al. Visual capacity of the hemianopic field following a restricted occipital ablation. *Brain*. 1974;97:709–728.

104. Kuyk J, Spinhoven P, van Dyck R. Hypnotic recall: a positive criterion in the differential diagnosis between epileptic and pseudoepileptic seizures. *Epilepsia*. 1999;40:485–491.

105. Fukudu M, Hata A, Niwa S, et al. Event-related potential correlates of functional hearing loss: reduced P3 amplitude preserved N1 and N2 components in a unilateral case. *Neuropsychiatry Clin Neurosci*. 1996;50:85–87.

106. Ludwig AM. Hysteria: a neurobiological theory. *Arch Gen Psychiatry*. 1972;27:771–777.

107. Brown RJ. Psychological mechanisms of medically unexplained symptoms: an integrative conceptual model. *Psychol Bull*. 2004;130:793-812.

108. Bendefeldt F, Miller LL, Ludwig AM. Cognitive performance in conversion hysteria. *Arch Gen Psychiatry*. 1976;33:1250–1254.

109. Horvath T, Friedman J, Meares R. Attention in hysteria: a study of Janet's hypothesis by means of habituation and arousal measures. *Am J Psychiatry*. 1980;137:217–220.

110. Roelofs K, van Galen GP, Keijsers GPJ, et al. Motor initiation and execution in patients with conversion paralysis. *Acta Psychol*. 2002;110:21–34.

Anxiety Disorders and Abnormal Movements: A Darkly Interface

17

Randolph B. Schiffer

ABSTRACT

The anxiety disorders are a heterogeneous group of neuropsychiatric syndromes characterized by nervousness, fearfulness, and psychomotor activation. Some are episodic (panic disorder), some are generalized and pervasive (generalized anxiety disorder), and some are conditioned to categories of environmental stimuli (phobias). Although a movement disorder dimension is not generally considered to be part of the phenomenology of the anxiety disorders, in fact, these patients often seem "fidgety" and "shaky." Anecdotal observations suggest that mild action and postural tremors are seen in these patients with some frequency, but also a variety of more elaborate psychogenic movement syndromes of the hyperkinetic sort. The neurochemical systems which are activated in the anxiety disorders are similar to those systems which become dysfunctional in Parkinson disease (PD) (noradrenergic, dopaminergic, serotonergic). There are no systematic reports, however, of movement disorders which occur in the course of the anxiety syndromes. Both episodic and generalized anxiety syndromes have been reported to occur in Parkinson patients prior to the first motor symptoms. When the anxiety disorders are successfully treated, the movement dimension of them improves.

INTRODUCTION

We do not currently know the causes of the psychogenic disorders. We do not know the neuropsychiatric conditions that confer vulnerability to the development of these disorders, although these vulnerabilities are generally considered to be psychological in some form or other. It is possible, however, that neurobiological variables also have some role in the genesis of the psychogenic movement disorders, even as Charcot believed over a century ago (1). It may also be true that the risk factors or vulnerabilities to the development of psychogenic movement disorders differ according to the type of movement mimicked by the psychogenic disorder. In this chapter, our current, limited knowledge of the interface between anxiety disorders and the parkinsonian movement disorders is reviewed, and some areas for future clinical and translational research are suggested.

MOVEMENT DISORDERS AMONG PATIENTS WITH ANXIETY SYNDROMES

The anxiety disorders are a heterogeneous group of neuropsychiatric syndromes characterized by clinical features

TABLE 17.1

ANXIETY DISORDERS IN THE *DIAGNOSTIC AND STATISTICAL MANUAL OF MENTAL DISORDERS*, FOURTH EDITION

Agoraphobia
Panic disorder
Specific phobia
Social phobia
Obsessive–compulsive disorder
Posttraumatic stress disorder
Acute stress disorder
Generalized anxiety disorder
Anxiety disorder due to substance abuse
Anxiety disorder due to general medical condition

of nervousness, fearfulness, and psychomotor activation (2). Some are episodic (panic disorder), some are generalized and pervasive (generalized anxiety disorder), and some are conditioned to certain discrete stimuli (the phobias, posttraumatic stress disorder). A listing of these disorders according to the American Psychiatric Association's *Diagnostic and Statistical Manual of Mental Disorders*, Fourth Edition (DSM-IV), is included here as Table 17.1 (3).

These disorders may be the most common of the Axis I psychiatric disorders, with lifetime prevalence rates exceeding 30% for women, and 19% for men (4). There is considerable comorbidity between the anxiety disorders and other psychiatric disorders, especially depression (5). Familial clustering is commonly seen in the anxiety disorders, and is considered to derive from a mix of not yet identified genetic risk factors, as well as environmental or psychosocial experiences (6). These disorders can occur across the lifespan of the individual, but most commonly symptoms first occur in the second and third decades of life.

The clinical symptomatology of the anxiety disorders crosses several neuropsychiatric functional domains (7). Subjective distress is common, including such symptoms as dread, nervousness, and fearfulness. Sometimes patients with anxiety disorders complain of cognitive changes, especially inattention and difficulty in concentrating. They may also present with a variety of somatic complaints, such as chest pain, shortness of breath, irritable bowel symptoms, and others. Occasionally, sleep disturbance is the most prominent complaint.

Patients with generalized anxiety disorders may also demonstrate a variety of hyperkinetic movement disorders. Action and postural tremulous movement disorders are observed according to anecdote in such patients. More overt hyperkinetic movement disorders can also be seen in such patients, occasionally mimicking parkinsonian syndromes.

The obsessive–compulsive disorders (OCD) are related neuropsychiatric disorders in which patients are bothered by recurrent, inappropriate thoughts or impulses, or compulsions to perform repetitive behaviors which are also perceived as inappropriate or alien (8). Imaging studies implicate various basal ganglion and medial temporal lobe structures in the generation of the OCD behavioral pathologies (9). Patients with OCD also demonstrate a spectrum of motor symptomatologies which are reminiscent of certain movement disorders, such as repetitive self-injurious behavior, hair pulling, and repetitive stereotypical behaviors such as "evening-up" and hand tapping (10).

The tic disorders and Tourette disorder, although not listed as anxiety disorders in DSM-IV, occur with considerable overlap alongside OCD symptomatology (11). The repetitive motor, vocalizations, and coprophenomena which occur in these disorders are also quite reminiscent of movement disorders. The overlap between OCD and these disorders is not fully understood, but is felt to be substantially genetic (12).

There are currently no systematic reports in the neuropsychiatric literature of movement disorders which occur in the course of the anxiety syndromes (13). It might be quite useful for one or two groups of clinical investigators to conduct a systematic survey of an anxiety disorders patient cohort to establish point prevalence rates and descriptive types of movement disorders in such a population.

CASE VIGNETTE

A 38-year-old married man was seen on urgent referral from an emergency room for evaluation of a recent-onset movement disorder. The emergency room physicians wondered if he might have "acute Parkinson disease."

He had been an anxious person since his teenage years. He described himself as "a chronic worrier," and "seeing the worst" that could conceivably emerge from every situation. His nervousness and low self-esteem had led him to feel self-conscious in social situations, where he acted shy and unassertive. By his late twenties, sudden attacks of palpitations and fear of death or suffocation had occurred, for which he saw several physicians in consultation. A diagnosis of panic disorder had been given, and he had been treated more or less continuously to the present with benzodiazepines. From time to time he had also experienced depressive symptoms, and he had seen a counselor for treatment of depression on at least one previous occasion.

Despite these difficulties, the patient had finished college, married, and had two children. He went to work for a truck rental agency, and he showed great stability in his loyalty to the company over a 10-year period. His family system was stable, although he described himself as "very dependent" on his wife, and feeling heightened anxiety whenever he had to be away from her.

A month prior to his evaluation, his employer had promoted the patient and transferred him from his home base in one city to another about 100 miles distant to manage the new company office. He had misgivings about this, but felt that he had to do it for the sake of the company. He was especially nervous because his wife remained behind with the children in their home city until the midpoint of the school year in January.

Once he arrived at his new work place, an abnormal shaking movement of his feet began almost immediately. It was worse at rest, irregular, and sometimes worsened when he walked. At first it was mild, but over his first month in the new city it escalated to the point that a co-worker asked if he might have "Parkinson disease." This comment frightened him, and was the occasion for his visit to the emergency room.

On examination, the subject displayed an exaggerated, irregular rocking motion of his feet at rest on the examination table, with some subtler, similar movements in his hands. When he was distracted, the movements diminished. He was able to write a sentence when told to "concentrate." With ambulation, the shaking movements ceased.

The initial treatment intervention was a labeling of the new movement disorder as psychogenic, "not Parkinson disease," and "not a sign of new brain disease." It was forecasted that he would gradually improve as he adjusted to his new living situation. No new psychotropic or neurotropic medications were prescribed. At the second clinical visit he was substantially improved. The anxiety symptoms still had not worsened.

In this vignette, although an anecdote, we see a psychogenic movement disorder in a man with chronic anxiety, which emerged during a time of heightened life stress. The abnormal movements were a remote imitation of some of the abnormal movements seen in Parkinson disease (PD). Interestingly, during the time of the abnormal movements, the subject did not report increased nervousness, suggesting a possible psychological "defensive" function for the psychogenic movement disorder, consistent with older, psychoanalytic theories about mechanisms of primary gain in conversion disorders. Clinical improvement seemed to derive from supportive but direct confrontation of the movement disorder as psychogenic, and reassurance that it would slowly improve.

ANXIETY SYNDROMES AMONG PATIENTS WITH MOVEMENT DISORDERS

Both episodic and generalized anxiety syndromes have been reported to occur frequently among populations with PD (14). A review by Richard et al. (15) found that generalized anxiety disorder (GAD), panic disorder, and social phobia have point prevalence rates of up to 40% in some cohorts of patients with PD. These rates are higher than those seen in normal populations, or in other chronic disease groups.

The anxiety symptoms in patients with PD do not seem to be clearly related to the timing of administration of antiparkinsonian medications (16), nor to the presence of on–off motor phenomena (15). There does seem to be common co-occurrence of anxiety symptoms and depressive disorders in PD patients, as in psychiatric patients generally (17). There does not seem to be any relationship between the presence of an anxiety disorder and any of the cognitive loss syndromes which occur in about 30% of Parkinson disease patients (18).

Certain clinical features surrounding the anxiety disorders which are seen in PD suggest that there may be a shared neurobiological vulnerability, both for Parkinson disease and for the psychiatric syndromes. Several studies indicate that the anxiety syndromes among patients with Parkinson disease often antedate the first motor symptoms of PD. Lauterbach and Duvoisin (19) described 12 patients in their movement disorders clinic who had suffered from social phobias prior to the onset of the motor symptoms of Parkinson disease. Stein et al. described nine PD patients with anxiety disorders, and reported that two had had the onset of anxiety symptoms prior to the diagnosis of PD, and seven after the diagnosis (20). A large case-control study from the Mayo Foundation showed a significant increased risk for PD patients to have shown both diagnosable anxiety and depressive syndromes at 10 and 20 years prior to first motor symptoms of PD (21). These clinical reports call to mind anecdotal stories from previous generations of psychiatrists and neurologists, to the effect that an anxious–phobic character style often antedated by many years the onset of motor symptoms in PD patients. The question emerges whether there could be an overlap, or sharing of vulnerability at a neurobiological level between risk for the development of PD and for the anxiety disorders.

SHARED NEUROBIOLOGY BETWEEN ANXIETY DISORDERS AND PARKINSON DISEASE

There may well be structural neuroanatomic circuits that subserve the reported clinical link between anxiety disorders and extrapyramidal movement disorders. From the work of Mogenson et al. in the 1970s, the nucleus accumbens has been described as an interactive neural relay, modulating striatal motor system output by ventral tegmental and temporal lobe limbic inputs (22). The shell of the accumbens is closely linked to or continuous with the anterior extension of the amygdala (23). Together, these structures provide circuitry linkage between the extrapyramidal motor system and limbic structures, which are activated in stress responses, reward, and fear (24,25). Brain imaging studies in a few psychiatric patients with anxiety have noted temporal lobe and basal ganglion metabolic changes (26,27).

The neurochemical systems which are activated in the anxiety disorders overlap considerably with those systems which become dysfunctional in Parkinson disease (noradrenergic, serotonergic) (28). The locus ceruleus-based norepinephrine system in the brainstem has an important role in the processing of fear-related stimuli (29). Abnormal regulation of presynaptic α2-adrenergic receptors has been described from evidence related to pharmacologic probes in panic disorder (28). A loss of noradrenergic locus ceruleus neurons has been described in PD, in addition to the dopamine-related cell loss in the substantia nigra (30). A functional hypersensitivity in these systems could be produced by such a neuropathologic process, and our group has reported a heightened susceptibility of some PD patients to yohimbine-induced panic attacks (31). Yohimbine is an α2-adrenergic antagonist that is capable of generating panic attacks in vulnerable individuals.

With regard to the psychogenic movement disorders, it may be that the overlapping neurobiology between panic and PD described above is of no consequence. Still, on the chance that Charcot may have been more correct than has been generally assumed, it might be worthwhile to review the cohorts of psychogenic parkinsonism that exist at some medical centers described in chapter 9 of this volume. Do these patients have co-occurring anxiety disorders? Do they respond therapeutically to antianxiety medications?

TREATMENT OF ANXIETY DISORDERS

The initial treatment of anxiety spectrum disorders associated with PD is not terribly different from that of anxiety disorders not associated with neurologic disease (32). We do not have controlled observations on this issue, but first-line agents by drug class include the sedative hypnotics, the antihistamines, the benzodiazepines, the beta blockers, buspirone, and zolpidem. The antidepressants, including the selective serotonin reuptake inhibitors, the tricyclics, and the monoamine oxidase inhibitors should be used with caution in PD patients (10). Many PD patients are on selegiline a monoamine oxidase B inhibitor, and there is some concern about combinations of this agent with any of the antidepressants.

REFERENCES

1. Trillat E. Conversion disorder and hysteria. In: Berrios G, Porter R, eds. *A history of psychiatric disorders.* Washington Square, NY: NYU Press, 1995:433–441.
2. Schiffer RB. Anxiety disorders in Parkinson's disease: insights into the neurobiology of neurosis. *J Psychosom Res.* 1999;47:505–508.
3. American Psychiatric Association *American psychiatric association, diagnostic and statistical manual of mental disorders,* 4th Ed. Washington, DC: APA Press, 1994.
4. Kessler RC, McGonagle KA, Zhao S, et al. Lifetime and 12-month prevalence of DSM-III-R psychiatric disorders in the United States. Results from the National Comorbidity Survey. *Arch Gen Psychiatry.* 1994;51:8–19.
5. Maser JD, Cloninger CR, eds. *Comorbidity of mood and anxiety disorders.* Washington, DC: American Psychiatric Press, 1990.
6. Hettema JM, Neale MC, Kendler KS. A review and meta-analysis of the genetic epidemiology of anxiety disorders. *Am J Psychiatry.* 2001;158:1568–1578.
7. Noyes R Jr, Hoehn-Saric R. *The anxiety disorders.* Cambridge: Cambridge University Press, 1998.
8. Jankovic J, De Leon ML. Basal Ganglia and Behavioral Disorders. In: Schiffer RB, Rao SM, Fogel BS, eds. *Neuropsychiatry,* 2nd ed. Philadelphia, PA: Lippincott Williams & Wilkins, 2003:934–946.
9. Rauch SL, Whalen PJ, Curran T. Probing striato-thalamic function in obsessive–compulsive disorder and Tourette syndrome using neuroimaging methods. In: Cohen DJ, Jankovic J, Goetz CG, eds. *Tourette syndrome. Advances in neurology.* Vol. 85. Philadelphia, PA: Lippincott Williams & Wilkins, 2001:207–224.
10. Hollander E, Twersky R, Bienstock C. The obsessive compulsive spectrum: a survey of 800 practitioners. *CNS Spectr.* 2000;5:61–64.
11. Eapen V, Yakeley JW, Robertson MM. Gilles de la Tourette syndrome and obsessive–compulsive disorder. In: Schiffer RB, Rao SM, Fogel BS, eds. *Neuropsychiatry,* 2nd ed. Philadelphia, PA: Lippincott Williams & Wilkins, 2003:947–990.
12. Eapen V, Pauls DL, Robertson MM. Evidence of autosomal dominant transmission in Tourette's syndrome. United Kingdom cohort study. *Br J Psychiatry.* 1993;162:593–596.
13. Neumeister A, Vythilingam M, Bonne O, et al. Anxiety. In: Schiffer RB, Rao SM, Fogel BS, eds. *Neuropsychiatry.* 2nd ed. Philadelphia, PA: Lippincott Williams & Wilkins, 2003:750–775.
14. Schiffer RB. Anxiety disorders in Parkinson's Disease: insights into the neurobiology of neurosis. *J Psychosomatic Research.* 1999;47:505–508.
15. Richard IH, Schiffer RB, Kurlan R. Anxiety and Parkinson's disease. *J Neuropsychiatry Clin Neurosci.* 1996;8:383–392.
16. Henderson R, Kurlan R, Kersun JM, et al. Preliminary examination of the comorbidity of anxiety and depression in Parkinson's disease. *J Neuropsychiatry Clin Neuroscience.* 1992;4:257–264.
17. Cummings JL. Depression and Parkinson's disease: a review. *Am J Psychiatry.* 1992;149:443–454.
18. Lauterbach EC. The locus ceruleus and anxiety disorders in demented and nondemented familial parkinsonism (ltr). *Am J Psychiatry.* 1993;150:994.
19. Lauterbach EC, Duvoisin RC. Anxiety disorders in familial parkinsonism (ltr). *Am J Psychiatry.* 1992;148:274.
20. Stein MB, Heuser IJ, Juncos JL, et al. Anxiety disorders in patients with Parkinson's disease. *Am J Psychiatry.* 1990;147:217–220.
21. Shiba M, Bower JH, Maraganore DM, et al. Anxiety disorders and depressive disorders preceding Parkinson's Disease: a case-control study. *Mov Disord.* 2000;15:669–677.
22. Mogenson GJ, Jones DL, Yim CY. From motivation to action: functional interface between the limbic system and the motor system. *Prog Neurobiol.* 1980;14:69–97.
23. Heimer L, Alheid GF, de Olmos JS, et al. The accumbens: beyond the core-shell dichotomy. *J Neuropsychiatry Clin Neurosci.* 1997;9: 354–381.
24. Abercrombie ED, Keefe KA, DiFrischia DS, et al. Differential effect of stress on *in vivo* dopamine release in striatum, nucleus accumbens, and medial frontal cortex. *J Neurochem.* 1989;52: 1655–1658.
25. Alheid GF, Heimer L. New perspectives in basal forebrain organization of special relevance for neuropsychiatric disorders: the striatopallidal, amygdaloid, and corticopetal components of substantia innominata. *Neuroscience.* 1988;27:1–39.
26. Wu JC, Buchsbaum MS, Hershey TG, et al. PET in generalized anxiety disorder. *Biol Psychiatry.* 1991;29:1181–1199.
27. Fontaine R, Breton G, Dery R, et al. Temporal lobe abnormalities in panic disorder: an MRI study. *Biol Psychiatry.* 1990;27:304–310.
28. Nutt D, Lawson C. Panic attacks; a neurochemical overview of models and mechanisms. *Br J Psychiatry.* 1992;160:165–178.
29. Goddard AW, Charney DS. Toward an integrated neurobiology of panic disorder. *J Clin Psychiatry.* 1997;58(Suppl 2):4–11.
30. German DC, Manaye KF, White CL, et al. Disease-specific patterns of locus ceruleus cell loss. *Ann Neurol.* 1992;32:667–676.
31. Kurlan R, Lichter D, Schiffer RB. Panic/anxiety in Parkinson's disease: yohimbine challenge (abst). *Neurology.* 1989;39:421.
32. Schiffer RB. Psychiatric disorders in medical practice. *Cecil textbook of medicine,* 22nd ed. Philadelphia, PA: WB Saunders, 2004: 2212–2222.

Depression

18

Valerie Voon   Mark Hallett

ABSTRACT

The prevalence of depression is high in psychogenic movement disorders (PMD), and there are multiple similarities between the two. However, the relationship between them is not clear: Depression may be secondary to PMD; pathophysiologic similarities could result in the simultaneous expression of these disorders; or depression may be a vulnerability to PMD. Depression is a disorder of multifactorial etiology presumed to be influenced by genetic predisposition, early and recent life stressors, gender, somatic disorders, and personality traits. An understanding of the pathophysiology behind depression may provide insights into the design of studies of "why" PMD occurs. In this chapter, we focus primarily on the biological mechanisms; the review is not meant to be exhaustive. Treatment of the underlying depression may be useful for patients with PMD.

INTRODUCTION

Patients with psychogenic movement disorders (PMDs) have a high prevalence of comorbid psychiatric disorders. Depression in particular is very common. For instance, in the series by Williams et al. (1), 71% of 24 patients had depression, and in the series by Feinstein et al. (2), the lifetime prevalence of major depression was 43%. Although the latter study did not utilize a control group, comparisons were made with the National Psychiatric Co-Morbidity study data, an epidemiologic survey of more than 8,000 respondents in the United States; this survey showed a much lower lifetime prevalence of depression in the general population, reported at 17.1%. The high prevalence of depression in PMD is in keeping with the prevalence of depression observed in other forms of conversion disorder (CD) (3). In this chapter, we explore the similarities

between the two disorders and postulate potential biological mechanisms underlying this relationship. We will refer to PMD and CD as if they had similar mechanisms, although differences between subtypes of CD are likely (4).

DEPRESSION

The pathophysiologic basis for depression has been postulated as a multifactorial model influenced by acute and chronic psychological stress, early adverse experiences, somatic disease, genetic factors, gender, and personality traits. The definition of a major depressive episode, according to the *Diagnostic and Statistical Manual of Mental Disorders*, Fourth Edition (DSM-IV), is that "a person must have experienced at least five of the nine symptoms below for the same two weeks or more, for most of the time almost every day, and this is a change from his/her prior level of functioning." One of the symptoms must be either (i) depressed mood, or (ii) loss of interest.

A. Depressed mood. For children and adolescents, this may be irritable mood.
B. A significantly reduced level of interest or pleasure in most or all activities.
C. A considerable loss or gain of weight (e.g., 5% or more change of weight in a month when not dieting). This may also be an increase or decrease in appetite. For children, they may not gain an expected amount of weight.
D. Difficulty falling or staying asleep (insomnia), or sleeping more than usual (hypersomnia).
E. Behavior that is agitated or slowed down. Others should be able to observe this.
F. Feeling fatigued, or having diminished energy.
G. Thoughts of worthlessness or extreme guilt (not about being ill).

H. Reduced ability to think, concentrate, or make decisions.
I. Frequent thoughts of death or suicide (with or without a specific plan), or attempt of suicide (5).

The category of mood disorders in the DSM-IV includes major depressive disorder, dysthymic disorder, bipolar disorder, cyclothymic disorder, mood disorder due to a general medical condition, and substance-induced mood disorder (5).

HOW ARE DEPRESSION AND CONVERSION DISORDER RELATED?

The comorbidity of depression is high in CD and there are multiple similarities between the two disorders as discussed below. The relationship between CD and depression can be conceptualized as follows: (i) depression may be secondary to CD; (ii) pathophysiologic similarities may result in the simultaneous expression of the disorders (e.g., genetic factors, abuse or stress, personality traits, HPA axis or neurotransmitter abnormalities); or (iii) depression may act as an underlying vulnerability to CD. With respect to the study of CD, depression can be conceptualized as a confounder, as a potential model for understanding the pathophysiology of conversion disorder, or as a potential mediator in the onset of conversion symptoms.

SIMILARITIES BETWEEN DEPRESSION AND CONVERSION DISORDER

Aside from the high comorbidity of depression in CD, the similarities between depression and CD include the association with multiple somatic symptoms, childhood abuse and stressors, female gender, and potentially personality traits.

Both depression and CD are highly associated with multiple somatic symptoms. Depression frequently has comorbid somatic symptoms, including those operationally defined within the DSM-IV such as bradyphrenia or fatigue (5), and other unexplained symptoms such as pain, gastrointestinal symptoms, and cardiovascular symptoms (6). Furthermore, the medically unexplained disorders or functional somatic syndromes such as fibromyalgia, irritable bowel syndrome, chronic fatigue syndrome, and chronic pain are also frequently comorbid with depression (7,8). Similarly, one of the supportive criteria in the operational definition of PMD is the presence of multiple somatic symptoms (1). Feinstein et al. (2) found that 38% of patients with PMD had developed other physical symptoms on follow-up, and Williams et al. (1) found that 12.5% of 24 PMD patients had somatization disorder. These findings are in keeping with the literature on CD (3). Whether these comorbid somatic symptoms in CD represent other undiagnosed somatoform disorders such as

somatization disorder, a greater propensity to develop somatic symptoms, or can be explained by the frequent comorbidity of depression is not known. The pathophysiologic link between these somatic symptoms and depression is not completely known. The frequent association of depression with unexplained chronic pain, for example, has been hypothesized neurochemically to be related to similar underlying abnormalities in serotonin, norepinephrine, substance P, and corticotrophin releasing factor (CRF) (9).

Both depression and CD have also been associated with childhood abuse (10,11). Other adverse childhood experiences such as parental loss (12) are associated with depression as well. Similarly, emotional neglect and family dysfunction have been associated with CD (11). It should be noted, however, that the incidence of childhood abuse may differ depending on conversion subtype. Most studies demonstrating an elevated incidence of childhood abuse have either mixed conversion disorders (11,13,14) or non-epileptic seizures (15). A recent study by Stone et al. (4) suggests that psychogenic paralysis, in comparison to non-epileptic seizures, may have a lowered association with childhood abuse. Similarly, Binzer et al. (16) noted a low incidence of childhood abuse in CD patients with motor symptoms, in contrast to expected findings, although the authors found increased perception of parental rejection, and lowered perception of affection and emotional warmth. Whether PMD, predominantly a disorder with hyperkinetic or positive symptoms, differs from that of psychogenic paralysis, a disorder with hypokinetic symptoms, is not known. A history of childhood abuse is also associated with an increased risk of medically unexplained somatic symptoms and high utilization of medical services (17). Dissociation and hypnotic susceptibility have been suggested as factors that mediate the relationship between abuse and conversion (11,15).

THE HYPOTHALAMIC–PITUITARY–ADRENAL AXIS

A potential biological link connecting depression and CD may lie in the regulation of the hypothalamic–pituitary–adrenal (HPA) axis. Hyperactivity of the HPA axis, as demonstrated by cortisol nonsuppression with the standard dexamethasone suppression test, has been consistently demonstrated in patients with severe depression or psychotic subtypes, and, in at least one study, in depressed patients with comorbid anxiety (18–20). The nonsuppression normalizes when the depression is remitted (21), whereas persistent nonsuppression is associated with recurrent episodes and risk of relapse (22). In addition to excessive cortisol secretion, the normal nocturnal decrease in cortisol was also lost in severely depressed patients (20). The presence of excessive cortisol itself and the glucocorticoid receptor have been implicated in mood disorders (23–25) as observed by the association of Cushing disease or exogenous steroid administration with depression.

Elevated CRF levels have also been demonstrated in depressed patients (26). Aside from its regulatory role in the HPA axis, CRF itself has been postulated to have a direct effect on the behavioral stress response. Administration of CRF to animals results in autonomic, anxious, and depressivelike behaviors. CRF increases the firing rate of noradrenergic neurons in the locus coeruleus, whereas serotonergic neurons in the raphe are inhibited (23,25). The elevated CRF release in depression has been suggested to be related to aberrant feedback inhibition from either the hippocampus or ventromedial prefrontal cortex (PFC), or from the permissive role of the amygdala (24,25). These neuroanatomic structures will be discussed in a subsequent section.

In addition to HPA axis abnormalities in depression, there is frequent suggestion in the literature that childhood abuse can lead to a dysfunction in the HPA axis which, as a primary regulator of the stress response, can lead to dysfunctional responses to further stressors (27–29). The HPA axis dysregulation secondary to childhood abuse has been hypothesized to play a role in the vulnerability to depression. Differences exist between the HPA axis dysregulation seen in that of abuse and in that of depression, and depression associated with childhood abuse has been suggested to be a subtype of depression (27–29).

As a potential link between depression and CD, one study demonstrated that the dexamethasone suppression test is abnormal in CD compared to healthy controls (30). In the study, 28% of CD patients were standard dexamethasone nonsuppressors in comparison to none in the control group. However, methodological problems limit the relevance of this study, which focused on patients with a range of conversion subtypes (change in consciousness, paraparesis, mutism, aphonia, and convulsions) compared with control subjects consisting of psychiatrists. The patient group had no other diagnosed psychiatric disorders including depression—an atypical finding with CD. Notably, the mean Hamilton Depression Rating score was 13.4 (SD 6.1), suggesting that a proportion of the patients may have been experiencing depressive symptoms. Although the findings of nonsuppression did not correlate with depression scores, the authors acknowledge that depression may still have mediated the abnormal HPA axis findings. Thus, the study does not necessarily help tease out the relationship between depression and CD.

Studying the HPA axis in PMD will be subject to the confounders of depression, remitted depression at high risk of relapse, and the effects of childhood abuse. Whether the depression-related HPA axis abnormalities predispose to PMD symptoms is not known. We are not aware of any associations between steroid or cortisol and movement symptoms, suggesting a direct association between cortisol and PMD may be less likely. Whether a direct relationship exists between CRF and PMD symptoms is not known. The

HPA axis abnormalities in depression may have bidirectional interactions with the fronto-temporo-limbic network as discussed in the following section, which could hypothetically predispose to PMD symptoms.

FRONTO-TEMPORO-LIMBIC NETWORK DYSFUNCTION

Fronto-temporo-limbic dysfunction may be involved in modulation of the HPA axis in depression (24,25). Abnormalities in the fronto-temporo-limbic network have been implicated in the pathophysiology of depression (31,32).

Hippocampus

Several meta-analyses have confirmed decreased left and right hippocampal volumes in depressed patients relative to control subjects (33,34). The elevated cortisol has been postulated to play a role in the decrease in hippocampal volume (24). Conversely, the hippocampus has a large number of glucocorticoid receptors and plays an inhibitory role in the HPA axis; as such, hippocampal dysfunction in depression has been suggested to play a role in the HPA axis abnormalities, resulting in a pathologic feedback loop (24).

Although the finding of decreased hippocampal volume is fairly consistent in depression, given the known function of explicit memory in the hippocampus, a relationship with CD cannot be postulated.

Amygdala

In contrast, functional and possibly volumetric abnormalities of the amygdala in depression may have a greater association with CD. Increased activity of the amygdala has been documented in patients with depression, which correlates with depression severity ratings and plasma cortisol levels (35). Two studies have documented either a decreased total (36) or a decreased core amygdala volume (37) on MRI in depressed women. The decrease was found only in depressed women and not in depressed men (36). One study documented a larger amygdala volume in depressed subjects, but studied both men and women (38). A postmortem histologic study suggests that lowered glial numbers in the amygdala, particularly on the left, account for these volumetric changes in depressed patients (39).

The amygdala has been extensively implicated in mood processing, particularly of negative affect and fear (31). The amygdala has extensive connections to the medial PFC; the amygdala also activates the HPA axis and increases norepinephrine release through the locus coeruleus (24,31). Hypercortisolism associated with depression has been suggested to increase amygdala activity, thus resulting in a pathologic positive feedback loop on the HPA axis (24,31).

Subgenual Medial Prefrontal Cortex

Functional activity of the subgenual medial PFC (the anterior cingulate ventral to the genu of the corpus callosum) is abnormal in depression (40). Postmortem histopathologic studies have demonstrated decreases in left-sided volume and decreases in glial number in the subgenual medial PFC in depressed patients (41,42). The subgenual PFC has extensive limbic, cortical, brainstem, and hypothalamic connections, which have been implicated in the mood, somatic, endocrine, cognitive, and motivation symptoms associated with depression (31,32).

Prefrontal Cortex

Abnormalities of other regions of the prefrontal cortex including increased functioning of the orbitofrontal cortex (OFC) and medial PFC, and decreased functioning of the dorsolateral PFC are reported (31,32). Decreased volumetric measurements of the OFC have been demonstrated (43,44) particularly in depressed men (44), although reports have not been consistent (36). Postmortem studies have demonstrated decreases in cortical thickness in the PFC including the dorsolateral PFC and OFC (45). A full discussion of the function of different regions of the PFC and of the PFC abnormalities in depression is not within the scope of this chapter.

Fronto-Temporo-Limbic Network and CD

Aside from the role of a dysfunctional fronto-temporo-limbic network in the regulation of emotion, specific neuroanatomic regions affected by depression may also contribute to CD. Changes in functioning and volume of the prefrontal cortex, subgenual cingulate, and amygdala associated with depression may play an important role in predisposing PMD patients to psychogenic movements. Abnormalities in prefrontal cortex functioning have been documented in psychogenic paralysis (46–48), anesthesia (49), and hypnotic paralysis (50) (which is presumed to be a paradigm for conversion paralysis). Frontal cortical regions have been implicated in the inhibition of motor or sensory processes (47). Impaired motor initiation as reflected in hypofunctioning of the dorsolateral PFC has been implicated in psychogenic paralysis (46). As only few studies are available and different paradigms and patient groups have been studied, limited conclusions can be drawn. A full discussion is beyond the scope of this chapter. Please see Chapter 26 for further details.

GENETICS

An underlying genetic diathesis may link the neural network abnormalities and stressful life events to depression. Genetic

vulnerability, in addition to other factors, has been well-established to play a role in depression (51).

The presence of the short "s" allele of the serotonin transporter gene promoter has recently been demonstrated to interact with stressful life events to increase the risk of depression (52) (i.e., a gene–environment interaction) and to be associated with increased coupling of the amygdala-prefrontal cortex (53) (i.e., functional neuroanatomic variations). The serotonin transporter is the protein inhibited by serotonin reuptake inhibitor antidepressants. The promoter of the serotonin transporter gene has two genetic variations. The short "s" allele is associated with lower transcription efficacy than the long "l" allele. The "s" allele has been associated with personality traits of harm avoidance and variably associated with neuroticism (54). Carriers of the "s" allele, as compared to those homozygous for the "l" allele, have been demonstrated to be more likely to develop depression and suicidal behaviors as a result of early childhood or recent stressful events (52). This effect of genetic variance, which moderates the influence of life stress on the development of depression, provides evidence for a gene–environment interaction.

Healthy individuals who are carriers of the "s" allele, in contrast to those homozygous for the "l" allele, have also been demonstrated to have greater amygdala activation to aversive, but not to pleasant visual stimuli (53,55). The basolateral amygdala is closely connected to the ventromedial PFC, both of which are activated in major depression. In healthy individuals, coupling of the amygdala and ventromedial PFC was demonstrated to be stronger in "s" carriers than in homozygous "l" subjects. The authors suggest that emotional salience for aversive events may be increased in the "s" carriers. Increased coupling was hypothesized to allow greater regulation of emotional states, but may also predispose to depression in the context of stressful states (53). This finding links together the association of a genetic variation with life stress and depression from the previous study with the same genetic variation in neuroanatomic coupling in regions relevant to depression.

Underlying genetic traits may explain a similar relationship between CD and early and recent stressors.

TREATMENT

Treatment of the underlying depression may improve the underlying PMD symptoms. Antidepressants may have effects on serotonergic or noradrenergic neurotransmission. Antidepressant effects on brain-derived nerve growth factor (56) or HPA axis normalization (25) have also been described. There are a number of biological treatment approaches to depression in the context of CD which range from antidepressants and electroconvulsive therapy (ECT) to repetitive transcranial magnetic stimulation (TMS). Psychotherapeutic approaches can also be utilized. Similar to the role of antidepressants in functional somatic syndromes and pain disorders, antidepressants may also play a role in the treatment of PMD. See Chapter 34 for further details on psychotropic treatment.

CONCLUSION

PMD, similar to depression, is likely a disorder of multifactorial etiology. These factors range from genetic predisposition, early and chronic life stressors, neuroanatomic network functional changes, HPA axis abnormalities, and potential neurotransmitter abnormalities. Understanding the relationship between depression and PMD, and particularly, drawing from the well-developed depression literature, may give us deeper insights into the "why" behind why conversion symptoms develop.

REFERENCES

1. Williams DT, Ford B, Fahn S. Phenomenology and psychopathology related to psychogenic movement disorders. *Adv Neurol.* 1995;65:231–257.
2. Feinstein A, Stergiopoulos V, Fine J, et al. Psychiatric outcome in patients with a psychogenic movement disorder: a prospective study. *Neuropsychiatry Neuropsychol Behav Neurol.* 2001;14: 169–176.
3. Binzer M, Anderson PM, Kullgren G. Clinical characteristics of patients with motor disability due to conversion disorder: a prospective control group study. *J Neurol Neurosurg Psychiatry.* 1997;63:83–88.
4. Stone J, Sharpe M, Binzer M. Motor conversion symptoms and pseudoseizures: a comparison of clinical characteristics. *Psychosomatics.* 2004;45(6):492–499.
5. American Psychiatric Association. *Diagnostic and statistical manual of mental disorders,* 4th ed. Washington, DC: American Psychiatric Association, 1994.
6. Haug TT, Mykletun A, Dahl AA. The association between anxiety, depression, and somatic symptoms in a large population: the HUNT-II study. *Psychosom Med.* 2004;66:845–851.
7. Wessely S, Nimnuan C, Sharpe M. Functional somatic syndromes: one or many? *Lancet* 1999;354:936–939.
8. Hudson JI, Mangweth B, Pope HG, et al. Family study of affective spectrum disorder. *Arch Gen Psychiatry.* 2003;60:170–177.
9. Campbell LC, Clauw DJ, Keefe FJ. Persistent pain and depression: a biopsychosocial perspective. *Biol Psychiatry.* 2003;54:399–409.
10. Nelson EC, Heath AC, Madden PA, et al. Association between self-reported childhood sexual abuse and adverse psychosocial outcomes: results from a twin study. *Arch Gen Psychiatry.* 2002; 59:139–145.
11. Roelofs K, Keijsers GP, Hoogduin KA, et al. Childhood abuse in patients with conversion disorder. *Am J Psychiatry.* 2002;159: 1908–1913.
12. Kendler KS, Neale MC, Kessler RC, et al. Childhood parental loss and adult psychopathology in women. A twin study perspective. *Arch Gen Psychiatry.* 1992;49:109–116.
13. Sar V, Akyuz G, Kundakci T, et al. Childhood trauma, dissociation, and psychiatric comorbidity in patients with conversion disorder. *Am J Psychiatry.* 2004;161:2271–2276.
14. Allanson J, Bass C, Wade DT. Characteristics of patients with persistent severe disability and medically unexplained neurological symptoms: a pilot study. *J Neurol Neurosurg Psychiatry.* 2002;73: 307–309.
15. Bowman ES, Markand ON. Psychodynamics and psychiatric diagnoses of pseudoseizure subjects. *Am J Psychiatry.* 1996;153: 57–63.
16. Binzer M, Eisemann M. Childhood experiences and personality traits in patients with motor conversion symptoms. *Acta Psychiatr Scand.* 1998;98:288–295.
17. Arnow BA. Relationships between childhood maltreatment, adult health and psychiatric outcomes, and medical utilization. *J Clin Psychiatry.* 2004;65(Suppl. 12):10–15.
18. Young EA, Abelson JL, Cameron OG. Effect of comorbid anxiety disorders on the hypothalamic-pituitary-adrenal axis response to a social stressor in major depression. *Biol Psychiatry.* 2004; 56:113–120.
19. Nelson JC, Davis JM. DST studies in psychotic depression: a meta-analysis. *Am J Psychiatry.* 1997;154:1497–1503.
20. Wong ML, Kling MA, Munson PJ, et al. Pronounced and sustained central hypernoradrenergic function in major depression with melancholic features: relation to hypercortisolism and corticotropin-releasing hormone. *Proc Natl Acad Sci U S A.* 2000;97:325–330.
21. Posener JA, DeBattista C, Williams GH, et al. Cortisol feedback during the HPA quiescent period in patients with major depression. *Am J Psychiatry.* 2001;158:2083–2085.
22. Ribeiro SC, Tandon R, Grunhaus L, et al. The DST as a predictor of outcome in depression: a meta-analysis. *Am J Psychiatry.* 1993;150:1618–1629.
23. Holsboer F. Stress, hypercortisolism and corticosteroid receptors in depression: implications for therapy. *J Affect Disord.* 2001;62: 77–91.
24. Gold PW, Drevets WC, Charney DS. New insights into the role of cortisol and the glucocorticoid receptor in severe depression. *Biol Psychiatry.* 2002;52:381–385.
25. Barden N. Implication of the hypothalamic-pituitary-adrenal axis in the physiopathology of depression. *J Psychiatry Neurosci.* 2004;29:185–193.
26. Nemeroff CB, Widerlov E, Bissette G, et al. Elevated concentrations of CSF corticotropin-releasing factor-like immunoreactivity in depressed patients. *Science.* 1984;226:1342–1344.
27. Heim C, Newport DJ, Heit S, et al. Pituitary-adrenal and autonomic responses to stress in women after sexual and physical abuse in childhood. *JAMA.* 2000;284:592–597.
28. Heim C, Newport DJ, Bonsall R, et al. Altered pituitary-adrenal axis responses to provocative challenge tests in adult survivors of childhood abuse. *Am J Psychiatry.* 2001;158:575–581.
29. Newport DJ, Heim C, Bonsall R, et al. Pituitary-adrenal responses to standard and low-dose dexamethasone suppression tests in adult survivors of child abuse. *Biol Psychiatry.* 2004;55:10–20.
30. Tunca Z, Fidaner H, Cimilli C, et al. Is conversion disorder biologically related with depression? A DST study. *Biol Psychiatry.* 1996;39:216–219.
31. Drevets WC. Prefrontal cortical-amygdalar metabolism in major depression. *Ann N Y Acad Sci.* 1999;877:614–637.
32. Mayberg HS. Limbic-cortical dysregulation: a proposed model of depression. *J Neuropsychiatry Clin Neurosci.* 1997;9:471–481.
33. Videbech P, Ravnkilde B. Hippocampal volume and depression: a meta-analysis of MRI studies. *Am J Psychiatry.* 2004;161: 1957–1966.
34. Campbell S, Marriott M, Nahmias C, et al. Lower hippocampal volume in patients suffering from depression: a meta-analysis. *Am J Psychiatry.* 2004;161:598–607.
35. Drevets WC. Neuroimaging abnormalities in the amygdala in mood disorders. *Ann N Y Acad Sci.* 2003;985:420–444.
36. Hastings RS, Parsey RV, Oquendo MA, et al. Volumetric analysis of the prefrontal cortex, amygdala, and hippocampus in major depression. *Neuropsychopharmacology.* 2004;29:952–959.
37. Sheline YI, Gado MH, Price JL. Amygdala core nuclei volumes are decreased in recurrent major depression. *Neuroreport.* 1998; 9:2023–2028.
38. Bremner JD, Narayan M, Anderson ER, et al. Hippocampal volume reduction in major depression. *Am J Psychiatry.* 2000;157: 115–118.
39. Bowley MP, Drevets WC, Ongur D, et al. Low glial numbers in the amygdala in major depressive disorder. *Biol Psychiatry.* 2002; 52:404–412.
40. Drevets WC, Price JL, Simpson JR, et al. Subgenual prefrontal cortex abnormalities in mood disorders. *Nature.* 1997;386:824–827.

41. Ongur D, Drevets WC, Price JL. Glial reduction in the subgenual prefrontal cortex in mood disorders. *Proc Natl Acad Sci U S A*. 1998;95:13290–13295.

42. Botteron KN, Raichle ME, Drevets WC, et al. Volumetric reduction in left subgenual prefrontal cortex in early onset depression. *Biol Psychiatry*. 2002;51:342–344.

43. Bremner JD, Vythilingam M, Vermetten E, et al. Reduced volume of orbitofrontal cortex in major depression. *Biol Psychiatry*. 2002; 51:273–279.

44. Lacerda AL, Keshavan MS, Hardan AY, et al. Anatomic evaluation of the orbitofrontal cortex in major depressive disorder. *Biol Psychiatry*. 2004;55:353–358.

45. Rajkowska G. Postmortem studies in mood disorders indicate altered numbers of neurons and glial cells. *Biol Psychiatry*. 2000; 48:766–777.

46. Spence SA, Crimlisk HL, Cope H, et al. Discrete neurophysiological correlates in prefrontal cortex during hysterical and feigned disorder of movement. *Lancet*. 2000;355:1243–1244.

47. Marshall JC, Halligan PW, Fink GR, et al. The functional anatomy of a hysterical paralysis. *Cognition*. 1997;64:1–8.

48. Tiihonen J, Kuikka J, Viinamäki H, et al. Altered cerebral blood flow during hysterical paresthesia. *Biol Psychiatry*. 1995;37: 134–137.

49. Mailis-Gagnon A, Giannoylis I, Downar J, et al. Altered central somatosensory processing in chronic pain patients with "hysterical" anaesthesia. *Neurology*. 2003;60:1501–1507.

50. Halligan PW, Athwal BS, Oakley DA, et al. Imaging hypnotic paralysis: implications for conversion hysteria. *Lancet*. 2000;355: 986–987.

51. Kendler KS, Thornton LM, Gardner CO. Genetic risk, number of previous depressive episodes, and stressful life events in predicting onset of major depression. *Am J Psychiatry*. 2001;158:582–586.

52. Caspi A, Sugden K, Moffitt TE, et al. Influence of life stress on depression: moderation by a polymorphism in the 5-HTT gene. *Science*. 2003;301:386–389.

53. Heinz A, Braus DF, Smolka MN, et al. Amygdala-prefrontal coupling depends on a genetic variation of the serotonin transporter. *Nat Neurosci*. 2005;8:20–21.

54. Munafo MR, Clark T, Flint J. Does measurement instrument moderate the association between the serotonin transporter gene and anxiety-related personality traits? A meta-analysis. *Mol Psychiatry*. 2004;10(4):415–419.

55. Hariri AR, Mattay VS, Tessitore A, et al. Serotonin transporter genetic variation and the response of the human amygdala. *Science*. 2002;297:400–403.

56. Hashimoto K, Shimizu E, Iyo M. Critical role of brain-derived nerve growth neurotrophic factor in mood disorders. *Brain Res Rev*. 2004;45:104–111.

19

Malingering/ Münchausen: Factitious and Somatoform Disorders in Neurology and Clinical Medicine

Hans-Peter Kapfhammer   *Hans-Bernd Rothenhäusler*

ABSTRACT

Beyond categoric diagnostic differentiation as factitious disorder and malingering on the one hand, and as somatoform disorders on the other, there is a clinical continuum/spectrum of somatization of mono-/oligosymptomatic somatoform disorder (e.g., conversion disorder) via polysymptomatic somatoform disorder (e.g., somatization disorder) to factitious disorder—all forms of abnormal illness behavior varying in severity of somatization and psychopathologic complications. With respect to such a uniform perspective, we carried out two prospective clinical studies on neurologic patients with pseudoneurologic symptoms, that is, conversion symptoms. We were able to show that, according to increasing somatization index, the rates of psychiatric comorbidity, personality disorders, traumatizing events in early development, autodestructive and other negative aspects of illness behavior resulting in remarkable psychosocial burden were escalating. From a reverse perspective, a sample of patients with the established diagnosis of factitious disorder showed frequent somatoform disorders and conspicuous transitions from somatoform disorders to factitious disorder in the psychiatric history. As a whole group, artifactual patients demonstrated quite identical problems in their early personality development as did patients with somatization disorder, with a high number of medically unexplained bodily symptoms on a spectrum of severity similar to that of the somatization patients. Therefore, it seems justified to study groups of patients with somatoform disorders on the one hand, and with factitious disorder on the other, within a uniform frame of reference.

INTRODUCTION

Despite diversified clinical and technical assessment, medically unexplained symptoms still account for a major subgroup of neurologic inpatients and outpatients (1). Pseudoneurologic symptoms may be viewed from various clinical and theoretic perspectives (2). A major psychiatric approach to put an order to this indeed heterogeneous class of symptoms is to differentiate between voluntary and involuntary symptom production, indicating conscious versus unconscious motivation. Malingering (i.e., intentionally feigning or producing somatic symptoms in order to obtain primary external gains) is the simple type of abnormal illness behavior. Purposeful deception is also an integral part of factitious disorder. As a rule, factitious disorder does not only comprise complex psychopathologic and psychodynamic factors, but also cannot be explained by obvious external influences. Self-harm, very often assuming alarming proportions, can sometimes result in life-threatening somatic conditions that seem to be in no reasonable relation to any secondary advantage. Münchausen syndrome may be considered as an extreme variant of chronic factitious disorder. Apart from patients falsely reporting symptoms or feigning states of illnesses by deliberately inducing self-harm to the body and thus deceiving doctors, Münchausen syndrome also includes pseudologia phantastica, itinerant behavior, and signs of social disintegration. On the other hand, there is a wide range of the so-called somatoform disorders, which are characterized by bodily symptoms that suggest a physical disorder but for which there are no demonstrable organic causes or known pathophysiologic mechanisms. These symptoms are, with high probability, linked to psychological factors, conflicts, or psychosocial stressors. Conversion disorder is the classic prototype of somatoform disorders. It involves a loss or change in sensory or motor functions, or in the regulation of consciousness accompanied by nonepileptic seizures. Conversion symptoms may also be part of somatization disorder, not only characterized by pseudoneurologic symptoms, but also by many functional disorders or pains in other organ systems. In contrast to malingering and factitious disorder, symptom production in somatoform disorder must be involuntary by definition. Official psychiatric classification systems such as the *Diagnostic and Statistical Manual of Mental Disorders*, Fourth Edition (DSM-IV), and the *International Classification of Diseases* (ICD-10) follow these categoric differentiations between somatoform disorders on the one hand, and factitious disorders and malingering on the other. This division into categoric diagnostic subgroups, however, causes many problems in clinical practice, so it sometimes seems to be very elusive to demonstrate unconscious motivation in cases of conversion disorder and not to stress a prevailing socially manipulative motive or to recognize an obvious secondary gain. And even if patients with factitious disorders are aware of the fact that they are deceiving their doctors by feigning a somatic condition, they may be totally unaware of the compulsory nature of self-harm which they may induce in a dissociative state. In addition, during individual courses of illness, there may be transitions from a somatoform disorder to a factitious disorder and vice versa (3–5). From a pragmatic standpoint of consultation/liaison (C/L) psychiatric activities, therefore, it is preferred to study all these pseudoneurologic conditions within one framework of analysis.

CONVERSION SYNDROMES IN NEUROLOGIC PATIENTS AS PART OF THE DIAGNOSTIC GROUPS OF CONVERSION DISORDER, SOMATIZATION DISORDER, AND FACTITIOUS DISORDER

In an initial *categoric* approach, we applied the diagnostic logic of DSM-III-R to patients with conversion syndromes referred to C/L service for psychiatric evaluation after a complete neurologic assessment had ruled out explaining neurologic disorders. In a prospective study lasting four years, 169 patients with pseudoneurologic signs of conversion were included (6). There was a typical majority of women (n = 121). From a clinical phenomenologic point of view, the following conversion syndromes were presented:

- Astasia/abasia: 27.2%
- Paresis/plegia: 24.3%
- Aphonia: 1.8%
- Hypesthesia: 1.8%
- Blindness: 5.3%
- Nonepileptic seizures: 19.5%

According to the diagnostic criteria of DSM III-R, three subgroups were differentiated: conversion disorder (n = 132), somatization disorder (n = 28), and factitious disorder (n = 9) (factitious disorder was diagnosed only if it was fortuitously discovered while a patient was engaged in factitious illness behavior, paraphernalia such as syringes or medications were detected among the patient's belongings, or laboratory tests suggested a factitious etiology). It must be stressed that clinical phenomenology of pseudoneurologic symptoms showed no differences among the three subgroups defined by psychiatric diagnostic categories.

A typical psychosocial stressor or intrapsychic conflict could be a decisive eliciting situation for the great majority of patients with conversion disorder. There were many types of conflicts, but any specificity of conflict could not be established regarding the special pseudoneurologic symptom produced in the process of conversion. The longer a conversion symptom persisted, the more important the secondary gains in the patients' social environment seemed to be. Outstanding, long-lasting psychosocial burdens and unsolvable chronic conflicts characterized the subgroup with somatization disorder. Conversion symptoms in this

TABLE 19.1

PRESENT PSYCHIATRIC AND SOMATIC COMORBIDITY IN DIAGNOSTIC SUBGROUPS OF NEUROLOGIC PATIENTS WITH CONVERSION SYMPTOMS[a]

	Conversion Disorder (n = 132)	Somatization Disorder (n = 28)	Factitious Disorder (n = 9)
Substance abuse	5%	61%[b]	22%
Major depression	2%	46%[b]	11%
Anxiety disorder	2%	25%[b]	11%
Obsessive–compulsive disorder	2%	11%[d]	—
Adjustment disorder	28%	14%	—
Personality disorder	10%	57%[b]	89%
Somatic disease	34%[d]	14%	22%
Psychosomatic illness[e]	—	8%[c]	33%

[a] Statistical comparison: conversion vs. somatization disorder.
[b] $p < 0.001$ (Fisher's exact, two-tail).
[c] $p < 0.01$ (Fisher's exact, two-tail).
[d] $p < 0.05$ (Fisher's exact, two-tail).
[e] e.g., M. Crohn, ulcerative colitis, eating disorders.

subgroup were in line with many other functional disorders and remarkable social disabilities. They were part of a highly complex abnormal illness behavior. Acute stressors or obvious secondary gains could not be detected in the small subgroup of patients with factitious disorder. Their sometimes serious self-induced injuries and covert dangerous self-harm rituals, in addition to a prominent conversion symptom, meant a dreadful contrast to what would be, at first glance, an otherwise unspectacular-looking superficial adaptation. Intermittent and acute courses of illness were prevailing in conversion disorder, whereas chronic courses predominated in the other two subgroups.

Considering the dimension of comorbidity, the splitting into the three diagnostic subgroups of patients with conversion symptoms was important. High rates of psychiatric comorbidity such as substance abuse, major depression, anxiety disorders, and so on were typical of patients with somatization disorder. Increasing frequency of additional axis II diagnoses (i.e., personality disorders) were obvious in the two subgroups of patients with somatization and factitious disorder, thus underlining the more complex determination of symptom production in both groups (Table 19.1).

Frequent autodestructive aspects (suicidality, deliberate and covert self-harm, chronic pain, high rates of obscure operations, and many invasive diagnostic procedures) in illness behavior were registered in somatization and factitious disorder. This dimension seemed to include important emotional conflicts also in the doctor–patient relationship, and hinted at a serious risk of iatrogenic harm during the course of illness (Table 19.2).

TABLE 19.2

SELF-DESTRUCTIVE ILLNESS BEHAVIOR IN DIAGNOSTIC SUBGROUPS OF NEUROLOGIC PATIENTS WITH CONVERSION SYMPTOMS[a]

	Conversion Disorder (n = 132)	Somatization Disorder (n = 28)	Factitious Disorder (n = 9)
Suicide attempt in history	5%	18%[d]	22%
Open self-harm	—	4%	33%
Deceptive self-harm	—	4%	100%
Chronic pain syndrome	25%	61%[c]	33%
Frequent invasive diagnostics/ operations (>5)	6%	89%[b]	78%

[a] Statistical comparison: conversion vs. somatization disorder.
[b] $p < 0.001$ (Fisher's exact, two-tail).
[c] $p < 0.01$ (Fisher's exact, two-tail).
[d] $p < 0.05$ (Fisher's exact, two-tail).

TABLE 19.3

EARLY PSYCHOSOCIAL DEVELOPMENT IN DIAGNOSTIC SUBGROUPS OF NEUROLOGIC PATIENTS WITH CONVERSION SYMPTOMS[a]

	Conversion Disorder (n = 132)	Somatization Disorder (n = 28)	Factitious Disorder (n = 9)
Psychiatric disorder in family	13%	43%[b]	33%
Somatic disease in family	10%	57%[b]	44%
Severe personal somatic disease	4%	11%	33%
Foster home	8%	11%[c]	33%
Early separations/losses	17%	11%	22%
Abnormal relations in family	17%	50%[b]	66%
Sexual/physical abuse	8%[c]	43%[b]	44%

[a]Statistical comparison: conversion vs. somatization disorder.
[b]$p < 0.001$ (Fisher's exact, two-tail).
[c]$p < 0.05$ (Fisher's exact, two-tail).

Both subgroups were characterized by frequent traumatic events during early psychosocial development. Among them, high rates of psychiatric disorders and serious somatic diseases within the family, personal experiences with serious health problems, painful early losses and separations, chronic family disharmonies, and frequent cases of devastating sexual and/or physical abuse were prevailing. Profound negative and traumatic influences in early personality development had to be assumed for patients with somatization and factious disorder, as well (Table 19.3).

Important socioeconomic aspects of illness behavior could be noticed for the diagnoses of somatization and factitious disorder. In this respect, especially the subgroup of patients with somatization disorder stood out. During the previous year of the C/L psychiatric evaluation at index term, these patients had been treated in various hospitals for more than two months, and had been off duty because of illness for more than 200 days. On the average, they reported five visits per month with a primary care doctor. In addition, they had been in contact with five special outpatient clinics (apart from neurology for pseudoneurologic symptoms, other special facilities such as for irritable bowel, chronic fatigue, atypical chest pain, multiple chemical sensitivities, etc.). Nearly one third of these patients (mean age in the thirties) had already been pensioned off due to their somatoform condition. Compared to patients with conversion disorder, patients with somatization, but also with factitious disorders, had to be considered as suffering from chronic psychiatric conditions and showing major social disabilities (measured by GAF scores). As a matter of fact, these alarming data do not only reflect the consequences of groups of patients with extreme psychopathology, but also show the consequences of the conditions of the German health delivery and social security systems (Table 19.4).

TABLE 19.4

OTHER ASPECTS OF ILLNESS BEHAVIOR DURING LAST YEAR IN DIAGNOSTIC SUBGROUPS OF NEUROLOGIC PATIENTS WITH CONVERSION SYMPTOMS[a]

	Conversion Disorder (n = 132)	Somatization Disorder (n = 28)	Factitious Disorder (n = 9)
Days in hospital	18 ± 6	76 ± 23[b]	62 ± 19
Days off duty	37 ± 18	214 ± 43[b]	187 ± 46
Contacts to doctors/month	0.4	4.8[b]	0.5
Other "special" outpatient clinics	—	5[b]	—
Pensioned off	3%	32%[b]	11%
Present GAF score	37 ± 16	31 ± 19	25 ± 7
Highest GAF score during recent year	74 ± 14[b]	42 ± 13	39 ± 8

[a]Statistical comparison: conversion vs. somatization disorder.
[b]$p < 0.001$ (Fisher's exact, two-tail).
[c]$p < 0.05$ (Fisher's exact, two-tail).

The results may be discussed in terms of psychiatric differential diagnosis and psychiatric comorbidity, psychodynamic evaluation, illness behavior, and therapeutic options in a C/L service. Although differentiation between categorically defined groups of psychiatric disorders may be useful to start an analysis with patients presenting conversion syndromes, our dimensional data seemed to confirm more of a standpoint stressing a spectrum of severity of somatization.

CONVERSION SYNDROMES OF NEUROLOGIC PATIENTS IN A SPECTRUM OF SEVERITY OF SOMATIZATION

Beyond a categoric diagnostic classification, the varying degrees of severity of somatization behavior as the number of "medically unexplained physical symptoms" over a specified time period may be the basis for dimensional differentiation of diverse somatization syndromes (7). A variable somatic index of symptoms helps to avoid conceptual and clinical difficulties which could arise in the process of diagnosing according to official categoric classification systems (8). A dimensional perspective may be a favorable background for studying more closely particular aspects of somatization behavior and how these are expressed in a continuum.

The process of somatization may be considered a very complex one, in which variables like psychosocial stress, personality, concept of the illness, psychopathologically relevant affective conditions, and illness behavior have a major influence (9).

In order to test this *dimensional* hypothesis regarding conversion syndromes, we prospectively studied 33 patients presenting with pseudoneurologic syndromes (psychogenic movement disorders) during a 6-month period (10). Complete clinical and neurologic diagnostics ruled out an underlying organic disease. According to the criteria of DSM-IV, the following diagnostic groups were differentiated: somatoform disorder (n = 29), factitious disorder (n = 4). According to a quantitative dimension of somatization (i.e., somatization index), three groups were then formed, showing a low (less than 4), an intermediary (4–12), and a high number (13 or more) of medically unexplained somatic symptoms. These groups presented with different profiles in anxiety (HAMA) and depression (HAMD) with accordingly increasing symptom severity. Hypochondria (Whiteley Index) did not discriminate between these groups. Pronounced hypochondriacal symptoms seemed to be clinically relevant for some patients in each group (Table 19.5).

There was a steady increase in the alexithymia scores (Toronto Alexithymia Scale) from subgroup I to subgroup III. The statistically significant difference had to be related first and foremost to differences in the factor I indicating difficulties in the differentiation between emotions and bodily sensations. Immature defense styles (Bond Defense Style Questionnaire) and discrete personality dimensions (excitability, strain, somatic complaints, emotionality) in the Freiburg Personality Inventory differentiated corresponding to a severity spectrum of somatization. The majority of patients with a factitious disorder demonstrated a psychological test profile which was quite similar to those patients showing a high number of somatoform symptoms.

TABLE 19.5

SOMATIZATION (SOMS-2Y), DEPRESSION (HAMD), ANXIETY (HAMA), AND HYPOCHONDRIA (WHITELEY INDEX) IN NEUROLOGIC PATIENTS WITH CONVERSION SYNDROMES

		Group I	Group II	Group III		I vs. III	I vs. II	II vs. III	
Somatization									
(SOMS-2y)	1-35	2.6 ± 1.3	10.7 ± 1.0	16.4 ± 2.9	a	+	+	+	f
	1-42	3.1 ± 2.0	13.0 ± 2.0	20.8 ± 3.6	b	+	+	+	f
Depression									
(HAMD)		16.2 ± 4.6	21.3 ± 4.7	29.5 ± 6.3	c	+		+	e
Anxiety									
(HAMA)		10.5 ± 3.0	11.5 ± 2.7	16.5 ± 1.6	d	+		+	e
Hypochondria									
(Whiteley-Index)		3.4 ± 3.8	6.3 ± 4.2	5.7 ± 2.9	n.s.e	—	—	—	—

Note: Groups I–III according to variable somatization index (SOMS-2 years) (I: <4, II: 4–12, III: ≥13 medically unexplained somatic symptoms).
[a] ANOVA one way: F = 125. 74, df = 2/27, $p < 0.001$
[b] ANOVA one way: F = 129. 37, df = 2/27, $p < 0.001$
[c] ANOVA one way: F = 18. 58, df = 2/27, $p < 0.001$
[d] ANOVA one way: F = 5. 02, df = 2/27, $p = 0.013$
[e] ANOVA one way: F = 1,57, df = 2/27, $p = 0.229$
[f] Student-Newman-Keuls Method for pairwise multiple comparisons: $p < 0.05$.

We concluded that severity of somatization may be a promising clinical approach to investigate the various dimensions of illness behavior in patients with conversion syndromes. In this respect, patients with factitious disorder seemed to have much in common with patients showing a high number of "medically unexplained symptoms" in addition to the prevailing symptom of "psychogenic movement disorder."

FACTITIOUS DISORDERS IN NEUROLOGY AND CLINICAL MEDICINE

Looking at a presumed common ground of somatoform and factitious disorders the other way around, we analyzed our data on patients with factitious disorders referred to our psychiatric consultation service at a university hospital in Munich (11).

During an 18-year period, 93 patients (women: n = 76, men: n = 12) with a factitious disorder were identified retrospectively and prospectively (0.62% of all C/L psychiatric contacts during the period of observation). Seventeen percent of patients were referred from the department of neurology, presenting with a variety of conversion and pain syndromes, most often in a dramatic state of emergency. No differences could be found between artifactual patients coming from neurology and patients having been referred from other departments of clinical medicine. Therefore, it seems justified to present the data from the whole sample.

In the whole sample, 50% of women were working in medical professions, whereas only 6% of men did so. Chronic courses of illness were prevailing, but at least one quarter of the women showed an intermittent type. "Pathologic peregrinating from hospital to hospital" (women: 51%, men: 47%) and "pseudologia phantastica" (women: 36%, men: 41%) were frequent single items both in men and women. In a stricter diagnostic sense, however, these cases still belonged to the general category of factitious disorder. There was a classic Münchausen syndrome only in 11% of patients (women: n = 1, men: n = 9). Depressive and anxiety disorders (10%, 4%) were to be respected as psychiatric comorbidity. Approximately 25% of the patients suffered from a somatic illness in addition to the factitious disorder, and one third of the women had symptoms of "psychosomatic" disorders, especially eating disorders. In addition, serious problems of substance abuse/dependency and sexual deviations were obvious. A high number of borderline personality disorders in women and of antisocial personality disorders in men had to be noted (Table 19.6).

Patients with factitious disorders had a remarkable history of several other psychiatric disorders. Above all, women frequently showed a series of somatoform disorders such as somatoform pain disorder or conversion disorder in their psychiatric history. In single cases, we observed

TABLE 19.6

PSYCHIATRIC AND SOMATIC COMORBIDITY IN A SAMPLE OF PATIENTS WITH OBJECTIFIED DIAGNOSIS OF FACTITIOUS DISORDER (N = 93)

	Women (n = 76)	Men (n = 17)
Major depression	10%	4%
Anxiety disorder	4%	—
Dependency of substance	40%	53%
Sexual disorders	43%	41%
Münchausen-by-proxy	4%	—
Münchausen syndrome	4%	41%[a]
Somatic morbidity	24%	29%
Psychosomatic illness	33%[b]	6%
Borderline	47%[a]	12%
Histrionic	15%	12%
Antisocial	4%	41%[a]

[a] p <0.001 (Fisher's exact, two-tail).
[b] p <0.05 (Fisher's exact, two-tail).

an ongoing transition among these syndromes. Rather than making a strict nosologic distinction, for example, between paralysis of a leg probably produced by unconscious motives, and in the further course of illness, an additional deliberate harming of this very same leg by self-induced infections, we assumed a dimensional spectrum of unconscious and conscious motives. A small number of patients with a current somatic factitious disorder gave evidence of previous periods in which they also feigned psychiatric disorders with prominent psychological symptoms (e.g. paranoid syndromes, Ganser syndrome, grief after feigning bereavement of a close relative, posttraumatic stress disorder after feigning rape), being admitted to a psychiatric hospital for these reasons. Either previously or during the time of factitious disorder, women and men also frequently tended to self-inflict injuries to their skin surface impulsively. This kind of deliberate self-harm seemed to fulfill a deceptive intent in the doctor–patient relationship only in rare cases. In addition, the psychiatric history of our patients' sample underlined a high risk of suicidality, with some patients repeatedly attempting to commit suicide (Table 19.7).

Once again here were found frequent traumatizing events (foster home, disturbing family disharmony, physical and sexual abuse, early losses, serious psychiatric and somatic disorders) in the early biography. The results were quite identical with the data presented in Table 19.3.

As a rule, the analysis of intrapsychic motives and/or psychosocial stressors turns out to be difficult in patients with factitious disorders. This is partly due to a time-limited assessment in psychiatric consultation services. Careful clinical explorations and consulting the often manifold clinical, social, and legal notes at hand from various sources,

TABLE 19.7

SOMATOFORM AND (PARA-) SUICIDAL BEHAVIOR IN PSYCHIATRIC HISTORY IN A SAMPLE OF PATIENTS WITH OBJECTIFIED DIAGNOSIS OF FACTITIOUS DISORDER (N = 93)

	Female (n = 76)	Male (n = 17)
Somatoform pain disorder	43%[a]	6%
Somatization disorder	7%	6%
Conversion disorder	31%	29%
Psychological factitious disorder	5%	2%
Open self-harm	33%	24%
Suicide attempt	37%	29%

[a]p = 0.004 (Fisher's exact, two-tail).

however, gave some insight into the actual psychodynamics of the artifactual patients in our sample. Conflicts and stressors of a varying structure were suggested:

- Prior to factitious self-harm, some patients were involved in partnership or family conflicts that obviously became extremely intense and out of personal control. These patients used their bodies in order to put their archaic feelings of jealousy, hatred, revenge, or envious rivalry into a concretized bodily form. They tended to express their self-harming and feigning behavior with a sense of superficial triumph. But in dynamic terms, this maneuver often served to defensively cover incestuous events tabooed within the family. Uncovering these incidents in front of medical or official authorities would have forced them to meet unbearable feelings of shame and guilt.
- A bereavement of a close relative or a relationship with a symbiotic partner having fallen seriously ill were some other important events preceding factitious self-harming. These incidents seemed to trigger a somatic self-punishment by means of introjecting aggressiveness. The self-induced somatic injuries enabled the patients to maintain a loving attachment to the lost or endangered partner via identification without self-exposure to painful feelings of bereavement and grief. Simultaneously, this mode of resolving conflicts made it obvious that the patients were not very secure about distinguishing between subject and object in certain areas of their bodily selves.
- Some patients had been demonstrating a highly narcissistic investment in their body, for example, engaging in extreme sports during late adolescent years. However, sometimes after minor accidents, they suddenly started to shift to a fierce bodily self-devaluation and to practice self-destructive behavior of a terrifying intensity. Other examples of serious narcissistic insults of the body self were seen in desires for having a baby completely associated with the person's self-esteem that remained

unfulfilled in spite of varied efforts, or a rape, all events triggering a factitious illness behavior.

- The cases of feigned illness in some women were rather considered as being interpersonal help-seeking behavior. These patients would otherwise not have escaped from an extreme family burden. In some men, we found what looked like an existential defense mechanism against complete social disintegration as an essential motive of the factitious disorder.

As a matter of fact, these important psychosocial stressors in the acute eliciting situation before hospital admission, such as insolvable conflicts in an incest family, pathologic grief reactions, narcissistic injuries to the body self, extreme intrafamiliar exhaustion, disharmony, or violence, must be evaluated against the background of a highly conflicted and traumatized personality development.

DISCUSSION

The frequency rates of factitious disorders observed in our psychiatric consultation service of a university hospital are highly comparable to those in analogously designed studies (12,13). Epidemiologically, however, it must be assumed that these figures probably represent only a small minority compared to much higher estimated rates of patients who self-destructively delay their curing process, for example, by intentionally taking the administered medication irregularly (14).

Sensational case reports on patients with Münchausen syndrome may lead to a distorted impression regarding the incidence and prevalence of this type of disorder. From a clinical point of view, these dramatic Münchausen cases are second to a factitious illness behavior presenting itself in a much less dramatic way. Only 11% of our sample could be classified as patients with a typical Münchausen syndrome. However, we should consider that a tendency for pseudologia phantastica and peregrinating from hospital to hospital existed in a much higher percentage among the sample as a whole. On the one hand, these items had to be discussed as particular psychopathologic and psychodynamic aspects of the fundamental feigning dimension; on the other hand, they had to be characterized as particular features of an illness behavior in a metropolitan health system supplying a great variety of outpatient and inpatient treatment facilities. A comparison of Münchausen patients with the more "secret self-harmers" yielded frequency rates and epidemiologic characteristics similar to the ones found in other studies (15). Our sample showed a high percentage of axis II diagnoses according to DSM-III-R. Women gave prevailing evidence of borderline personality disorder, while antisocial personality disorder dominated in men. Accordingly, a predominating secret self-abuse on the one hand and classic

Münchausen syndrome on the other had to be differentiated between the sexes. The long history of illness with the features of a fragile self-awareness and of complete lack of or at most very unstable relationships could best be considered as traits of a seriously impaired personality (16). Suicidality, impulsivity, deliberate self-harm, addiction, and sexual disturbance had to be regarded as frequent coexisting problems associated with this personality disorder. The particular role of self-destructively exploiting one's body was worth being picked out as a central theme.

Etiopathogenesis of factitious disorder must be considered in a multifactorial way. It certainly cannot be approached adequately by a single theoretic model only. The most important etiologic-pathogenetic arguments, however, are still oriented to psychodynamics and traumatology (17). Common psychodynamic themes are about dependency, masochism, and mastery over the trauma. In fact, paternal cruelty with traumatizing physical and sexual abuse, emotional deprivation, separation, and bereavement events, periods of personal serious illnesses or those of close family members, of hospitalizations, and so on were very frequent characteristics in the patients' early development in our sample. These traumatic experiences may be associated with a basic disturbance of the body self, a pathologic regulation of self-esteem, and highly conflicted patterns of personal relationships (18). It must be observed that the two fundamental psychopathologic dimensions of "self-harm" and "feigning," which also characterize the relationship between artifactual patient and doctor, reflect these basic dynamics. We agree with Kooiman (19) that factitious disorders may not only be associated with regular somatic diseases, but even quite often represent the primary medium of secretly self-harming and interpersonally manipulative behavior. In addition, reflecting on the coexisting "psychosomatic disorders," especially of the gastrointestinal system and eating disorders seen surprisingly often in women, important additional signs of equivalents of factitious disorder according to Plassmann (18) turned out. In this respect, we should not only consider the aggressive conflict topics of dependency and autonomy so typical of borderline patients, but also the unconscious fantasies relating to the body and the attempts to concretisize them in bodily symptoms. The high rate of operations associated with factitiously self-harming and interactionally feigning behavior underlines a decisive involvement of medical doctors in the self-destructive body dialogue among these patients.

In our 15-year survey of patients with factitious disorder, careful psychiatric assessment yielded a high rate of somatoform disorders in the previous psychiatric history. These somatoform disorders were quite often seen in the women; however, a quarter of the men had been treated for pseudoneurologic functional symptoms, as well. Transitions from conversion disorder to somatoform pain, and finally to factitious self-harm, as verified in some single cases,

present a dimensional perspective as a more reasonable way of looking at factitious disorders rather than an exclusive categorization.

Assuming a global spectrum of malingering, factitious disorder and somatoform disorder seem to be confirmed also by the clinical data of our two other prospective studies on neurologic patients presenting with pseudoneurologic symptoms (conversion symptoms). It turned out that patients with factitious disorder regularly formed a subgroup of patients with conversion symptoms. With respect to the course of illness, psychiatric comorbidity, personality disorders, autodestructive motives, and other dimensions of illness behavior, these artifactual patients shared many characteristics especially with patients of the diagnostic subgroup of somatization disorder, respectively, with patients showing a high number of medically unexplained bodily symptoms on a spectrum of severity of somatization. Therefore, it seems to be justified to stress a common ground of somatoform and factitious disorders too often considered as separate clinical entities.

CONCLUSION

From a clinical standpoint, it may be more useful to assume a spectrum of severity of somatization rather than postulating exclusive categories of somatoform disorders on the one hand, and of factitious disorders and malingering on the other. Differentiating several dimensions of illness behavior, psychopathology, psychodynamics, and so on seems to be a more promising approach to recognizing and managing this group of sometimes difficult, but nevertheless fascinating, patients in neurology.

REFERENCES

1. Akagi H, House A. The epidemiology of hysterical conversion. In: Halligan P, Bass C, Marshall JC, eds. *Contemporary approaches to the study of hysteria. Clinical and theoretical perspectives.* Oxford: Oxford University Press, 2001:73–87.
2. Halligan P, Bass C, Marshall JC, eds. *Contemporary approaches to the study of hysteria. Clinical and theoretical perspectives.* Oxford: Oxford University Press, 2001.
3. Cramer B, Gershberg MR, Stern M. Münchausen syndrome. Its relationship to malingering, hysteria, and the physician-patient relationship. *Arch Gen Psychiatry.* 1971;24:573–578.
4. Fink P. The use of hospitalizations by persistent somatizing patients. *Psychol Med.* 1992;22:173–180.
5. Taylor S, Hyler SE. Update on factitious disorders. *Int J Psychiatry Med.* 1993;23:81–94.
6. Kapfhammer HP, Dobmeier P, Mayer C, et al. Conversion syndromes in neurology. A psychopathological and psychodynamic differentiation of conversion disorder, somatization disorder and factitious disorder. *Psychother Psychosom Med Psychol.* 1998a; 48:463–474.
7. Katon W, Lin E, von Korff M, et al. Somatization: a spectrum of severity. *Am J Psychiatry.* 1991;148:34–40.
8. Hiller W, Rief W, Fichter MM. Further evidence for a broader concept of somatization disorder using the somatic symptom index. *Psychosomatics.* 1995;36:285–294.

9. Mayou R, Bass C, Sharpe M. Overview of epidemiology, classification, and aetiology. In: Mayou R, Bass C, Sharpe M, eds. *Treatment of functional somatic symptoms.* Oxford, New York, Tokyo: Oxford University Press, 1997:42–65.

10. Kapfhammer HP, Ehrentraut S, Wittbrodt M, et al. Conversion Syndromes in Neurology—a differentiation by psychological tests. *Gen Hosp Psychiatry (submitted).*

11. Kapfhammer HP, Rothenhäusler HB, Dietrich E, et al. Artifactual disorders–between deception and self-mutilation. Experiences in consultation psychiatry at a university clinic. *Nervenarzt.* 1998b;69:401–409.

12. Krahn LE, Li H, O'Connor MK. Patients who strive to be ill: factitious disorder with physical symptoms. *Am J Psychiatry.* 2003; 160:1163–1168.

13. Sutherland AJ, Rodin GM. Factitious disorders in a general hospital setting: clinical features and a review of the literature. *Psychosomatics.* 1990;31:392–399.

14. Freyberger H, Nordmeyer JP, Freyberger HJ, et al. Patients suffering from factitious disorders in the clinico-psychosomatic consulta-tion liaison service: psychodynamic processes, psychotherapeutic initial care and clinicointerdisciplinary cooperation. *Psychother Psychosom.* 1994;62:108–122.

15. Fink P, Jensen J. Clinical characteristics of the Münchausen syndrome. A review and 3 new case histories. *Psychother Psychosom.* 1989;52:164–171.

16. Nadelson T. The Münchausen spectrum: borderline character features. *Gen Hosp Psychiatry.* 1979;1:11–17.

17. Ford CV, Feldman MD. Factitious disorders and malingering. In: Wise MG, Rundell JE, eds. *Textbook of consultation-liaison psychiatry. Psychiatry in the medically ill.* 2nd ed. Washington, DC, London: American Psychiatric Publishing, 2002:519–531.

18. Plassmann R. Inpatient and outpatient long-term psychotherapy of patients suffering from factitious disorders. *Psychother Psychosom.* 1994;62:96–106.

19. Kooiman CG. Neglected phenomena in factitious illness: a case study and review of literature. *Compr Psychiatry.* 1987;28:499–507.

Treatment of Hypochondriasis and Psychogenic Movement Disorders: Focus on Cognitive–Behavioral Therapy

20

John R. Walker *Patricia Furer*

ABSTRACT

Hypochondriasis is a form of abnormal illness behavior often seen in the clinic and the community. Factor analytic studies suggest three important aspects of this problem: bodily preoccupation, disease phobia, and disease conviction. Bodily preoccupation describes the tendency of individuals high in the hypochondriasis or somatization dimensions to focus attention on bodily symptoms and to be alarmed by unusual or unpleasant symptoms. Disease phobia is a fear that one will develop a serious disease, usually life-threatening or severely disabling. Disease conviction is the belief that one has a serious disease (such as cancer or heart disease), even though the physician does not provide a diagnosis consistent with this disease. It is likely that bodily preoccupation and disease conviction are high among individuals presenting various forms of psychogenic movement disorder (PMD).

There is little information on the extent to which health anxiety or disease phobia are factors in the development or maintenance of psychogenic movement disorders. This chapter describes cognitive–behavioral therapy, the most well-developed approach to understanding, assessing, and treating the various aspects of hypochondriasis, using a case example. We emphasize aspects of the approach that may be applicable to PMDs.

INTRODUCTION

We were surprised at first when we were invited to give a presentation at a conference focusing on psychogenic movement disorders. Our challenge was to consider the connection between psychogenic movement disorders and hypochondriasis or, more broadly, health anxiety. It became clear that there are many common issues, and that research and clinical experience with hypochondriasis may be helpful in understanding psychogenic movement disorders. Some of the common issues are as follows:

- The problems are not well-understood in the community or in the health care system.
- Patients who experience these problems may be anxious or perplexed about their symptoms and may be concerned about the implications of the symptoms for their future health.
- The patient may expect a clear explanation of the symptoms, but on the other hand, the patient's scientific understanding of the symptoms may be limited.
- The patient may expect a definitive treatment that will remove the symptoms, but the treatment may not be clear and it may not completely remove the symptoms.
- The symptoms may be very distressing and disabling.
- The problems are costly for the health care system and often for the patient and the family.
- Some strategies patients use to cope with the symptom may be very useful, while other strategies may make the symptoms or the patient's situation worse.

DEFINITIONS

Somatization

The clinical language we use to discuss the experiences of our patients is based on common agreement about definitions. Definitions used by specialists evolve over time, and the general public may not have the same understanding or interpretation. Sometimes, applying circular reasoning, we may come to believe that applying a label explains a phenomenon. As a simple example, if a woman has difficulty getting to sleep almost every night and is worried about this problem, we might say she has insomnia. If someone asks why she has difficulty getting to sleep, she could explain, "I have insomnia." The label for the experience becomes an explanation for the phenomenon. In thinking about problems such as health anxiety, somatization, and hypochondriasis, we will want to be aware of the interpretation and definitions of our terms, and not use circular reasoning to explain phenomena.

The most widely accepted terminology related to diagnosis in the mental health field in North America has been developed in the process of publication of the fourth edition of the *Diagnostic and Statistical Manual of Mental Disorders*, Fourth Edition, Text Revision (DSM-IV-TR) by the American Psychiatric Association (1). The definitions of the disorders outlined in this manual are derived from the work of expert committees who consider scientific evidence on the characteristics of the problem, when seen in the clinic or the community. Although evidence available to these committees is often limited, the definition of hypochondriasis has remained consistent through the latest editions of this manual, where it is grouped with the somatoform disorders. The manual describes somatoform disorders as follows:

> The common feature of the Somatoform Disorders is the presence of physical symptoms that suggest a general medical condition (hence, the term somatoform) and are not fully explained by a general medical condition, by the direct effects of a substance, or by another mental disorder (e.g., Panic Disorder). The symptoms must cause clinically significant distress or impairment in social, occupational, or other areas of functioning. In contrast to Factitious Disorders and Malingering, the physical symptoms are not intentional (i.e., under voluntary control) (1).

Note that individuals with somatoform disorder may also have related medical conditions, but their reaction to the symptoms is beyond what would normally be expected in that condition. In addition to hypochondriasis, the somatoform category includes somatization disorder, undifferentiated somatoform disorder, conversion disorder, pain disorder, body dysmorphic disorder, and somatoform disorder not otherwise specified.

The term "somatoform disorder" is related to the concept of somatization. Lipowski (2) promoted the recent use of the term "somatization" and published a clear review of the concept in 1988. He wrote:

> Somatization is defined here as a tendency to experience and communicate somatic distress and symptoms unaccounted for by pathological findings, to attribute them to physical illness, and to seek medical help for them. It is usually assumed that this tendency becomes manifest in response to psychosocial stress brought about by life events and situations that are personally stressful to the individual. This interpretation represents an inference on the part of outside observers, since somatizing persons usually do not recognize, and may explicitly deny, a causal link between their distress and its presumed source. They respond primarily in a somatic rather than a psychological mode and tend to regard their symptoms as indicative of physical illness and hence in need of medical attention (2).

This definition includes experiential, cognitive, and behavioral aspects. Lipowski (2) described several important dimensions of somatization, including its duration, the degree of hypochondriasis accompanying the symptoms, the degree of overt emotionality or distress, and the individual's ability to describe feelings or emotion states. Individuals having difficulty with somatization may vary a great deal along these dimensions.

Each of the DSM-IV-TR somatoform disorders has detailed criteria to be met in applying the definition. The criteria for somatization disorder are very demanding, requiring that the individual have several years' history of many physical complaints starting before the age of 30 and resulting in treatment being sought or significant impairment in functioning. Further, the individual must have, at some time, experienced at least four different pain symptoms, at least two gastrointestinal symptoms, at least one sexual symptom, and at least one pseudoneurologic symptom. The criteria for undifferentiated somatoform disorder are less demanding, requiring one or more physical complaints lasting for at least 6 months that cause clinically significant distress or impairment in functioning. The most common symptoms are fatigue, loss of appetite, and gastrointestinal or urinary complaints.

Hypochondriasis

The DSM-IV-TR criteria for a diagnosis of hypochondriasis are shown in Table 20.1. The criteria for hypochondriasis used in the tenth edition of the *International Classification of Diseases* (3) differ significantly from the DSM-IV-TR criteria. These differences in the two major diagnostic systems may cause difficulty in comparing results in studies using the different criteria.

Categoric versus Dimensional Views

The definition of hypochondriasis in DSM-IV-TR assumes a categoric view: An individual either has or does not have the condition. In contrast, a dimensional view measures the extent of hypochondriacal or somatization symptoms. An individual may have a high level or a low level of the symptoms. The categoric view has the advantage of simplicity in producing a relatively stable definition that may be used in research. The disadvantage is that for every individual with a full-blown expression of the condition, there are others who meet some but not all the criteria and may have similar levels of distress and disability. For example,

several studies indicate that hypochondriacal symptoms are common in many of the anxiety and depressive disorders (4). The dimensional view may allow for differing levels of symptom severity in individuals and for more clear consideration of the waxing and waning of symptom intensity often seen in individuals with hypochondriacal concerns. Dimensional measures also allow for better evaluation of changes in response to treatment and may allow for more detailed assessment of different aspects of the problem.

Adopting a dimensional view of hypochondriasis, Pilowsky (5) carried out a factor analytic study of hypochondriacal symptoms in 200 patients in a psychiatric setting. Half were included because they were judged to have a high level of hypochondriacal symptoms and the other half were selected for having low levels of these symptoms. Pilowsky (5) had developed a 20-item scale of items (later reduced to 14), scored as true or false, descriptive of hypochondriasis based on definitions provided by a large number of hospital staff. Three dimensions of hypochondriasis were identified: bodily preoccupation, disease phobia, and disease conviction. Bodily preoccupation describes the tendency of individuals high in the hypochondriasis or somatization dimensions to focus attention on bodily symptoms and to be alarmed by unusual or unpleasant symptoms. Disease phobia is a fear that one will develop a serious disease, usually life-threatening or severely disabling. Disease conviction is the belief that one has a serious disease (such as cancer or heart disease) even though the physician does not provide a diagnosis consistent with this disease.

A more recent factor analytic study with a larger sample and broader range of measures (6) confirmed the importance of these three factors in hypochondriasis. Further, the researchers found that the best subscales for discriminating among hypochondriasis, somatization, and psychiatric control groups (with depressive and anxiety disorders)

TABLE 20.1

THE *DIAGNOSITIC AND STATISCAL MANUAL OF MENTAL DISORDERS*, FOURTH EDITION, TEXT REVISION, CRITERIA FOR HYPOCHONDRIASIS

A. Preoccupation with fears of having, or the idea that one has, a serious disease based on the person's misinterpretation of bodily symptoms.
B. The preoccupation persists despite appropriate medical evaluation and reassurance.
C. The belief in Criterion A is not of delusional intensity (as in Delusional Disorder, Somatic Type) and is not restricted to a circumscribed concern about appearance (as in Body Dysmorphic Disorder).
D. The preoccupation causes clinically significant distress or impairment in social, occupational, or other important areas of functioning.
E. The duration of the disturbance is at least 6 months.
F. The preoccupation is not better accounted for by Generalized Anxiety Disorder, Obsessive–Compulsive Disorder, Panic Disorder, a Major Depressive Episode, Separation Anxiety, or another Somatoform Disorder.

Specify if: **With poor insight:** if, for most of the time during the current episode, the person does not recognize that the concern about having a serious illness is excessive or unreasonable.

From the *Diagnostic and Statistical Manual of Mental Disorders*, Fourth Edition, Text Revision Copyright © 2000 American Psychiatric Association, with permission.

were measures of disease phobia. This study also compared categoric and dimensional measures and revealed that dimensional measures were effective in identifying individuals likely to meet categoric criteria.

Escobar et al. (7) described a dimensional measure of somatic symptoms based on part of a structured epidemiologic interview. The Somatic Symptom Index (6,7) identified individuals who demonstrate a high level of disability and high use of health care services with a lower threshold than that required for the conservative DSM-IV-TR Somatization Disorder.

What's in a Term?

It has been challenging to find terms that are acceptable to both clinicians and patients for the phenomena observed in the somatoform disorders in general and hypochondriasis in particular. The history of the term "hypochondriasis" has been reviewed by Berrios (8). While the term "hypochondria" dates back to the time of the Greeks, it was used originally to describe different phenomena from what we consider with our current definition. The term "hypochondriac" in the sense we use it today was first used by medical writers in the 1600s. As Berrios (8) notes, even the writers describing this condition in the 16th to 19th centuries indicate the term had negative connotations among the public, and patients were not happy when it was used to describe the problems they experienced. Patients continue to fear being labeled as a hypochondriac and interpret the concept to imply that "the symptoms are all in your head." Patients may jokingly acknowledge that family members tell them they are hypochondriacs, but they would prefer this term not appear in consultation reports concerning their treatment. Several alternative terms have been considered for problems with hypochondriasis. The terms we have used in our clinic for hypochondriasis include "intense illness worry" or "severe health anxiety." These terms are well-accepted by patients. Clearly, the term "health anxiety" is much broader and could be applied to a wide range of situations and conditions, not only to hypochondriasis or other somatoform disorders.

Terms that have been used in describing problems with somatization have been "medically unexplained physical symptoms" (9) and "functional somatic symptoms" (10). One can imagine the challenges in treatment management that could arise from announcing to patients that they have "medically unexplained symptoms," or that perhaps they have a psychiatric diagnosis such as undifferentiated somatoform disorder. They are likely to respond with frustration and disappointment, and perhaps by continuing to seek a reasonable explanation. The term "functional somatic symptom" has the advantage of having fewer negative connotations.

HOW COMMON IS HYPOCHONDRIASIS?

Assessment of hypochondriasis and other somatoform disorders usually has not been included in large-scale studies of mental disorders in the community. This may have been because of the limited research focused on somatoform disorders and the broad range of other mental disorders typically assessed in these interviews. As noted above, the number of cases identified is strongly related to the restrictiveness of the diagnostic criteria and the specific definitions applied. Clearly, however, the conditions frequently comorbid with hypochondriasis, particularly anxiety and depressive disorders, are very common in the community (4).

The most comprehensive community study of the epidemiology of somatoform disorders was carried out by Faravelli et al. (11) in Florence, Italy. A random sample of 800 residents of two health districts was identified and 84% agreed to participate in a structured interview (using DSM-III-R criteria) (12). Several unique features of this study make it especially important. The structured interviews were carried out by physicians providing services to these catchment areas. These physicians had access to the participants' health records and undertook further investigations to rule out organic causes of symptoms. Among the respondents, 31.6% reported physical symptoms that were explainable by medical pathology, and 33.3% reported physical symptoms apparently not due to organic factors. The mean number of physical symptoms reported by respondents with symptoms but no demonstrable somatic illness was 6.24 (S.D. 3.58), and respondents with a physical illness reported an average of 2.99 (S.D. 2.24) symptoms. The study found one-year prevalence rates of 4.5% for hypochondriasis, 0.7% for somatoform disorder, 13.8% for undifferentiated somatoform disorder, 0.6% for somatoform pain disorder, 0.3% for conversion disorder, and 0.7% for body dysmorphic disorder. Symptoms related to movement were frequently reported by the subgroup who met the diagnostic criteria for hypochondriasis: difficulty swallowing, 6.7%; loss of voice, 13.3%; double vision, 3.3%; blurred vision, 13.3%; fainting, 6.7%; trouble walking, 10%; and paralysis, 23.3%. In this sample, a high proportion of those meeting the criteria for somatoform disorders were women. For example, 67.7% of those with hypochondriasis were women, as were 75% of those with undifferentiated somatoform disorder. The rate of mood and anxiety disorders was three to four times higher among those with hypochondriasis compared to the overall population. Considering use of medical services in the year covered by the study, among those with hypochondriasis, 3.3% had sought no medical services, and 66.7% saw a GP, 3.3% a public psychiatrist, 40% a private psychiatrist, and 3.3% a psychologist/psychotherapist.

Noyes et al. (13) describe a community study of illness fears in a random sample of 500 residents in a county in the Midwestern United States. Respondents were asked a series of 14 questions about illness fears, fear of medical care, fear of blood or needles, and fear of aging or death. The researchers found that 5% of respondents reported much more nervousness than did most people in relation to at least four of six illness/injury items, 4% indicated that such fears interfered with obtaining medical care, and 5% reported some negative effect of these fears on their lives.

In a review of the occurrence of hypochondriasis in general medical settings, Noyes (14) reported a range of 2.2% to 6.9%. Rates were higher in psychiatric populations and specialty medical clinics.

WHAT IS THE RELATIONSHIP BETWEEN HYPOCHONDRIASIS AND PSYCHOGENIC MOVEMENT DISORDERS?

The factor analytic studies of hypochondriacs described above identify three aspects of hypochondriasis, varying across individuals, identified by self-report measures: bodily preoccupation, disease phobia, and disease conviction. Disease phobia was the characteristic that most clearly differentiated individuals with hypochondriasis from those with other common psychiatric disorders (anxiety and depression). On the other hand, a group with hypochondriasis would be higher than individuals in the general population on all these measures. It is likely that many individuals with psychogenic movement disorders are also high on these dimensions, particularly disease conviction and bodily preoccupation. It is not clear to what extent these individuals would report disease phobia—the fear that their symptoms are related to a serious or life-threatening disease—but this may be one of the factors that motivates people to seek assessment and treatment. A variety of anxiety and mood disorders is common in the backgrounds of patients with hypochondriasis and psychogenic movement disorders. This suggests there may be some common factors in the development of these disorders.

Another framework that has been helpful in understanding hypochondriasis has been to consider and assess three systems where anxiety symptoms are seen: bodily sensations, thoughts, and behavior. Just as individuals with hypochondriasis typically have symptoms in each of these areas, many individuals with psychogenic movement disorders also present with symptoms in these areas. The treatment approach applied most consistently in understanding and treating these problems has been cognitive–behavioral therapy (CBT).

SOMATIC SYMPTOMS AND THE SICK ROLE

Specialists in child development and parents have often noted that somatic symptoms are a major way in which children experience and express problems with stress and distress. Most of us are familiar with the tendency of many children to report stomachaches and headaches, or more broadly, to feel sick and want to avoid difficult situations when they are experiencing stress. Most adults have had some experience with somatic symptoms, and with reducing or avoiding activities when we are feeling unwell, that dates back to childhood years.

The development of the concept of the sick role in sociology (15) has been one of the most thorough considerations of common expectations concerning health and illness in our society. With his description of the sick role, Parsons (16) had a strong impact on the development of a sociological understanding of illness behavior. He described the rights and duties conferred on individuals in the sick role and the impact on their functioning in society. In Parson's view, the sick role was conferred on the individual by a medical practitioner.

Segall (15) described later criticisms of Parson's concept of the sick role as being overly medicalized and argued for a broader view of health behavior. He maintained that much of the assessment and management of sickness takes place outside the formal health care system. The most common forms of health care are self-care and care by members of the individual's support system. He suggested:

> A sick role concept would consist of the following rights: the right to make decisions about health-related behavior (Right 1), the right to be exempt from performing usual well roles (Right 2), and the right to become dependent on lay others for care and social support (Right 3).... [The] sick role concept would also consist of the following duties: the duty to maintain health and overcome illness (Duty 1), the duty to engage in routine self-health management (Duty 2), and the duty to make use of a range of health care resources (Duty 3).

These rights and duties will vary with the nature and severity of the illness (exemption from some responsibilities vs. all responsibilities) and duration (temporary vs. permanent). Depending on the nature of the condition, some individuals rely heavily on the health care system in negotiating these rights and duties, and others rely extensively on their own resources and those of their social system. Given that so much happens outside the formal health care system, it is very important to understand the beliefs (and theories) about the health condition that guide decision-making and health (or illness) behavior.

Most people will move into the sick role when dealing with episodic bouts of illness (e.g., influenza or severe back pain), but for some individuals, the sick role becomes a central part of their larger role in their social network for extended periods of time. This is certainly the case for many patients with psychogenic movement disorders, but it is also true of individuals with other forms of severe chronic illness. Patients' beliefs about their role in coping with their health problems will be influenced by their experience with, and understanding of, the sick role. For some individuals, the sick role is a way of escaping from very stressful situations or from life problems that seem insoluble.

Our society looks to medical practitioners to provide information and advice concerning the sick person's rights and responsibilities. As an example, the physician is often required to provide information concerning an individual's request to be excused from work responsibilities. Many sources of assistance to those who are ill (unemployment or disability income, home care) require the recommendation of a physician. A physician's recommendation is frequently sought concerning an appropriate course of assessment and treatment. Finally, the opinion of the physician is frequently sought concerning whether the patient is following his or her duty to care for the health problem and striving to return to a state of good health.

MANAGEMENT OF SOMATIZATION AND HYPOCHONDRIASIS IN PRIMARY CARE

As noted above, individuals with high levels of somatic concern and hypochondriasis are frequently seen in primary care. Several clinicians and researchers with a special interest in this area have developed recommendations for primary care providers in helping these patients. Arthur Barsky (17) has been particularly influential in this area with his recommendations for medical management of hypochondriasis and his work on a cognitive-educational treatment (18).

Goldberg and colleagues developed a model of treatment for somatization appropriate for use in primary care during brief medical consultations (15 minutes) that may occur over a series of visits (19). This model has undergone extensive development and been evaluated in a cost-effectiveness analysis in primary care settings (20). The most common physical complaints involved pain or fatigue. After primary care providers received training in the treatment model, costs of referrals outside the primary health care team decreased by 23% with little overall change in primary care costs. Total direct health care costs were reduced by 15% even when the cost of training was considered.

Smith, Monson, and Ray (21) studied a structured psychiatric consultation for individuals with somatization disorder receiving services in primary care. After a thorough assessment, a consultation letter was sent to the primary care physician, describing somatization disorder, including its chronic relapsing course and low morbidity and mortality rates. The letter encouraged the physician to continue to serve as the primary care physician for the patient, to schedule regular visits (possibly every 4 to 6 weeks), and to carry out a physical examination each visit. It was suggested the physician avoid hospitalization, diagnostic procedures, surgery, and the use of laboratory procedures

unless they were clearly indicated. Finally, physicians were encouraged not to tell patients "it's all in your head." No other psychiatric services were provided. Quarterly health care charges in the consultation group declined by 53%, and there was no change in the average charges for control patients. The number of outpatient visits remained the same in both groups but a decrease in hospital days for the consultation group was the major factor in the reduction in cost. There were no changes in health status or patient satisfaction with health care.

The primary care interventions discussed above are very compatible with the CBT approaches described in the following sections.

COGNITIVE BEHAVIORAL APPROACHES

CBT has been a very influential approach in the psychosocial treatment of a wide range of health and mental health problems. It has the advantage of a close relationship to an extensive body of research in the behavioral sciences on environmental influences on behavior and cognition, and the development over many years of methodologies for evaluating behavior and cognitive change strategies. Clinical scientists developing CBT approaches have a strong allegiance to the development and evaluation of evidence-based treatments. This approach has been applied to problems of hypochondriasis and other somatoform disorders, and has the largest body of research of any approach to these problems.

Case Study

The best way to illustrate this approach is with a case example, a young man seen in our clinic recently. This man had problems with hypochondriasis with high levels of disease conviction, bodily preoccupation, and disease phobia.

Derek was a 29-year-old draftsman who worked in the construction industry. He contacted us at the suggestion of a friend who had been seen previously in our clinic. He was skeptical about seeing a psychologist as he had a wide variety of physical symptoms and wanted to have a clear medical diagnosis. He acknowledged that having the symptoms and trying to obtain the diagnosis were stressful, and he was very worried about his health. In fact, he felt that his death was imminent. He described the onset of symptoms as being about a year earlier. He noticed changes in his vision first and eventually was bothered by black blotches in his vision with lines coming from them. He saw two ophthalmologists and one optometrist. According to his report, "none of them could see any floaters and they told me that my eyes were okay." He said his vision often seemed to shimmer as if he was looking through a heat wave. At other times he had difficulty focusing and experienced double vision. Later he was troubled by ringing in his ears, which later turned to buzzing, and then the sound of his heartbeat. His right ear was popping constantly. In December he finished playing hockey and noticed that both of his legs were tingling from the knees down. Later this feeling moved up to his thighs and eventually to his arms. These symptoms were very disturbing and he went to a hospital emergency department. They offered reassurance but no specific diagnosis or treatment. Two days later he consulted another physician, who noted these symptoms and his neck pain and mentioned there was a chance he had multiple sclerosis. He was very upset about this news. At one point he was sitting and having a cigarette (feeling very worried) and he suddenly felt dizzy and fell off to the right. He did not lose consciousness, according to his account, but he felt "like he had been hit in the head with a shovel." An MRI was arranged, with negative results and a recommendation for another one in three months. He was unable to wait and went to another city within a few weeks to have another MRI, with no abnormal findings again.

A few weeks later, he was frequently experiencing burning sensations in both legs and one arm and through the groin area. It seemed the burning got worse after he exercised so he stopped his regular visits to the gym. He noticed twitching and trembling in his leg, particularly when he woke up at night. This problem evolved into pain in the calves and back of the legs that seemed worse when he walked. Frequent urination and a change in consistency of his stool were also concerns.

When it was clear he did not have MS, he decided, based on the wide range of symptoms and the episode of dizziness and unsteadiness after he had a cigarette, that he had suffered a small brainstem stroke and was at risk for another stroke. He was very frustrated that he had not received a specific diagnosis. He was concerned that with his background of extensive medical tests and the use of an antidepressant medication, doctors would not take his symptoms seriously.

Assessment

In CBT, a careful assessment of the problem is the essential first step. We consider bodily symptoms, thoughts related to the problem, emotion, and behavior and its relation to the external environment. In the following section, we discuss these aspects separately. In practice, these aspects are intertwined and are explored simultaneously in interactions with the patient.

Bodily Symptoms

Patients experiencing health anxiety and somatic concerns often present with a wide array of perplexing symptoms. Symptom diaries can develop a better understanding of the experience of symptoms in the patient's life. A diary may be used to obtain information concerning frequency and intensity of symptoms, antecedents or provoking factors for symptoms, coping strategies—adaptive and maladaptive—thoughts and emotional reaction to symptoms, and response of others in the environment. A symptom diary kept over a week or two tends to produce much more detailed and accurate reports concerning symptoms than do retrospective reports. We typically provide a diary sheet for each day and have space for date, time of day, symptom experienced, activity in the period before the symptom occurred, response to the symptom, and thoughts at the time about the symptom. Patients generally respond well to using a diary because they feel that their symptoms and concerns are being taken seriously. We make it clear that the diary is for assessment and it may take some time to identify an approach to cope with the symptoms. In Derek's case, we started to use a diary of sleep patterns after the first contact because he was very concerned about difficulty with sleep. During the treatment phase we used diaries to keep track of coping activities.

Thoughts about the Problem (Cognition)

In typical medical assessment, there is often a great deal of emphasis on the evaluation of signs and symptoms related to the problem and how they have evolved over time. Little time may be spent on the person's thoughts about the problem. Behavioral scientists who have studied health and illness behavior argue that patients' understanding of the problem is crucial in determining their reaction to the problem, and later, their response to treatment (22). Howard Leventhal, in his "common sense model of health and illness behavior" places the process of symptom perception in the context of self-regulatory behavior. Symptoms often elicit fear and anxiety, leading the sufferer to engage in ameliorative behaviors. Simultaneously, the layperson evaluates the set of symptoms and develops a naïve theory (or common-sense model) of what the symptoms mean and how best to respond" (23). Often the patient's understanding of the problem is very different from the physician's understanding, and this may result in coping behavior that is different from what the clinician would recommend. Evaluating the patient's beliefs about the problem and about how to treat it will help the clinician to develop appropriate interventions.

Here are examples of questions we use to evaluate the patient's understanding of the symptoms:

- What do you think has been causing [the symptoms]?
- How has the medical evaluation of your symptoms gone?
- How has the medical care for your symptoms been? How has the medical advice for managing your symptoms been?
- Many people who experience this type of symptom worry about it being a sign of something really serious. When you notice [the symptom], do you worry about its being the sign of something really serious? What things have you worried about since this symptom developed?

■ Have you worried about the symptom's getting worse?
■ Have you worried about the impact on your everyday life?
■ Have you worried about other people's reactions?
■ What treatment do you think might be necessary to help with the problem?

Many of Derek's thoughts about his symptoms are covered in the case description above. He felt that the wide range of symptoms he was experiencing was clear evidence of problems in the brainstem, since the brainstem is crucial to many basic human functions such as breathing, sleeping, elimination, and perception. He thought about dying every day and felt that each day might be his last. He felt he was not being taken seriously by the doctors he saw, and that due to this lack of concern a serious diagnosis was likely to be missed.

Behavior

Patients attempt to cope with their symptoms, and their coping strategies are based on their understanding of the problem and what might help. A high degree of focus on bodily symptoms is the central aspect of hypochondriasis. Frequent checking of symptoms is common and it is not unusual to see patients who check their weight, blood pressure, pulse, or some other aspect of bodily functioning several times a day. Many patients attempt to reassure themselves by repeatedly discussing the symptoms with family members, friends, or health professionals. Excessive visits to medical services and frequent medical tests are common. Often, people reduce their normal activities because of discomfort or distraction caused by the symptoms. Some patients are reluctant to engage in their normal activities because they fear the symptoms will get worse. Patients with a high degree of disease phobia may avoid activities they feel will put them at risk of illness or death. Many patients are fearful about taking medication because of unrealistic concerns about dangerous side effects (e.g., addiction or an increased risk of cancer). Here are some of the questions we ask to clarify the behavioral aspects of the problem:

■ What things have you tried to cope with [the symptoms]? What else? [Look for multiple examples of coping strategies.]
■ Have you had to cut down or change your usual routine because of [the symptoms]?
■ Are there activities you have avoided because of [the symptoms]?
■ Could you tell me about the doctors you have seen to evaluate this problem?
■ What types of medical tests have you been through?
■ What have been the findings in the examinations and the tests?
■ Do you check your body to evaluate your symptoms or to see if some symptoms are getting worse? Could you tell me about how you do that and how often you do that?

■ Do you check your bodily fluids to see if something is wrong? If yes, how often?
■ Do you talk to your family and friends about your symptoms to get their opinion or their reassurance? If yes, how often?
■ Do you spend time reading about health problems or looking up medical information on the Internet? Could you tell me about that?

Derek had seen a number of medical specialists and had a range of tests—all with normal findings. He had started on sick leave from his job a few weeks before our initial consultation. Due to concerns about his vision, he had given up driving and arranged for friends and family members to drive him to his frequent medical appointments. Although he had been very physically active in the past, he was currently getting little physical activity. In fact, he would often go to bed early and spend time resting in bed. He would frequently attend to areas of his body where he had been experiencing symptoms to evaluate the intensity of the symptoms (vision, pain or burning in his legs, etc.). He paid close attention to patterns of elimination and was concerned about weakness in the flow of his urine and about changes in his bowel movements and the consistency of his stool. He consulted the Internet about the symptoms of stroke. At times, he felt he had to get a clear diagnosis of his condition or he would not be able to go on living. He arranged for a very extensive and expensive diagnostic evaluation at a clinic in another region, which was not covered by his health insurance. No specific diagnosis was provided by the clinic. He had extensive discussions with family members, friends, and co-workers about his symptoms and experiences with the health care system.

Emotion

An evaluation of the emotional response to problems with symptoms is essential in treatment planning.

Derek felt a high degree of anxiety about the risk of disability or death. He also reported a considerable amount of frustration and anger that doctors did not believe him (in his view) and about not receiving a definitive diagnosis or treatment. (At least, he had not received a diagnosis he was willing to accept.) He was angry about the implication that people thought the problem was "all in his head"—even though no one had said this to him. Finally, he felt a great sense of guilt with the view that his illness had been precipitated by his own behavior—smoking, having high levels of stress, and drinking at times. We have found each of these emotions to be common in hypochondriasis, especially in individuals with a high degree of disease conviction.

History and Case Formulation

Case formulation is another essential step in developing an effective treatment plan for hypochondriasis and other somatoform disorders. A thorough review of the patient's history is critical. It is important to consider the predisposing, precipitating, and perpetuating factors in the development of the problem. Many individuals report an extensive history of difficult life experiences of illness and death, often dating from childhood. Unresolved grief is also common. The onset or exacerbation of the disorder at a stressful time in the person's life is characteristic of these problems. Once the disorder is established, there are often perpetuating factors that make it difficult to break out of the pattern of health anxiety and related disability. A thorough understanding of these factors will help the clinician to develop an intervention approach that fits well with the experiences of that individual. These are major areas we explore in the patient's history:

- Life situation in the months before and after the onset of the problem. Exploration of any particularly stressful experiences or situations around this time.
- Any influence of the problem in allowing the patient to escape from a very stressful situation.
- Evolution of the symptoms and thoughts, behaviors, and emotions as the symptoms evolved.
- Past experiences with illness and death. Particular experiences with the illness that is the focus of the patient's concern.
- Past experiences with, anxiety, and depression, both in adult years and in childhood.

Derek indicated that life had been going quite well for him before the onset of the problem. He enjoyed his job, had been promoted to a more senior position, and was viewed as a productive employee. This employer put an emphasis on having a balanced life, in contrast to previous employers, where he had coped with work demands and a desire to be financially successful by working excessive hours. During his college years he was very focused on studying and getting good marks. He would even vomit before exams because of his high level of anxiety. He would experience strong symptoms of anxiety when he encountered situations that were difficult for him.

As a youngster, he was very anxious. He recalled that at one point a teacher told him that if he did not get his anxiety under control, he would be dead of a heart attack by the time he was 30. When he was 10 years old, his father died suddenly of a heart attack when he was on a business trip. His father was overweight, smoked, and had high blood pressure, but he had not been ill previously. An aunt and uncle came over to his house during the night to explain his father's death and told him he should not cry in front of his mother as this would be upsetting to her. He experienced three other deaths of family members in the six months after his father's death. One paternal uncle died of a stroke at age 56, another of a heart attack at age 64. His grandmother, who lived with Derek's family, also became very ill and died shortly after they took her to the hospital. When he was 12, his mother had an unusual loss of consciousness on two occasions that was thought to be a seizure. It was explained to him later that she did not have

epilepsy but had experienced some sort of stress attack. She lost her driver's licence for a period of time but she was able to get it back with the help of a neurologist. Derek was very worried that he would lose his mother just like he had lost his father. He had a strong fear of death after these difficult experiences.

Cognitive–Behavioral Therapy

There is not a single form of CBT but, rather, a range of approaches based on a common set of principles. This form of treatment has generated more controlled trials than any other psychosocial approach. Studies have used various populations, and the specific cognitive–behavioral procedures have differed somewhat from study to study. The treatment strategies have generally been drawn from previous work on anxiety disorders, particularly work on panic disorder, obsessive–compulsive disorder, and generalized anxiety disorder. At this point there is not sufficient research to suggest which of the CBT procedures are most essential in treatment.

The pioneering group in this area (Warwick, Salkovskis, Clark and Wells) is from Oxford University (24,25). This group has applied a range of behavioral procedures commonly used with anxiety disorders to treat hypochondriasis: education about the problem (patients are given an individualized written formulation of their problem from a cognitive–behavioral framework); education on the meaning of previous symptoms, medical interventions, and medical opinions; induction of symptoms through bodily focusing; use of diaries to record negative thoughts and rational responses; behavioral experiments to clarify the development of symptoms; response prevention for bodily checking and reassurance seeking; the participation in treatment of significant others involved in providing reassurance; and exposure to previously avoided illness-related situations. The Oxford group has completed two randomized clinical trials demonstrating a high degree of improvement over 16 weeks of treatment (25,26). Treatment gains were maintained over a follow-up period. Similar positive results have been found by a research group in Holland over two randomized clinical trials (27,28).

When we began our work in this area, we had some concern that psychological treatments would not be well-accepted by individuals with hypochondriasis. Our group surveyed 23 volunteers from the community with a DSM-IV-TR diagnosis of hypochondriasis, seeking help with problems with worries about illness (29). The survey included balanced descriptions of a medication treatment and CBT. Respondents viewed CBT as more effective in both the short and long term and rated CBT as more acceptable overall. Psychological treatment was indicated as the first choice by 74% of respondents, medication by 4%, and 22% indicated an equal preference. Forty-eight percent of respondents would only accept the psychological treatment.

Cognitive–Behavioral Therapy for Conversion Disorder

Speed (30) provides an excellent description of the use of behavior therapy in a case series with conversion disorder. The ten patients in the study all presented with serious gait problems and were treated in an inpatient rehabilitation setting. The treatment approach was based on previous work by Trieschmann et al. (31). Speed gives a detailed description of the treatment protocol, including the roles of various health professionals involved. Briefly, once conversion disorder was diagnosed, no further diagnostic tests or physical examinations were done. A pseudoscientific explanation for the symptoms was given to the patient, that tests and examination established that the brain, spinal cord, nerves, and muscles were intact, and that the messages allowing normal muscle movement were being blocked. It was explained that appropriate physical therapy can reestablish the normal flow of messages, and that sometimes certain stressors can make the problem worse, opening the door to psychological evaluation of the patient once the treatment regimen is underway. The patient was confined to a wheelchair at all times, except during therapy, and there was no discussion with patients about their abnormal gait. The program emphasizes the development and reinforcement of normal motor behaviors and withdrawal of attention for abnormal behaviors. Duration of the treatment was short (4 to 22 days, average 11.8 days). All ten patients had appropriate ambulation at the end of the program, one was lost to follow-up immediately after leaving, seven maintained their gains over the follow-up period (6 to 36 months), and two experienced a return of symptoms. Teasell and Shapiro (32) describe successful treatment, using a strategic–behavioral intervention, of three patients who were unsuccessful in a traditional behavioral physical rehabilitation approach.

Treatment Example: Hypochondriasis with High Disease Conviction

We will provide an example of the use of CBT in our clinic in the case described above, with a particular focus on aspects of treatment that may be useful in some forms of psychogenic movement disorder. While the application of the CBT techniques to different aspects of the problem will be described, in practice these approaches are integrated as they are applied over the course of the treatment.

Anxiety, Avoidance, and Exposure to Feared Situations

A scientific understanding of anxiety underlies the CBT approach to anxiety problems. Fear and anxiety are normal emotions, present in all higher organisms. From the perspective of evolution, having a behavioral system with some hard-wired fears (e.g., fears of heights, large animals, and the unfamiliar) and the capacity to develop new fears based on unpleasant experiences would have important survival value. Two of the common ways of coping with feared situations are escape and avoidance. Unfortunately, consistently avoiding feared situations sustains a fear even when it does not have survival value or is not realistic. For example, fears of flying or public speaking can be maintained over the entire course of a person's life by avoiding these situations. On the other hand, repeated and prolonged exposure to the feared situation in a context where there are not negative consequences will typically result in habituation or desensitization. During prolonged exposure, the individual learns that the feared situation is actually safe. Over time, exposure to feared situations reduces all aspects of the anxiety response—physiological arousal, the behavioral tendency to avoid, negative or catastrophic thoughts, and the unpleasant emotions that accompany these reactions.

Just as individuals may avoid feared environmental situations, they may also avoid verbal and cognitive representations of those situations. So individuals with fears of illness and death may avoid media depictions of illness and death, hospital visits, and funerals, and they may try to avoid thinking and talking about illness and death. When anxiety becomes severe, however, individuals with health anxiety often begin to have intrusive thoughts concerning illness and death. They may be very preoccupied by their fears and struggle to feel safe by remaining vigilant for danger (signs of illness), by seeking out tests that will provide reassurance that the danger is not severe (a CAT scan or MRI), or by finding medical interventions that will remove the threat of illness and death. The reassurance provided by medical tests or interventions may be temporary and the fears of illness and death may re-emerge.

In CBT for anxiety problems, the clinician works to assist the individual in the process of exposure to feared situations (related to symptoms, illness, and death). There is also a focus on eliminating unrealistic safety behaviors (such as always remaining close to a hospital) that provide temporary relief but maintain the anxiety in the longer run. Both the cognitive and the behavioral components of CBT described below emphasize the exposure process.

Cognitive Approach

When focusing on cognitive aspects of the hypochondriasis, CBT is directed at helping the patient to move from unrealistic to more realistic thoughts and beliefs. The patient may not state these beliefs spontaneously until there is a discussion of beliefs related to health and coping. Note that this process of cognitive reappraisal is not the same as the more simplistic approach of "changing negative thinking to positive thinking." Studies of the changes that occur with successful cognitive–behavioral interventions suggest that over time there is a gradual reduction in negative and catastrophic thoughts and an increase in neutral thoughts. There is not a dramatic increase in the level of positive thoughts. This represents a movement toward patterns of cognition seen in people without problems with anxiety or depression as they deal with everyday life challenges.

The work on changing thoughts usually does not involve a head-on attack on the core belief ("I have a severe illness") but, rather, involves a process of considering other possible ways to understand the patient's experiences. This exploration of other possibilities may take place through a discussion of other ways of looking at people's experiences and through *behavioral experiments* aimed at helping people consider other possible explanations for their experiences and different ways of behaving in relation to their health concerns. These approaches will be illustrated in Derek's situation. We will start by considering a whole series of unrealistic beliefs that Derek held (beliefs are the ideas and views that lie behind one's thoughts) and more realistic beliefs the clinician was working toward.

■ *Unrealistic Belief:* My symptoms indicate I have had a brainstem stroke or they are signs of brainstem malfunction that will lead to a brainstem stroke.
More Realistic Belief: My symptoms can be caused by many different factors, including stress. The tests and examinations so far do not indicate any neurologic disease. Any person can develop a stroke or a neurologic disease, but these are more common later in life.

■ *Unrealistic Belief:* If the doctors tell me I do not have a neurologic problem, it means my symptoms are not serious and are imaginary (all in my head). If I do not have a neurologic problem, doctors will not take me seriously.
More Realistic Belief: My symptoms are real and distressing, even if they are not caused by a neurologic problem. Doctors have taken my problem seriously by arranging a wide variety of tests. They will try to help me with my symptoms in the future.

■ *Unrealistic Belief:* I cannot go on with life until I have a clear diagnosis of the problem and a treatment that will remove the symptoms.
More Realistic Belief: Many people go on with life in spite of symptoms that do not have a clear diagnosis or treatment. An active lifestyle often improves symptoms and makes it easier to cope.

■ *Unrealistic Belief:* I should rest and avoid vigorous activity in order to preserve my health.
More Realistic Belief: I can improve my health by staying as physically active as possible. Exercise can strengthen the body, increase flexibility, reduce stress, and reduce pain.

■ *Unrealistic Belief:* Negative test results are very threatening because they mean the doctors do not understand the reason for my symptoms. The problem is even more dangerous because the doctors do not understand it.
More Realistic Belief: Negative test results are good news because they mean the doctors have removed a number of serious illnesses from the list of possible explanations for my symptoms.

■ *Unrealistic Belief:* I must watch my symptoms closely so I can respond immediately if they become worse.
More Realistic Belief: It is normal for symptoms to wax and wane. Symptoms will be less of a problem if I accept them but do not focus on them excessively.

Understanding Symptoms

After obtaining a detailed description of the symptoms, it is helpful to discuss with the patient what makes the symptoms seem more or less intense. It is often easier for patients to identify factors that make the symptoms worse than factors that make the symptoms better. They are more attentive to increasing symptoms as this is a stronger sign of danger. Many patients are able to identify some environmental factors that have these effects. Symptom diaries, such as those discussed in the assessment section, may be useful in identifying factors that make symptoms worse. Symptoms often increase during periods of increased stress, anxiety, conflict, fatigue, or when the person is less occupied with daily activities, such as during the evening, when they are relaxing alone or lying in bed getting ready to sleep. It is also helpful to evaluate whether anything can be done during the office visit to make the symptom more intense. A procedure that may be applied to almost any symptom is to focus increased attention on the symptom and then reduce that attention to evaluate the effect of attention on the symptom. Observing factors that make a symptom more or less intense often helps to make it more understandable and less frightening. This also helps to develop alternative explanations—that symptoms may be related to stress, fatigue, and increased attention, as opposed to a failing brainstem. We applied this approach with Derek in our second appointment.

"Derek, we were talking earlier about the burning and pain you feel in your legs. I was wondering if you could rate how that has been feeling over the last few minutes on a 0 to 100 scale with 0 being not at all present and 100 being the strongest it has ever been?" [Derek gives a rating of 60.] "Now I would like you to close your eyes as you are sitting there and focus on your legs and describe the symptoms in your legs in as much detail as you can.... Good. Could you describe it a bit more...? Good. Now I wonder if we could sit here for a minute or two and have you focus on the feelings you are having in your legs...? Now could you rate the level of symptoms you are having in your legs on the 0 to 100 scale again." [Derek gives a rating of 75.] The clinician goes on to discuss a different topic, unrelated to symptoms, for 5 or 10 minutes, ensuring that the patient is very engaged in the topic. The clinician then returns to the symptoms. "Derek, I want to return to the feelings in your legs again. I wonder if you would rate how strong the symptoms have been for the last few minutes, before I asked this question." [Derek gives a rating of 50.] "That's interesting. Other people find the same thing—if their attention is more focused on the symptoms, they feel them more strongly. If there is less focus, they are less strong." The key thing about a behavioral experiment is that it is interesting however it turns out. So if Derek rates 75, you might say, "It seems like when you focus on your symptoms that feeling of greater intensity lasts for some time." Or if he rates 90, you could say: "That's interesting; even when we were talking about something else, the intensity of your symptoms was increasing. What are your thoughts about that? After we focused on your legs that first time, did you notice any particular thoughts about that?" (Some people report a feeling of anxiety, frustration, or anger when they notice that their symptoms are more intense.)

An approach we used later in Derek's treatment was to learn to provoke unpleasant symptoms (stronger visual symptoms and feelings of being off-balance) intentionally in the office and at home. This approach has been found to be very useful in the treatment of panic disorder. Symptoms can be provoked by procedures to produce light-headedness and other symptoms of arousal (hyperventilation), dizziness and feeling off-balance (spinning while standing or seated in an office chair), or rapid heart rate (running on the spot or using a stepper). In Derek's case, we used a brief period of hyperventilation (60 to 120 seconds) with the clinician hyperventilating along with the patient. These procedures are often presented to the client as a behavioral experiment. ("I was wondering if we could do a little experiment to see how your symptoms are influenced by a change in your breathing for a few minutes. I would like you to breathe very rapidly along with me for a minute or two and then we will notice what feelings you are having.") The clinician carefully reviews the symptoms they both experience, then changes the focus of conversation. Ten or 15 minutes later, the clinician asks the patient to focus on the areas where there had been symptoms earlier and to describe the intensity of symptoms compared to just after the period of hyperventilation. Using the 0 to 100 rating scale, the patient usually notes a very significant drop in symptoms over 10 to 15 minutes. If the patient indicates that the intensity of symptoms has reduced, the clinician may ask the following question: "I was wondering what you did to reduce the symptoms?" This is a very useful behavioral experiment because it can illustrate that in many cases, it is easy to increase the intensity of bodily symptoms, but they then diminish by just switching the focus of attention to something else and allowing time to pass.

In addition to the use of focusing on symptoms and symptom induction to demonstrate how symptoms can be increased and decreased by small environmental changes, these procedures can also be used later in treatment in an exposure therapy approach. Patients are instructed to practice inducing symptoms or focusing on them for 30 to 40 minutes daily for a week or two in order to produce a process of desensitization where the symptom becomes so familiar (and is not avoided) that the negative emotion (anxiety, anger, frustration) associated with the symptom is reduced.

This fits well with the approach of learning to *accept* the symptom and get on with life, rather than struggling to eliminate the symptom.

Understanding Medical Management

Patients often have unrealistic expectations concerning medical assessment and management, and about the normal course of common illnesses. Derek was focused on his fear of having a brainstem stroke in spite of his limited knowledge about this condition. We spent some time exploring his understanding of the processes involved in a brainstem stroke. He was not aware that a stroke involves an interruption of the blood supply to the brain, related to a blood clot or a bleed that typically produces a sudden and lasting (at least over days) change in function. He was aware that his CAT and MRI results indicated no signs of the damage caused by a stroke. He had the view, however, that a stroke could also involve a subtle deterioration in the functioning of the neurons in an area and that this was causing his symptoms. We provided corrective information about this. At his request, we also provided reading material concerning brainstem strokes from a rehabilitation manual that described the dramatic effects of a brainstem stroke. Over time, with this information, Derek's concerns changed from the view that he had experienced a stroke to fear that he was going to have a stroke, and that the symptoms he was experiencing were early signs of this.

We also spent time exploring the usual medical management of a stroke. Again, he was not aware that the approach involves conservative measures to manage the clot or the bleed. If a person does not die from the acute event, the longer-term approach emphasizes rehabilitation and return to functioning. Derek had the sense that his concerns were not being taken seriously when in fact he was already taking one of the main treatments for prevention (a small daily dose of aspirin) recommended by his physician. He had expected that some high-technology medical solution might be possible when this did not exist. We emphasized that many of the measures we were recommending would be the same things he would be doing if he did have a stroke: gradually increasing exercise, keeping active and involved, and returning to the maximum function possible. Rather than reassuring Derek that he would never have a stroke, we informed him that young people do have strokes and that either one of us could have a stroke any day. If this happened, we would have to use our resourcefulness to manage the situation. In the meantime, the most effective approach is to maintain a healthy lifestyle with an emphasis on exercise, healthy food, and control of weight and blood pressure.

We find that people experiencing difficulty with anxiety and depression often feel they do not receive the same consideration in the health care system, the workplace, and the family as someone with a clear physical diagnosis. To address this concern, we tell people that a working adult with a first heart attack is typically back to work within 4 to 6 weeks. Following a heart attack, patients are encouraged to start a gradual exercise program shortly after the acute recovery period is finished.

Decreasing Reassurance Seeking and Checking

When Derek became upset about his symptoms, he often consulted a new medical practitioner to request an evaluation of his symptoms. In each case, he was hopeful the new evaluations would finally provide an answer about his symptoms. Each time, he was disappointed and angry about the results. We pointed out this pattern and described how the examinations, tests, and checking actually feed the problem with anxiety.

In this discussion we also spent some time on the meaning of normal or negative test results. Rather than being relieved by normal test results, Derek felt the problem was even more threatening. We pointed out that the evaluations eliminated many, very serious, potential causes of the problem that have few or limited treatment options (multiple sclerosis, brain tumor, etc.). This is good news. A high proportion of the people receiving these tests have normal results because the tests are being used to rule out even rare problems. Negative tests do not mean his symptoms cannot be understood. In fact, these types of symptoms are common in stress-related situations and health anxiety. We reviewed the symptoms covered on a common measure used in our clinic to evaluate psychological distress—the Symptom Checklist 90, Revised (33). Many of the symptoms he had been experiencing were included in the checklist.

Given that numerous medical visits and tests had not resolved his problems, we encouraged Derek to limit himself to scheduled medical visits (rather than rushing off for consultations when he was feeling upset about his symptoms). We encouraged him to hold off any further tests and evaluations unless these were recommended to him by someone who knew his situation well. Finally, we also recommended he move away from excessive discussion of his symptoms and worries with family members and co-workers because this would distract them from their normal relationship with him. They were unlikely to have any new information about the situation. Derek was receptive to this suggestion because he felt that people at work and in the family were reacting differently to him because of his many health concerns.

Another form of checking is when patients repeatedly focus on their symptoms to evaluate their intensity at a particular time. As an example, Derek would look at vertical lines of buildings to see how much they moved due to disturbances in his vision. In the approach of reducing checking, patients are encouraged to reduce the amount of time they spend checking their symptoms. This may seem to contradict the treatment approach involving exposure to body symptoms, but the difference is that exposure takes place at planned times for longer periods of time

(e.g., 45 minutes). The longer period of time involved in exposure assignments allows for a decrease in arousal over a period of time. Checking, on the other hand, tends to take place repeatedly over the course of the day for short periods of time and has a different purpose: looking for signs of danger rather than focusing on acceptance.

Returning to Normal Functioning and Focusing on Life Goals

When patients experience problems with anxiety or depression, they often give up some of their normal activities and are less involved in activities that bring a sense of competence, satisfaction, or enjoyment. Typically, we review the patient's current activities and compare them to activities at a time when life was going well. We also explore the short-, medium-, and long-term goals the patient would have in life if they were not experiencing health problems. We emphasize working toward goals in spite of difficulties with health problems. In reviewing the unrealistic beliefs above, we noted Derek's unrealistic beliefs that he could not go on with life until he had a clear resolution of his health concerns and that avoiding vigorous activity is important to improving health. We pointed out that even people who are dealing with very serious health problems find it helpful to stay involved with life and focused on their personal goals.

Derek had recently given up driving because of concerns about his vision. He had extensive investigations of his vision without serious problems being identified. We explored whether the visual disturbances made it difficult to see other cars or pedestrians or to judge distances between cars. He indicated that even though he found the visual disturbances distracting and emotionally upsetting, they did not interfere with his ability to make normal driving decisions. In fact, he noticed the visual disturbances less when he was involved in an activity (such as driving) and more when he focused specifically on his vision. After discussing this at some length, we agreed it would be appropriate to start driving again with a focus initially on driving during daylight hours and close to home. Driving was an important aspect of his job so it would be helpful in the long run if he could maintain this ability. His return to driving went smoothly and allowed him to be less dependent on others.

Physical activity had previously been enjoyable for Derek. His informal observation had been that the pain and trembling feelings were worse after exercise. We pointed out that exercise has a positive effect on a range of health problems and is routinely recommended after strokes or heart attacks, and also helps in the management of pain. Cardiovascular exercise also helps prevent these problems. We recommended he start with moderate exercise, considering his level of exercise recently, and then gradually increase the duration and intensity of his workouts. We agreed it would be useful to use a symptom diary to evaluate the extent to which the symptoms changed during and after exercise, and how long this change lasted after a period of exercise. After a week or two of keeping a diary, he found that exercise had only a temporary effect of increasing his symptoms and that he generally felt better on a day when he exercised.

Work had been a source of satisfaction and a sense of competence for Derek over the years. His co-workers and especially his manager were very friendly and supportive. Once he was driving and more physically active, we agreed that returning to work on a phased-in basis would be helpful for his morale. We pointed out that even people with very severe illness—multiple sclerosis, heart attack, and cancer—usually benefit from working as much as they are able. The return to work went fairly smoothly, although there was a period when excessive discussion of his health concerns in the workplace became a problem. We agreed on a strategy of focusing on work issues in the workplace and limiting talk about health concerns to after work hours and with appropriate health professionals.

We also noticed that Derek was less involved in enjoyable leisure activities when he was concerned about his health. During some of the early sessions, we focused on his returning to his normal leisure activities, also, and planning enjoyable activities every week.

Derek was more enthusiastic about returning to former activities than were many patients. The therapist encourages the patient to target activities that fit with the patient's interests and preferences, and that are likely to bring some positive results and satisfaction in the short term. In cases where return to more normal functioning can be difficult or painful, the clinician works with the patient and others in the environment to increase the likelihood of immediate positive consequences for efforts at behavior change. Areas where negative consequences are possible (such as a return to a family situation or job that were unpleasant) have to be handled with much more strategic planning so that the patient does not move into situations where the sick role may be reinforced.

Exposure to Fears of Illness, Disability, and Death

Fear of illness, disability, and death is a central aspect of hypochondriasis. Patients may agree that a stroke or heart attack is a low-probability event for people of their age, but they still fear this unlikely and very frightening event will happen to them. They engage in activities to try to prevent it from happening, including excessive seeking of medical attention. The media is full of accounts of unlikely events that have suddenly killed or disabled people similar in age and personal characteristics to the patient. We approach this problem by an exposure or face-your-fear approach. The clinician acknowledges that severe illness or death may come suddenly to any one of us. The time could come for our next scheduled appointment and one of us could arrive only to find that the other has died or is gravely ill.

Facing the reality of death is an important aspect of having a good life. Philosophers have argued that an awareness of the shortness of life and the reality of death would help any person to have a better life. We approach this task by having patients write an *illness story* (working independently using a sample story, or with the help of the therapist). The story should include all their worst fears about negative health outcomes, and should not have a happy ending, such as being rescued somehow by medical care. Once the story is completed, patients are instructed to spend 45 to 60 minutes a day over two or three weeks using the story to help them face their worst fears about illness and death. Rather than trying to reassure themselves that they will avoid the illness or receive medical help that will bring a cure, they should work to accept that illness may come any day and take away their life or quality of life.

Many patients have difficulty at first understanding the approach of facing their fears and worries head-on like this. They may say, "I worry all day about my health so this isn't any different from what I already do. How will this help me to deal with the problem?" The clinician explains that typically when people worry about something, they are often searching for ways to get out of the problem—to obtain treatment for their illness, to avoid death, and to try to get the unpleasant worries out of their mind. This is different from really facing and accepting fears; it is trying to get away from fears. The approach of facing your fears directly has been found to help people reduce their worrying and anxiety about some future threatening event.

Here is Derek's story about his fear of having a stroke:

Brainstem Stroke
 Today I was walking down the street, having problems walking a straight line, feeling the deep pain in my knees and hamstrings. As always, swallowing is a problem. As usual, I have nystagmus and double vision. No one can explain this. This alone tells me I am about to have a brainstem stroke. Sure enough, I drop on the street, losing consciousness.

 I am now bound to a wheelchair, unable to communicate or share my life with someone. This has been my greatest fear: never making a difference. Never making an impact in this world. I have run with fear and smoked myself into sickness. Why didn't I see it earlier? You idiot, you wasted 29 years of your life, broken relationships because of personal inadequacies, and being ashamed of yourself as a person. Now you are wheelchair-bound, not being able to speak, run, or play hockey again.

 The build-up of pressure to this point has been pure terror. Unexplained changes in my body, some people thinking I am looking for attention, some saying it's all in my head, what a legacy for the family. I was told in grade three that my demise would occur before 30. She was better than dead-on…29 none-the-less. You can't make your family proud of you with a stress-induced disease. A son who has been obsessive, completely stressed out, and smoking himself to death until two years ago. Two years ago, I changed; but the change came too late.

Look at what my mother has to live with. Everyone knows her son couldn't control his thoughts. He was successful in school and work, but as much as put a gun to his head with his lifestyle. The doctors shake their heads in amazement. How could a guy this young, without doing street drugs, manage to ruin himself like this? Reckless disregard for his life!

Will anyone care, will anyone care, or come see me? I mean, I have treated people poorly, because I don't treat myself well. Now that the stroke has occurred, no woman will want me. In short, I don't fear being missed, I fear being forgotten. That no one will really care.

In Derek's situation, it was also helpful to discuss his experiences with death as a youngster (the deaths of his father and grandmother) and his reactions to these events. As an adult, he had questions about how people cope with life-threatening illness and death. We discussed the specifics of what patients experience in the first stages of a stroke and what it might be like to die from a stroke. He found it helpful when the therapist could explain that people are able to cope with these events with dignity in most cases and still maintain some quality of life. For example, people with terminal cancer still find it helpful to focus on personal goals and to plan activities to enjoy life while life is still with them. We often recommend personal accounts of experience with illness and death in books and movies as a way of facing fear of death. We may also have people prepare an obituary for themselves at their current age, plan funeral arrangements, and prepare a will as ways of facing the reality of death in concrete terms.

The exposure approach can also be used to come to terms with particularly upsetting symptoms. In this approach, the patient uses symptom induction or focusing on the symptom (as described above) for 45 to 60 minutes a day for a week or two to become desensitized to the symptom and more able to accept it. The symptoms then tend to be experienced less often and with lower levels of distress.

Cognitive Reappraisal

Rather than insisting the patient give up strongly held beliefs about the meaning of symptoms at the start of treatment, we take the approach of monitoring thoughts about the symptoms and encouraging patients to consider other possible explanations of the symptoms. We emphasize that we believe the symptoms are real and very distressing, but there may be a variety of different explanations for the symptoms. Over the course of treatment, we encourage patients to observe what factors will make symptoms stronger and weaker. As part of this approach, we encourage patients to develop an awareness of their own thoughts about their symptoms and how these thoughts can change over time. Symptom diaries that include thoughts about symptoms are very helpful to identify common patterns in thinking. During the treatment phase, we provide diaries and examples to use in practicing developing more realistic thoughts. Here are questions we use to explore thoughts about illness:

- What are the most common frightening thoughts you have about your symptoms? For each of the major thoughts note the following:
  - When does this thought tend to come to you?
  - What is the probability this negative event will happen? (In considering this, if you have had this negative thought before, how often has the negative outcome happened in the past?)
  - Do not ask whether this negative event will happen in your lifetime (we are all likely to have serious illnesses in our lifetime). How likely is it that it will happen today? This year?
  - How often does this negative event happen to other people of your age? (Patients are often very far off on their estimates of the probability of specific illnesses at particular ages. The clinician may help by providing estimates of the number of people in 10,000 who will experience a particular illness by a particular age.)
  - If this negative outcome did happen, how would you cope with it? Negative events happen to people throughout their lifetime, often not when they are worrying about them, but at an unexpected time. If the negative event did happen, how would you cope?
  - This negative or catastrophic thought will occur again in the future. What are some coping thoughts you could use when this thought happens again?

Problem Solving

Another approach frequently used in CBT is problem solving concerning symptoms. Developing approaches to manage symptoms more effectively makes them seem less threatening and distressing.

Sleep concerns were prominent and Derek would often spend long periods lying in bed, trying to get to sleep. He felt the sleep disruption was an indication of the brainstem problems. A sleep diary indicated he was spending unusually long times in bed each day. When his time in bed was reduced and some CBT sleep strategies were introduced, he found the quality of his sleep was improved.

Bowel symptoms were also a concern and taken as evidence of difficulties in brainstem functioning. His main concern was that his stool was smaller and harder than it had been in the past and he often had to strain to have a bowel movement. As a behavioral experiment, we agreed he would increase the amount of fiber in his diet each day by substituting a high-fiber food (beans, peas, lentils) for meat in one of his meals each day. He had frequently eaten these foods when he was growing up and he did not think it would be too difficult to make this change. He was asked to keep a diary concerning his food consumption and bowel functioning. After a few weeks of this approach, bowel problems were of less concern.

Patients frequently have interpersonal or workplace problems that are a source of stress. Problem-solving assistance for these issues often helps patients move to a higher level of functioning with a lower level of life stress (34).

Summary
The CBT techniques outlined above are used in an integrated approach. The timing of the interventions is very important, and experienced therapists become skilled at evaluating the patient's life situation and intervening first in areas where the patient is likely to experience reasonable progress. Specific approaches have been developed to deal with the wide range of symptoms seen in the somatoform disorders.

PHARMACOTHERAPY FOR HYPOCHONDRIASIS AND SOMATIZATION

Early descriptions of pharmacologic treatments of hypochondriasis in the psychiatric literature were not optimistic. In 1985, a major psychiatric textbook, Kaplan and Sadock's *Comprehensive Textbook of Psychiatry* (35), indicated that unless hypochondriasis is part of a depressive disorder with an overt affective disturbance, medications and electroconvulsive therapy (ECT) are without effect. Subsequently, a number of case reports have described more favorable results with hypochondriasis with and without delusional psychotic features [reviewed by Enns et al. (36)]. To date, there have been only three reports of open-label trials of treatment of hypochondriasis with generally positive effects (37–39). Open-trial evaluations of antidepressants with somatoform disorder have also been reported with generally favorable results (40,41). Only a single randomized placebo-controlled trial for hypochondriasis has been reported with eight of 12 patients who received fluoxetine being classed as responders, as compared to 4 of 8 on placebo over a 12-week trial. The sample size in this study was small, and statistical comparison did not reveal a statistically significant difference (42).

In spite of the limited research on pharmacologic treatment of these disorders, this is the most widely available treatment and probably the most frequently used with both hypochondriasis and other somatoform disorders (43). Enns et al. (36) point out that many of these individuals have comorbid anxiety or depressive disorders, and these pharmacologic treatments (usually selective serotonin reuptake inhibitors or serotonin–norepinephrine reuptake inhibitors) have been shown to be effective in these comorbid disorders.

RESEARCH QUESTIONS CONCERNING THE RELATIONSHIP BETWEEN HEALTH ANXIETY AND PSYCHOGENIC MOVEMENT DISORDERS

Our understanding of both hypochondriasis and psychogenic movement disorders (PMD) is at an early stage.

In spite of this, experience in assessing and treating hypochondriasis and related problems with health anxiety may add to our understanding of the management of psychogenic movement disorders. We outline below some research questions concerning the relationship between these groups of conditions. The term "psychogenic movement disorder" covers a wide range of conditions (as illustrated by the chapters in this book). It is likely that the relationship with health anxiety varies among the different types of psychogenic movement disorder.

- Preliminary studies suggest that many people with PMD have current or past anxiety or depressive disorders. Do some individuals with PMD have a history of health anxiety?
- Does health anxiety have a role in the development of some forms of PMD?
- Do patients with PMD give up more activities and functions than do patients with comparable organic disorders?
- Do patients with PMD experience more difficulties in interpersonal relationships than do patients with comparable organic disorders?
- Do patients with PMD report more mood disturbance and loss of enjoyment in life than do patients with comparable organic disorders?
- In both hypochondriasis and PMD, the actions of health care providers may feed into the development of the problem. Are there strategies health care providers could use to reduce the development of PMD or chronic forms of the disorder?
- Can early identification of patients with unclear diagnosis but high levels of health care utilization improve health, reduce disability, and decrease unnecessary health care consumption (20,44)?
- Would more attention and support to the patient's role in health care and recovery from disability reduce the degree of disability related to PMD? (Our current health care system is very oriented to diagnosis and cure. Less energy is spent educating and informing patients about their role in self-care and recovery.)
- Would closer monitoring and more effective support of people who leave the workplace because of injuries and illness reduce the development of maladaptive ways of coping and the long-term disability associated with them?
- Could the development of serious health anxiety or movement disorders following traumatic experiences or injuries be reduced through better support after exposure to these experiences?

REFERENCES

1. American Psychiatric Association. *Diagnostic and statistical manual of mental disorders*, 4th ed. Washington, DC: American Psychiatric Association, 2000.
2. Lipowski ZJ. Somatization: the concept and its clinical application. *Am J Psychiatry.* 1988;145:1358–1368.

3. World Health Organization. *The ICD-10 classification of mental and behavioural disorders: diagnostic criteria for research.* Geneva: World Health Organization, 1993.

4. Noyes R Jr. Hypochondriasis: boundaries and comorbidities. In: Asmundson G, Taylor S, Cox B, eds. *Health anxiety: clinical and research perspectives on hypochondriasis and related conditions.* London: John Wiley and Sons, 2001:132–160.

5. Pilowsky I. Dimensions of hypochondriasis. *Br J Psychiatry.* 1967;113:89–93.

6. Hiller W, Rief W, Fichter MM. Dimensional and categorical approaches to hypochondriasis. *Psychol Med.* 2002;32:707–718.

7. Escobar JI, Rubio-Stipec M, Canino G, et al. Somatic symptom index (SSI): a new and abridged somatization construct. Prevalence and epidemiological correlates in two large community samples. *J Nerv Ment Dis.* 1989;177:140–146.

8. Berrios G. Hypochondriasis: history of the concept. In: Starcevic V, Lipsett D, eds. *Hypochondriasis: modern perspectives on an ancient malady.* Oxford: Oxford University Press, 2001:3–20.

9. Melville DI. Descriptive clinical research and medically unexplained physical symptoms. *J Psychosom Res.* 1987;31:359–365.

10. Kellner R. Hypochondriasis and somatization. *JAMA.* 1987;258:2718–2722.

11. Faravelli C, Salvatori S, Galassi F, et al. Epidemiology of somatoform disorders: a community survey in Florence. *Soc Psychiatry Psychiatr Epidemiol.* 1997;32:24–29.

12. American Psychiatric Association. *Diagnostic and statistical manual of mental disorders.* 4th ed. Washington, DC: American Psychiatric Association, 2000.

13. Noyes R Jr, Hartz AJ, Doebbeling CC, et al. Illness fears in the general population. *Psychosom Med.* 2000;62:318–325.

14. Noyes R Jr. Epidemiology of hypochondriasis. In: Starcevic V, Lipsitt DR, eds. *Hypochondriasis: modern perspectives on an ancient malady.* Oxford: Oxford University Press, 2001:125–154.

15. Segall A. Sick role concepts and health behaviour. In: Gochman D, ed. *Handbook of health behaviour research I: personal and social determinants.* New York: Plenum Press, 1977:289–301.

16. Parsons T. *The social system.* New York: Free Press, 1951.

17. Barsky AJ. Hypochondriasis. Medical management and psychiatric treatment. *Psychosomatics.* 1996;37:48–56.

18. Barsky AJ, Geringer E, Wool CA. A cognitive-educational treatment for hypochondriasis. *Gen Hosp Psychiatry.* 1988;10:322–327.

19. Goldberg D, Gask L, O'Dowd T. The treatment of somatization: teaching techniques of reattribution. *J Psychosom Res.* 1989;33:689–695.

20. Morriss R, Gask L, Ronalds C, et al. Cost-effectiveness of a new treatment for somatized mental disorder taught to GPs. *Fam Pract.* 1998;15:119–125.

21. Smith GR, Monson RA, Ray DC Jr. Psychiatric consultation in somatization disorder. A randomized controlled study. *N Engl J Med.* 1986;314:1407–1413.

22. Leventhal H, Meyer D, Nerenz D. The common sense representation of illness danger. In: Rachman S, ed. *Contribution to medical psychology.* Oxford: Pergamon Press, 1980:7–30.

23. Martin R, Lemos K, Leventhal H. The psychology of physical symptoms and illness behaviour. In: Asmundson G, Taylor S, Cox B, eds. *Health anxiety: clinical and research perspectives on hypochondriasis and related conditions.* London: John Wiley and Sons, 2001:22–45.

24. Warwick HM, Marks IM. Behavioural treatment of illness phobia and hypochondriasis. A pilot study of 17 cases. *Br J Psychiatry.* 1988;152:239–241.

25. Warwick HM, Clark DM, Cobb AM, et al. A controlled trial of cognitive-behavioural treatment of hypochondriasis. *Br J Psychiatry.* 1996;169:189–195.

26. Clark DM, Salkovskis PM, Hackmann A, et al. Two psychological treatments for hypochondriasis. A randomised controlled trial. *Br J Psychiatry.* 1998;173:218–225.

27. Bouman TK, Visser S. Cognitive and behavioural treatment of hypochondriasis. *Psychother Psychosom.* 1998;67:214–221.

28. Visser S, Bouman TK. The treatment of hypochondriasis: exposure plus response prevention vs cognitive therapy. *Behav Res Ther.* 2001;39:423–442.

29. Walker J, Vincent N, Furer P, et al. Treatment preference in hypochondriasis. *J Behav Ther Exp Psychiatry.* 1999;30:251–258.

30. Speed J. Behavioral management of conversion disorder: a retrospective study. *Arch Phys Med Rehabil.* 1996;77:147–154.

31. Trieschmann RB, Stolov WC, Montgomery ED. An approach to the treatment of abnormal ambulation resulting from conversion reaction. *Arch Phys Med Rehabil.* 1970;51:198–206.

32. Teasell RW, Shapiro AP. Strategic-behavioral intervention in the treatment of chronic nonorganic motor disorders. *Am J Phys Med Rehabil.* 1994;73:44–50.

33. Derogatis LR. *SCL-90-R: administration, scoring, and procedures manual–II for the revised version and other instruments of the psychopathology rating scale series.* Towson, MD: Clinical Psychometric Research, 1975.

34. D'Zurrilla T, Nezu A. *Problem-solving therapy. A social competence approach to clinical intervention.* New York: Springer, 1999.

35. Kaplan BJ, Sadock VA, eds. *Comprehensive textbook of psychiatry,* 4th ed. Baltimore, MD: Williams & Wilkins, 1985.

36. Enns MW, Kjernisted K, Lander M. Pharmacological management of hypochondriasis and related disorders. In: Asmundson G, Taylor S, Cox B, eds. *Health anxiety: clinical and research perspectives on hypochondriasis and related conditions.* London: John Wiley and Sons, 2001:193–219.

37. Fallon BA, Liebowitz MR, Salman E, et al. Fluoxetine for hypochondriacal patients without major depression. *J Clin Psychopharmacol.* 1993;13:438–441.

38. Kjernisted KD, Enns MW, Lander M. An open-label clinical trial of nefazodone in hypochondriasis. *Psychosomatics.* 2002;43:290–294.

39. Wesner RB, Noyes R Jr. Imipramine an effective treatment for illness phobia. *J Affect Disord.* 1991;22:43–48.

40. Menza M, Lauritano M, Allen L, et al. Treatment of somatization disorder with nefazodone: a prospective, open-label study. *Ann Clin Psychiatry.* 2001;13:153–158.

41. Noyes R, Happel RL, Muller BA, et al. Fluvoxamine for somatoform disorders: an open trial. *Gen Hosp Psychiatry.* 1998;20:339–344.

42. Fallon BA, Schneier FR, Marshall R, et al. The pharmacotherapy of hypochondriasis. *Psychopharmacol Bull.* 1996;32:607–611.

43. Escobar JL. Overview of somatization: diagnosis, epidemiology, and management. *Psychopharmacol Bull.* 1996;32:589–596.

44. Cummings N. A new vision of health care for America. In: Cummings N, O'Donahue W, Hayes S et al., eds. *Integrated behavioral healthcare.* San Diego, CA: Academic Press, 2001:1–18.

Somatization Disorder: Briquet's Hysteria

21

Michael Trimble

INTRODUCTION

The term "hysteria" is as old as the earliest medical writings, and classic descriptions of symptoms we now refer to as conversion disorder are found in the texts of the Egyptians, Greeks, and Romans. However, it is also clear that there were early descriptions of polysymptomatic patients, with chronic somatic symptoms outlined. Edward Jorden (1569–1632), a physician of London and Bath, in his treatise, *A Briefe Discourse of a Disease called the Suffocation of the Mother* described the case of a charwoman, Elizabeth Jackson, who was accused of bewitching the 14-year-old Mary Glover. The latter had convulsions, episodes of loss of speech, periodic blindness, paralysis, and loss of sensation down the left side of the body. Also noted were aggressivity and personality changes. Jorden recognized not only the polymorphous nature of the symptoms, but also a link of such a profile to the female sex and the importance of perturbations of the mind as a cause of the disorder (1).

Sydenham (1624–1689), who considered hysteria to be one of the commonest medical conditions in his practice, also recognized the chronic nature of the disorder and noted the personality contributions, which included capriciousness, and labile moods and affections (2).

Robert Brudenell Carter (1828–1918) divided hysteria into two main forms: the simple and the complicated. The former manifests mainly as hysterical seizures, but the latter was a foreboding of the later Briquet's form. It "generally involves much moral and intellectual, as well as physical derangement, and when it is fully established, the primary convulsion, the *fons et origo mali* is sometimes suffered to fall into abeyance . . . being arrested by the urgency of new maladies (3)." He was writing in the19th century, which saw an explosion of interest in the condition of hysteria, particularly from the German and French physicians. It was in this context that Pierre Briquet embarked upon his writings.

BRIQUET AND HIS SYNDROME

Pierre Briquet (1796–1881) became chief physician to the Paris Charité, and he readily admitted that he undertook to study hysteria as a matter of duty, on account of the frequency of cases that he reluctantly had to examine.

His book *Traité Clinique et Thérapeutique de L'Hystérie* (4) reported on the results of personal examinations of nearly 450 patients, and is a 19th-century landmark in hysteria studies. It was to have a considerable influence on Charcot and his school, and then later on the development of today's concept of somatization disorder. Briquet, in contrast to a number of other theorists, rejected uterine theories of causation of the condition, and clarified the presentation of hysteria in men. He outlined the multifarious symptoms, including the spasms, anesthesias, convulsions, paralyses, and contractures, which have become familiar in descriptions of patients diagnosed with hysteria over time.

Briquet referred to the length of time that the symptoms lasted. Of 418 patients, 179 had the condition for between 6 months and 4 years, 81 between 5 and 10 years, and of the rest, it lasted a longer time. Thus, in 59 patients the condition had continued more than 20 years, and in five patients for 55 years. These patients were polysymptomatic, and were clearly forerunners of the later-christened Briquet's hysteria. Briquet incidentally opined that hysteria was a condition of that portion of the brain which received sensations and affective impressions, and he described hysteria as a nervousness of the encephalon.

The notion of chronic hysteria fell into some abeyance with the writings of Charcot and Janet, who became more interested in the underlying personality structure of patients who might be susceptible to suffering from hysteria and the precipitating mental events. Freud, too, was more concerned with the psychological traumas involved, although clearly he treated patients with multiple physical symptoms, many of which persisted for years, and included neuralgias and anesthesias of various kinds, contractures and paralyses, hysterical attacks and other kinds of seizures, anorexia, vomiting, and disturbances of vision. Freud commented, "the disproportion between the many years' duration of the hysterical symptom and the single occurrence which provoked it is what we are accustomed invariably to find in traumatic neuroses (5)."

A renewed interest in Briquet's hysteria, rechristened chronic hysteria, and evolving to the rather clumsy, inelegant term "somatization," occurred in the mid-20th century (6). The term somatization was originally introduced to neuropsychiatry through the writings of the psychoanalyst Stekel (1868–1940), who used the term "somatizieren" to refer to neurotic patients who expressed their mental states symbolically as somatic symptoms (7). The term "somatization" made a limited appearance in America in the 1940s, but the concept seems to have been crystallized by three influential authors some 3 decades later. Lipowski (7) considered somatization to be, rather as the concept of conversion was becoming at that time, a disorder as well as a process. Kleinman (8) defined somatization as an expression of distress in the idiom of bodily complaints and medical help seeking, thus placing the concept firmly in a cultural setting. Then, in 1983, Ford wrote his book *The Somatizing Disorders*, which was subtitled *Illness as a Way of Life*. This was a landmark contribution to the field, and somatization was defined as follows: "... a process by which the body (the soma) is used for psychological purposes or for personal gain. Any one symptom or constellation of symptoms may concurrently serve more than one function, including issues related to intrapsychic conflicts, intrapersonal relationships, and social or environmental problems (9)."

Contemporary research into patients with somatization disorder evolved from the work of Cohen et al. at Harvard and Guze, at St Louis. Purtell et al. (10) described a group of patients, mainly women, who presented with a chronic disorder manifesting a wide variety of unexplained medical complaints. In this paper, they refer to the condition as hysteria, but use the soubriquet Briquet to name the syndrome.

CONTEMPORARY CLASSIFICATIONS

In the *Diagnostic and Statistical Manual of Mental Disorders*, Second Edition (DSM-II), there are hysterical neuroses—conversion type (300.13) and hysterical neuroses—dissociative type (300.14). In conversion disorder, the special senses of the voluntary nervous system are affected, while in the dissociative type, alterations to the state of consciousness are seen.

Further editions of the DSM retain a similar division. However, in DSM-III, the term "somatoform disorders" emerges with various subtypes including somatization disorder (300.81). The use of the subcategory somatization relates back to the studies of the St. Louis group and essentially incorporates their concept of Briquet's hysteria. It was seen as separate from conversion disorder, but sadly, the eponym was seen as superfluous and was discarded.

However, the concept of Briquet's hysteria is to be found both in DSM-IV and The International Classification of Diseases (ICD-10). Referred to as somatization disorder in DSM-IV (300.81), and the same in the ICD-10 (AF 45.0), it represents a chronic condition, and the patients by definition are polysymptomatic. This is seen in contrast to conversion disorder, with a much more restricted symptomatology, which tends to run a shorter course.

The original criteria for Briquet's hysteria, as given by Perley and Guze (11), required the patient to have 25 out of 59 possibly medically unexplained symptoms, coming from nine out of ten possible symptom groups. However, over time, a fewer number of complaints have been included, such that in DSM-III, the requirements were 14 symptoms for women and 12 for men from a list of 37, and in DSM-III-R, 13 symptoms from a list of 35 were needed.

The full criteria given in DSM-IV are shown in Table 21.1. The requirements are a history of many physical complaints over a period of several years, but with rather specific numbers of complaints from four main areas, namely, pain symptoms, gastrointestinal and pseudoneurologic symptoms, and sexual complaints.

The diagnosis of somatization disorder comes under the overall category of somatoform disorders, and corresponds well with the original concept of Briquet's hysteria.

The essential features are the development of medically unexplained symptoms, usually before the age of 30, for which the patient seeks medical advice and treatment, or which causes significant social and occupational impairment. Sometimes symptoms occur in association with some relevant somatic pathology, but in such settings, the complaint exceeds that which would normally be expected.

According to DSM-IV, patients often describe their complaints in "colorful, exaggerated terms," they are often inconsistent historians, and their lives can be as chaotic as their medical history.

The ICD-10 refers to somatization disorder as describing a patient who presents "multiple recurrent, and frequently changing physical symptoms, which have usually been present for several years before the patient is referred to a psychiatrist. Many patients have a long and complicated history of contact with primary and specialist medical services, during which many negative investigations or fruitless operations may have been carried out (12)." Central features, in addition to longstanding multiple and variable physical symptoms which carry no physical explanation, are

TABLE 21.1

SOMATIZATION DISORDER: *DIAGNOSITIC AND STATISTICAL MANUAL OF MENTAL DISORDERS, FOURTH EDITION*, CRITERIA

A. A history of many physical complaints beginning before age 30 years that occur over a period of several years and result in treatment being sought or significant impairment in social, occupational, or other important areas of functioning.

B. Each of the following criteria must have been met, with individual symptoms occurring at any time during the course of the disturbance:

  (i) *four pain symptoms:* a history of pain related to at least four different sites or functions (e.g., head, abdomen, back, joints, extremities, chest, rectum, during menstruation, during sexual intercourse, or during urination)

  (ii) *two gastrointestinal symptoms:* a history of at least two gastrointestinal symptoms other than pain (e.g., nausea, bloating, vomiting other than during pregnancy, diarrhea, or intolerance of several different foods)

  (iii) *one sexual symptom:* a history of at least one sexual or reproductive symptom other than pain (e.g., sexual indifference, erectile or ejaculatory dysfunction, irregular menses, excessive menstrual bleeding, vomiting throughout pregnancy)

  (iv) *one pseudoneurologic symptom:* a history of at least one symptom or deficit suggesting a neurologic condition not limited to pain (conversion symptoms such as impaired coordination or balance, paralysis or localized weakness, difficulty swallowing or lump in throat, aphonia, urinary retention, hallucinations, loss of touch or pain sensation, double vision, blindness, deafness, seizures; dissociative symptoms such as amnesia; or loss of consciousness other than fainting)

C. Either (i) or (ii):

  (i) after appropriate investigation, each of the symptoms in Criterion B cannot be fully explained by a known general medical condition or the direct effects of a substance (e.g., a drug of abuse, a medication)

  (ii) when there is a related general medical condition, the physical complaints or resulting social or occupational impairment are in excess of what would be expected from the history, physical examination, or laboratory findings

D. The symptoms are not intentionally produced or feigned (as in factitious disorder or malingering).

---

a persistent refusal to accept the advice or reassurance of doctors that there is no physical explanation for the symptoms, and some degree of impairment of social and family functioning attributable to the behavior.

ABNORMAL ILLNESS BEHAVIOR

The latter features often reflect upon what is referred to as abnormal illness behavior (AIB). Thus, one elegant attempt to bring uniformity to and to unite the various categories of behavior in which patients present with medically unexplained symptoms was that of abnormal illness behavior defined by Pilowsky (13). This concept evolved from the term "illness behavior," used initially by Mechanic. Illness behavior described "the manner in which persons monitor their bodies, define and interpret their symptoms, take remedial actions, and utilise the health care system."

Mechanic pointed out how ethnic variations, and cultural and developmental experiences determine a person's reaction to the threat of illness, and, what to a doctor may not seem rational behavior, to patients with symptoms may seem a logical approach to their problems.

Presentations to doctors, and the manner of the presentation, are essentially culturally and socially determined, and not directed primarily by underlying diseases. Thus, there is always a conceptual and obvious gap between the patient's signs and symptoms, and any underlying disease process. However, in these settings, that is, patients presenting with medically unexplained symptoms, causes of the disorder are not explicable in pathologic terms; what

is outstanding is the syndromic presentation, and the patient's illness (as opposed to disease). In order to describe this chasm between disease and apparent illness, physicians use epithets such as supratentorial or functional overlay. However, the concept of abnormal illness behavior is founded on the simple principle that there is a normal illness behavior (which can theoretically be measured), and a normal "sick role" which a person with disease adopts, usually temporarily, which defines certain privileges, but it also carries with it obligations. Amongst the latter are an obligation to comply with treatments and to attempt to get better, leaving the sick role behind. Thus, normal illness behavior has given parameters, and it is therefore possible to define abnormal illness behavior. Pilowsky defines it as follows: ". . . the persistence of an inappropriate or maladapted mode of experiencing, evaluating, or acting in relation to one's own state of health (13)." It is noted by patients' ways of behaving and responding with respect to their symptoms, and by their interactions with physicians and other helpers. Abnormal illness behavior can be illness affirming (continuing to insist on the presence of a disease when it is not possible to confirm it), or illness denying (refusing to accept the presence of a disease which has been diagnosed) (Table 21.2). Often, this abnormal illness behavior is noted by the way the patients behave in respect to presentation, investigations, and diagnosis, and their attitude toward their physicians and other caregivers. The abnormal illness behavior is a key to the diagnosis of not only somatoform disorders in general, but to somatization disorder in particular.

TABLE 21.2

A CLASSIFICATION OF ABNORMAL ILLNESS BEHAVIOR

Somatic focus

A. Illness affirming	(a) Motivation conscious, e.g., Münchausen syndrome, malingering
	(b) Motivation unconscious, e.g., conversion phenomena, hypochondriasis (neurotic)
	(c) Schizophrenia, monosymptomatic psychosis (psychotic)
B. Illness denying	(a) Motivation conscious, e.g., to avoid insurance penalty or therapy
	(b) Motivation unconscious, e.g., denial (neurotic or psychotic)
	(c) Neuropsychiatric, e.g., anosognosia

Psychological focus

A. Illness affirming	(a) Motivation conscious, e.g., Ganser states, malingering
	(b) Motivation unconscious, e.g., amnesia, dissociative behavior (neurotic)
	(c) Delusions of amnesia (psychotic)
B. Illness denying	(a) Motivation conscious, e.g., to avoid psychiatric consultation or hospitalization
	(b) Motivation unconscious, e.g., denial in the presence of neurotic or psychotic illness with lack of insight

(After Pilowsky I. *Abnormal illness behaviour.* Chichester: John Wiley and Sons, 1997.)

CLINICAL PRESENTATIONS

The incidence and prevalence of unexplained medical symptoms have been reviewed by a number of authors (14,15). However, little information is provided in these reviews, or indeed on the follow-up studies that have been performed on somatization disorder *per se*. In population surveys, Robins and Regier (16) reported a prevalence of somatization disorder of 0.01%, Deighton and Nicol (17) of 0.2%, and Escobar et al. (18) of 0.3 to 0.7%. However Kroenke et al. (19) in a study of 1,000 primary care patients, reported multisomatoform disorder (falling short of somatization disorder) in 8%. Gureje et al. (20) reported the prevalence of abridged form of somatization to be up to 19%. Whatever, the incidence of this disorder in clinical practice is certainly higher than generally thought or discussed, and in certain settings, particularly in neurologic practice, the prevalence is most likely to be amongst the highest.

A key to a diagnosis is the patient's illness history. The latter is so often poorly documented, especially in somatization disorder, which after all is a chronic disorder. A past history of a conversion symptom is reported in about 20%. Patients should always be asked if they have had other illnesses which have not been well-clarified or diagnosed, or which have led to an unclear diagnosis. Those of childhood and adolescence are important, especially illnesses that have led to a prolonged time away from school or any other evidence of school refusal. A propensity to seek surgery, or at least persuade surgeons to operate, seems a feature of many patients. Appendectomy, hysterectomy, cholecystectomy, operations on adhesions, laparoscopies, tonsillectomy, and the like are so often noted in the history. An appendix operation should always be held with suspicion. When examined pathologically, about 50% of removed appendices are

normal. In effect, the surgeon has operated on a case of abdominal pain, which still remains unexplained after the operation. Such people usually give a history of grumbling abdominal pain rather than acute appendicitis.

The hysterectomy reflects most often on the gynecologic history, with menorrhagia and dysmenorrhea, while operations on "adhesions" suggest ongoing abdominal problems after index operations.

An essential part of the workup and the diagnosis is the collection of information about this past medical history, preferably through other medical records. In the United States, this is a much more difficult enterprise than in Europe, particularly in the United Kingdom, where patients tend to have general practitioners for stable and prolonged periods of their lives. The general practitioner records contain a wealth of biographic information that allows the current illness symptoms to be evaluated in the context of past symptoms, and past episodes of possible medically unexplained symptoms can be noted.

The response of patients to a medical inquiry may give away the obvious abnormal illness behavior. There may be an immediate hostility to psychological inquiry, a rejection to explore even superficial personal details. Answers are not so much evasive, but more in the mold of "What is the relevance of ...?" It should be noted that such attitudes are not necessarily unfounded or unexpected. It is not an unfamiliar scenario that patients who have been examined and referred for specialist opinion by their general practitioners have a battery of investigations carried out in the hospital, the results of which turn up nothing positive, but at which point the patient is discharged or referred to other specialists. Further referrals and examinations follow, and, at the end of a long trail through negative findings, the patient is triumphantly given the news that nothing abnormal can be found.

The immediate assumption, often encouraged by the medical messenger, is that if it is not in the body, it must be in the mind, and if it is in the mind, then the patient must be putting it on. This, of course, may be a valid conclusion in some cases. However, many patients become quite defensive about such conclusions, and express this through their interaction with doctors.

On examination of patients with somatization disorder, the medical exchange has embedded within it the signs of the abnormal illness behavior. The patient's insistence that the doctor, along with a dozen other doctors, has got it wrong, reveals a failure of the normal mechanisms of reassurance. The patient's insistence on yet more tests, or on yet another scan, or even worse, another operation, reflects the tendency to procure medical attention. There may be obvious signs of a breakdown in the relationships between patients and the staff responsible for their management. The patient becomes referred to as "difficult," or "noncompliant." Sometimes patients put unreasonable limits on what they can and cannot do. An obvious one is, "I will do anything to get well, doctor, except see a psychiatrist." Resistance to absolutely any form of psychological exploration is nearly always a reflection of abnormal illness behavior.

In patients with somatization disorder, it is important to let patients know that their reported symptoms are being taken seriously, and a physical examination should be conducted when the patient is first assessed or when obvious new symptoms arise. However, repeated requests for examinations, a reflection of the abnormal illness behavior, should be declined, and invasive investigations should be avoided. One of the serious complications of medically unexplained symptoms is iatrogenic damage that stems from physically invasive tests.

It is important to ascertain that the symptoms complained of, and the signs revealed, do not obey anatomic and physiologic laws, and do not fit the pattern of an alternative medical diagnosis. In neurologic practice, common signs are the demonstration of obvious muscle contraction in supposedly paralysed muscles, the finding of nonphysiologic anesthetic patches, anomalous visual eye fields, with tubular vision or spiral vision, or simply a bizarre presentation. A number of signs are easily distinguishable, such as the typical hysterical gait. One feature of such gaits, including *astasia-abasia*, in which the patient struggles deftly to maintain an upright posture, virtually stumbling along the way, is that they reveal quite intact neuromuscular co-ordination and balance mechanisms.

The classic patient with somatization is hard to miss in clinical practice, and it is astonishing how often the diagnosis is not made. In part this is attributable to patients' abnormal illness behavior, which leads them off to several different specialists, who all fail to take an adequate illness history and concentrate exclusively on their own particular specialist signs, symptoms, and investigations. Further, it reflects on an ignorance of psychiatry generally amongst nonpsychiatrists,

and a failure to come to terms with the fact that for some patients, illness simply is "a way of life" (9). After all, in medical school, the conventional teaching is that most people are well most of the time, but when they fall sick they do so with disorders that, over several centuries, have been empirically charted, and that they come to doctors to get diagnosed, treated, and made well again. The idea that patients may develop nonillnesses, present with anomalous signs and symptoms, and seek illness rather than wellness not only makes little sense, but to some it is simply repugnant.

A TYPICAL PATIENT

The typical patients are women, usually between the ages of 20 and 30 years old by the time they present to neurologic specialists. They will have come from a turbulent background, perhaps with a family history of sociopathy or alcoholism, and often from broken homes. There may be a hint or acknowledgement of some form of early abuse, sexual or otherwise. School refusal for some minor childhood complaints may be noted. Often this is recurrent abdominal pain, but headaches and "growing pains" may be documented in the general practitioner notes (which are so important in unearthing such early histories, since these symptoms are often simply not related, or perhaps not even recalled by the patient). The patient may just have been "a sickly child." The abdominal pains lead to the first operation (although the tonsils may already have been extracted), and a normal appendix is removed. Further abdominal pains may follow, although there may be a medically quiescent phase. There may be conduct problems at school, some truancy, perhaps an early pregnancy or marriage. Then other medical problems arise, but exactly when is often difficult to tie down. The symptom history is imprecise, often dramatized, and invariably complicated.

Visits to gynecologists, neurologists, and other specialists are common, and a glance at the general practitioner records will reveal that the use of medical facilities is above average. Seventy percent of these people will have had an appendectomy, and nearly 50% will have had a gynecologic procedure. In the controlled study of Cohen et al. (1953), the operative procedures of 50 patients with somatization disorder were compared to healthy controls, and a comparison group of patients from the same hospital who had other nonpsychiatric illnesses was charted. Dilatation and curettage occurred nearly five times more frequently in the hysteria group, hysterectomy four times, and by the age of 35, 20% of the hysteria patients were rendered sterile, compared with none in the controls. It was estimated that three times the weight of body organs were removed from patients diagnosed as having hysteria compared with controls.

The illness history progresses, but who knows in what direction? Classic chronic hysteria tends, as noted, to end up in gynecologic or neurologic hands, and certainly the contractures, seizures, and inevitable loss of muscle power leads to neurologic referral at some stage.

The state of dependency often increases, encouraged by physicians who make pseudodiagnoses such as rheumatism, which leads to the prescription of steroids, or myalgic encephalomyelitis, which encourages patients to languish in bed. This is further encouraged by paramedical staff, who make suggestions such as; "Perhaps you have a touch of multiple sclerosis." It is encouraged by local authorities who adapt patients' homes to become cocoons of illness, with all kinds of special aids, often provided at considerable expense. It is encouraged by spouses who give up their jobs to become full-time caregivers.

In time, the patient often becomes bed-bound, probably wheelchair-bound, and usually requiring full-time care. Patients wear splints for orthopaedic complaints, dark glasses for visual problems, and carry other insignias of the sick role. In more severe cases, the urinary symptoms lead to self-catheterization, or even worse, to operations to provide false bladders. Eating difficulties can lead to abdominal pegs, and painful dystonias and recurrent infections to amputation. Patients take a compendium of medications, usually with opiates somewhere in their regimen, the latter on which they have become dependent. It is estimated that some 10% of these patients become wheelchair-bound, and the average patients spend about a quarter of their time in bed (21).

CONCLUSIONS

Somatization disorder is a form of chronic hysteria, eponymously referred to as Briquet's hysteria, which essentially reflects on a lifelong pursuit of illness rather than wellness. Symptoms begin in childhood, and are slowly cumulative and progressive, and patients end up with multiple diagnoses, although careful dissection of the signs and symptoms reveals that they simply do not hang together, except as a case of somatization disorder.

Once seen, this is one of the most recognizable disorders in neuropsychiatry, but it is often missed in clinical practice. There are a number of reasons for this that not only relate to the microscopic view of many specialists, but also to the patients' abnormal illness behavior, and, quite frankly, to a failure of medical education.

The prognosis is inevitably poor, although some benefit can be obtained by treating patients on specialist units that emphasize a multidisciplinary approach to management.

REFERENCES

1. Jorden E. *A brief discourse of a disease called the suffocation of the mother.* London: Windet, 1963.
2. Sydenham T. *The works of Thomas Sydenham.* London: Sydenham Society, 1850.
3. Carter RB. *On the pathology and treatment of hysteria.* London: Churchill Livingstone, 1853.
4. Briquet P. *Traité Clinique et Thérapeutique de L'Hystérie.* Paris: J-B Bailliere & Fils, 1859.
5. Breuer J, Freud S. *Studies in hysteria.* New York: New York Nervous Mental Diseases Publishing Company, 1893.
6. Berrios GE, Mumford D. Somatoform disorders: clinical section. In: Berrios GE, Porter R, eds. *A history of clinical psychiatry.* London: The Athlone Press, 1995:384–409.
7. Lipowski ZJ. Somatization: the experience and communication of psychological distress as somatic symptoms. *Psychother Psychosom.* 1987;47:160–167.
8. Kleinman A. Depression, somatization and a new cross cultural psychiatry. *Soc Sci Med.* 1977;11:3–10.
9. Ford CV. *The somatizing disorders—illness as a way of life.* New York: Elsevier Science, 1987.
10. Purtell JJ, Robins E, Cohen LE. Observations on clinical aspects of hysteria. *J Am Med Assoc.* 1951;146:902–909.
11. Perley MG, Guze SB. Hysteria: the stability and usefulness of clinical criteria. *N Engl J Med.* 1962;266:421.
12. American Psychiatric Association. *Diagnostic and statistical manual of mental disorders,* 4th ed. Washington, DC: APA Press Washington World Health Organisation, 1994.
13. Pilowsky I. *Abnormal illness behaviour.* Chichester: John Wiley and Sons, 1997.
14. Akagi H, House A. The epidemiology of hysterical conversion. In: Halligan PW, Bass C, Marshall JC, eds. *Contemporary approaches to the study of hysteria.* Oxford: Oxford University Press, 2001:73–87.
15. Trimble MT. *Somatization disorder in medicolegal practice.* Cambridge: Cambridge University Press, 2004.
16. Robins LN, Regier D. *Psychiatric disorders in America. The epidemiologic catchment area study.* New York: Free Press, 1991.
17. Deighton CM, Nicol AR. Abnormal illness behavior in young women in a primary care setting: is Briquet's syndrome a useful category. *Psychol Med.* 1985;15:515–520.
18. Escobar JI, Burnam MA, Karno M, et al. Somatization in the community. *Arch Gen Psychiatry.* 1987;44:713–718.
19. Kroenke K, Spitzer RL, De Gruy FV, et al. Multisomatoform disorder. An alternative to undifferentiated somatoform disorder of the somatizing patient in primary care. *Arch Gen Psychiatry.* 1997;54:352–358.
20. Gureje O, Simon GE, Ustun TB, et al. Somatization in cross cultural perspective: a WHO study in primary care. *Am J Psychiatry.* 1997;154:989–995.
21. Bass C, Murphy M. Somatisation disorder in a British teaching hospital. *Br J Clin Pract.* 1991;45:237–244.

Pathophysiology

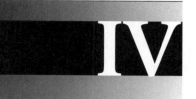

22

Voluntary and Involuntary Movements in Humans

Mark Hallett

ABSTRACT

Psychogenic movements may be voluntary or involuntary. If voluntary, the mechanism is factitious or malingering and the patient is lying. Most commonly, the movements are conversion or somatization in origin, and are involuntary. The movements look voluntary, however, and the fact that they are preceded by a normal-looking Bereitschaftspotential suggests that they share some brain mechanisms with normal voluntary movement. Perhaps there is an unconscious force that initiates these movements. More likely, the brain just does not interpret them as being voluntary. There is good evidence that the brain generates movements as a result of all the inputs to the motor system, and that the sense of voluntariness is a perception. Physiologic studies are providing information on how this can happen.

INTRODUCTION

Psychogenic movement disorders may be factitious or malingering. In these circumstances, the movement is voluntary, but the patient says it is involuntary. The patient is lying. The task for the physician is to determine that the patient is lying, and this is not necessarily easy. All agree that the lie detector test is not foolproof. There has been some work in this area using electroencephalogram (EEG) and functional magnetic resonance imaging (fMRI) (1–4), but there is nothing

definitive yet, certainly on the individual level. More work is needed in this area of investigation, and this problem will not be considered further in this chapter. However, whether the patient is lying or not is really the first consideration when faced with a patient with psychogenic movements.

Most patients with psychogenic movement disorders have a conversion etiology. The mechanism of somatization is thought also to be conversion. Patients with conversion exhibit movements that look voluntary and even share some physiologic aspects with voluntary movements, but the patients say that the movements are involuntary. In general, we believe this to be true. Indeed, if the patient was lying, and the movements were actually voluntary, we would make a different diagnosis. These considerations raise a number of questions. Are the patients just lying to themselves, and if so, what does that mean? What makes a movement voluntary? What separates voluntary and involuntary movements?

Clearly the critical aspect of voluntary movement is that a person believes that he or she has chosen to make the movement. This is the general view of free will, the decision to make (or not make) movements. The brain is certainly responsible for all movements that the body makes. Only a subset is thought to be voluntary. The "thought of voluntariness" is a qualia of consciousness (5), an element of which a person is aware. The nature of consciousness is a difficult matter and dealt with elsewhere in this book (see Chapter 24). Is it the case that movements are actually "chosen," or is the "choosing" just a perception of consciousness? This issue will be addressed here, but also elsewhere in this book (see Chapters 23 and 24).

ARGUMENTS IN FAVOR OF FREE WILL AS A PERCEPTION

One possibility is that there is some mechanism in the brain that chooses the movement to be made. This is certainly the commonly held view. On the other hand, there are several arguments that can be made that the brain's motor system produces a movement as a product of its different inputs, consciousness is informed of this movement, and it is perceived as being freely chosen. It is controversial which of these is correct, but there are some good arguments in favor of the latter.

The Brain Initiates a Movement before Awareness of Volition

The clever experiment that showed this was reported by Libet et al. in 1983 (6). Subjects sat in front of a clock on which a rapidly moving spot was projected and were told to move at will. Subsequently, they were asked to say what time it was (where the spot was) when they had the first subjective experience of intending to act (this time was called W). They also were asked to specify the time of awareness of actually moving (this time was called M). There were two types of voluntary movements: one type was thoughtfully initiated and a second type was "spontaneous and capricious." As a control for the ability to successfully subjectively time events, subjects were also stimulated at random times with a skin stimulus and they were asked to time this event (called S). At the same time, EEG was being recorded and movement-related cortical potentials (MRCPs) were assessed to determine timing of activity of the brain.

The MRCP has a number of components (7). An early negativity preceding movement has two phases: an initial, slowly rising phase lasting from about 1,500 ms to about 400 ms before movement [the Bereitschaftspotential (BP), also called the readiness potential in translation of the German], and a later, more rapidly rising phase lasting from about 400 ms to approximately the time of movement onset, the negative slope, or NS'. (These two components could also be called the BP1 and the BP2.) The NS' peaks about 90 ms before the onset of EMG activity and is followed often by a brief decline in the negativity, called the premotor positivity. The next component is the motor potential or MP which begins before movement, peaks after movement onset, and produces the highest negativity in the recording. The topography of the BP is generalized with a vertex maximum. With NS', the negativity begins to shift to the central region contralateral to the hand that is moving. The main contributors to the BP are the primary sensorimotor cortex and premotor cortex, and the supplementary motor area, both bilaterally (8). With the appearance of NS', the activity of the contralateral motor cortical regions predominate. With thoughtful, preplanned movements, the BP begins about 1,050 ms prior to electromyogram (EMG) onset (the type 1 of Libet), and with spontaneous movements, the BP begins about 575 ms prior to movement (the type 2 of Libet) (9). The type 2 may consist mainly of the NS' component.

While the MRCP clearly is indicative of movement preparatory processes in the brain, its exact meaning is not clear. In particular, a relatively normal-looking MRCP precedes unconscious movements as well as conscious movements. This was studied by looking at the brain events preceding unrecognized movements made by subjects at rest or engaged in a mental task (10).

Subjects were reasonably accurate in determining the time of S, indicating that this method of timing of subjective experience was acceptable. W occurred about 300 ms prior to EMG onset, and M occurred about 90 ms prior to EMG onset. The onset of the BP type 1 occurred about 800 ms prior to W, and the onset of the BP type 2 occurred about 350 ms prior to W (Fig. 22.1). The authors concluded that

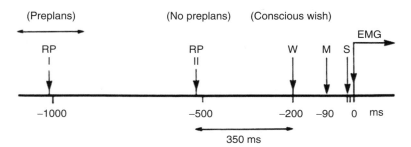

Figure 22.1 Timing of subjective events and the Bereitschaftspotential (readiness potential, RP) with data from Libet et al. (1983). RP1 is the onset of the Bereitschaftspotential with ordinarily voluntary movements and RP2 is the onset with movements made quickly with little forethought. W, the subjective timing of the will to move; M, the subjective timing of the onset of movement; S, the timing of a shock to the finger. Electromyogram (EMG) onset is set at 0 ms. (From Libet et al. Readiness-potentials preceding unrestricted "spontaneous" vs. preplanned voluntary acts. *Electroencephalogr Clin Neurophysiol.* 1982;54:322–335.)

"cerebral initiation of a spontaneous, freely voluntary act can begin unconsciously, that is, before there is any (at least recallable) subjective awareness that a 'decision' to act has already been initiated cerebrally"(6).

Voluntary Movements Can Be Triggered with Stimuli That are Not Perceived

To understand the experiments here, the phenomenon of backward masking is a prerequisite. By itself, a small stimulus would be easily recognized. If the small stimulus is followed quickly by a large stimulus, then only the large stimulus is appreciated; the small one has been masked. This phenomenon is robust and has been demonstrated in the visual and tactile modes. Its physiology is not completely understood, although there is some speculation (11).

Taylor and McCloskey (12) looked to see if voluntary movements could be triggered by backwardly masked stimuli. Large and small visual stimuli were presented to normal human subjects in two different experiments. In some trials, the small stimulus was followed 50 ms later by the large stimulus. In perception experiments, the researchers demonstrated in this circumstance that the small stimulus was not perceived even with forced-choice testing showing the phenomenon of "backward masking." In reaction time (RT) experiments, the RTs for responses to the masked stimulus were the same as those for responses to the easily perceived, nonmasked stimulus. Hence, subjects were reacting to stimuli not perceived. In this circumstance, the order of events was stimulus-response-perception, and not stimulus-perception-response that would seem necessary for the ordinary view of free will.

Sense of Volition Depends on Sense of Causality

Wegner and Wheatley (13) point out that the experience of will depends on the relationship between one's thought and the movement itself. The thought must occur before the movement, it must be consistent with the movement, and there must not be another obvious cause for the movement. These features that are aspects of causality imply that the thought led to the movement. Thus, the fact that Libet's W precedes M is mentally consistent with W producing M. In one experiment, Wegner and Wheatley performed (13), they showed that subjects thought they caused an action, actually caused by someone else, by leading them to think about the action prior to its occurrence. The subject and an experimenter together manipulated a mouse that drove a cursor on a computer screen. The screen showed many objects. The object names were occasionally given in an auditory signal to the subject followed by the experimenter stopping the cursor on the named object. Subjects often had the sense that they had decided to stop the cursor on that object. Wegner has expanded on these ideas elsewhere (14).

NEUROLOGIC DISORDERS OF WILL

In neurology, there are many disorders in which the issue of will arises. There are patients who have movements that are commonly held as being involuntary. Myoclonus is such an example. The brain makes the movement, yet the patient interprets the movement as involuntary. Why should this be so? Chorea is another example. Yet, early in the course of their illness, patients with chorea often do not recognize that there are any involuntary movements. Why not? Are their brains interpreting everything that is done as voluntarily chosen at that time? Why does that change?

Although tics are generally considered involuntary, patients with tics often cannot say whether their movements are voluntary or involuntary. This may not be a relevant distinction in their minds. It is perhaps a better description to say that they can suppress their movements or they just let them happen. Tics look like voluntary movements in all respects from the point of view of EMG and kinesiology (15). Interestingly, they are often not preceded by a BP or only a brief BP (consistent with only an NS' component), and hence the brain mechanisms for their production clearly differ from ordinary voluntary movement (16,17). The presence of a premovement potential was not correlated with the patient's sense of voluntariness (17). The term "unvoluntary" has been suggested (18), but it is not clear how that helps us understand the physiology. If forced to choose voluntary or involuntary, patients will more commonly say that the movements were voluntarily performed.

The symptom of loss of voluntary movement is often called abulia or, in the extreme, akinetic mutism (19). The classic lesion is in the midline frontal region affecting areas including the supplementary motor area (SMA) and cingulate motor areas (CMA). Recent studies have further detailed these regions to the SMA, the pre-SMA, and rostral and caudal cingulate motor areas (CMAr, CMAc), with perhaps further division of the caudal cingulate area into the dorsal and ventral (caudal) cingulate areas (CMAd, CMAv). Which of these regions is the most critical is not yet clear. Lesions in other areas may give rise to similar symptoms including particularly the basal ganglia. The bradykinesia and akinesia of Parkinson disease is a symptom complex of the same type.

The alien hand phenomenon is characterized by unwanted movements that arise without any sense of their being willed. In addition to simple, unskilled, quasireflex movements (such as grasping), there can also be complex, skilled movements such as intermanual conflict or interference (20). There appears to be a difficulty in self-initiating movement and excessive ease in the production of involuntary and triggered movements. In cases with discrete lesions, this seems to have its anatomic correlation in the territory of the anterior cerebral artery.

In patients with amputations, there can often be the phantom limb phenomenon. In this situation, patients can have the sense of moving their phantom limb, but there is, of course, no actual movement. This seems to indicate that there can be a sense of volition without feedback from an actual movement.

In schizophrenia, there is often the subjective impression of patients that their movements are being externally (or alien) controlled. Their movements typically look normal, are goal directed, and are clearly generated by the patients' brains, but do not get associated with a sense that the patients themselves have willed the movements (21).

Conversion psychogenic movements are movements interpreted by the patient as involuntary. Their etiology is actually obscure since the physiology of conversion is really unknown. EEG investigation of these movements shows a normal-looking MRCP preceding them (22,23). As noted above, some patients with tics describe their movements as voluntary and there is no MRCP. Hence, the MRCP does not indicate "voluntariness." The normal MRCP, however, does indicate that there must be substantial sharing of brain voluntary movement mechanisms. There have been several recent neuroimaging studies of psychogenic paralysis that have given disparate results (24,25), and are discussed in Chapter 26, but no investigations of psychogenic movements. There are some physiologic differences between psychogenic myoclonus and epileptic myoclonias, and differences between psychogenic tremor and "organic" tremors that can be useful for diagnosis (26–28); these will also be discussed in other chapters.

HOW CAN THERE BE (VOLUNTARY) MOVEMENT WITHOUT FREE WILL?

Humans do not appear to be purely reflexive organisms, simple automatons. A vast array of different movements are generated in a variety of settings. Is there an alternative to free will? Movement, in the final analysis, comes only from muscle contraction. Muscle contraction is under the complete control of the α motoneurons in the spinal cord. When the α motoneurons are active, there will be movement. Activity of the α motoneurons is a product of the different synaptic events on their dendrites and cell bodies. There is a complex summation of EPSPs and IPSPs, and when the threshold for an action potential is crossed, the cell fires. There are a large number of important inputs, and one of the most important is from the corticospinal tract which conveys a large part of the cortical control. Such a situation likely holds also for the motor cortex and the cells of origin of the corticospinal tract. Their firing depends on their synaptic inputs. And a similar situation must hold for all the principal regions giving input to the motor cortex. For any cortical region, its activity will depend on its synaptic inputs. Some motor cortical inputs come via only a few synapses from sensory cortices, and such influences on motor output are clear. Some inputs

will come from regions, such as the limbic areas, many synapses away from both primary sensory and motor cortices. At any one time, the activity of the motor cortex and its commands to the spinal cord will reflect virtually all the activity in the entire brain. Is it necessary that there be anything else? This can be a complete description of the process of movement selection, and even if there is something more—like free will—it would have to operate through such neuronal mechanisms.

There have been some demonstrations that movements occur when cellular activity in specific regions of the brain achieve a certain level of firing. One such nice example is saccadic initiation in the primate in a reaction time experiment. Saccades are initiated when single cell activity in the frontal eye field reaches a certain level; more rapid reaction times occur when the cellular activity reaches the threshold level more rapidly (29–31). This has also been demonstrated in the motor cortex for skeletomotor movements (32). Moreover, electrical stimulation within a nuclear region can raise firing rates and influence behavior. Electrical stimulation within the supplementary eye field can speed up the initiation of smooth pursuit initiation (33). In another situation, monkeys discriminated among eight possible directions of motion while directional signals were manipulated in visual area MT (34). One directional signal was generated by a visual stimulus and a second signal was introduced by electrically stimulating neurons that encoded a specific direction of motion. The monkeys made a decision for one or the other signal, indicating that the signals exerted independent effects on performance and that the effects of the two signals were not simply averaged together. The monkeys, therefore, chose the direction encoded by the largest signal in the representation of motion direction, a "winner-take-all" decision process. This topic is expanded on in Chapter 23.

If the sense of will arises in part as a deduction about causality, it is critical that "awareness" of the movement be prior to the movement itself. Not only the sense of willing the movement, W in Libet's terminology, but also the sense of the movement having occurred, M in Libet's terminology, occurs prior to the actual movement. The awareness of M could well derive from the feedforward signal for the movement since it certainly occurs prior to movement feedback, and movement feedback is not necessary, anyway (21,35).

WHERE IS MOVEMENT SELECTION LOCATED IN THE BRAIN?

Can we use the tools of neurology and neuroscience to locate movement selection? Lesion studies can reveal situations in which voluntary movements are lacking or diminished, and some of these have been noted above. Functional imaging studies can reveal what regions are active with movement selection.

Using blood flow positron emission tomography (PET), Deiber et al. (36) have investigated the issue of movement selection in a series of studies. In the first study, normal subjects performed five different motor tasks consisting of moving a joystick on hearing a tone. In the control task, they always pushed it forward (fixed condition), and in four other experimental tasks, the subjects had to select among four possible directions of movement depending on instructions, including one task in which the choice of movement direction was to be freely chosen and random. The greatest activation was seen in this latter task with significant increases in regional cerebral blood flow most prominently in the SMA. In a second study, normal subjects were asked to make one of four types of finger movements depending on instructions (37). The details here were better controlled and included a rest condition. Of the numerous comparisons, the critical one for the discussion here is between the fully specified condition and the freely chosen, random movement. The anterior part of the

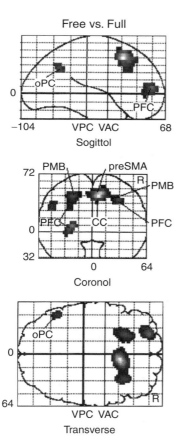

Figure 22.2 Positron emission tomography (PET) study with different finger movements showing the difference in activation between the fully specified condition and the freely chosen, random movement. Areas activated indicate brain activity associated with the choosing of what movement to make. (From Deiber M-P, Ibanez V, Sadato N, et al. Cerebral structures participating in motor preparation in humans: a positron emission tomography study. *J Neurophysiol.* 1996;75:233–247, with permission.)

SMA was the main area preferentially involved (Fig. 22.2). Both of these studies addressed specifically the issue of the choice of *what* to do at a designated time.

The other side of the coin in movement selection is the choice of *when* to move. This was approached by Jahanshahi et al. (38) using PET. Normal subjects, in a first task, were asked to make self-initiated right index finger extensions on average once every 3 seconds. A second task was externally triggered finger extension with the rate yoked to that of the self-initiated task. Greater activation of the right dorsolateral prefrontal cortex (DLPFC) was the only area that significantly differentiated the self-initiated movements from the externally triggered movements. In a follow-up PET experiment, measurements of regional cerebral blood flow were made under three conditions: rest, self-initiated right index finger extension at a variable rate of once every 2 to 7 seconds, and finger extension triggered by pacing tones at unpredictable intervals (at a rate yoked to the self-initiated movements). Compared with rest, unpredictably cued movements activated the contralateral primary sensorimotor cortex, caudal SMA, and contralateral putamen. Self-initiated movements additionally activated rostral SMA, adjacent anterior cingulate cortex, and bilateral DLPFC.

A similar experiment was conducted by Deiber et al. using fMRI focusing on the frontal mesial cortex (39). There were two types of movements, repetitive or sequential, performed at two different rates, slow or fast. Four regions of interest (pre-SMA, SMA, CMAr, CMAc) were identified anatomically on a high-resolution MRI of each subject's brain. Descriptive analysis, consisting of individual assessment of significant activation, revealed a bilateral activation in the four mesial structures for all movement conditions, but self-initiated movements were more efficient than visually triggered movements. The more complex and more rapid the movements, the smaller the difference in activation efficiency between the self-initiated and the visually triggered tasks, which indicated an additional processing role of the mesial motor areas involving both the type and rate of movements. Quantitatively, activation was more for self-initiated than for visually triggered movements in pre-SMA, CMAr, and CMAc.

Stephan et al. used neuroimaging to identify structures that were activated with consciously made movements more than subconscious ones. Subjects were asked to tap their right index finger in time with different rhythmic tone sequences. One sequence was perfectly regular and others had deviations of the timing of the tones by 3%, 7%, and 20%. Only with the 20% variance were subjects aware of having to alter the timing of the tapping. When done at a subconscious level (3%), movement adjustments were performed employing bilateral ventral mediofrontal cortex. Awareness of change without explicit knowledge of the nature of the change (7%) led to additional ventral prefrontal and premotor, but not dorsolateral prefrontal activations. Only fully conscious motor adaptations (20%)

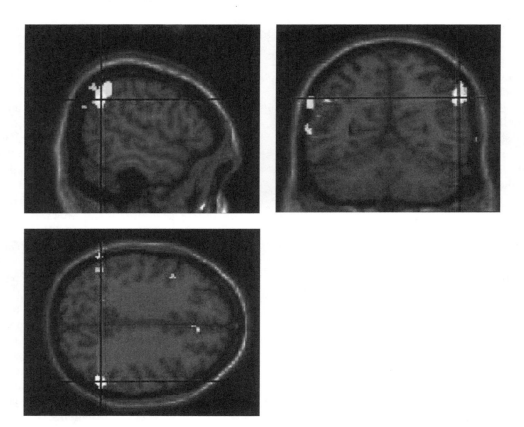

Figure 22.3 Positron emission tomography (PET) study with variable amounts of the sense of agency of hand movements. This figure shows the areas of the brain that were more active with less sense of agency. (From Farrar C, Frank N, Georgieff N, et al. Modulating the experience of agency: a positron emission tomography study. *NeuroImage.* 2003;18:324–333, with permission.)

showed prominent involvement of anterior cingulate and dorsolateral prefrontal cortex. The authors proposed that "these results demonstrate that while ventral prefrontal areas may be engaged in motor adaptations performed subconsciously, only fully conscious motor control which includes motor planning will involve dorsolateral prefrontal cortex."

The self-initiation of movement and conscious awareness of movement appear to involve mesial motor structures and the DLPFC. As pointed out by Paus (40), the mesial motor structures, and the anterior cingulate cortex in particular, is a place of convergence for motor control, homeostatic drive, emotion, and cognition.

An imaging study has investigated "agency," the feeling of being causally involved in an action, the feeling that leads us to attribute an action to ourselves rather than to another person (41). The investigators used a device that allowed them to modify the subject's degree of control of the movements of a virtual hand presented on a screen. During a blood-flow PET study, they compared four conditions: (i) a condition in which the subject had full control of the movements of the virtual hand, (ii) a condition in which the movements of the virtual hand appeared rotated by 25 degrees with respect to the movements made by the subject, (iii) a condition in which the movements of the

virtual hand appeared rotated by 50 degrees, and (iv) a condition in which the movements of the virtual hand were produced by another person and did not correspond to the subject's movements. In the inferior part of the parietal lobe, specifically on the right side, the less the subject felt in control of the movements of the virtual hand, the higher the level of activation (Fig. 22.3). In the insula, the more the subject felt in control, the more the activation. Hence, there are activation correlates to the sense of agency.

We are far from being able to interpret these imaging findings unequivocally. It may be that the basic decision processes that lead to "voluntary" movement are generated in frontal lobe structures, including the mesial motor areas. On the other hand, the perception, the qualia, that the movement is generated in a voluntary fashion, is processed in the parietal lobe.

CONCLUSION

Disorders of will are common in neurology. Because the issue of free will raises philosophical considerations, neurologists and physiologists have often been afraid to investigate or even discuss it. The situation is now evolving and progress can be anticipated. Conversion psychogenic movements appear to share some brain mechanisms with voluntary movements, but their genesis is largely mysterious. There may be a pathologic unconscious influence on movement production. Another aspect of conversion movement is that there is a disconnection between movement production and sense of volition. We are making strides in understanding the production of movement by the brain and in understanding how the brain decides whether something is voluntary or not. This basic information should help clear up the physiology of conversion and, hopefully, lead to better diagnostic methods and therapy.

ACKNOWLEDGMENT

This paper is extensively modified from a syllabus written for the American Academy of Neurology. As work of the United States Government, it has no copyright.

REFERENCES

1. Langleben DD, Schroeder L, Maldjian JA, et al. Brain activity during simulated deception: an event-related functional magnetic resonance study. *Neuroimage.* 2002;15:727–732.
2. Ganis G, Kosslyn SM, Stose S, et al. Neural correlates of different types of deception: an fMRI investigation. *Cereb Cortex.* 2003;13:830–836.
3. Lee TM, Liu HL, Tan LH, et al. Lie detection by functional magnetic resonance imaging. *Hum Brain Mapp.* 2002;15:157–164.
4. Spence SA, Farrow TF, Herford AE, et al. Behavioural and functional anatomical correlates of deception in humans. *Neuroreport.* 2001;12:2849–2853.
5. Searle JR. How to study consciousness scientifically. *Philos Trans R Soc Lond B Biol Sci.* 1998;353:1935–1942.
6. Libet B, Gleason CA, Wright EW, et al. Time of conscious intention to act in relation to onset of cerebral activity (readiness-potential). The unconscious initiation of a freely voluntary act. *Brain.* 1983;106:623–642.
7. Deecke L. Electrophysiological correlates of movement initiation. *Rev Neurol (Paris).* 1990;146:612–619.
8. Toma K, Matsuoka T, Immisch I, et al. Generators of movement-related cortical potentials: fMRI-constrained EEG dipole source analysis. *Neuroimage.* 2002;17:161–173.
9. Libet B, Wright EW Jr, Gleason CA. Readiness-potentials preceding unrestricted "spontaneous" vs. pre-planned voluntary acts. *Electroencephalogr Clin Neurophysiol.* 1982;54:322–335.
10. Keller I, Heckhausen H. Readiness potentials preceding spontaneous motor acts: voluntary vs. involuntary control. *Electroencephalogr Clin Neurophysiol.* 1990;76:351–361.
11. Macknik SL, Livingstone MS. Neuronal correlates of visibility and invisibility in the primate visual system. *Nat Neurosci.* 1998;1:144–149.
12. Taylor JL, McCloskey DI. Triggering of preprogrammed movements as reactions to masked stimuli. *J Neurophysiol.* 1990;63:439–446.
13. Wegner DM, Wheatley T. Apparent mental causation. Sources of the experience of will. *Am Psychol.* 1999;54:480–492.
14. Wegner DM. *The Illusion of conscious will.* Cambridge, MA: MIT Press, 2002.
15. Hallett M. Neurophysiology of tics. In: Cohen DJ, Goetz CG, Jankovic J, eds. *Tourette syndrome.* Philadelphia, PA: Lippincott Williams & Wilkins, 2000:237–244.
16. Obeso JA, Rothwell JC, Marsden CD. Simple tics in Gilles de la Tourette's syndrome are not prefaced by a normal premovement potential. *J Neurol Neurosurg Psychiatry.* 1981;44:735–738.
17. Karp BI, Porter S, Toro C, et al. Simple motor tics may be preceded by a premotor potential. *J Neurol Neurosurg Psychiatry.* 1996;61:103–106.
18. Lang A. Patient perception of tics and other movement disorders. *Neurology.* 1991;41:223–228.
19. Fisher CM. Honored guest presentation: abulia minor vs. agitated behavior. *Clin Neurosurg.* 1983;31:9–31.
20. Fisher CM. Alien hand phenomena: a review with the addition of six personal cases. *Can J Neurol. Sci* 2000;27:192–203.
21. Frith CD, Blakemore S, Wolpert DM. Explaining the symptoms of schizophrenia: abnormalities in the awareness of action. *Brain Res Brain Res Rev.* 2000;31:357–363.
22. Toro C, Torres F. Electrophysiological correlates of a paroxysmal movement disorder. *Ann Neurol.* 1986;20:731–734.
23. Terada K, Ikeda A, Van Ness PC, et al. Presence of Bereitschaftspotential preceding psychogenic myoclonus: clinical application of jerk-locked back averaging. *J Neurol Neurosurg Psychiatry.* 1995;58:745–747.
24. Vuilleumier P, Chicherio C, Assal F, et al. Functional neuroanatomical correlates of hysterical sensorimotor loss. *Brain.* 2001;124:1077–1090.
25. Spence SA, Crimlisk HL, Cope H, et al. Discrete neurophysiological correlates in prefrontal cortex during hysterical and feigned disorder of movement. *Lancet.* 2000;355:1243–1244.
26. Brown P, Thompson PD. Electrophysiological aids to the diagnosis of psychogenic jerks, spasms, and tremor. *Mov Disord.* 2001;16:595–599.
27. Deuschl G, Koster B, Lucking CH, et al. Diagnostic and pathophysiological aspects of psychogenic tremors. *Mov Disord.* 1998;13:294–302.
28. Thompson PD, Colebatch JG, Brown P, et al. Voluntary stimulus-sensitive jerks and jumps mimicking myoclonus or pathological startle syndromes. *Mov Disord.* 1992;7:257–262.
29. Schall JD. Neural basis of deciding, choosing and acting. *Nat Rev Neurosci.* 2001;2:33–42.
30. Stuphorn V, Schall JD. Neuronal control and monitoring of initiation of movements. *Muscle Nerve.* 2002;26:326–339.
31. Schall JD. The neural selection and control of saccades by the frontal eye field. *Philos Trans R Soc Lond B Biol Sci.* 2002;357:1073–1082.
32. Lecas JC, Requin J, Anger C, et al. Changes in neuronal activity of the monkey precentral cortex during preparation for movement. *J Neurophysiol.* 1986;56:1680–1702.
33. Missal M, Heinen SJ. Facilitation of smooth pursuit initiation by electrical stimulation in the supplementary eye fields. *J Neurophysiol.* 2001;86:2413–2425.
34. Salzman CD, Newsome WT. Neural mechanisms for forming a perceptual decision. *Science.* 1994;264:231–237.
35. Frith C. Attention to action and awareness of other minds. *Conscious Cogn.* 2002;11:481–487.
36. Deiber M-P, Passingham RE, Colebatch JG, et al. Cortical areas and the selection of movement: a study with positron emission tomography. *Exp Brain Res.* 1991;84:393–402.
37. Deiber M-P, Ibañez V, Sadato N, et al. Cerebral structures participating in motor preparation in humans: a positron emission tomography study. *J Neurophysiol.* 1996;75:233–247.
38. Jahanshahi M, Jenkins IH, Brown RG, et al. Self-initiated versus externally triggered movements. I. An investigation using measurement of regional cerebral blood flow with PET and movement-related potentials in normal and Parkinson's disease subjects. *Brain.* 1995;118:913–933.
39. Deiber MP, Honda M, Ibanez V, et al. Mesial motor areas in self-initiated versus externally triggered movements examined with fMRI: effect of movement type and rate. *J Neurophysiol.* 1999;81:3065–3077.
40. Paus T. Primate anterior cingulate cortex: where motor control, drive and cognition interface. *Nat Rev Neurosci.* 2001;2:417–424.
41. Farrer C, Franck N, Georgieff N, et al. Modulating the experience of agency: a positron emission tomography study. *Neuroimage.* 2003;18:324–333.

23

The Neurophysiology of Voluntary Movement in Nonhuman Primates: Accumulator Models of Decision and Action in Relation to Psychogenic Movement Disorders

Steven P. Wise   *Jerald D. Kralik*

ABSTRACT

According to some recent models of decision, choice, and action, distinct neural networks accumulate evidence in favor of making a potential movement. Voluntary movements arise when one of these "accumulator networks" reaches its threshold for producing an output. Sluggish operations in these networks could prevent an intended movement or make one difficult. Hyperactive accumulators might generate unintended movements. Other networks operate through similar accumulator mechanisms to "veto" movements, and hyperactive operations in these networks could also prevent intended movements. Taken together with the idea that people might be aware of some of the "evidence" for making or vetoing a movement, but not all of it, these models provide useful insights into psychogenic movement disorders.

INTRODUCTION

"Accumulator–racetrack models" of decision and choice have gained support from recent neurophysiologic experiments in monkeys. According to these models, voluntary movements occur when certain premotor neural networks reach a threshold for producing an output. These networks, which we call "commanding accumulators," act like leaky integrators, gathering evidence in favor of the action that they command. Their output leads to a cascade of events that ends in the generation of a movement, either by triggering activity in motor pattern generators or releasing them from tonic inhibition. Commanding accumulators work in parallel and in competition with each other, with the one (or ones) reaching threshold first, controlling movement in a winner-take-all manner.

Any pathology that undermines the ability of these networks to reach their threshold could either prevent an intended movement entirely or require that the accumulators receive unusually large or abnormally sustained inputs to reach their threshold. The former possibility might be relevant to psychogenic paralysis, the latter to psychogenic weakness. A different kind of accumulator network has outputs that serve to prevent or "veto" movements. Undesired or uncontrolled output from these networks, which we call "countermanding accumulators," could also lead to negative psychogenic movement disorders such as paralysis or weakness.

Conversely, a pathologic increase in the output of commanding accumulators, the failure of countermanding accumulators, or some dysfunction of the winner-take-all mechanism might lead to unintended movements, as in positive psychogenic movement disorders such as dystonia, tremor, or myoclonus.

This chapter presents these concepts and then develops them in the context of two ideas about the functional organization of primate brains: (i) Primate brains have separate neural systems for perception and action, and (ii) their prefrontal cortex mediates a form of behavioral inhibition. The first idea holds that many apparently voluntary actions are actually controlled subconsciously by automatic sensorimotor transforms called "autopilot mechanisms." The second holds, by analogy, that the process of vetoing or suppressing movements may also proceed without conscious mediation. Our goal is to provide a conceptual "toolbox" for thinking about the pathophysiology of psychogenic movement disorders and discussing their potential causes with patients and family members. (Some readers may choose to pass over most of the next section, which deals with philosophic and conceptual issues that arise in studying voluntary movements in monkeys or other nonhuman animals. For such readers, the subsection entitled "Terminology," which defines the terms used here, picks up the presentation from this point.)

WHAT IS A VOLUNTARY MOVEMENT AND DO MONKEYS MAKE ANY?

Are Studies in Monkeys Relevant to Psychogenic Motor Disorders?

Monkeys never appear in a clinic complaining of a psychogenic movement disorder; they neither claim nor deny making voluntary movements. So one might reasonably doubt the relevance of behavioral neurophysiology, as studied in monkeys, to disorders of voluntary movement.

Fundamental biologic principles suggest, however, that the insights gained from behavioral neurophysiology in monkeys have some bearing on understanding voluntary movements in humans. We share with monkeys approximately 500 million of our 530 million years of vertebrate history. From the inception of vertebrates, our common ancestors made movements based on decisions about what to do, when to do it, and whether it should be done at all. The vertebrate brain may have evolved specifically for this function (1). Much later, 55 to 65 million years ago, our most distant primate ancestors built on that heritage by evolving mechanisms for grasping fruit, nectar, and leaves from the distal end of branches (2). These "aboreal graspers" eventually gave rise to monkeys, apes, and humans. New World monkeys—which include three kinds of monkeys that will be mentioned in this chapter: cotton-top tamarins, squirrel monkeys, and common marmosets—went their separate way from the ape–human lineage approximately 35 million years ago. Another group of monkeys, Old World monkeys, includes the mainstay of behavioral neurophysiology, the rhesus monkey. Old World monkeys diverged from the ape–human lineage about 30 million years ago. That lengthy period saw the evolution of upright posture, bipedal gait, language, and extensive tool use. So a lot happened in those 30 to 35 million years. Nevertheless, the ape–human lineage inherited many of the mechanisms for choosing and guiding actions that both we and monkeys retain. Still, our separate history and the taciturn nature of our fellow primates raises questions about whether monkeys make voluntary movements in the same sense that we do—or, at least, in the same sense that we *think* we do (3).

What Is a Voluntary Movement?

In his seminal monograph on *The Frontal Lobes and Voluntary Action*, Passingham (4) defined voluntary movements as actions that are learned, attended, and based on a comparison among alternatives. We will use his definition in this chapter, but not without explicitly recognizing its problems.

The biggest problem is that for people, we usually accept a symbolic report—usually, but not necessarily, verbal—about whether a movement is voluntary. Alternatively, we see that a person does as he or she is instructed, again usually verbally. So how could anyone know if a monkey, which cannot make such reports or comprehend verbal instructions, is making a voluntary movement? Using Passingham's definition solves the problem operationally but not satisfyingly. To appreciate the source of this dissatisfaction, imagine that a person sees some "thing"—so far away that it could be either a person or a robot—reach to an object. On the assumption that the "thing" is a person, most people would suppose that he or she had just made a conscious decision to reach to the object and was, therefore, making a voluntary movement. On the assumption that the "thing" is a robot, however, most people would be reluctant to draw the same conclusion. They might imagine that the robot guides those movements through a complex computation of sensorimotor transforms, but they would not think that the robot had made a conscious decision, and they would not consider it to have made a voluntary movement.

But what if the person made a movement in a "robot-like" way, using "autopilot" control mechanisms divorced from conscious awareness? As discussed later in this chapter and by Zeman (Chapter 24), people perform many complex, purposive behaviors without awareness, including sleepwalking, reaching to objects in "blindsight" (5), and performing sequences of movement (6). These actions look just like voluntary movements. So how could anyone verify the voluntary nature of a monkey's movement?

The answer is that it cannot be done, at least not for certain. The problem is, of course, that of animal consciousness. To say that expert opinion remains divided on the topic of animal consciousness is to say the least. There are books in which the author of one chapter obsesses about whether chimpanzees have anything remote like human consciousness, while the author of another chapter discusses his or her studies of conscious knowledge in rats without the slightest hint that the issue might be controversial. Without a verbal or symbolic report, there is no straightforward way of telling whether a movement is voluntary in the sense used in ordinary conversation. For this reason and others—some of which stem from the continuing legacy of radical behaviorism in contemporary neuroscience—many neuroscientists are "afraid to discuss" topics related to consciousness, including voluntary movement (Chapter 22). Indeed, most discussions of knowledge and goal-oriented action in nonhuman animals keep the problem of consciousness securely in the closet and use a broad array of proxy terms instead. Conscious knowledge is called "declarative" when applied to memory systems or "explicit" when applied to tasks. By exclusion, information that has no access to conscious awareness is often termed implicit or procedural. Some psychologists use the term "habit" interchangeably for procedural knowledge, even though they often do so in a way that is inconsistent with the concept as defined in formal animal learning theory (7). Unfortunately, the evidence for explicit knowledge in

nonhuman primates is, as yet, inconclusive (8). Despite more than a decade of research into imitation, ape "language," deception, theory of mind, and related issues, opinion remains divided on whether nonhuman primates, in general, or monkeys, in particular, show any of these traits. So while we can accept Passingham's (4) definition of voluntary action for the purposes of discussion, the problem of animal consciousness needs to be acknowledged, and, for the present purposes, this means being as explicit as possible (no pun intended) about the terminology used here.

Terminology

We have defined the "voluntary" part of voluntary movement above, following Passingham (4), subject to the inherent limitations on speculating about the conscious life of monkeys. The "voluntary" part implies a movement that is learned, attended, and based on an evaluation of alternative actions and their potential outcomes. Involuntary movements are thus defined, by exclusion, as movements that are either unattended (and are thus on "autopilot" control), do not have to be learned or are learned virtually automatically (and are thus "prepotent responses"), or require no evaluation of potential outcomes (and are thus "habits"). The "movement" part of voluntary movement also deserves some elaboration. We usually think of voluntary movement as a positive act, depending on muscle activity. However, deciding to *do* something inevitably means deciding *not* to do many other things. Not only does decision-making require the selection of one voluntary movement instead of others, but it also requires the inhibition of competing involuntary actions. And the decision *not* to do something—or anything—may be as voluntary as the decision to make a movement. So for the purposes of this chapter we construe "movement" very broadly to include stable posture and, therefore, the withholding, suppression, or vetoing of movement. And we also use the term "perception" in a particular way in this chapter, which differs from common usage. We restrict use of the term perception to instances of conscious awareness and do not use it as a synonym for sensation or sensory input, as is often the case.

THE NEUROPHYSIOLOGY OF DECISIONS: ACCUMULATOR–RACETRACK MODELS

Accumulator–Racetrack Models in Theory

Although studies of cognition in nonhuman primates and other animals to date have not resolved the question of whether they have explicit knowledge, awareness, or consciousness, their capacity for expectation and prediction is not in question. Accordingly, animal learning theory—which depends on the concepts of expectation and prediction—has contributed importantly to the understanding of voluntary behavior (although many of its practitioners would be reluctant to call it that). In animal learning theory, voluntary action is considered to result from a "decision-making" process. Animals appear to make responses based on a choice among a (large) set of possible responses, and this decision appears to be based on a comparison of the expected outcomes, in terms of biologic value, of alternative actions. The assessed value of each response alternative can be quantified, including the relative influence of variables such as reinforcement rate, reward magnitude, certainty, effort, and delay. These ideas have recently been successfully applied to behavioral neurophysiology in monkeys (9,10). In this section, therefore, we describe some key results and ideas coming from this work, and, in the final section of this chapter, we attempt to place these ideas in the context of psychogenic movement disorders.

Significant progress has been made toward understanding the neurophysiology of decisions that monkeys make about the stimuli they see and the actions that they perform. Recent findings indicate that neural networks called *accumulators*, which act something like leaky integrators, gather evidence about the world or gather evidence for making a given response. Because both of these processes involve accumulating information, these theories of decision have been termed accumulator models. In some accumulator models, competing accumulators generate different decisions, and the first accumulator to reach a threshold for producing its output "wins." For that reason such models are also called racetrack models. To capture both ideas, we call them *accumulator–racetrack models*. (In other versions, the accumulator that gets "far enough" ahead of the others wins, or a given accumulator weighs both the evidence for and against a particular decision.)

Accumulator–racetrack models posit that neural integrators accumulate evidence; if this evidence eventually reaches a threshold, the accumulators generate a decision. The evidence is usually considered to be of a sensory nature, but these models can be extended to include internally generated signals, as well. Decisions can relate to the nature of the sensory evidence alone, as in sensory perception, or to a choice among potential responses, as in voluntary movement. Motor decisions can be both positive and negative: They can lead to a chosen movement or to the inhibition of unchosen ones. Typically, accumulator–racetrack models divide decisions and choices into phases, as illustrated in Figure 23.1, with the early phases dealing primarily with the evaluation of sensory evidence, and later phases, usually thought to overlap in time with the earlier ones, dealing with decisions about and choices of potential actions (11). According to these models, the central nervous system makes decisions at both stages: first deciding what the sensory inputs represent and somewhat later choosing what action to perform.

The model illustrated in Figure 23.1 has a "front end" component that corresponds to the several related concepts that are usually subsumed by the term "attention" (11). Consider a task in which someone must respond to a number, presented on a screen, by saying whether it is odd or even. In the model depicted in Figure 23.1, a bias parameter (also known as a response set) might push decisions toward a response in terms of "odd versus even" numbers, as opposed to other response rules or "sets," such as "prime versus nonprime," "larger versus smaller" than 5, and so forth. Another attentional factor involves which features are extracted from the environment. And a third attentional factor is a priority parameter, sometimes called a stimulus set.

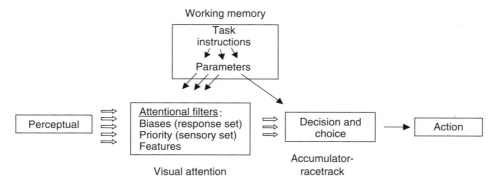

Figure 23.1   An accumulator model of decision. Decisions involve accumulating evidence about sensory inputs (and, by extension, internal neural signals) and making a decision about a response. Although construed as occurring in stages, beginning with perception and proceeding to action, one stage need not finish before the next begins. In the model of Logan and Gordon, the requirements of some task, such as its rules, relevant features, favored responses, and a difference threshold, are passed to an attention system and accumulator networks as parameters. Decisions occur when the accumulator for a given decision or choice reaches its threshold or gets sufficiently "far ahead" of other accumulators, which receive evidence in favor of competing decisions and choices. (From Logan GD, Gordon RD. Executive control of visual attention in dual-task situations. *Psychol Rev.* 2001;108.)

For example, imagine that someone needs to say whether a number is odd or even, but there are two odd numbers on a screen, one above the other. According to the model in Figure 23.1, a priority parameter predisposes the system to assign its response, oddity, to the top number, for example. Together, these attentional factors modulate the influence of evidence on the accumulators involved in decisions and choices.

Although accumulator–racetrack models might seem highly theoretical, recent neurophysiologic research has provided evidence for these mechanisms. Accordingly, we next consider neurophysiologic evidence for neurons (i) accumulating evidence for a movement, (ii) accumulating sensory evidence, (iii) accumulating equivocal evidence, and (iv) accumulating evidence against a movement.

Neurophysiology of Accumulator–Racetrack Models

To understand the neurophysiologic data, it is important to bear in mind that the vast majority of neurons in the cortex are "tuned" for a particular region of space or some other set of stimulus parameters. The concept of a receptive field captures this idea for the sensory system. One way of looking at spatial tuning is that, due to their synaptic inputs, neurons "monitor" some region of space. Sometimes this takes the form of a circumscribed region of space, and such cells often show neuronal tuning that approximates a Gaussian function of the central point in that space. In other instances, spatial tuning involves only one dimension, such as direction (independent of amplitude) from the current location of the hand, for example.

Figure 23.2 illustrates some of the first neurophysiologic evidence for accumulator–racetrack models; it shows the activity of a neuron in the frontal eye field (FEF) of a monkey. This cell changed its firing rate 50 to 100 ms before the onset of a saccadic eye movement up and to the right. Schall et al. (12) studied its activity when they presented several stimuli of one type in the visual field (e.g., seven green squares), along with one stimulus of a different type (e.g., a red square). In their experiment, the red stimulus served as the target for a saccadic eye movement. The representation of the target emerged gradually as neural signals progressed through the visual system, from occipital to frontal cortex. When the target appeared up and to the right from the monkey's fixation point, the FEF neuron illustrated in Figure 23.2 accumulated inputs up to its threshold for generating a saccade to that target (13). When the neuron reached its threshold quickly, the movement began with a relatively short reaction time (left arrow in Fig. 23.2). If the neuron took longer to reach its threshold, a slower response resulted (middle and right arrows in Fig. 23.2). Thus, accumulator models accord well with classic reaction-time theories (14), as extended to include neurophysiologic concepts, which hold that variation in reaction time depends upon stochastic variability in a neural integrator.

The same ideas apply to the accumulation of sensory evidence, even when that evidence is less directly linked to movement. Neurons in visual, posterior parietal (15), and prefrontal (16) areas appear to accumulate evidence about sensory inputs. Figure 23.3 illustrates neuronal activity in the middle temporal area (MT), which subserves motion vision. To study the activity of MT neurons, Roitman and

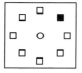

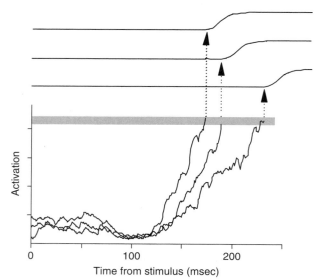

Figure 23.2 Accumulation of evidence for a saccadic eye movement. The activation level of a neuron in the frontal eye field (FEF) is shown for three different reaction times. The inset at the **top left** shows the monkey's task. The monkey began by fixating the central light spot *(circle)*. Then eight stimuli appeared, seven green *(unfilled squares)*, one red *(filled square)*. The monkey's task was to make a saccadic eye movement to fixate the red stimulus. For the shortest reaction times, the neuron's activity rose with the greatest slope and reached a threshold *(shaded horizontal line)* fastest *(leftmost arrow)*. (Reproduced from Schall JD, Thompson KG. *Annual Review of Neuroscience.* 1999:22, with permission, copyright by Annual Reviews.)

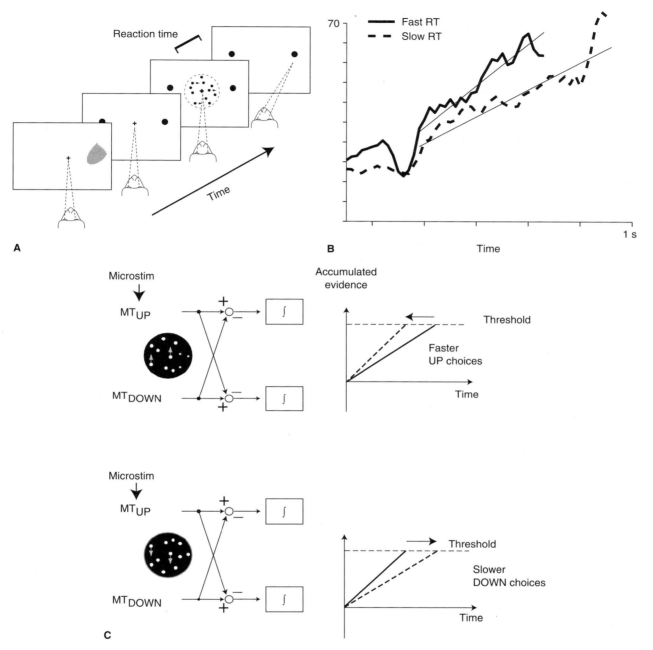

Figure 23.3 Accumulation of sensory evidence. **A**: Four images seen by the monkey, which occurred in order, from left to right. As a monkey fixated *(dashed lines)* the center of a screen, it viewed a central display of dots, which moved coherently (i.e., in the same direction at the same speed) or randomly, as determined by the experimenter. The monkey "reported" whether the dots, in aggregate, moved to the right by making a saccadic eye movement to fixate the right "report target" *(right filled circle)*. **B**: Discharge of a neuron in the middle temporal area (MT). The solid line shows the accumulation of neuronal activity during trials in which the monkey responded relatively quickly *(fast RT)*. The dashed line shows the neuronal activity when the monkey responded relatively slowly *(slow RT)*. **C**: A model of mutual inhibition among competing accumulators. Electrical stimulation *(microstim.)* near the site of cells responding to upward dot motion caused a decrease in reaction time to upward motion **(top right)** and an increase in reaction time to downward motion **(bottom right)**. (**A, B** from Roitman JD, Shadlen MN. *Journal of Neuroscience* 2002:22, with permission, copyright 2002 by the Society for Neuroscience; **C** reproduced from Ditterich J, Mazurek ME, Shadlen MN. *Nature Neuroscience*. 2003:6, with permission, copyright 2003 by the Nature Publishing Group.)

Shadlen (17) used an experimental paradigm pioneered by Newsome and his colleagues (18). In these experiments, a monkey viewed a screen that has a small field of moving light spots (Fig. 23.3A). For people, if many light spots move in the same direction at the same speed, they can easily detect the coherent motion. If only a small proportion of the spots move coherently, with the rest moving randomly, detecting the coherent motion becomes more difficult. In that case, it takes longer to accumulate evidence and the reaction time increases. In applying this experiment to monkeys, the investigators made the reasonable assumption that the stimuli look the same to the monkey as to human observers. In monkeys, however, the report required some kind of movement, typically an eye movement, so the experiment could not distinguish perceptions, *per se*, from sensorimotor transforms. The monkey observed the stimuli for as long as necessary to make a decision, then initiated a "report" in the form of a saccadic eye movement. Near the perceptual threshold of 6% to 7% coherence, the monkeys took up to a second to respond, but with substantial variation (17,19). The experimenters later divided the trials into those that had faster reaction times (solid line in Fig. 23.3B) and those that had slower ones (dashed line). In accord with accumulator–racetrack models, a more rapid increase in neuronal activity was found to correspond to the faster reaction times, and vice versa, much like the cell activity illustrated in Figure 23.2.

Also in accord with accumulator–racetrack models, experimental results from monkeys show that sensory evidence for making a given decision acts against alternative decisions. In an experiment by Ditterich et al. (20), electrical stimulation was used to activate cells near an electrode that also recorded neuronal activity. As the monkey viewed a spot display with a moderate amount of either upward or downward motion, small amounts of current were injected in the vicinity of neurons that accumulated evidence for upward motion. The stimulation speeded up the monkey's "report" of upward motion (Fig. 23.3C, top right). Thus, by exciting neurons thought to accumulate evidence for upward motion, the threshold of the network was attained more quickly than occurred without such artificial excitation. Importantly, the same stimulation also had an effect on the reaction time for downward motion. Excitation of neurons accumulating evidence for upward motion slowed reports of downward motion (Fig. 23.3C, bottom right). The results from this experiment show that accumulator networks appear to inhibit each other. Such inhibition would promote a winner-take-all system, in which evidence for one decision counts as evidence against others.

Figures 23.2 and 23.3 show that when accumulator networks reach their threshold for producing an output faster, reaction time decreases and vice versa. Figure 23.4 presents data showing that sometimes, in the presence of equivocal evidence, the accumulators fail to reach threshold, and therefore no movement occurs. To study these properties, Schall et al. (21) trained a monkey to make a saccadic eye movement from a fixation spot at the center of a screen to a light spot (the target) that appeared somewhere else on the screen (and quickly disappeared). On any given trial, the target could have appeared in any one of eight locations,

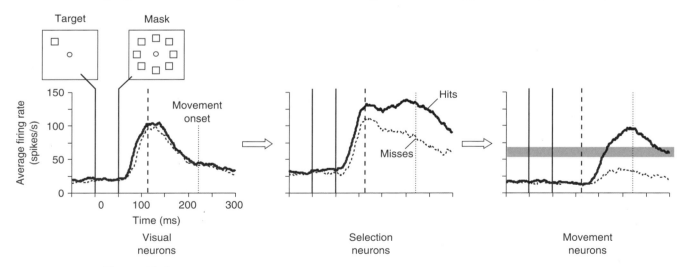

Figure 23.4 Failure to move in the presence of evidence for that movement. The two insets at the **top left** show the monkey's task. The monkey fixated a central fixation point *(circle)*. At the time labeled as 0 ms, a saccade target appeared *(square)*, in this case up and to the left from center. After a carefully adjusted period of time, a mask appears, which consisted of stimuli *(squares)* at eight locations, including that of the target. When the delay between the target and the mask had a critical value, the monkey responded to the target correctly on many trials *(hits)*, but failed to respond on other trials *(misses)*. Note that the sensory evidence was precisely the same in both cases. Nevertheless, neuronal activity differed for hits and misses. The dashed vertical lines mark the same time point in all three plots. (From data obtained by Thompson KG, Schall JD. *Vision Research.* 2000;40, replotted, with permission.)

arranged in a circle around the central fixation point. On some trials, a masking stimulus appeared 50 ms after the target. At this critical interval, the monkey responded on some trials (called "hits"), but not on others (called "misses"), despite the fact that the sensory evidence was identical in both. As Figure 23.4 shows, the investigators found several classes of neurons in the FEF. Two of these classes showed rapid increases in activity after the target appeared. One of these classes, called visual neurons, showed little difference in activity during hits versus misses, and the activity decayed rather quickly in either case. In another class, called selection neurons, the activity increased at the same rate as in visual neurons, but decayed much less overall, and decayed less for hits than misses. These neurons seemed to accumulate information about a stimulus in the location that they monitored. A third class, called movement neurons, showed activity increases that began later (after the dashed vertical line in all parts of Fig. 23.4). These cells seemed to accumulate information about whether to make a movement to the region of space they monitored. Note that qualitatively similar neural processing occurred for hits and misses; the activity was similar in many ways when the monkey made a movement and when it did not. Accumulator–racetrack models assume that when the network's activity fails to reach threshold, no movement occurs. In the "misses," the evidence for making the movement was present and identical to that in "hit" trials, but for some reason the activity of the movement neurons did not reach the threshold. In looking at these cell classes, one can imagine that the influence of selection neurons on movement neurons depended on the maintenance of activity seen for "hit" trials, and without it, the activation level of the movement neurons remained subthreshold. Unfortunately, no direct evidence exists for this idea. But subthreshold decisions clearly exist. For example, stimulation of cells in the FEF evokes eye movements that deviate systematically in the direction of a subthreshold decision (19,22). A failure of such subthreshold decisions-in-the-making to reach threshold could have some relevance to negative psychomotor disorders.

Movements might be prevented when decisions-in-the-making fail to reach threshold, but they can also be vetoed by subsequent decisions. Accumulator–racetrack models account for this (negative) behavior, as well. Schall et al. (23) studied this phenomenon in an experiment with a "stop" signal called a *countermanding* task. In their experiment, every trial began with the monkey looking at a fixation point in the center of a screen (Fig. 23.5A, top). On most trials, a target appeared somewhere at the same time as the fixation point disappeared, never to appear again on that trial. On those trials, the monkey reliably made a saccadic eye movement to fixate the new target. On other trials (Fig. 23.5A, bottom), the fixation point reappeared at some variable time after it had gone off. This signaled the monkey to "stop"—that is, cancel or veto—the saccade. If the stop signal appeared soon after the target, the monkey

reliably canceled the saccade. As the interval between the target's appearance and the stop signal increased, it became progressively more difficult for the monkey to veto the movement. Figure 23.5B shows the activity of a representative FEF neuron in a difficult condition, one in which the duration of the interval between the target ("go" cue) and the stop signal made it difficult, but not impossible, to veto the movement. The thin line shows the activity for trials on which the stop signal occurred but the monkey failed to veto the saccade. In accord with accumulator–racetrack models, the neuron seemed to integrate evidence for a movement to the location that it monitored, and the movement was executed shortly after it reached a threshold. On trials in which the monkey successfully vetoed the saccade, as shown by the thick line in Figure 23.5B, the activity began to decrease shortly after the stop signal, and (presumably) the accumulator never reached threshold. Note that the sensory evidence did not differ in any way between these two situations.

The pattern of single-neuron activity in the FEF has a remarkable resemblance to the shape of the readiness potential, recorded by Libet et al. (24), as illustrated in Figure 23.5C. They asked people to make a movement when a rotating dot reached a certain location, called the triggering point. When they did so, the readiness potential built to the time of movement onset (Fig. 23.5C, left). At another time, they asked participants to go through the same process of preparing to execute the movement, but when the dot got to a certain place prior to the triggering point, to veto the planned movement. During the vetoed-movement trials, the readiness potential appeared to level off and, in some people (arrows in Fig. 23.5C), it began to decrease prior to the time that the movement would have occurred. Of course, the decrease was not as dramatic as in the single FEF neuron (Fig. 23.5B), presumably because these scalp potentials measure the activity of many synapses and neurons. The general similarity in the two effects remains intriguing, nevertheless.

Figure 23.6 illustrates the theory behind the countermanding of a movement. The theory holds that accumulator networks of the countermanding type ("stop" activity in Figs. 23.6B,C) compete with accumulators of the commanding type ("go" activity). A reaction-time distribution can always be divided into fast responses (the shaded region in Fig. 23.6A) and slow ones. According to accumulator–racetrack models, if the movement was destined to have a relatively fast reaction time, then the commanding accumulator reached its threshold before the countermanding accumulator reached its own (Fig. 23.6B), and the movement was executed. If, on the other hand, the movement was destined to be have a relatively slow reaction time, the countermanding accumulator "won" (Fig. 23.6C), and the movement was canceled or vetoed.

Accumulator–racetrack models of decision-making and voluntary movement have several implications for the

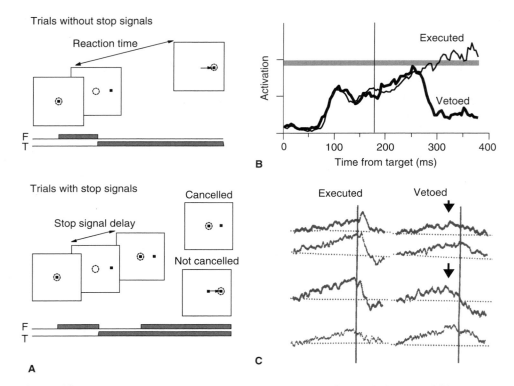

Figure 23.5 The countermanding task. **A:** On some trials the fixation light *(central filled square)* turned off as a saccade target *(right filled square)* appeared and the fixation light never came back on **(top)**. On other trials **(bottom)**, the fixation light came back on after a variable delay, called the stop-signal delay. At a critical stop-signal delay, the monkey canceled (or vetoed) some movements, but not others. The gray bars show the times during a trial that the fixation *(F)* and target *(T)* lights were on. The dotted circle surrounds the stimulus fixated by the monkey at any given time (time runs from left to right). **B:** After the instruction stimulus appeared at time 0, the activity of an FEF neuron showed an accumulation of activity that began after a latency of about 70 ms. At the time of the solid vertical line (at 175 ms), a veto signal appeared. The activity on trials in which the monkey executed the movement *(thin solid line)* and those with vetoed movements (thick solid line) diverged shortly before the activity reached threshold *(gray horizontal bar)*. **C:** Readiness potentials for a self-generated veto of a movement **(right)** and the executed movement **(left)** for four people. Note the decrease in the readiness potential at the arrows. (**A, B** reproduced from Schall JD, Thompson KG. *Annual Review of Neuroscience.* 1999:22, with permission, copyright by Annual Reviews. **C** reproduced with permission from Libet B, Wright EW, Gleason CA, *Electroencephalography and Clinical Neurophysiology.* 1983:56, copyright Elsevier.)

pathophysiology of psychogenic movement disorders, which we take up last. First, we consider their place in larger neural systems. Broadly construed, sensory inputs appear to have two different functions—perception and the guidance of action—and there is evidence that partially separate neural systems mediate them. For visual inputs, these functions depend on a "vision-for-perception" system and a "vision-for-action" system (25).

VISION FOR PERCEPTION VERSUS VISION FOR ACTION

Koch and Crick (26) refer to the vision-for-action system as "the zombie within." As they point out, people:

 . . . perform complex yet routine tasks without direct conscious input . . . , which is why we call them "zombie"

agents. One can become conscious of the actions of one's own zombie, but usually only in retrospect. The best evidence comes from studying dissociation of "vision for perception" and "vision for action. . . ."

Ideas of this nature contrast starkly with the traditional view of the relation between perception and action. Rather than viewing perception as a necessary intermediate to action (Fig. 23.7A), an alternative view holds that as evidence accumulates for perception (in the sense of that word implying awareness), it also accumulates—in parallel—for guiding action. As one consequence of this parallel organization, the awareness of one's own actions might come primarily from efference copy, reafference, or both (Fig. 23.7B). According to this view, first championed by Milner and Goodale (27), vision contributes in parallel to both visual perception and subconscious visuomotor control mechanisms often called "autopilots."

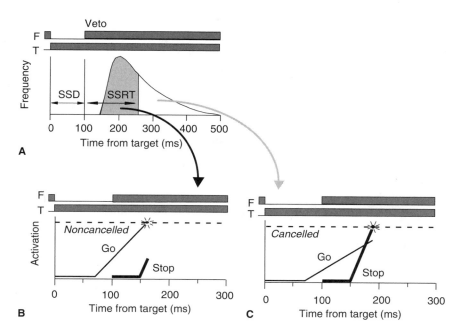

Figure 23.6 Veto of an instructed movement: theory. **A:** After the stop-signal delay *(SSD)*, movements destined to be made quickly *(shaded)* were within the stop-signal reaction time *(SSRT)* and could not be cancelled **(B)**. Those destined to occur at a longer response latency *(unshaded)*, were cancelled successfully **(C)**. Format of fixation *(F)* and target *(T)* lights as in Figure 23.5A. **B:** On trials in which the monkey made the saccade, the accumulation of activity in commanding *(go)* accumulators reached its threshold (dashed horizontal line) prior to the countermanding *(stop)* accumulators reaching theirs. **C:** On canceled trials, the countermanding accumulators won the "race." Note that the thresholds for the two kinds of accumulator networks need not be, as depicted, the same. (Reproduced from Hanes DP, Patterson WF, Schall JD. *Journal of Neurophysiology.* 1998:79, copyright by the American Physiological Society.)

Illusions can distinguish vision-for-perception from vision-for-action. One such illusion relies on the relative sizes of disks in a scene (28). A disk surrounded by smaller disks appears larger than the same sized disk surrounded by larger ones. By adjusting the sizes of the two central disks, disks of slightly different sizes can be made to appear the same (Fig. 23.8A). Although the perceptual system fails to detect the true difference in the disks' diameters, the vision-for-action system does not lose this information: When people reach to grasp the central disks, their fingers move farther apart for the larger one (Fig. 23.8B).

This same kind of dissociation between vision-for-perception and vision-for-action also occurs for eye movements. In one experiment, an illusion was caused by a discrete, instantaneous shift of a background frame that surrounded a light spot (29). When the central light spot jumped 1 degree left, but the background frame remained

stationary (Fig. 23.9A), people reported the spot's shift with ease and could also make a saccadic eye movement to fixate the spot's new location. When asked to make a saccade back to the remembered, initial location of the light spot, then 1 degree to the right of fixation, people did so accurately. However, when the central light spot jumped 1 degree to the right, but the background frame jumped in the same direction, at the same time, by twice as much (Fig. 23.9B), people reported that the spot had moved to the left. Presumably because there was no other frame of reference other than this background frame, they did not detect the frame's shift. Instead, the frame captured their perception and the central light spot appeared to have jumped to the left, although it had actually moved to the right. However, when asked to make a saccadic eye movement to fixate the light spot, people made an accurate saccade to the right, even though they had reported that they

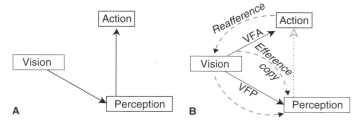

Figure 23.7 Perception and action in decision-making. **A:** A traditional view of the relationship between vision, perception, and action. **B:** A modified view of the relationship between vision, perception, and action. Sensory inputs, in this case visual ones, have privileged access to the motor-control system and form part of a vision-for-action system *(VFA)*. Sensory inputs also contribute to perception via the vision-for-perception system *(VFP)*. The perception of action results either from efference copy or the sensory effects of action (reafference). (Adapted from Lebedev MA, Wise SP. *Behavioral and Cognitive Neuroscience Reviews.* 2002:1, with permission, copyright by Sage Publications.)

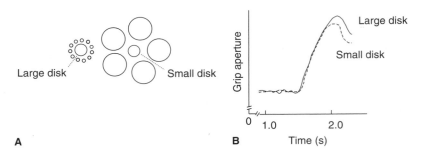

Figure 23.8 A size-contrast illusion that demonstrates a dissociation between the vision-for-action and vision-for-perception systems. **A:** The central disks had different diameters, but people perceived them as being of the same size because of the surrounding disks (28). **B:** The degree of hand opening during a reach to grasp the central disks. (Adapted from Lebedev MA, Wise SP. *Behavioral and Cognitive Neuroscience Reviews.* 2002:1, with permission, copyright by Sage Publications.)

had seen the spot jump to the left. Furthermore, when asked to look back to the spot's original location, they made a second rightward saccade. The "look-back" saccade required them to remember the spot's initial location. Because memory is based on perception and because they had perceived that the spot had jumped to the left, they made a rightward saccade in the "look-back" condition.

The experiments illustrated in Figures 23.8 and 23.9 provide examples of a behavioral dissociation between two neural systems: one for perceptual reports, the other for sensorially guided movements. The latter computations have, collectively, been called autopilot mechanisms, and Figure 23.10A attempts to place them in an anatomical context. Milner and Goodale (27) proposed that the ventral visual processing stream, consisting in part of inferior temporal areas, subserves the vision-for-perception system and that the dorsal stream, consisting in part of posterior parietal areas, underlies the vision-for-action system. The evidence that the posterior parietal cortex plays an important

role in autopilot control includes deficiencies in such control after damage to that region, disruption of autopilot control by transcranial magnetic stimulation of parietal cortex, and results from neuroimaging studies (30–32). The situation is probably more complex than suggested by Milner and Goodale, with a mixture of functions in both "streams" (33). Nonetheless, it is reasonable to conclude that the predominant function of both the dorsal and ventral stream is more or less as Milner and Goodale suggested. A review of the literature by Lebedev and Wise (33) produced the scheme presented in Figure 23.10A. The posterior parietal cortex is depicted as playing a larger role in the vision-for-action system (shaded parts of the box labeled "posterior parietal") than the vision-for-perception system (unshaded parts of the box). By contrast, the inferior temporal cortex is depicted as playing a larger role in the perceptual system. Based on some neurophysiological data (33) and anatomical considerations (34), the prefrontal cortex, and the rostral premotor areas with which it is

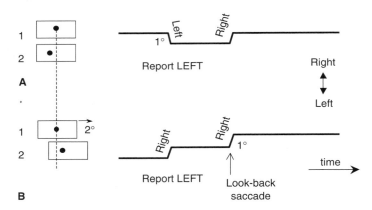

Figure 23.9 A frame-shift illusion that demonstrates a dissociation between the vision-for-action and vision-for-perception systems. **A: Left:** A frame *(rectangle)* and light spot *(filled circle)* originally appear in the configuration shown in *A1*. The frame and the light spot then disappeared and reappeared in the configuration shown in *A2*, after which the participants responded with a saccade to the light spot and reported its shift direction. **Right:** Facsimile eye-position record and reports about light-spot shifts. In **A**, the frame does not shift location from *A1* to *A2* and, accordingly, no illusion results. **B:** The light spot shifts 1 degree to the right, but the frame shifts 2 degrees to the right. People reported an illusory leftward movement of the target spot, but made a saccade in the (correct) rightward direction to fixate it. When instructed to look back to the spot's original location, they made an additional saccade to the right. (Modified from Lebedev MA, Wise SP. *Behavioral and Cognitive Neuroscience Reviews.* 2002:1, with permission, copyright by Sage Publications.)

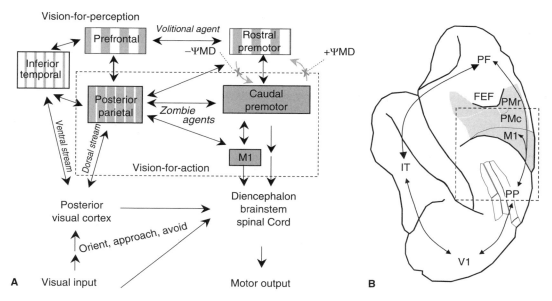

Figure 23.10 Perception and action: anatomical correlates. **A:** The principal components of the vision-for-action system are located in the dashed box. Positive psychogenic symptoms (+ΨMD) and negative ones (−ΨMD) might result from disruption of communication between the areas within the box and those outside it. **B:** A drawing of the brain of a macaque monkey, rotated so that the frontal pole is at the top and the inferior aspect is to the left. This orientation corresponds roughly to the configuration of the boxes in (**A**). (**A:** Modified from Lebedev MA, Wise SP. *Behavioral and Cognitive Neuroscience Reviews.* 2002:1, with permission. **B:** From Kalaska JF, Cisek P, Gosselin-Kessiby N. *The Parietal Lobe.* Siegel AM, Andersen RA et al., editors. Philadelphia: Lippincot Williams & Wilkins, 2003.)

allied, are depicted as having roughly equal contributions to the vision-for action and vision-for-perception systems. The core of the vision-for-action system, the parts that function mainly or exclusively in that system, appears inside the dashed box. It consists of posterior parietal areas, which receive visual inputs from lower-order (posterior) visual areas and interact with the caudal parts of premotor cortex and the primary motor cortex (M1) to guide movements.

Figure 23.10 raises a number of issues that extend beyond the scope of this chapter. Of some note, however, is the fact that the figure was not developed with psychogenic movement disorders in mind; neither author had ever heard of them at the time. Nevertheless, it captures the idea that the vision-for-action system might need to communicate with a partially separate system, involving different cortical areas, for the normal experience of agency and, for those who believe in such things (cf.3), the translation of thoughts into action.

In the previous section we discussed evidence for accumulator–racetrack mechanisms. These mechanisms of decision function in both the vision-for-action and vision-for-perception systems. We also discussed the existence of two kinds of accumulator: commanding accumulators and countermanding accumulators. Are they, too, concentrated in different neural systems?

PREFRONTAL INHIBITION OF PREPOTENT RESPONSES

A voluntary behavior is something a person can do when asked. [footnote] It is also something a person can *not do* when asked not to do it. The ability to inhibit voluntary acts . . . is sometimes described as a hallmark of voluntary behavior. . . . (3).

Automatic, involuntary responses are often called prepotent responses to emphasize the idea that they are either unlearned (i.e., innate) or subject to very rapid, virtually automatic learning (35). The ability to refrain from making prepotent responses—such as refraining from choosing an immediate reward in favor of a delayed, but larger, one—appears to require inhibitory-control mechanisms. There may be a number of different inhibitory control processes (36), but one that appears particularly relevant to psychogenic movement disorders involves inhibiting responses that are often aimed at obtaining highly desirable rewards, such as, for people, a large sum of money, or, for monkeys, a large amount of food. A clear example of the role of the prefrontal cortex in inhibitory control of behavior is the performance of monkeys with lesions of the orbitofrontal cortex on a food-retrieval task. In this task, a large piece of food is placed inside a transparent box, with the food item being placed directly in front of the monkey, just behind the transparent front wall of the box. Furthermore, in plain view of the monkey, the box has an opening in one of its side walls, allowing the monkey to grab the desired object by reaching through the side. Common marmosets—a New World monkey—quickly learn to reach the food through this side entrance to the box. By contrast, marmosets with lesions of the orbitofrontal cortex perseveratively reach directly for the food, even though they continue to hit their hand against the front wall of the box, and even though they can see the opening in the side of the box (37–41). This result has been attributed to their inability to inhibit the prepotent response of reaching directly for the food. Because intact marmosets inhibit their prepotent response, the experiment provides evidence that the orbitofrontal cortex mediates the inhibitory control of that behavior.

Another demonstration of inhibitory control comes from studies of nonhuman primates as they perform what is called a reversed-contingency task. In the original experiment, chimpanzees were offered a smaller quantity of food on one plate and a larger quantity of food on another plate (42). If the chimpanzees pointed to the plate with the larger quantity of food, they were given the smaller quantity; if they pointed to the smaller quantity of food, they were given the larger amount. Thus, the chimpanzees had to learn to select the smaller amount of food to receive the larger amount. None of the chimpanzees tested in this experiment could learn the task, even after hundreds of trials. Surprisingly, when the quantities of food were replaced with Arabic numerals (in previous experiments the chimpanzees had learned the associations of the numerals with the quantities), the chimpanzees *immediately* performed the task successfully. Because the chimpanzees could perform the task immediately, it appears that they had in fact learned the rule that should guide performance of the reversed-contingency task ("choose the smaller quantity to receive the larger one") in the original condition, but when seeing the actual food items, they were unable to inhibit reaching for the larger quantity of food.

Since that first experiment, other chimpanzees (43), Japanese macaques (44), cottontop tamarins (45), squirrel monkeys (46), and children (47) have all been tested on the task, and, until very recently, only humans over the age of four years performed the original task successfully (47). Recently, however, Murray et al. (48) found that rhesus macaques were able to learn the reversed-contingency task successfully when given enough trials to do so. It is clear from an analysis of the learning rates that the previous results on monkeys (44), which led to the conclusion that they could not learn the task, resulted from insufficient testing. Thus, rhesus monkeys can learn to inhibit the prepotent response and choose the smaller quantity of food. It appears that at least some Old World monkeys, such as rhesus monkeys, can learn the reversed-contingency task, but New World monkeys, such as squirrel monkeys and tamarins cannot, at least not in the form described here.

It is not too farfetched to imagine that the pronounced evolutionary expansion of the frontal lobe (49–51)—first in ancestors common to Old World monkeys and the human–ape lineage, then dramatically in the human–ape lineage—enabled the full development of inhibitory control abilities in humans (40). Indeed, areas throughout prefrontal cortex appear to be involved in inhibitory control processes. Perhaps the most evidence has implicated orbitofrontal and medial prefrontal cortex (36–41,52–54), including the anterior cingulate cortex (36,54). However, some evidence also indicates that other prefrontal areas, including dorsolateral prefrontal areas (37,38,41,55,56), play a role in behavioral inhibition. In accord with these findings, an excess of prefrontal inhibition has been implicated in negative psychogenic movement disorders (57,58) (see Chapters 25 and 26).

Thus, it appears that the prefrontal cortex has some specialization for the inhibitory control of behavior. Perhaps it evolved, in part, in response to adaptive pressures to enhance the proportion of countermanding accumulators in the cerebral cortex. Taken together, then, the conceptual tools developed to this point in the chapter include the idea of commanding and countermanding accumulators, the partial separation of a vision-for-action system from a vision-for-perception system, and the specialization of prefrontal cortex for countermanding accumulators. The next and final section addresses what might happen when these accumulator mechanisms—and the neural systems that depend upon them—malfunction.

FAILURE MODES OF ACCUMULATOR–RACETRACK MECHANISMS AND THE NEURAL SYSTEMS THEY COMPOSE

If one accepts the idea that data on sensorially guided movements in monkeys has relevance to voluntary movement in humans, then accumulator–racetrack models of decision and choice offer hints about how the mechanisms of voluntary movement can go wrong. Application of these models to voluntary movement in humans requires generalizing them from a form in which accumulators gather sensory evidence to one in which both internal and sensory signals can guide decision-making and choice. But with that extension, these ideas might contribute to a general conceptual framework for understanding psychogenic movement disorders and discussing those disorders with patients and their families.

Murphy's Law holds that what can go wrong, will, and many processes underlying accumulator–racetrack mechanisms could go wrong. At the pathophysiological level, accumulators might have two main failure modes (Fig. 23.11A). In one, either the threshold for the accumulator network's

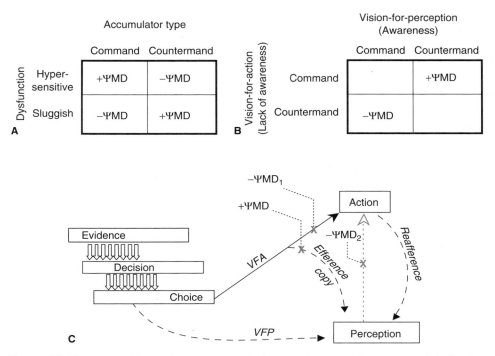

Figure 23.11 **A:** Possible psychogenic motor dysfunctions by accumulator type and dysfunction mode (+ΨMD, positive psychogenic symptoms; −ΨMD, negative psychogenic symptoms). **B:** Evidence for either commanding or countermanding accumulators can have access to conscious awareness (*columns*) or not (*rows*). **C:** The model of Fig. 23.7B in the context of accumulator models of decision and choice. On the assumption that the perception of agency relies upon efference copy from the VFA system to the perceptual system, note that a disconnection at different points of the system (*gray X*) might cause either positive psychogenic symptoms (ΨMD) or negative ones (−ΨMD$_1$ and −ΨMD$_2$).

output is set too low or the rate of neural integration proceeds at a much higher rate than normal. Perhaps, for accumulator networks in the cerebral cortex, deficient GABAergic mechanisms could cause such a defect, which we call "hypersensitive accumulators." In those instances, decisions that normally take much longer to come to threshold would do so very quickly, on the basis of minimal evidence for a given action, and perhaps merely on the basis of neural noise.

Conversely, accumulators could become activated too slowly, their threshold might be set too high, or their neural integrator circuits might leak too much. Excessive GABAergic inhibition or insufficient excitatory neurotransmission might cause such defects, which we call "sluggish accumulators." These kinds of dysfunction might lead to a complete inability of accumulators to reach threshold. More likely, in order to get such leaky, overinhibited, or high-threshold networks to produce an output would require enormously greater and more persistent input, which could require a Sisyphean effort for internally generated decisions and choices (Fig. 23.11A).

Regardless of the cause at the neuropharmacological level, hypersensitive accumulators of the commanding type might lead to positive psychogenic movement disorders, as

might sluggish accumulators of the countermanding type (Fig. 23.11A). Conversely, hypersensitive accumulators of the countermanding type and sluggish accumulators of the commanding type might lead to psychomotor paralysis or weakness. If no commanding accumulator reaches threshold, then no movement takes place, although many of the same underlying neural processes might occur (Fig. 23.4). Similarly, if unwanted processes drive countermanding accumulators to threshold before those for producing a movement can reach their threshold (Fig. 23.6C), intended movements might be unintentionally vetoed.

Accumulator models of decision become especially relevant to psychogenic movement disorders when considered in the broader context of the separate vision-for-action and vision-for-perception systems, which the accumulator mechanisms presumably compose. As discussed above, vision plays two different and dissociable roles, mediated by at least partially separate neural networks. One function, performed by the vision-for-perception system, involves the detection of "what is out there" and emphasizes relative judgments. The other, the role of the vision-for-action system, guides movements through autopilot mechanisms and emphasizes the accurate transduction of information needed for physical interaction with the world. Accumulator–racetrack models posit that accumulators gather evidence, in parallel. On the assumption that some of this evidence has access to awareness in humans, but much of it does not, the situations tabulated in Figure 23.11B become possible. Evidence can drive either commanding or countermanding accumulators, and the evidence could be accessible to the vision-for-perception system, and therefore to conscious awareness, or not. Inputs unnoticed by the perceptual system might be sufficient to drive commanding accumulators to threshold, and in that situation the movement might seem unintended (Fig. 23.11B, upper right). And when similarly unnoticed inputs drive countermanding accumulators to threshold, intended movement might not occur (Fig. 23.11B, lower left).

The concept of partially separate vision-for-perception and vision-for-action systems has an additional important consequence. It suggests that the perception of agency might depend on communications between the two systems. As Wegner (3) argues in his Theory of Apparent Mental Causation, the perception of agency might depend upon the precise temporal relationship between the awareness of a thought or intention and the occurrence of an action consistent with that thought or intention. One idea about how this might work involves efference copy. According to this idea, when the accumulator network for a given movement reaches its threshold, the resulting motor command—in the form of efference copy—is communicated to the systems mediating awareness (Fig. 23.11C). This efference copy might lead to the appreciation of agency in the same (unknown) way that sensory signals cause the qualia of phenomenal consciousness of sensory perceptions.

What if communication between the autopilot-control systems and the perceptual system breaks down (Figs. 23.11C and 23.10A)? A blockade of information flow from the vision-for-action system to the perception system would block perceptual accumulator networks from receiving efference copy. This might lead to the misperception, as in positive psychomotor disorders ($+\Psi$MD), that a movement lacks intention. According to this idea, if a person's perceptual system does not receive a copy of the motor command from the action system, he or she might fail to recognize the authorship of his or her own movement or intention (Figs. 23.11C and 23.10A). Likewise, blockade of information flow at some point distal to the link between evidence and perception would lead to the failure to make an intended movement (Fig. 23.11C), as in negative psychogenic motor disorders ($-\Psi$MD) and, if it exists [contrary to (3)], so would a blockade between perception and action (Fig. 23.11C). According to this idea, all of the information processing that usually accompanies a consciously intended (and attended) movement would occur, which would produce the perception of one's intention, but the movement would not occur.

Although admittedly speculative, these ideas about accumulator–racetrack models provide some insight into how competing, winner-take-all networks could lead to actions without intention or a difficulty in executing intended movements. We have proposed the following: (i) Some of these accumulators are of the commanding type, whereas others are of the countermanding type; (ii) they could become hypersensitive or sluggish; (iii) some cortical areas may be specialized for countermanding accumulators (e.g., medial and orbital prefrontal cortex), whereas others may be specialized for commanding accumulators (much of premotor and primary motor cortex); (iv) both sensory inputs and internal intentional signals could drive accumulators; (v) both kinds of driving signals could be available to conscious awareness—or not; (vi) the signals available to awareness are those that drive accumulator networks in the vision-for-perception system; (vii) those unavailable to awareness drive accumulators in the "autopilot," vision-for-action system; and finally (viii), a breakdown in communication between these two neural systems could interfere with the perception of agency or cause a paucity of intended action.

REFERENCES

1. Shadmehr R, Wise SP. *The computational neurobiology of reaching and pointing: a foundation for motor learning.* Cambridge, MA: MIT Press, 2004.
2. Bloch JI, Boyer DM. Grasping primate origins. *Science* 2002;298: 1606–1610.
3. Wegner DM. *The illusion of conscious will.* Cambridge, MA: MIT Press, 2002.
4. Passingham RE. *The frontal lobes and voluntary action.* Oxford: Oxford University Press, 1993.
5. Stoerig P, Cowey A. Blindsight in man and monkey. *Brain.* 1997; 120:535–559.
6. Willingham DB, Koroshetz WJ. Evidence for dissociable motor skills in Huntington's disease patients. *Psychobiology.* 1993;21: 173–182.
7. Dickenson A, Balleine B. Motivational control of goal-directed action. *Anim Learn Behav.* 1994;22:1–18.
8. Wise SP, Murray EA. Role of the hippocampal system in conditional motor learning: mapping antecedents to action. *Hippocampus.* 1999;9:101–117.
9. Platt ML, Glimcher PW. Neural correlates of decision variables in parietal cortex. *Nature.* 1999;400:233–238.
10. Glimcher PW. *Decisions, uncertainty, and the brain: the science of neuroeconomics.* Cambridge, MA: MIT Press, 2002.
11. Logan GD, Gordon RD. Executive control of visual attention in dual-task situations. *Psychol Rev.* 2001;108:393–434.
12. Hanes DP, Schall JD. Neural control of voluntary movement initiation. *Science.* 1996;274:427–430.
13. Schall JD, Thompson KG. Neural selection and control of visually guided eye movements. *Annu Rev Neurosci.* 1999;22:241–259.
14. Luce RD. *Respone times: their role in inferring elementary mental organization.* New York: Oxford University Press, 1986.
15. Shadlen MN, Newsome WT. Neural basis of a perceptual decision in the parietal cortex (area LIP) of the rhesus monkey. *J Neurophysiol.* 2001;86:1916–1936.
16. Kim JN, Shadlen MN. Neural correlates of a decision in the dorsolateral prefrontal cortex of the macaque. *Nat Neurosci.* 1999; 2:176–185.
17. Roitman JD, Shadlen MN. Response of neurons in the lateral intraparietal area during a combined visual discrimination reaction time task. *J Neurosci.* 2002;22:9475–9489.
18. Newsome WT, Britten KH, Movshon JA. Neuronal correlates of a perceptual decision. *Nature.* 1989;341:52–54.

19. Gold JI, Shadlen MN. Representation of a perceptual decision in developing oculomotor commands. *Nature.* 2000;404:390–394.

20. Ditterich J, Mazurek ME, Shadlen MN. Microstimulation of visual cortex affects the speed of perceptual decisions. *Nat Neurosci.* 2003;6:891–898.

21. Thompson KG, Schall JD. Antecedents and correlates of visual detection and awareness in macaque prefrontal cortex. *Vision Res.* 2000;40:1523–1538.

22. Gold JI, Shadlen MN. The influence of behavioral context on the representation of a perceptual decision in developing oculomotor commands. *J Neurosci.* 2003;23:632–651.

23. Hanes DP, Patterson WF, Schall JD. Role of frontal eye fields in countermanding saccades: visual, movement, and fixation activity. *J Neurophysiol.* 1998;79:817–834.

24. Libet B, Wright EW, Gleason CA. Preparation- or intention-to-act, in relation to pre-event potentials recorded at the vertex. *Electroencephalogr Clin Neurophysiol.* 1983;56:367–372.

25. Boussaoud D, di Pellegrino G, Wise SP. Frontal lobe mechanisms subserving vision for action vs. vision for perception. *Behav Brain Res.* 1996;72:1–15.

26. Koch C, Crick F. The zombie within. *Nature.* 2001;411:893.

27. Milner AD, Goodale MA. *The visual brain in action.* Oxford: Oxford University Press, 1996.

28. Aglioti S, DeSouza JFX, Goodale MA. Size-contrast illusions deceive the eye but not the hand. *Curr Biol.* 1995;5:679–685.

29. Wong E, Mack A. Saccadic programming and perceived location. *Acta Psychol.* 1981;48:123–131.

30. Grea H, Pisella L, Rossetti Y, et al. A lesion of the posterior parietal cortex disrupts on-line adjustments during aiming movements. *Neuropsychologia.* 2002;40:2471–2480.

31. Pisella L, Grea H, Tilikete C, et al. An "automatic pilot" for the hand in human posterior parietal cortex: toward reinterpreting optic ataxia. *Nat Neurosci.* 2000;3:729–736.

32. Desmurget M, Epstein CM, Turner RS, et al. Role of the posterior parietal cortex in updating reaching movements to a visual target. *Nat Neurosci.* 1999;2:563–567.

33. Lebedev MA, Wise SP. Insights into seeing and grasping: distinguishing the neural correlates of perception and action. *Behav Cogn Neurosci Rev.* 2002;1:108–129.

34. Picard N, Strick PL. Imaging the premotor areas. *Curr Opin Neurobiol.* 2001;11:663–672.

35. Changizi MA, McGehee RM, Hall WG. Evidence that appetitive responses for dehydration and food-deprivation are learned. *Physiol Behav.* 2002;75:295–304.

36. Fuster JM. *The prefrontal cortex: anatomy, physiology, and neuropsychology of the frontal lobe.* Philadelphia, PA: Lippincott–Raven, 1997.

37. Roberts AC, Wallis JD. Inhibitory control and affective processing in the prefrontal cortex: neuropsychological studies in the common marmoset. *Cereb Cortex.* 2000;10:252–262.

38. Dias R, Robbins TW, Roberts AC. Dissociable forms of inhibitory control within prefrontal cortex with an analog of the Wisconsin card sort test: restriction to novel situations and independence from "on-line" processing. *J Neurosci.* 1997;17:9285–9297.

39. Santos LR, Ericson BN, Hauser MD. Constraints on problem solving and inhibition: object retrieval in cotton-top tamarins (*Saguinus oedipus oedipus*). *J Comp Psychol.* 1999;113:186–193.

40. Hauser MD. Perseveration, inhibition and the prefrontal cortex: a new look. *Curr Opin Neurobiol.* 1999;9:214–222.

41. Diamond A, Goldman-Rakic PS. Comparison of human infants and rhesus monkeys on Piaget's AB task: evidence for dependence on dorsolateral prefrontal cortex. *Exp Brain Res.* 1989;74:24–40.

42. Boysen ST, Berntson GG. Responses to quantity: perceptual versus cognitive mechanisms in chimpanzees (*Pan troglodytes*). *J Exp Psychol Anim Behav Proc.* 1995;21:82–86.

43. Boysen ST, Berntson GG, Hannan MB, et al. Quantity-based interference and symbolic representations in chimpanzee (*Pan troglodytes*). *J Exp Psychol Anim Behav Proc.* 1996;22:76–86.

44. Silberberg A, Fujita K. Pointing at smaller food amounts in an analogue of Boysen and Berntson's (1995) procedure. *J Exp Anal Behav.* 1996;66:143–147.

45. Kralik JD, Hauser MD, Zimlicki R. When inhibitory mechanisms fail: cotton-top tamarin (*Saguinus oedipus*) performance on a reversed contingency task. *J Comp Psychol.* 2002;116:39–50.

46. Anderson JR, Awazu S, Fujita K. Can squirrel monkeys (*Saimiri sciureus*) learn self-control? A study using food array selection tests and reverse-reward contingency. *J Exp Psychol Anim Behav Process.* 2000;26:87–97.

47. Russel J, Mauthner N, Sharpe S, et al. The "windows task" as a measure of strategic deception in preschoolers and autistic subjects. *Brit J Dev Psychol.* 1991;9:331–349.

48. Murray EA, Kralik JD, Wise SP. Learning to inhibit prepotent responses: successful performance by rhesus macaques on the reversed-contingency task. *Anim Behav.* 2005; 69: 991–998

49. Semendeferi K, Lu A, Schenker N, et al. Humans and great apes share a large frontal cortex. *Nat Neurosci.* 2002;5:272–276.

50. Passingham RE. The frontal cortex: does size matter? *Nat Neurosci.* 2002;5:190–192.

51. Preuss TM. What's human about the human brain? In: Gazzaniga MS, ed. *The new cognitive neurosciences.* Cambridge, MA: MIT Press, 2000:1219–1234.

52. Iversen SD, Mishkin M. Perseverative interference in monkeys following selective lesions of the inferior prefrontal convexity. *Exp Brain Res.* 1970;11:376–386.

53. Rolls ET, Critchley HD, Mason R, et al. Orbitofrontal cortex neurons: role in olfactory and visual association learning. *J Neurophysiol.* 1996;75:1970–1981.

54. Bechara A, Tranel D, Damasio H, et al. Failure to respond autonomically to anticipated future outcomes following damage to prefrontal cortex. *Cereb Cortex.* 1996;6:215–225.

55. Spence SA, Crimlisk HL, Cope H, et al. Discrete neurophysiological correlates in prefrontal cortex during hysterical and feigned disorder of movement. *Lancet.* 2000;355:1243–1244.

56. Konishi S, Jimura K, Asari T, et al. Transient activation of superior prefrontal cortex during inhibition of cognitive set. *J Neurosci.* 2003;23:7776–7782.

57. Marshall JC, Halligan PW, Fink GR, et al. The functional anatomy of a hysterical paralysis. *Cognition.* 1997;64:B1–B8.

58. Halligan PW, Athwal BS, Oakley DA, et al. Imaging hypnotic paralysis: implications for conversion hysteria. *Lancet.* 2000;355: 986–987.

Consciousness

24

Adam Zeman

ABSTRACT

The topic of consciousness is relevant to psychogenic movement disorders, both because of close conceptual links between consciousness and volition, and because our understanding of psychogenesis is intertwined with our understanding of consciousness. The etymologic root of consciousness in Latin implied the *sharing* of knowledge. In colloquial English, the term can refer either to wakefulness or to awareness. Self-consciousness can refer to self-detection, self-recognition, the "awareness of awareness" and self-knowledge broadly construed. Over the 20th century, work in neurology and neuroscience has greatly extended our knowledge of the neural basis of both wakefulness and awareness. Research contrasting brain activity in conscious and unconscious states suggests that several factors influence the likelihood that local processing will give rise to awareness; these factors include the amplitude and duration of processing, the degree of synchronization of neuronal activity, the brain regions involved, and the details of their connectivity. There is a growing consensus that the neurology of awareness involves the operation of a "global workspace" which allows local activity to be broadcast widely through the brain. Whether theories framed in these terms can solve the "hard problem" of consciousness—why neural processing should cause subjective awareness at all—is controversial. Work on a variety of forms of disordered movement and action provide potential analogies for psychogenic movement disorders: Several types and levels of explanation are likely to be required to understand these fully.

WHY IS CONSCIOUSNESS RELEVANT TO PSYCHOGENIC MOVEMENT DISORDERS?

A chapter devoted to the problem of consciousness may seem out of place in a volume concerned with movement disorders. However, it soon became clear at the meeting which this book commemorates that any attempt to make sense of psychogenic movement disorders (PMDs) compels one to take account of consciousness. In this introductory section I shall outline two reasons why this should be so, before reviewing relevant aspects of the contemporary state of consciousness science. The chapter will conclude by exploring themes and models from the study of awareness which may help us to understand PMDs. Although I will not explore the historical background here, I note in passing that the history of thinking about consciousness over the past 200 years has been intertwined with thinking about PMDs; Charcot's writings on hypnosis, Janet's concept of dissociation, and Freud's views on the unconscious all owed much to their encounters with these puzzling disorders.

The first link between consciousness and PMDs goes by way of the concept of will or volition. Roughly speaking, willed or volitional acts are those which flow, or seem to flow, from conscious intentions. Conscious intentions, in turn, are those of which we are aware, which we are prepared to acknowledge as our own, or which were, or might have been, the outcome of a process of reflection. Will is therefore, in a sense, the active face of consciousness, the expression of consciousness in action. Now the will is clearly relevant to PMDs, for the following reason: PMDs are typically disorders which appear at first glance to resemble neurologically more straightforward organic disorders, like Parkinson disease or paralysis due to stroke, but which on further assessment turn out to (i) have no basis in pathologically defined neurologic disease and (ii) have a plausible psychological explanation of some kind. That is, they turn out to resemble willed or volitional actions at least as closely as they resemble orthodox neurologic disorders; it is *as if* the patient is "acting" the role of a patient with parkinsonian tremor or stroke-induced paralysis. Yet, by and large, patients with PMDs deny that they are willing or consciously producing their symptoms— and we are, by and large, inclined to believe them (I shall return to the difficult issue of malingering). This state of affairs obliges us to come up with an explanation of how actions, which closely resemble those that we will, can occur in the absence of normal volition, by way of unconscious or subconscious routes which somehow bypass awareness. This train of thought makes it clear that if we are to understand PMDs, we will have to take an interest in both the concept and the neurology of consciousness, and of its counterpart, volition.

The second link between consciousness and PMDs is fundamental. It relates to a dilemma which surfaced with great regularity at our meeting, particularly in connection with our choice of terminology for the disorders under discussion: the relationship between the body and the mind. The central problem of consciousness, much discussed in recent work in which it is sometimes termed the "hard problem," is how the 10^{11} intricately organized neurons within our brains give rise to our mental lives: to sensations, emotions, intentions, or, in a word, to our *experience*. This is an ancient problem in modern disguise—the problem of how mind and body, psyche or soma, the functional and the organic are related. These dichotomies are deeply entrenched in our everyday thought, and we find them seductive. We use them to carve up intellectual and professional territories. We want a clear answer to the question of whether a movement disorder is organic or psychogenic: If organic, it belongs to the neurologist, if psychogenic, to the psychiatrist. This is a pragmatic approach with which most medical readers will be thoroughly familiar. Yet, in our reflective moments, few if any of us believe that these apparent *oppositions*—mind versus body and the like—are anything of the kind. All our scientific knowledge of experience, behavior, and the brain insists that the mind is a function of the brain, psyche a function of soma, the functional a vital aspect of the living organism. We are, in other words, saddled with a set of time-honored distinctions in which we do not believe, yet cannot do without; in time, this will have to change.

Imagine for a moment that it has changed. Accept, as I think most of us believe, that all illness—indeed all normal human behavior—has both a physiologic and a psychological dimension. We would surely still need some way of distinguishing the kinds of movement disorders under consideration here from their organic cousins, for example, psychogenic tremor from the tremor of Parkinson disease. If a biopsychosocial (or psychobiologic) approach is appropriate to both, then what's the difference between them? I suggest that, first, to reiterate the argument of the previous paragraph, this approach reminds us that the differences between these two kinds of disorders are less fundamental than we normally tend to suppose. But second, accepting that there are indeed some important differences, they lie in two main areas: (i) most PMDs have the potential to be brought under voluntary control to a greater extent than most orthodox neurologic movement disorders, although this difference is one of degree rather than kind, and (ii) the etiologic explanation of PMDs will

mostly be at a different level from the etiologic explanation of organic disorders. The explanation of the latter will appeal largely to a chain of neuropathologic events, while the explanation of the former will appeal largely to life events, personality, and mood; different kinds of stories most readily make sense of the different classes of disorder. But once again the difference is of degree, not kind, and there will be numerous points of contact between physical and psychological factors in both organic and functional movement disorders.

WHAT DO WE MEAN BY "CONSCIOUSNESS"?

The word "consciousness" originates from the elision of two Latin words: *cum*, meaning "with," and *scio*, meaning "know" (1). To be conscious of information in the original Latin sense was to share the knowledge of it with another person: The knowledge in question was often secret or shameful, the kind one would share with a co-conspirator. But, of course, knowledge that can be shared literally with another person can also be shared metaphorically with oneself, as in this 17th-century example: "I am conscious to myself of many failings." As the use of the term evolved in the English language, it weakened, so that being conscious sometimes meant simply "knowing." But the original sense of *shared* knowledge lives on in the background of our thoughts, coloring our use of consciousness. As we shall see, it still resonates in current scientific theories of consciousness.

In contemporary colloquial and scientific use, consciousness is used in two key senses: wakefulness and awareness (2,3). The first is relatively straightforward. In emergency rooms all over the world it is important to establish whether patients are or are not conscious in the sense of being able to perceive and respond to events around them in the well-integrated fashion which characterizes a normal state of alertness. The use of objective criteria, such as those brought to bear by the Glasgow Coma Scale (GCS)—which considers eye opening, and verbal and motor behavior—generally allows an accurate assessment of consciousness in this first sense. Such criteria allow us to distinguish both degrees of consciousness, for example, GCS 10/15 versus 15/15, or drowsy versus wide awake, and states of consciousness, for example, wakefulness versus sleep or coma.

The second sense of consciousness, awareness, is less obviously exhausted by objective descriptors and much more controversial in consciousness science. However, it is clear enough that while we are conscious in the first sense I have distinguished, we are normally conscious *of* something; awareness refers to the contents of consciousness. Numerous authors (4–10) have drawn attention to features of these contents which most agree call out for explanation: The contents of consciousness are stable over short periods, of a few hundred milliseconds, but typically changeful over longer periods. They have a limited capacity at any one time, often combining a sharply focused background with a less highly specified background, but over time they can range right across the spectrum of our cognitive capacities. We can be conscious of sensations, thoughts, memories, emotions, plans, and so on, and our awareness from moment to moment often combines elements from several of these sources. Awareness of the present is usually connected with awareness of the past by means of memory. Our awareness is perspectival, always afforded by a particular, necessarily limited, point of view. Our capacity for awareness is fundamental to the value we place upon our lives; most of us would not wish to be kept alive if it were clear that we had lost this capacity forever. The distinction between wakefulness and awareness is exploited in the familiar description of the vegetative state as one of wakefulness without awareness, a condition in which some objective signs of wakefulness—eye opening and a (very limited) degree of responsiveness to environmental stimuli—are present, but there is no evidence of any sophisticated form of awareness, of any "inner life."

Discussions of consciousness often touch on its close relative, self-consciousness. This term, also, has a complex web of senses, probably an even more tangled web than does consciousness itself. At least five senses can be distinguished: (i) proneness to embarrassment: a colloquial sense in which the term refers to excessive sensitivity to the attention of others; (ii) self-detection: a relatively impoverished sense in which the term refers to the ability to detect stimuli directly impinging on the subject (an ant crawling over one's hand) or actions which the subject has performed; (iii) self-recognition: a sense in which it refers to the more demanding ability to recognize oneself, for example, in a mirror, an ability which apes possess but monkeys do not, and which human children acquire at around the age of 18 months; (iv) awareness of awareness: a sense in which it refers to our ability to interpret our own behavior and that of others in terms of mental states, recognizing ourselves and others not merely as objects—which might be reflected in a mirror—but also as *subjects* of experience; (v) self-knowledge: a sense in which it refers to our view of ourselves as, for example, members of a particular profession or society, and to our developing understanding, over the course of a lifetime, of ourselves and our reasons for behaving as we do.

THE SCIENCE OF CONSCIOUS STATES

The scientific understanding of wakefulness, sleep, and pathologically altered states of consciousness has been transformed over the 20th century by physiologic, anatomic, and pharmacologic advances.

Hans Berger's demonstration in 1929 illustrated that it was possible to record the brain's electrical activity from the

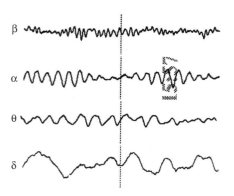

Figure 24.1 The rhythms of the EEG. Records from diagnostic encephalograms performed in four different patients, exemplifying β rhythm (greater than 14 Hz); α rhythm (8–13 Hz); θ rhythm (4–7 Hz); and δ rhythm (<4 Hz). In each case the dotted line bisects a 2-second sample (2).

scalp provided a tool—the EEG—with which to track the concerted shifts in cerebral activity which accompany changes in conscious state (11). Berger and others soon described the fundamental rhythms of the EEG (Fig. 24.1): β, at greater than 14 Hz, which accompanies mental effort; α, at 8–13 Hz, the signature of relaxed wakefulness; θ (4–7 Hz) and δ (less than 4 Hz), which predominate in deep sleep. In the 1950s, Kleitman et al. in Chicago discovered that sleep itself has an internal architecture (12,13). Over the first hour of sleep, the sleeper descends through a series of deepening stages into stage III and IV sleep in which slow waves predominate (slow wave sleep, SWS, known as non–REM, NREM, sleep), only to ascend back through these stages into a state resembling wakefulness in its EEG appearance, accompanied by rapid eye movements, profound muscular atonia, and vivid mentation—dreaming, and paradoxic or rapid eye movement sleep (REM) (Fig. 24.2). This cycle repeats itself four or five times in the course of the night, with decreasing amounts of SWS and increasing amounts of REM as the night proceeds. Recent work on the brain's electrical rhythms has highlighted the potential importance of rapid, widely synchronized, high frequency γ oscillations (25–100 Hz) in wakefulness and REM (14), although their true significance is not yet clear.

The anatomic and pharmacologic mechanisms which control these cycling states have also been clarified over the past 100 years. Moruzzi and Magoun's proposal (15) that the brainstem and thalamus are home to an activating system which maintains arousal in the hemispheres has stood the test of time. However, the notion of a monolithic system has given way to a pharmacologically complex picture of multiple interacting activating systems innervating the cerebral hemispheres widely from the brainstem and diencephalon (16) (Fig. 24.3). These systems are defined by their neurotransmitters, which include acetylcholine, serotonin, noradrenaline, dopamine, histamine, hypocretin, and glutamate. The normal succession of conscious states

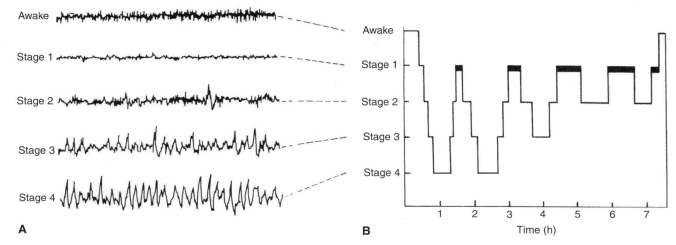

Figure 24.2   The architecture of sleep. An example of sleep staging over the course of a single night. **(A)** The sleeper passes from wakefulness to deep sleep and then ascends to REM sleep (dark bars). Five similar cycles occur in the course of the night. The EEG tracings **(B)** show the EEG appearances associated with the stages of sleep; the EEG in REM resembles the "awake" trace. (Kandel ER, Schwartz JH, Jessell TM, eds. *Principles of Neural Science*. Prentice Hall, 1991.)

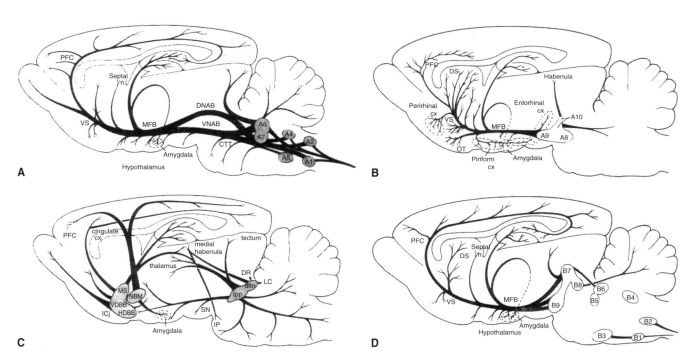

Figure 24.3   The pharmacology of the brainstem activating systems. The figure shows **(A)** the origin and distribution of the central noradrenergic pathways in the rat brain; **(B)** the dopaminergic pathways; **(C)** the cholinergic pathways; **(D)** the serotonergic pathways. CTT, central tegmental tract; dltn, dorsolateral tegmental nucleus; DNAB, dorsal noradrenergic ascending bundle; DR, dorsal raphe; DS, dorsal striatum; HDBB, horizontal limb nucleus of the diagonal band of Broca; Icj, islands of Calleja; IP, interpeduncular nucleus; LC, locus ceruleus; MFB, medial forebrain bundle; MS, medial septum; NBM, nucleus basalis magnocellularis (Meynert in primates); OT, olfactory tubercle; PFC, prefrontal cortex; SN, substantia nigra; tpp, tegmental pedunculopontine nucleus; VDBB, vertical limb nucleus of the diagonal band of Broca; VNAB, ventral noradrenergic ascending bundle; VS, ventral striatum.
(Robbins TW, Everitt BJ. Arousal systems and attention. *The cognitive neurosciences*. Cambridge: MIT Press 1995;703–720.)

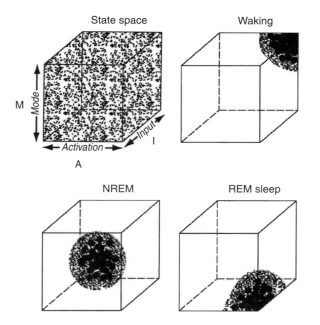

State space

Waking

M — Mode

Activation

Input

A

I

NREM

REM sleep

Figure 24.4 The AIM model. Hobson's AIM model locates the three principal states of healthy consciousness in a "state space" defined by input (I: external in wakefulness, internal during REM), activation (A: high in REM and wakefulness, low in NREM sleep), and mode (M: during REM prefrontal regions involved in regulation of waking behaviour and encoding of memories are deactivated). (Hobson JA. Consciousness, sleep and dreaming. In: Nadel L, ed. *Macmillan encyclopaedia of cognitive science*. Nature Publishing, 2002.)

is regulated by these systems (17). For example, in SWS, all these systems become relatively quiescent; in REM periods, the ascending cholinergic system becomes disproportionately active. REM periods are eventually brought to an end by rising levels of activity in noradrenergic and serotonergic neuronal groups which had fallen silent at REM onset. Hobson's AIM model attempts to integrate several lines of evidence on the genesis and nature of conscious states (Fig. 24.4).

The practical upshot of these advances is a useful taxonomy of states of healthy and disordered consciousness. In health, we cycle between wakefulness, SWS, and REM. Pathologic states include coma (Glasgow Coma Score <7, eyes closed), the vegetative state mentioned above, brain death, and the locked-in syndrome (18) (Table 24.1). While wakefulness, SWS, and REM are as a rule mutually exclusive, overlaps between these states occasionally occur (19) (Fig. 24.5). For example, sleepwalking reflects motor activation of the kind seen during wakefulness, occurring at a time when much of the brain is deactivated, as during SWS (20); REM sleep behavior disorder, in which sufferers enact their dreams, results from a failure of the normal atonia of REM sleep, allowing dream mentation to give rise to behavior, like self-defense, of a kind which would normally be confined to wakefulness (21,22).

TABLE 24.1

THE DIFFERENTIAL DIAGNOSIS OF IMPAIRED AWARENESS

Condition	Vegetative State	Minimally Conscious State	Locked-in Syndrome	Coma	Death Confirmed by Brainstem Tests
Awareness	Absent	Present	Present	Absent	Absent
Sleep–wake cycle	Present	Present	Present	Absent	Absent
Response to pain	+/−	Present	Present (in eyes only)	+/−	Absent
Glasgow Coma Score	E4, M1-4, V1-2	E4, M1-5, V1-4	E4, M1, V1	E1,M1-4,V1-2	E1, M1-3, V1
Motor function	No purposeful movement	Some consistent or inconsistent verbal or purposeful motor behavior	Volitional vertical eye movements or eyeblink preserved	No purposeful movement	None or only reflex spinal movement
Respiratory function	Typically preserved	Typically preserved	Typically preserved	Variable	Absent
EEG activity	Typically slow wave activity	Insufficient data	Typically normal	Typically slow wave activity	Typically absent
Cerebral metabolism (positron emission tomography)	Severely reduced	Insufficient data	Mildly reduced	Moderately severely reduced	Severely reduced or absent
Prognosis	Variable: if permanent, continued vegetative state or death	Variable	Depends on cause but full recovery unlikely	Recovery, vegetative state, or death within weeks	Already dead

(Working party of the Royal College of Physicians. *The vegetative state: guidance on diagnosis and management*. London: Royal College of Physicians of London, 2003.)

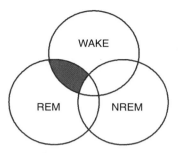

Figure 24.5 State boundary dissociation. The states of wakefulness, REM, and NREM sleep are normally distinct. Many parasomnias can be understood as the result of a fusion of two or more states. For example, overlap between the phenomena of REM sleep and wakefulness *(shaded)* gives rise to REM sleep behavior disorder; overlap between NREM sleep and wakefulness occurs during sleepwalking and night terrors. (Mahowald MW, Schenck CH. Dissociated states of wakefulness and sleep. *Neurology.* 1992; 42:44–51.)

THE SCIENCE OF AWARENESS

Much of the groundbreaking work of the 20th century on the biology of cognition, exploring the neurology of perception, language, memory, emotion, and intention, is relevant to understanding the neural basis of awareness. Awareness, as mentioned earlier, ranges over these processes: Its neural underpinnings must overlap with theirs. For example, the existence of highly selective deficits of visual awareness, such

as central achromatopsia (23) (loss of color vision) and akinetopsia (24) (loss of visual motion perception) is substantially explained by the existence of visual cortical areas— V4 and V5—which specialize in processing information about color and visual motion, respectively.

However, it is clear that only certain kinds of neural processes give rise to conscious awareness. For example, visual stimuli presented very briefly to normal subjects with backward masking (i.e., followed rapidly by a second item) (25), visual stimuli presented in the neglected visual fields of subjects with hemispatial neglect (26), and stimuli presented to subjects in the vegetative state (27), or under anesthesia (28,29), can all be shown to trigger content-specific neural activity without having any reportable impact on awareness. This suggests that there is an important distinction between conscious and unconscious neural processes. A similar contrast is evident when only one of two simultaneously presented stimuli gives rise to awareness, for example, during binocular rivalry (when different stimuli are presented to the two eyes but only one stimulus is perceived at a time) (30) or as a result of focused attention. The main aim of current research on the neurology of awareness is to clarify the underlying differences between those neural processes which do and those which do not give rise to awareness. Bernard Baars, one of the founders of consciousness science, has termed this the method of "contrastive analysis" (31).

Table 24.2 lists some illustrative examples of studies of this kind from a variety of contexts. The comparisons

TABLE 24.2
CONTRASTIVE ANALYSIS: STUDIES COMPARING CONSCIOUS AND UNCONSCIOUS BRAIN ACTIVITY

Study (context)	Comparison	Results
Laureys (32) (Vegetative state)	Vegetative state vs. recovery	Increase in cortical metabolic rate and restoration of connectivity with recovery
John (33) (Anesthesia)	Anesthesia vs. awareness	Loss of γ band activity and cross-cortical coherence under anesthesia
Sahraie (34) (Blindsight)	Aware vs. unaware mode of perception in blindsight patient GY	Aware mode associated with DLPF and PS activation, unaware with medial F and subcortical
Dehaene (25) (Backward masking)	Perceived numbers vs. backward masked but processed numbers	Unreported numbers underwent perceptual, semantic, and motor processing similar but less intense to reported numbers
Kanwisher (30) (Binocular rivalry)	Attention to face or place when stimuli of both kind are simultaneously in view, or perception of face or place during binocular rivalry	Activity in FFA and PPA locked to presence or absence of *awareness* of face and place
Moutoussis (35) (Invisible stimuli)	Perceived vs. "invisible" but processed faces/houses	Similar but less intense activation of FFA and PPA by invisible stimuli
Engel (36) (Binocular rivalry)	Perception of one or other of a pair of rivalrous stimuli	Firing of cells processing currently perceived stimulus better synchronized than firing of cells processing suppressed stimulus
Tononi (37) (Binocular rivalry)	Perception of high vs. low frequency flicker during binocular rivalry	More widespread and intense activation by perceived stimulus
Petersen (38) (Task automatization)	Effortful verb generation task vs. performance after training	LPF, ant cing, and cerebellar activation shifts to left perisylvian activation with training

Ant cing, anterior cingulate; DLPF, dorsolateral prefrontal cortex; FFA, fusiform face area; LPF, lateral prefrontal cortex; medial F, medial frontal cortex; PPA, parahippocampal place area; PS, prestriate.

drawn in these studies point to several factors which can influence whether local, modular brain activity becomes conscious: its amplitude and duration, the degree of synchronization of the relevant neuronal firing, the brain regions involved, and the reach or connectivity of the processing into other brain areas (see Table 24.2). Locally appropriate activity which is intense, subserved by synchronized neuronal firing, which involves cortical and perhaps especially prefrontal regions, and which excites widely distributed cerebral regions, is more likely to be conscious than low intensity, poorly synchronized, subcortical, or purely local processing.

THEORIES AND FUNCTIONS OF AWARENESS

It is too early in the development of consciousness science to expect a single firmly based, fully articulated account of its neural basis. However, the evidence outlined in the previous two sections has given rise to a growing consensus (10,31,39) which holds that awareness results when information which is being processed locally is broadcast widely through the brain, capturing the focus of attention, and thereby gaining access to the neural equipment required for such purposes as report, reflection, and planning. Baars (31) and Dehaene (39) have described this model of consciousness in terms of a global workspace, a theatre of operations which allows the brain to pool its modular resources to meet a range of cognitive challenges. Such a model need not invoke a dedicated consciousness system. The global workspace might consist of temporary coalitions between systems of which many or all can also function in the absence of awareness. According to this model, while local cortical modules operate unconsciously, automatically, swiftly, and in parallel, the global workspace allows for a different mode of conscious, flexible, or voluntary serial operation to occur. Baars argues that this mode of activity is, in fact, required for many cognitive purposes, including the comprehension of novel information, working memory, several types of learning, and voluntary control of our actions. In broad terms, such theories hold that consciousness permits the flexible selection of actions from a wide potential repertoire on the basis of fine perceptual distinctions. Interestingly, with their implication that the neural essence of awareness is the sharing of information with oneself, these theories echo the etymology of consciousness discussed at the start of this chapter.

Some readers will experience a sense of disappointment at this juncture. They will feel that I have sketched an explanation of awareness which says something about the kind of neural information processing with which it is associated, but nothing about awareness *itself*, about why or how this style of information processing should give rise to experience. Why should activity in the global workspace

feel like this, or like anything at all? How does the observable, objective brain create the invisible, subjective features of awareness? The distinction at issue here has been described in terms of the contrast between the easy and hard problems of consciousness (8), and between explanations of access and phenomenal consciousness (40). The idea is that biologic and information processing theories address the (relatively) easy problem of what distinguishes conscious processes, with their wide access to the brain's resources, from unconscious ones, but fail to touch the really hard question of why such processes cause phenomenal experience. I sympathize with the disappointed reader, but cannot follow this fascinating train of thought further here, except to comment that there is continuing debate about whether these distinctions—hard versus easy, access versus phenomenal—mark a real difference or signpost a philosophic mirage (3,41).

DISORDERS OF CONSCIOUSNESS/ VOLITION AND MODELS OF FUNCTIONAL MOVEMENT DISORDER

This review of consciousness science has taken us some way from our point of departure. But the journey may have been worthwhile if we can plunder consciousness science for some insights into PMDs. Whether we can do so fruitfully depends on whether we can find informative analogies between disorders of awareness we understand relatively well and the PMDs which are puzzling us. Table 24.3 lists some possible candidates which I will discuss briefly in turn.

1. *Automatisms and habits:* Automatisms are more or less complex actions which we do not intend and are not aware of performing at the time. Examples include sleepwalking, semipurposeful behavior during complex partial seizures, parapraxias, like spooning tea leaves

---

TABLE 24.3

ROUTES TO QUASIVOLITIONAL ACTION

- Automatic "action"
  - Habit, automatism (unintended, unaware)
- Unintended "action"
  - Alien limb (unintended, aware)
- Passive or forced "action"
  - Hypnosis (suggested, aware)
  - Delusion of control (enforced, aware)
  - Psychomotor retardation/agitation (mood congruent, aware)
- Misinterpreted action
  - Self-deception (misunderstood, aware)
- Duplicitous action
  - Deception of others (calculated, aware)

Note: Parentheses indicate whether each type of action is intended and whether the agent is aware of performing it; the quotation marks around the first three types of action acknowledge that some authors would not regard them as actions at all.

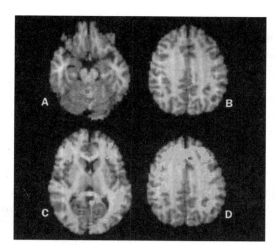

Figure 24.6 SPECT scan during sleepwalking. This figure illustrates the activation *(dark shading)* of cerebellum and posterior cingulate cortex during sleepwalking in the face of widespread cortical deactivation *(light shading)*. (Bassetti C, Vella S, Donati F, et al. SPECT during sleepwalking. *Lancet.* 2000;356:484–485.)

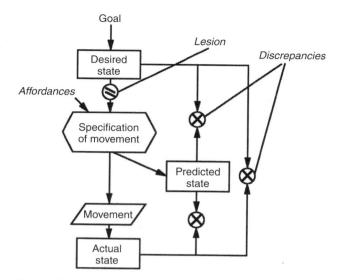

Figure 24.7 A motor control model of the anarchic limb. During normal movement, a motor command, issued to achieve a desired state, both gives rise to the movement and to a corollary discharge which allows the brain to predict the result of the movement. Comparisons can be made between the desired and predicted states, actual and predicted states, and desired and actual states. The anarchic limb is the result of a disconnection between the specification of the desired state and the specification of movement. (Frith CD, Blakemore S-J, Wolpert DM. Abnormalities in the awareness and control of action. *Philos Trans R Soc Lond B Biol Sci.* 2000;355:1771–1788.)

into the kettle instead of the teapot, and, sometimes at least, habits, such as picking at our fingernails.

We know something of the neural basis of automatisms. As mentioned earlier, sleepwalking is an example of state boundary dissociation, with evidence, from functional imaging, of activation of motor regions in the face of deactivation across much of the cerebral cortex, including frontal executive regions (20) (Fig. 24.6). Studies tracking changes in brain activation as novel tasks are gradually automatized provide some insight into the neurology of habits; they reveal a shift from dorsolateral and cerebellar activation to more local processing in regions associated with the type of motor activity involved (42). These studies suggest that automatisms result from a dissociation of activity in brain regions directly governing movement from those regions which normally govern and monitor our behavior.

It is doubtful that this group of phenomena offers a close analogy to PMDs. Patients with PMDs are usually all too well-aware of their disordered movements or failure to move, and features such as diminution of psychogenic tremor on distraction suggests that they are in some sense attending to them, too. If both automatisms and PMDs involve dissociation, it seems that different sets of processes must be dissociated.

2. *Alien or anarchic limbs:* These terms describe behavior in a limb of which the agent is aware but which he or she does not intend (43). This behavior can involve stereotyped actions, like putting a hand repeatedly in a pocket, involuntary utilization of objects, magnetic groping after the examiner's hand, and sometimes apparently concerted interference with the activities of another limb.

These movements can result from at least two kinds of pathology (44): First, damage to the corpus callosum,

which presumably allows the hemispheres to develop independent motor goals; second, damage to medial frontal regions, in particular, the supplementary motor cortex, which is thought to inhibit motor programs activated by stimuli currently present—for example, the "drinking program" elicited by the sight of a glass of water—but not consistent with current motor goals. Frith et al. (45) have developed an engineering systems model of motor control which locates the lesion responsible for this second type of anarchic limb in the pathway connecting the desired state with the specification of movement (Fig. 24.7).

Anarchic limbs offer a slightly more promising model for PMDs than do automatisms. Like the owner of an anarchic limb, patients with a PMD may complain that their limbs are moving outside their conscious control. But the kind of movements to which anarchic limbs are prone—such as utilization behavior—are rare in PMDs, suggesting that the analogy is loose at best.

3. *Passive or forced "action" in hypnosis, delusions of control, and depression:* I have grouped together three somewhat different phenomena here. In all cases, the agents are aware of their behavior, but they attribute it to factors which are, for different reasons, outside their control. The hypnotized subjects say simply that they do not know why they placed their hands on their heads at the striking of the clock; the psychotic subjects say that

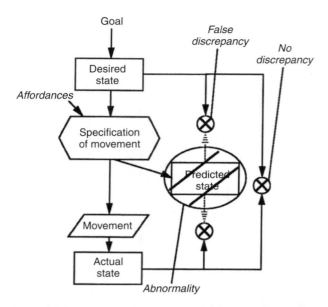

Figure 24.8 A motor control model of delusions of control. See the legend to Figure 24.6. In this case, a lesion preventing normal prediction of the outcome of movement leads to a loss of the sense of ownership of action. (Frith CD, Blakemore S-J, Wolpert DM. Abnormalities in the awareness and control of action. *Philos Trans R Soc Lond B Biol Sci.* 2000;355:1771–1788.)

their limbs were maneuvered there by an alien force; the depressed subjects say that their limbs are motionless because they can no longer see any point in moving them.

These examples might provide analogies for at least some PMDs. Unfortunately, we understand them less well than we do the examples already mentioned. The nature of hypnosis is as controversial as the nature of PMDs themselves, although there is a growing body of interesting work on the neurobiology of hypnotic states. Frith et al. have adapted their engineering model of motor control to explain delusions of control in terms of a failure in the system which normally predicts our actions via feedforward pathways from motor "controllers" (Fig. 24.8). The motor retardation of depression is presumably an expression of a neurochemically altered brain state. It is at least a well-established and uncontroversial example of a psychogenic movement disorder.

4. *Misinterpreted action:* The examples given so far relate to pathologic or unusual states. The two examples which follow are closer to everyday life. The first reflects the insight that our reasons for action are not transparent to the agent, that is to say, when we explain our behavior to ourselves or others, we are developing hypotheses which can be false—we can be mistaken about why we behave as we do.

There are several possible explanations for such mistakes. Sometimes we act as we do because of remote episodes of learning which exert their influence on our behavior long after we have forgotten they occurred, if indeed we ever remembered them. At other times, we act

on the basis of strong motivating forces, like fears or desires, which we may not have fully acknowledged to ourselves, or which we may not have linked, consciously, to our behavior. Sometimes behavior of this kind amounts to self-deception. A number of such examples were cited during the meeting (Rosebush, Stone), for instance, the case of the child who became quadraparetic after witnessing a terrifying assault committed by a parent on one of her schoolmates. The relationship between this event and the resulting PMD was not at all obvious at first to either the patient or her mother. There may be potential for understanding some of these cases in terms of the global workspace model of awareness outlined in the previous section. The idea would be that the information relevant to explaining a subject's behavior can exert its effects without entering the workspace. Whether this metaphor can be made to do really useful work in explaining or treating such symptoms remains to be seen.

5. *Duplicitous action:* People sometimes simulate symptoms deliberately to attract medical attention (factitious disorder) or for various forms of material gain (malingering). In such cases, people are aware of their behavior and of their reasons for acting as they do: They intend to deceive. Some might argue that *all* PMDs are of this kind, but this seems very unlikely. It ignores the extremely complex determination of human behavior, influenced by factors ranging from mood through early learning to the effect of life events which may be understood poorly by the agent. It relies on a misleading view of human action as wholly rational.

In assessing these potential analogies, we need to bear in mind that PMDs are far from uniform. They vary, among other respects, in the nature of the motor disorder, the chronicity of symptoms, the presence of comorbid psychopathology, especially mood disturbance, of pain, deconditioning, secondary gain, and insight. The explanations of PMDs will have to take account of this variety; it is likely that several levels of explanation, and several of the analogies I have listed, will be required to understand them. Functional imaging is beginning to explore some of these possible analogies, including those hypnotically induced or simulated, and those involving feigned weakness (see Chapter 26). It is encouraging that, while we still have much to learn about the mechanisms of PMDs, we are at least breaking free from the constraints of a false opposition between the organic and the functional, the body and the mind.

REFERENCES

1. Lewis CS. *Studies in words.* Cambridge: Cambridge University Press, 1960.
2. Zeman A. Consciousness. *Brain.* 2001;124:1263–1289.
3. Zeman Adam. *Consciousness: a user's guide.* London: Yale University Press, 2003.

4. James W. *The principles of psychology*. New York: Henry Holt, 1890.
5. Shallice T. *Information-processing models of consciousness*. Consciousness in contemporary science 1988;350–433.
6. Searle JR. *The rediscovery of the mind*. Cambridge, MA MIT Press, 1992.
7. Crick F. *The astonishing hypothesis*. New York: Simon & Schuster, 1994.
8. Chalmers DJ. *The conscious mind*. New York: Oxford University Press, 1996.
9. Greenfield S. *How might the brain generate consciousness?* In: Roses, ed. From brains to consciousness. London: Allen Lane 1998; 210–227.
10. Tononi G, Edelman GM. Consciousness and the integration of information in the brain. *Adv Neurol*. 1998;77:245–279.
11. Berger H. Uber das elektrenkephalogramm des menschen. *Arch Psychiat*. 1929;87:527–570.
12. Aserinsky E, Kleitman N. Two types of ocular motility occurring during sleep. *J Appl Physiol*. 1955;8:1–10.
13. Dement W, Kleitman N. Cyclic variations in EEG during sleep and their relation to eye movements, body motility, and dreaming. *Electroencephalogr Clin Neurophysiol*. 1957;9:673–690.
14. Llinas R, Ribary U. Coherent 40-Hz oscillation characterizes dream state in humans. *Proc Natl Acad Sci U S A*. 1993;90:2078–2081.
15. Moruzzi G, Magoun HW. Brainstem reticular formation and the activation of the EEG. *Electroencephalogr Clin Neurophysiol*. 1949; 1:455–473.
16. Robbins TW, Everitt BJ. Arousal systems and attention. *The cognitive neurosciences*. Cambridge: MIT Press 1995;703–720.
17. Hobson JA, Pace-Schott EF. The cognitive neuroscience of sleep: neuronal systems, consciousness and learning. *Nat Rev Neurosci*. 2002;3:679–693.
18. Working party of the Royal College of Physicians. *The vegetative state: guidance on diagnosis and management*. London: Royal College of Physicians of London, 2003.
19. Mahowald MW, Schenck CH. Dissociated states of wakefulness and sleep. *Neurology*. 1992;42:44–51.
20. Bassetti C, Vella S, Donati F, et al. SPECT during sleepwalking. *Lancet*. 2000;356:484–485.
21. Schenck CH, Bundlie SR, Ettinger MG, et al. Chronic behavioral disorders of human REM sleep: a new category of parasomnia. *Sleep*. 1986;9:293–308.
22. Olson EJ, Boeve BF, Silber MH. Rapid eye movement sleep behaviour disorder: demographic, clinical and laboratory findings in 93 cases. *Brain*. 2000;123:339.
23. Zeki S. A century of cerebral achromatopsia. *Brain*. 1990;113(Pt 6): 1721–1777.
24. Zeki S. Cerebral akinetopsia (visual motion blindness). A review. *Brain*. 1991;114(Pt 2):811–824.
25. Dehaene S, Naccache L, Le Clec' HG, et al. Imaging unconscious semantic priming. *Nature*. 1998;395:595–600.
26. Rees G, Wojciulik E, Clarke K, et al. Unconscious activation of visual cortex in the damaged right hemisphere of a parietal patient with extinction. *Brain*. 2000;123(Pt 8):1624–1633.
27. Laureys S, Berre J, Goldman S. Cerebral function in coma, vegetative state, minimally conscious state, locked-in syndrome and brain death. In: Vincent JL (ed) *Yearbook of intensive care and emergency medicine*. Berlin: Springer, 2001:386–396.
28. Jones JG. Perception and memory during general anaesthesia. *Br J Anaesth*. 1994;73:31–37.
29. Schwender D, Kaiser A, Klasing S, et al. Midlatency auditory evoked potentials and explicit and implicit memory in patients undergoing cardiac surgery. *Anesthesiology*. 1994;80:493–501.
30. Kanwisher N. *Neural correlates of changes in perceptual awareness in the absence of changes in the stimulus*. Towards a science of consciousness Thorverton: Imprint Academic 2000; Abstr. No. 164.
31. Baars BJ. The conscious access hypothesis: origins and recent evidence. *Trends Cogn Sci*. 2002;6:47–52.
32. Laureys S, Faymonville M-E, Degueldre C, et al. Auditory processing in the vegetative state. *Brain*. 2000;123:1589–1601.
33. John ER, Prichep LS, Kox W, et al. Invariant reversible QEEG effects of anesthetics. *Conscious Cogn*. 2001;10165–83.
34. Sahraie A, Weiskrantz L, Barbur JL, et al. Pattern of neuronal activity associated with conscious and unconscious processing of visual signals. *Proc Natl Acad Sci U S A*. 1997;94:9406–9411.
35. Moutoussis K, Zeki S. The relationship between cortical activation and percpetion investigated with invisible stimuli. *Proc Natl Acad Sci U S A*. 2002;99:9527–9532.
36. Engel AK, Fries P, Roelfsema PR, et al. Temporal binding, binocular rivalry, and consciousness. Available from: http://www.phil. vt.edu/ASSC/engel/engel.html 2000.
37. Tononi G, Edelman GM. Consciousness and complexity. *Science*. 1998;282:1846–1851.
38. Petersen SE, van Mier H, Fiez JA, et al. The effects of practice on the functional anatomy of task performance. *Proc Natl Acad Sci U S A*. 1998;95:853–860.
39. Dehaene S, Naccache L. Towards a cognitive neuroscience of consciousness: basic evidence and workspace framework. *Cognition*. 2003;79:1–37.
40. Young AW, Block N. *Consciousness*. In: Bruce J, ed. Unsolved mysteries of the mind. Hove, East Sussex: Erlbaum (UK), Taylor & Francis, 1996.
41. O'Regan JK, Noe A. A sensorimotor account of vision and visual consciousness. *Behav Brain Sci*. 2001;24:939–973.
42. Raichle ME. The neural correlates of consciousness: an analysis of cognitive skill learning. *Philos Trans R Soc Lond B Biol Sci*. 1998;353:1889–1901.
43. Della Sala S, Marchetti C, Spinnler H. The anarchic hand: a fronto-mesial sign. *Handbook Neuropsychol*. 1994;9:233–255.
44. Zaidel E, Jacoboni M, Zaidel DW. The callosal syndromes. In: Heilman KM, Valenstein E, eds. *Clinical Neuropsychology*. Oxford: Oxford University Press, 2003:404–446.
45. Frith CD, Blakemore S-J, Wolpert DM. Abnormalities in the awareness and control of action. *Philos Trans R Soc Lond B Biol Sci*. 2000;355:1771–1788.

The Cognitive Executive Is Implicated in the Maintenance of Psychogenic Movement Disorders

25

Sean A. Spence

ABSTRACT

Psychogenic movement disorders (PMDs) comprise a range of functional abnormalities characterized by motor inconsistencies and differentiated, diagnostically, by varying degrees of inferred conscious causation (on the part of the patient). At one extreme is conversion disorder ("hysteria"), in which patients are thought to be unaware of the mechanism of their impairments; at the other extreme is feigning (malingering), in which patients are suspected of consciously, deliberately, deceiving the physician. These alternatives are difficult to differentiate reliably and, to be valid, their diagnoses would require that the physician either know what the patient is thinking or else demonstrate some pathognomonic physical sign or investigative finding (currently lacking). The characteristic physical features of PMD tend to be those of inconsistent motor dysfunction, which may remit with distraction or sedation. Though these features may help to distinguish PMD from organic pathology, they are less helpful in distinguishing conversion from feigning. Here, we consider the evidence that subcategories of PMD share the following feature: reliance upon the cognitive executive. The executive comprises those control processes engaged in the production of nonroutine, nonautomated behaviors—behaviors that require attention to action. It is because executive resources are constrained that they may decompensate with sufficient distraction or sedation, thereby revealing a "normal" motor system. In this regard, PMDs behave differently to most exemplars of organic movement disorder.

INTRODUCTION

Psychogenic movement disorders (PMDs) present obvious difficulties for the clinician. The absence of demonstrable organic pathology is accompanied by inconsistent motor signs, and although the operations of the motor system manifesting disorder are those over which a conscious agent has a degree of control, the patient who expresses these abnormalities denies producing them (consciously, at least). Such a situation may be difficult to manage clinically. The physician wishes to be certain that no organic pathology has been missed, thereby risking overinvestigation. The patients wish to establish the veracity of their symptoms, thereby risking exaggeration. They may swap one doctor for another, transferring their care at the very point at which continuity is most crucial—when physical investigations have excluded organic pathology. Failure to obtain appropriate psychiatric evaluation at this point may lead to further unnecessary (and perhaps even dangerous) investigations. In the background, impending litigation may complicate matters: the patient perhaps feels wronged because of a causal injury sustained at work, while the physician may be sensitive to the possibility of being duped for financial gain.

Likewise, there are conceptual problems. The diagnosis of conversion disorder relies upon Freudian notions of the psychodynamic unconscious, which have been superseded in some contemporary psychoanalytic accounts of hysteria (1–3). Clinically, physicians are required to infer unconscious processes in the patient, which are essentially theoretic abstractions. They are hard to demonstrate reliably. There is also ample risk of dualism: splitting the mind (psychogenic) from the body (organic, "real" disease); the conscious (feigning) from the unconscious (conversion); the dishonest from the sincere. It is all too easy for the patient to be construed as either a victim or a villain, hysteric or deceiver on the basis of inferences drawn from inconsistent physical findings (4).

In this chapter, we adopt an agnostic position on the differentiation between conversion disorder and feigned symptomatology, recognizing that clinically there is little which might objectively sustain such a distinction (4,5). Instead, we shall regard PMD as a heterogeneous entity, which nevertheless exhibits certain unifying features. We will argue that PMD is differentiated from organic movement disorders by the way in which it relies upon the engagement of the cognitive executive for the maintenance of its clinical expression (motor phenomenology).

COGNITIVE ARCHITECTURE: THE ROLE OF THE EXECUTIVE

In cognitive neuropsychological accounts of brain function, a distinction is often made between processes (and behaviors) that occur automatically and those that require the intervention of higher centers or systems, to generate novelty or complexity. Examples of the former may be drawn from everyday life, in which much of our behavior may be relatively overlearned, routine, and automated, requiring very little of our conscious attention, for example, the movements we execute while driving a car. We *can*

attend to these movements (if necessary), but in general, because their demands are low, we are able to attend to other behaviors as well, for example, conversing while driving. However, when the task demands change or a nonroutine occurrence intervenes, we are able to redirect our attention to the task in hand, for example, we change our motor routines when we realize that there is fog on the road ahead. The motor behaviors that we have automated through overuse may be inappropriate in certain new situations. For instance, if I am used to driving along a particular route to work and have to travel part of that same journey on an errand on the weekend, I may, if distracted, continue driving toward my place of work instead of turning off onto the new route. In this context, my routine behavior has become inappropriate. It has intruded into the new motor program.

A number of authors have conceptualized cognitive architectures that might support such changes in emergent behavior (6–9). Commonly, these architectures privilege the prefrontal cortex, with it serving to modulate lower, "slave" systems within the brain (Fig. 25.1). Within such a model, the premotor, motor, and sensory cortices, together with specific subcortical regions (such as the basal ganglia and cerebellum), are hypothesized to be sufficient for the performance of routine cognitive/motor procedures. Much automated behavior can be conceptualized as programs run on such subordinate brain systems. However, in nonroutine situations, the intervention of prefrontal systems is required. Hence, the prefrontal cortex is involved in such executive tasks as planning, selecting, initiating, and inhibiting behavior; the programming and execution of such behaviors being delegated to posterior, lower systems (10,11).

An example of this cognitive architecture is provided by a simple protocol that we have used to study the functional anatomy of mouth movements (12). We utilized positron emission tomography (PET) to study healthy subjects under three conditions:

A. Rest: Lying in the scanner listening to a pacing tone emitted by a computer metronome at a rate of one tone every 3 seconds (0.33 Hz).
B. Stereotypic responding, in which subjects responded with one vocal articulation each time they heard the pacing tone (0.33 Hz), specifically enunciating the following repetitive sequence: "Lah, bah, bah, lah, lah, bah, bah, lah . . . ," one syllable at a time.
C. Freely selected responding, in which subjects responded to each tone (0.33 Hz) by saying either "lah" or "bah" in a sequence of their own choosing, the instruction being that they make the sequence as *random* as possible.

The stereotypic response condition requires that subjects perform behaviors that are totally determined by the experimenter. In response to a tone, the subjects have only one response to make that is appropriate (lah or bah,

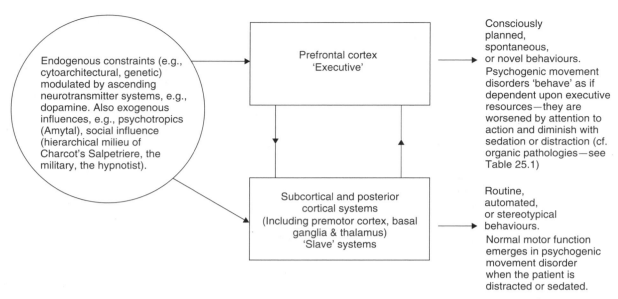

Figure 25.1 Schematic diagram illustrating the neural basis of behavioral control. Prefrontal systems are implicated in control of complex and novel behavior patterns, modulating lower brain systems (such as basal ganglia and premotor cortices). However, constraints are imposed by endogenous and exogenous factors **(left)**. While genetic and neurodevelopmental factors constrain anatomy and function is modulated by neurotransmitters, social influences may facilitate certain behaviors and constrain others. Together, these endogenous and exogenous constraints impose limits on the envelope of possible responses generated by the organism **(right)**. Psychogenic movement disorders behave as if they are the products of prefrontal executive systems, as attention to action is required for their execution. Distraction leads to improved motor performance, the emergence of normal motor function.

depending upon their progress through the stereotypic sequence). When we compared brain activity during this condition with that of the resting state, we found bilateral premotor and motor cortex activation, together with cerebellar activity (Fig. 25.2). Hence, the motor system was activated during performance of the task, but there was no significant activation in prefrontal regions. Lower brain areas were sufficient to produce stereotypic responding.

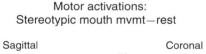

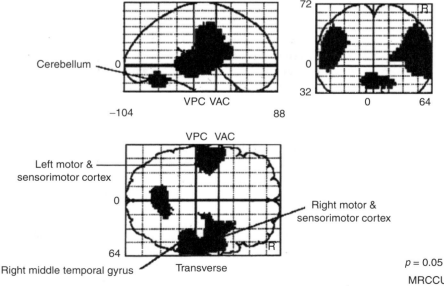

Figure 25.2 Brain regions exhibiting a significant neural response to the stereotypic performance of mouth movements (reciting "lah, bah, bah, lah, lah" in a repetitive cycle). These figures show statistical parametric maps thresholded at $p < 0.05$, corrected for multiple comparisons. There is prominent activation of bilateral premotor and motor cortices (and cerebellum).

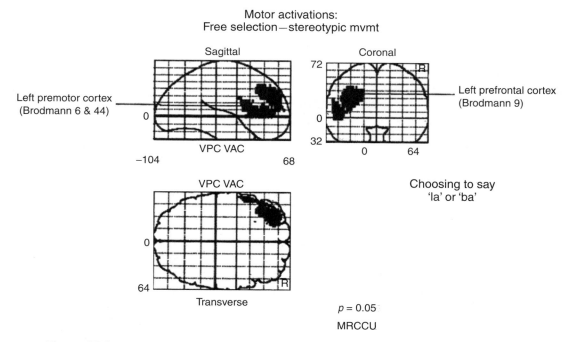

Figure 25.3 Brain regions exhibiting a significant neural response to the free selection of mouth movements (saying "lah" or "bah" in a random, self-determined sequence). These figures show statistical parametric maps thresholded at $p < 0.05$, corrected for multiple comparisons. There is prominent activation of regions in left prefrontal cortex. (Adapted from Spence SA, Hirsch SR, Brooks DJ, et al. Prefrontal cortex activity in people with schizophrenia and control subjects: evidence from positron emission tomography for remission of "hypofrontality" with recovery from acute schizophrenia. *Br J Psych.* 1998;172:316–323.)

When subjects were allowed a degree of choice in their response, albeit constrained to two possible exemplars (lah or bah), there was increased activation in left prefrontal cortex. Figure 25.3 shows those brain regions exhibiting greater activation during freely selected response compared with the stereotypic condition (12).

Hence, when there is choice over the selection of motor response, there is greater activation in prefrontal cortex (particularly left dorsolateral prefrontal cortex, DLPFC) (11,12). Similar results have been found when subjects choose which finger to move (13) or which direction to move a joystick (12). The commonality among these findings is that prefrontal activation is necessary when subjects are called upon to *choose* their response to the environment. Subordinate brain regions (e.g., premotor and motor cortices) are no longer sufficient for the production of such behavior.

PROBING THE EXECUTIVE

In the clinical setting, we are often concerned with assessing the cognitive executive. Implicit in such assessment is the acknowledgement that the executive is central to independent living, its dysfunction impacting upon patients' day-to-day lives (14).

Part of the mental state examination used by psychiatrists comprises the performance of orthographic verbal fluency. The patient is asked to produce a sequence of verbal responses on the basis of an arbitrary letter rule, for example, "say as many words as you can in the next minute, beginning with the letter 's'" (excluding proper nouns and numbers). These sorts of tasks are used to probe prefrontal function. Subjects are allowed to generate self-selected responses, although they are, of course, constrained to selecting them from a specified category of exemplars (e.g., words beginning with the letter "s"). When verbal fluency has been studied using functional neuroimaging [PET or functional magnetic resonance imaging (fMRI)], it has been shown to activate left DLPFC and anterior cingulate cortex (13,15,16). Such findings are congruent with a neuropsychiatric literature implicating lesions or functional abnormalities of the left DLPFC in expressive and dynamic, or transcortical motor, aphasia (17) and the alogia seen in schizophrenia and depression (18).

However, healthy subjects may also be made to exhibit decrements in executive performance if cognitive demands are increased sufficiently. Hence, if subjects perform the verbal fluency task while also attempting to generate random sequences of movements with a joystick, the randomness of the latter will be less than when they perform such movements alone (19). Therefore, having to generate self-chosen words at the same time as self-chosen movements (dual tasking) impairs the subject's ability to generate novelty. The normal executive system is subject to demonstrable processing constraints (20). (Various authors have demonstrated that the threshold for such decompensation may be lower in neuropsychiatric disorders.) (6)

This principle is borne out in another context when healthy subjects generate a sequence of single responses under increasing task demands. If subjects are asked to respond faster, then there is a demonstrable fall off in the degree of randomness they can generate (i.e., their numeric responses become more stereotypic) (6). Similarly, if the set of possible response exemplars is increased, for example, from digits between 1 and 4 to digits between 1 and 32, then the subjects require longer to respond. Hence, the cognitive substrate of their ability to generate random response sequences is doubly constrained by processing speed and capacity. If time to respond decreases, then performance diminishes. If cognitive load (the set of exemplars) increases, then processing time increases. The cognitive executive is constrained by finite resources, and its constraint is manifest in performance decrements (6).

Do similar principles apply in the clinic? There is evidence that they do. Indeed, as other chapters (Chapters 4, 6, 13, and 31) in this book will demonstrate, the inability of the executive to maintain a psychogenic dysfunction in the face of increasing cognitive demands is one plank upon which neurologists build their diagnosis of PMD. The patient exhibiting psychogenic movements of one limb cannot sustain them when asked to move the other. The diagnostic "tricks" that neurologists deploy often exploit such processing decrements, even if they are not conceptualized in this way (4,21).

THE EXECUTIVE IN THE CLINIC

If cognitive executive resources are being utilized in the maintenance of one form of behavior (or its suppression), then we might predict that asking a subject to perform a second executive task will affect the performance of the first. In other words, the first behavior, which the executive facilitates, will be diminished if the executive is stressed. Alternatively, a target behavior that the executive suppresses may be "released" under the same conditions, as the executive's resources are diverted toward the second task. Clinically, psychiatrists exploit this decompensation of the executive when they assess patients for the presence of tardive dyskinesia. The patient with schizophrenia may exhibit abnormal movements of the mouth and tongue, which may be attributable to neuroleptic medication or schizophrenia itself (22). At rest, such movements may be hard to discern; indeed, patients themselves may not be aware that they make any abnormal movements. However, if they are asked to perform a distracting task, the effect may be to reveal abnormalities, previously latent. Commonly, the task might involve performing complex hand movements while standing. Patients may be asked to alternately oppose the palmar and dorsal surfaces of one hand against their other hand (or to oppose the thumb of their left hand with each of its fingers in sequence). When such behaviors are performed, the dyskinetic tongue may start to protrude from the mouth of the patient. Such movements may not be noticed by the patient, but the role of his or her executive system in suppressing them is implied by the fact that distraction with a demanding task reveals them (i.e., the executive "cannot do two things at

TABLE 25.1

SOME DIFFERENTIATING CHARACTERISTICS OF ORGANIC AND PSYCHOGENIC MOVEMENT DISORDERS

Disorder	Behavioral Features
Akathisia secondary to neuroleptic medication	Although patients may be unaware of their abnormal movements, they may suppress them nevertheless. Evidence that cognitive resources are used in suppressing abnormal movements. They become *more pronounced* (i.e., more abnormal) when the patient is *distracted* (22), cf. PMD.
Tardive dyskinesia secondary to neuroleptic medication	Although patients may be unaware of their abnormal movements, when aware of them they may suppress them. Evidence that cognitive resources are used in suppressing abnormal movements. They become *more pronounced* when the patient is *distracted* (22), cf. PMD.
Parkinson disease	Although undoubtedly organic, movement abnormalities may be ameliorated by *attention to action* (23), cf. PMD (24).
Organic tremor	Tremor may be suppressed consciously (25). Amplitude decreases as extremity is loaded with additional weights (cf. psychogenic tremor; 32). Tremor persists during contralateral limb tapping sequences (cf. psychogenic tremor; 26).
Tic disorder	A forced quality to the intention to act; patients report an "urge" to act (27) but behaviors may be resisted or suppressed by attentional strategies, at least temporarily (25).
Psychogenic movement disorder	In contrast to all of the above, performance may be improved by distraction (24,28). Similarly, sedation has been found to ameliorate symptoms (21,29–31). Psychogenic tremor increases in amplitude with addition of load to extremity (cf. organic tremor; 32). Psychogenic tremor frequency is not maintained while tapping the contralateral limb (26).

PMD, psychogenic movement disorder.

once," so the movements emerge from their former suppression). A similar rationale is used to elicit signs of akathisia (Table 25.1) (22).

THE ROLE OF THE EXECUTIVE IN PSYCHOGENIC MOVEMENT DISORDER

In the case of people with schizophrenia exhibiting tardive dyskinesia (above), we noted that their abnormal movements emerged (or became more pronounced) when they were distracted. This implies involvement of the cognitive executive in normalizing their motor function. When not distracted they were able (consciously or unconsciously) to suppress abnormal movements. However, when distracted by the requirement to perform a complex manual task, their dyskinesia became apparent. Hence, distraction revealed *greater* functional impairment. By implication, a decompensation in the function of the executive released such motor abnormalities. Other organic movement disorders share this feature: People with Parkinson disease may use attentional strategies to improve their performance (23), and patients with organic tremors or tics may consciously suppress these movements, at least temporarily (25).

This brings us to an interesting contrast between PMDs and movement disorders that are regarded as organic (Table 25.1). In general, attention to action seems to improve performance in organic movement disorders, whereas its opposite, *distraction*, seems to improve motor function in PMDs (28). Is this principle not at the root of the late John Campbell's (24) "shortest paper"? He wrote:

> Organic tremor is aggravated by taking the attention away from the area involved and usually improves when attention is directed toward the involved limb. . . . Functional or psychogenic tremor disappears when attention is withdrawn from the limb or area involved. I will give $25.00 to the first MD who can prove me wrong.

It seems that in PMD, distraction releases *normal* function (Fig. 25.1). One implication is that *the executive serves to maintain dysfunction*.

There are several clinical, anecdotal examples that might be used to defend the above hypothesis. On clinical examination, the (PMD) patients who cannot extend an affected leg upon examination do so when the contralateral limb is flexed (21). The patient with psychogenic aphonia or paresis recovers when administered a general anesthetic, barbiturate, or benzodiazepine (29–31,33). Hence, distraction by contralateral limb movement or sedation with a drug seems to release the normal function of the affected anatomic domain (congruent with Campbell's observation above).

An elegant experimental demonstration of this principle is supplied by O'Suilleabhain and Matsumoto's (26) study of organic and psychogenic tremors, using time-frequency analysis of EMG data. Studying people with Parkinson disease, essential tremor, and psychogenic tremor, the investigators demonstrated distinct differences between the two former conditions and PMD. While patients with organic tremors exhibited variations in their frequencies across affected limbs, those with PMD did not. While those with organic disorders continued to exhibit their tremors when carrying out a tapping task (with the contralateral limb), those with PMDs lost their tremor (while performing the same task). The suggestion of the authors is that organic tremors are generated by multiple oscillator systems within the nervous systems of those affected (although a possible exception has been identified in orthostatic tremor) (32), while a single oscillator is responsible for those seen in PMD (26). Psychogenic tremor behaves more like *voluntary* rhythmic behavior (26). O'Suilleabhain and Matsumoto write:

> In psychogenic tremor . . . we propose that the motor system *per se* is intact, and that rhythmic contractions are mediated by top-down synchronization involving a common oscillator system, perhaps at a higher cerebral level. The tendency for psychogenic tremor to attenuate when patients are distracted could be explained by a requirement for such high-level involvement. . . ."

The cerebral production of PMDs is also supported by findings in psychogenic myoclonus. Terada et al. (34) demonstrated that in five out of six patients with this form of myoclonus, a Bereitschaftspotential, indicative of voluntary causation, preceded the abnormal movement. "Therefore, it is most likely that the jerks in these patients were generated through the mechanisms common to those underlying voluntary movement" (34).

The expression of PMDs diminishes when patients are distracted—when they do not attend to their symptoms—and utilizes similar cognitive resources to voluntary acts.

IS PSYCHOGENIC MOVEMENT DISORDER THE SAME AS FEIGNING?

The purpose of this chapter has been to consider the evidence for the contribution of the cognitive executive to the maintenance of psychogenic abnormalities of movement. We stated at the outset that we would remain agnostic with regard to the hypothesized distinction between conversion disorder and deliberately feigned dysfunction. Nevertheless, it may be tempting to equate one with the other and to collapse all PMDs into one diagnosis. This would be premature for several reasons:

A. Although the contents of the cognitive executive may gain access to consciousness (as they do when we consider future plans or manipulate the contents of working memory in our heads), they need not do so (35). We saw this with the schizophrenia patients who were unaware of their (suppressing) tardive dyskinesia, yet manifested such movements when consciously diverted toward a complex task (above). Just because the maintenance of PMDs requires the resources of the cognitive executive does not *necessarily* mean that patients "know what they are doing."

B. A mechanism by which complex behaviors may occur without their host being aware of them has been proposed by Oakley (36). Essentially, this relies upon dissociation among components of the executive. Hence, quite complex behaviors might be initiated and maintained by one component of the executive, while another, identified with subjective awareness, might not know or recognize the origin of those behaviors. Oakley's account proposes a similar mechanism for hysterical and hypnotic phenomena. Other, philosophical accounts have been provided in attempts to explain individuals' apparent antagonism of themselves (e.g., self-deception or disavowal) (4,33).

C. The retention of the potentially nebulous concept of PMD (or similarly "hysteria"), though it may seem unsatisfactory, has one distinct advantage: It spares the patient from automatic attributions of deception, or deceit (37). It may be pragmatic to retain such a space for diagnoses that are currently uncertain, either because they cannot be proven (in the cases of conversion and deception) or because they have yet to be understood (there may come to light, in the future, organic diagnoses currently unknown).

D. The literature on human deception serves to demonstrate that humans are generally rather poor at detecting deception (38), and physicians are no better than other groups who have been studied. Hence, it may be wise to refrain from diagnosing deception (malingering), in the clinical arena, as one may well be mistaken.

E. Though there are preliminary neuroimaging studies distinguishing between conversion and feigning (5), and examining the functional anatomy of deception *per se* (39–42), these remain exploratory. Indeed, there may be ethical obstacles to ever applying these techniques in the clinical setting; their application, to detect whether a patient is "lying," might clearly undermine any chance of a therapeutic relationship. Nevertheless, *understanding* the brain systems required to sustain deception may provide valuable insight into social cognition, human volition, responsibility, and mitigation (43).

F. The assumption that deception is meant for others (including the physician), overlooks the concept of self-deception (9,33) and the real possibility that patients may deceive themselves. Following conduct of which they are ashamed, patients may assume the sick role to protect the ego or self-esteem (4). In the words of the medical anthropologist Brent Wenegrat (44), "the difference between the malingerer and the patient who sincerely acts an illness role may be less a matter of the latter's relative honesty than his relative lack of insight."

This is a complex area that has received scant attention in the context of PMD.

The whole area of deception in the clinical arena is one which deserves careful study, especially in those areas of medicine where pathognomonic physical findings are lacking (PMD remains a case in point). The hinterland of psychiatry encompasses a number of such disorders, in which it can be very difficult to establish subjective veracity (i.e., whether patients *really* believe what they are saying). The psychoses retain an essentially subjective phenomenology: Though grossly disordered behavior and thought disorder may be easy to identify much of the time, the clinician interprets verbal reports. We must retain a truth bias in our clinical relationships, since our role is essentially for the patient, yet accuracy demands that we consider veracity when appropriate. Even the portrayal of psychosis may be used to instrumental ends (45). Likewise, the language of threatened self-harm often appears compelling, linguistically and emotionally, but may be accompanied by features which seem to contradict its stated intent (e.g., the overdose once taken is reported immediately and an ambulance called). The Ganser syndrome patient's "approximate answers" (*vorbeigehen*) seem to betray a knowledge of the correct answer so prominent that it may be hard to believe that the patient is not being disingenuous. When asked how many legs a cow has, a patient may reply "five." In Ganser's original report he stated: "In the choice of answers the patient appears to pass over deliberately the indicated correct answer and to select a false one (46)." The latter reminds one of a psychological test, the Hayling Test, in which subjects are deliberately asked to complete a sentence with a word that is out of context. When examining the functional anatomy associated with giving such deliberately incongruent sentence completions, Nathaniel-James and Frith (47) found activation of left DLPFC. This suggests a hypothesis—that the executive may likewise be engaged when patients provide misleading answers—as in the Ganser syndrome, though further work is needed in this area.

CONCLUSION

It may be posited that the key program for future studies of psychogenic movement disorder is the principled investigation of executive brain processes during the expression of these behaviors and the re-examination of such systems over time as symptoms remit. Functional neuroimaging provides a means by which the nature of psychogenic brain states may be objectively determined.

REFERENCES

1. David-Menard M. *Hysteria from Freud to Lacan: body and language in psychoanalysis (transl. C. Porter)*. Ithaca, NY: Cornell University Press, 1989.

2. Zizek S. *Looking awry: an introduction to Jacques Lacan through popular culture.* Cambridge, MA: October Books, MIT Press, 1991.
3. Mitchell J. Sexuality and psychoanalysis: hysteria. *Br J Psychother.* 1996;12:473–479.
4. Spence SA. Hysterical paralyses as disorders of action. *Cognit Neuropsych.* 1999;4:203–226.
5. Spence SA, Crimlisk HL, Cope H, et al. Discrete neurophysiological correlates in prefrontal cortex during hysterical and feigned disorder of movement. *Lancet.* 2000a;355:1243–1244.
6. Baddeley A, Della Sala S. Working memory and executive control. *Philos Trans R Soc Lond B.* 1996;351:1397–1404.
7. Shallice T, Burgess P. The domain of supervisory processes and temporal organization of behavior. *Philos Trans R Soc Lond B.* 1996;351:1405–1412.
8. Shallice T. Fractionation of the supervisory system. In: Stuss DT, Knight RT, eds. *Principles of frontal lobe function.* Oxford: Oxford University Press, 2002:261–277.
9. Spence SA. Disorders of willed action. In: Halligan PW, Bass C, Marshall JC, eds. *Contemporary approaches to the study of hysteria: clinical and theoretical perspectives.* Oxford: Oxford University Press, 2001:235–250.
10. Passingham RE. Attention to action. *Philos Trans R Soc Lond B.* 1996;351:1473–1479.
11. Spence SA, Frith CD. Towards a functional anatomy of volition. *J Conscious Stud.* 1999;6:11–29.
12. Spence SA, Hirsch SR, Brooks DJ, et al. Prefrontal cortex activity in people with schizophrenia and control subjects: evidence from positron emission tomography for remission of "hypofrontality" with recovery from acute schizophrenia. *Br J Psych.* 1998; 172:316–323.
13. Frith CD, Friston K, Liddle PF, et al. Willed action and the prefrontal cortex in man: a study with PET. *Proc R Soc Lond B.* 1991;244:241–246.
14. Velligan DI, Bow-Thomas C, Mahurin RK, et al. Do specific neurocognitive deficits predict specific domains of community function in schizophrenia? *J Nerv Ment Dis.* 2000;188:518–524.
15. Spence SA, Liddle PF, Stefan MD, et al. Functional anatomy of verbal fluency in people with schizophrenia and those at genetic risk: focal dysfunction and distributed disconnectivity reappraised. *Br J Psych.* 2000b;176:52–60.
16. Hunter MD, Thiyagesh SN, Wignall EL, et al. Overt letter fluency investigated using fMRI and an interleaved verbal response/ imaging paradigm. Presented at the *9th International Conference on Functional Mapping of the Human Brain,* June 19-22, 2003, New York, NY. Available on CD-Rom *in Neuroimage.* 2003;19(2).
17. Robinson G, Blair J, Cipolotti L. Dynamic aphasia: an inability to select between competing verbal responses? *Brain.* 1998;121: 77–89.
18. Dolan RJ, Bench CJ, Liddle PF, et al. Dorsolateral prefrontal cortex dysfunction in the major psychoses: symptom or disease specificity? *J Neurol Neurosurg Psychiatr.* 1993;56:1290–1294.
19. Passingham RE. Functional organization of the motor system. In: Frackowiak RSJ, Friston KJ, Frith CD, et al., eds. *Human brain function.* San Diego, CA: Academic Press, 1997:243–274.
20. Spence SA, Hunter MD, Harpin G. Neuroscience and the will. *Curr Opin Psych.* 2002;15:519–526.
21. Merskey H. *The analysis of hysteria: understanding conversion and dissociation.* London: Gaskell, 1995.
22. Barnes TRE, Spence SA. Movement disorders associated with antipsychotic drugs: clinical and biological implications. In:

Reveley MA, Deakin JFW, eds. *The psychopharmacology of schizophrenia.* London: Arnold, 2000:178–210.
23. Morris ME, Iansek R, Matyas TA, et al. Stride regulation in Parkinson's disease. Normalisation strategies and underlying mechanisms. *Brain.* 1996;119:551–568.
24. Campbell J. The shortest paper. *Neurology.* 1979;29:1633.
25. Lang AE. Clinical phenomenology of tic disorders: selected aspects. In: Chase TN, Friedhoff AJ, Cohen DF, eds. *Advances in neurology.* New York: Raven Press, 1992;58:25–32.
26. O'Suilleabhain PE, Matsumoto JY. Time-frequency analysis of tremors. *Brain.* 1998;121:2127–2134.
27. Bliss J. Sensory experiences of Gilles de la Tourette syndrome. *Arch Gen Psych.* 1980;37:1343–1347.
28. Lempert T, Brandt T, Dieterich M, et al. How to identify psychogenic disorders of stance and gait: a video study in 37 patients. *J Neurol.* 1991;238:140–146.
29. Adrian ED, Yealland LR. The treatment of some common war neuroses. *Lancet.* 1917;I:867–872.
30. Ellis SJ. Diazepam as a truth drug. *Lancet.* 1990;336:752–753.
31. Keating JJ, Dinan TG, Chua A, et al. Hysterical paralysis. *Lancet.* 1990;336:1506–1507.
32. Deuschl G, Raethjen J, Lindemann M, et al. The pathophysiology of tremor. *Muscle Nerve.* 2001;24:716–735.
33. Fingarette H. *Self-deception.* London: Routledge and Kegan Paul, 1969.
34. Terada K, Ikeda A, Van Ness PC, et al. Presence of Bereitschaftspotential preceding psychogenic myoclonus: clinical application of jerk-locked back averaging. *J Neurol Neurosurg Psychiatr.* 1995;58:745–747.
35. Badgaiyan RD. Executive control, willed actions, and nonconscious processing. *Hum Brain Mapp.* 2000;9:38–41.
36. Oakley DA. Hypnosis and suggestion in the treatment of hysteria. In: Halligan PW, Bass C, Marshall JC, eds. *Contemporary approaches to the study of hysteria: clinical and theoretical perspectives.* Oxford: Oxford University Press, 2001:312–329.
37. Mace CJ. Hysterical conversion: 1. A history. *Br J Psych.* 1992; 161:369–377.
38. Vrij A. *Detecting lies and deceit: the psychology of lying and the implications for professional practice.* Chichester: Wiley, 2001.
39. Spence SA, Farrow TFD, Herford AE, et al. Behavioural and functional anatomical correlates of deception in humans. *Neuroreport.* 2001;12:2849–2853.
40. Spence SA, Hunter MD, Farrow TFD, et al. A cognitive neurobiological account of deception: evidence from functional neuroimaging. *Philos Trans R Soc Lond B.* 2004;359:1755–1762.
41. Langleben DD, Schroeder L, Maldjian JA, et al. Brain activity during simulated deception: an event-related functional magnetic resonance study. *Neuroimage.* 2002;15:727–732.
42. Lee TMC, Liu H-L, Tan L-H, et al. Lie detection by functional magnetic resonance imaging. *Hum Brain Mapp.* 2002;15:157–164.
43. Spence SA. The deceptive brain. *J R Soc Med.* 2004;97:6–9.
44. Wenegrat B. *Theatre of disorder: patients, doctors, and the construction of illness.* Oxford: Oxford University Press, 2001.
45. Tyrer P, Babidge N, Emmanuel J, et al. Instrumental psychosis: the Good Soldier Svejk syndrome. *J R Soc Med.* 2001;94:22–25.
46. Sims A. *Symptoms in the mind.* London: Balliere-Tindall, 1988.
47. Nathaniel-James DA, Frith CD. The role of the dorsolateral prefrontal cortex: evidence from the effects of contextual constraint in a sentence completion task. *Neuroimage.* 2002;16:1094–1102.

Neuroimaging of Hysteria

26

Gereon R. Fink   Peter W. Halligan   John C. Marshall

ABSTRACT

The potential of imaging the functional neuroanatomy of hysteria was first recognized in the closing decades of the 19th century. Charcot argued that patients without apparent structural injury to the brain who nonetheless manifested clinical symptoms that mimicked organic paralysis, sensory loss, or aphasia should have "dynamic" or "functional" lesions in the regions in which structural damage could give rise to the same symptomatology. The advent of modern functional neuroimaging methods such as single photon emission computed tomography (SPECT), positron emission tomography (PET), or functional magnetic resonance imaging (fMRI) have now made it possible to detect *in vivo* regionally specific changes in cerebral blood flow and task-related changes in neural activity associated with sensorimotor or cognitive processes. Charcot's hypothesis can thus be tested. Here we review the recent, but still comparatively few, attempts to elucidate the functional neuroanatomy underlying hysterical symptoms. We suggest that the data available are difficult to reconcile with a single neural mechanism, but do reliably implicate anterior cingulate cortex and dorsolateral prefrontal cortex in many cases of sensorimotor hysteria reported to date. The specific contribution of these areas to the neuropsychology underlying hysteria, however, remains to be elucidated. We conclude that hysteria as clinically diagnosed is a protean disorder. Furthermore, future studies of the neural mechanisms associated with hysteria should also take into account the high probability that functional specialization may not be a fixed property of brain regions as previously supposed, but may rather depend on the neural context. Accordingly, functional neuroimaging studies of hysteria should analyze the functional interaction ("dynamics") between the brain regions involved in normal and defective task performance.

INTRODUCTION

The two international systems of diagnostic classification for psychiatric disorders, namely, the *International Classification of Diseases* (ICD-10) and the *Diagnostic and Statistical Manual of Mental Disorders*, Fourth Edition (DSM-IV), summarize a variety of syndromes as "conversion disorders" (DSM-IV) or "dissociative disorders" (ICD-10). These disorders are unified by the assumption that they have in common the presence of positive physical symptoms (e.g., tremor, tonic-clonic convulsion), or negative symptoms (e.g., organic paralysis, sensory loss, or aphasia) without evidence of any discernable "organic" correlate. Since these diagnoses refer to a "psychological" conflict preceding the onset of physical symptoms, conversion or dissociative disorders are considered to be related to the older concept of "hysteria" (1). Although earlier references to hysteria (Hippocrates, 460?–377 BCE) restricted the diagnostic label to a gynecologic context, the etiology of this protean disorder has "migrated over time from the uterine to the cerebral to the psychodynamic" (2) and remains to be fully elucidated. Unsurprisingly, the medical concept of hysteria (conversion disorder, dissociative disorders, etc.) has always been controversial (3), and despite its recognition in current psychiatric taxonomies, many physicians still regard hysterical disorders as either feigned or as a failure to find the responsible organic cause for the patient's symptoms.

The concept of hysteria evokes considerable interest because, as a putative disorder of willed action or intention (4), the underlying mechanisms are supposed to be of a "psychological" nature and, if not feigned, the product of unconscious processes. A major problem with the current concept of hysteria is that the diagnosis can only be put forward if the physician's best guess, or, in fact, belief, is that the patient is not consciously/intentionally producing or feigning dysfunction (5). Thus, a key issue when distinguishing conversion disorder from malingering is the clinician's ability to make inferences about the patient's intentions when much of the evidence relies on the patient's subjective report. Accordingly, the issue of an impairment to the volitional system becomes the focus of interest once any explanatory organic disorder has been excluded.

This chapter summarizes the findings obtained using functional imaging [single photon emission computed tomography (SPECT), positron emission tomography (PET), or functional magnetic resonance imaging (fMRI)] in cases of hysteria and related disorders. Unfortunately, functional neuroimaging studies of hysteria are still very rare and the few data available are difficult to reconcile with a single neural mechanism. The results promise, however, new insights into the neural mechanisms associated with hysteria, as they allow for the testing of hypotheses about the pathophysiology underlying hysterical conditions.

HYSTERICAL PARESTHESIA OR ANESTHESIA

One of the first studies to investigate conversion disorders using functional neuroimaging was concerned with altered cerebral blood flow in a single case of hysterical paresthesia (6). The patient was a nurse who had no history of psychiatric or neurologic treatment, but developed symptoms of depressed mood and a panic disorder when she was in a state of extreme stress due to her current marital and domestic situation. Eleven months after the first attack, she was hospitalized for left-sided paresis and paresthesia associated with mild apathic symptoms. Her somatosensory-evoked potentials (SEP) and motor-evoked potentials were normal, and her symptoms disappeared within a week. In contrast to the normal electrophysiologic examinations of her long sensory and motor tracts, SPECT during electrical stimulation of the left median nerve at the time of paresthesia showed associated alterations in cerebral blood flow. Prior to recovery from paresthesia there was increased perfusion in the right frontal lobe, but hypoperfusion in the right parietal region (compared to the equivalent left hemisphere regions).

After recovery, the perfusion in the right parietal region was greater than in the left parietal region during left

median nerve stimulation, as one would expect. These results suggested that psychogenic paresthesia may have arisen from the simultaneous activation of frontal inhibitory areas and the associated inhibition of somatosensory cortex. Tiihonen et al. (6) hypothesized that "distressing psychological events may alter the neurophysiology of the human brain in a specific way and trigger symptoms such as . . . paresthesia through activating or inhibiting critical areas of the brain." More importantly, this first imaging study of hysteria suggested that hysteria was indeed amenable to investigation by functional imaging.

Using fMRI, Mailis-Gagnon et al. (7) studied altered central somatosensory processing in four chronic pain patients with hysterical anesthesia. Patients with chronic pain frequently present with nondermatomal somatosensory deficits (NDSD) to various cutaneous sensory modalities (touch, pinprick, cold) ranging from mild sensory loss to complete anesthesia. These changes of somatosensory processing are often considered to be of psychogenic origin as they typically occur in the absence of substantial structural pathology. Interestingly, NDSD may occur with variable motor abnormalities including complete motor paralysis (7). Mailis-Gagnon (7) tested their hypothesis that central factors may underlie NDSD by using fMRI to measure brush and noxious stimulation-evoked brain responses. They observed altered somatosensory-evoked responses in forebrain areas: Unperceived (unreported) stimuli failed to activate areas that were activated with perceived touch and pain, including the thalamus, the posterior part of the anterior cingulate cortex (ACC), and Brodmann area 44/45. Rather, these unperceived (i.e., unreported) stimuli were associated with deactivations in primary and secondary somatosensory areas (SI, SII), posterior parietal cortex, prefrontal cortex, and rostral parts of the ACC. Application of the same stimuli to the unaffected side of the four patients resulted in the normal patterns of activations and awareness commonly associated with somatosensory stimulation. In contrast to these fMRI results, tests using cortical evoked potentials found no changes in function (8).

The results of Tiihonen et al. (6) and Mailis-Gagnon et al. (7) suggest that functional neuroimaging is a sensitive tool for examining afferent function in cases of hysterical anaesthesia, as both show evidence of altered cerebral activity in the neural networks known to support sensory information processing. In both studies, increases as well as decreases in neural activations in response to somatosensory stimulation were observed. Reduced processing of sensory information was associated with attenuated neural activity in parietal areas in both studies (comprising SI, SII, and posterior parietal cortex), while increased neural activity was observed in frontal areas. With respect to this latter activity, however, the results of the two studies differed substantially. While the data of Tiihonen et al. implicated prefrontal areas and supervisory inhibitory processes (6), Mailis-Gagnon et al. (7) observed increased neural activity in a region of the anterior cingulate cortex that may be involved in aspects of divided attention, response inhibition, and possibly emotion (9).

The role of striatothalamocortical circuits involved in sensorimotor processing was stressed in another SPECT study of the functional correlates of unilateral hysterical sensorimotor loss in seven patients (10). Passive vibratory stimulation was given to each hand when the deficit was present and 2 to 4 months later when the patients had recovered. SPECT blood flow measurements consistently detected a decrease in rCBF in the thalamus and basal ganglia (contralateral to the deficit) which resolved after recovery. The data thus converge with the study by Tiihonen et al. (6) which also reported, using a similar paradigm, that abnormal blood flow patterns may be reversible upon recovery from hysterical sensory loss. The study by Vuilleumier et al. (10), however, extended these findings by showing that reduced activation of the contralateral caudate predicted poor recovery at follow-up (10). The authors speculated that the basal ganglia, and in particular the caudate nucleus, "might be well suited to modulate motor processes based on emotional and situational cues from the limbic system" (10).

HYSTERICAL PARALYSIS

Marshall and co-workers reported a woman with left-sided paralysis (and without somatosensory loss) in whom no organic disease or structural lesion that could have explained the paralysis was found after intensive investigation (11). By contrast, psychological trauma was associated with the onset and recurrent exacerbation of her hemiparalysis. Using PET, no activation of primary motor cortex was observed when the patient attempted to move her affected leg (as might be expected from the lack of any observed actual movement), though there was increased neural activity in right orbitofrontal cortex and anterior cingulate cortex (11). In contrast, preparing to move or moving her good leg, and also preparing to move her paralyzed leg, activated motor and/or premotor areas previously described with movement preparation and execution. Marshall et al. (11) suggested that the right orbitofrontal and right anterior cingulate cortex inhibited prefrontal (willed) brain areas with the resultant effect on right primary motor cortex [when the patient tried (i.e., willed) to move her affected left leg]. While orbitofrontal cortex had not been described in previous studies of motor imagery, or motor execution (or hysteria), activation of the anterior cingulate cortex (11) has been conjectured to reflect a "meeting place for interactions between cognitive and motivational processes, particularly related to the generation of motor output (12)."

Spence et al. used PET to examine the neural correlates of hysterical motor loss versus a feigned disorder of movement (13). They postulated that the pathophysiology of "genuine" hysterical motor symptoms would differ from that involved in feigning. Two men with hysterical motor symptoms that substantially affected their left arms were investigated while they performed joystick movements (moving the left hand or the right hand) and at rest. In addition, two healthy individuals were instructed to "feign" difficulty in moving their left arm. For control, six healthy individuals were asked to perform the joystick movements normally. Comparing brain activations during movement of the left hand (relative to rest) in patients with hysteria versus controls and feigners showed that the two patients exhibited relative *hypo*activation of the left dorsolateral prefrontal cortex (DLPFC). In contrast, the two feigners exhibited *hypo*function of the right anterior prefrontal cortex.

Subsequently, Spence et al. studied a right-handed man with hysterical weakness of the right upper limb and two healthy volunteers who feigned abnormality of their right upper limb (13). A combined data analysis showed that the observed left prefrontal hypoactivation was common to all three patients with hysteria when they moved the affected limb, irrespective of symptom-lateralization, while the feigners were characterized by right prefrontal hypofunction, again irrespective of the side for which they feigned malfunction. Spence et al. suggested that "taken together" their data support the hypothesis that hysteria involves the left DLPFC and differs from feigning with respect to its neural mechanisms (13).

ASTASIA-ABASIA

Five patients with psychogenic astasia-abasia were investigated by Yazící and Kostakoglu using SPECT (14). Somatosensory evoked potentials (SEPs) of the posterior tibial nerve were abnormal in two of the five patients. In these latter patients, SEPs returned to normal after 6 months (despite incomplete clinical remission). Two patients showed decreased perfusion of the left parietal lobe. Four patients showed temporal hypoperfusion (bilateral n = 1, unilateral left n = 3). Interestingly, although clinical symptoms were bilateral in the patient group, the observed effects of hypoperfusion were mostly unilateral and in the dominant (left) hemisphere. Only one patient showed a right-sided temporal hypoperfusion in addition to a left-sided temporal defect. The ongoing right-sided perfusion defect was thought to underlie the symptom of paresis in his left leg, which persisted during imaging.

HYPNOTIC PARALYSIS

A relationship between hysteria and hypnosis has been postulated by many in the history of psychiatry and psychology, and hypnotic induction of motor paralysis has been used since the 19th century to mimic hysterical symptoms (15). Hypnotic phenomena and conversion symptoms, particularly in the acute stage, share many clinical, cognitive, and neurophysiologic features. Accordingly, hypnotic states are often considered as a kind of "controlled state of hysteria" (16). Unsurprisingly, experiments on hypnosis have thus developed into an experimental analogue for studying hysterical symptoms. The concept of a relationship between hysteria and hypnosis is based on the assumption that both hysteria and hypnosis are abnormal states of behavior and experience influenced by "ideas," whether these ideas emerge from the outside (as in hypnosis) or from the inside (as in hysteria). The view that conversion symptoms can be usefully thought of as an "autosuggestive disorder" (17) gained support from a functional imaging study of a single case of hypnotic paralysis (18) where similar brain areas were activated during hypnotic paralysis [right orbitofrontal cortex, right anterior cingulate cortex (ACC)] as in the study by Marshall et al. of a patient with longstanding hysterical paralysis (see above). Halligan et al. (18) suggested that their findings were consistent with the hypothesis that hysterical and hypnotic paralysis might share common neural mechanisms involving the right (in both cases, contralateral) prefrontal region.

Using a within-subject design in 12 normal, hypnotized subjects, Ward et al. approached the neurophysiologic basis of hypnosis-based paresis more systematically (19). Subjects were tested under two paralysis conditions during the same PET-scanning session. Half of the PET scans were performed under the suggestion that the left leg was paralyzed (subjectively experienced paralysis condition), while for the other half of the PET scans, subjects had the instruction to feign the paralysis (intentionally simulated paralysis condition). Thus, two versions of the same motor behavior (or neurologic symptom) were created in the same subject, but these behaviorally indistinguishable versions differed in their subjective characteristics and in the subjects' intentions to deceive an observer. During the subjectively experienced paralysis condition (relative to the intentionally simulated paralysis condition), differentially increased neural activity was observed in the right orbitofrontal but not the ACC. Further differential increases in neural activity were observed in the right cerebellum, left thalamus, and left putamen. The reverse contrast (i.e., intentionally simulated paralysis condition greater than subjectively experienced paralysis condition) revealed differential increases in brain activity in the left ventrolateral prefrontal cortex and also right posterior temporoparietal cortex (including the parietal operculum, the posterior superior temporal sulcus, the intraparietal sulcus, and the medial parietal cortex). These results thus only in part replicate the findings by Halligan et al. (18), which is not too surprising, given the differences in the study design and behavioral paradigm applied. For instance, in the Halligan et al. case study (18), actual (restrained) movement was compared to preparation to move, whereas in the Ward et al. study (19), attempted (unrestrained) movement was compared to rest. Furthermore, both baseline and active tasks differed. More importantly, however, the data lend support to the previous study by Spence et al. (13) in that they provide further evidence that subjectively experienced paralysis (as a result of either hypnosis or hysteria) has a different neural basis from intentionally simulated paralysis. This finding has implications for our understanding of both malingering and hysteria (18).

HYPNOTICALLY INDUCED PAIN

Cerebral activation during hypnotically induced versus imagined pain was studied by Derbyshire et al. (20). In their fMRI study, brain areas were identified that were directly involved in the generation of pain induced by hypnotic suggestion (i.e., in the absence of any noxious stimulus). When contrasted to imagined pain, significant changes during hypnotically induced pain were observed within the thalamus bilaterally, the left ACC, left posterior insula, and bilateral prefrontal and right parietal cortices. On the contrary, imagining pain resulted in only minimal activations of the pain network. The authors concluded that the observed pattern of activation fit well with the activation patterns observed during pain from nociceptive sources and thus provided direct evidence for linking specific neural activity with the generation of the experience of pain. Furthermore, the data support the possibility of a direct central involvement in functional pain disorders.

PSYCHOGENIC AMNESIA

Markowitsch et al. studied a patient with psychogenic amnesia (21) who had lost his personal identity 8 months prior to the PET investigation. Neuropsychological testing detected normal anterograde memory abilities, no retrograde amnesia for factual knowledge, but severe persistent amnesia for personal events prior to the psychogenic fugue (retrograde episodic amnesia), while postfugue episodic memory was well-preserved. The patient was studied during the following conditions: "rest" (control), "prefugue" (during which sentences containing episodic information of the patient's past prior to the fugue were presented), and "postfugue" (where episodic information concerned with personal experiences following the fugue were presented) (21). In the patient, the two activation conditions both led to increased neural activity in the left ACC, the left lateral temporal cortex, and the left supplementary motor area. In contrast, a group of healthy control subjects tested with a similar paradigm showed increased neural activations predominantly in the right hemisphere (21,22).

The same group studied another case of probable psychogenic amnesia with impaired episodic memory retrieval (23). Like the other patient, this patient showed no anterograde amnesia but severe, selective retrograde amnesia for personal material. SPECT performed 3 weeks after the onset of symptoms demonstrated right temporal and right frontal hypoperfusion, that is, reduced blood flow, in areas which have been suggested as critical for episodic memory retrieval (22). Six months after the onset of symptoms, a PET study of episodic memory retrieval was performed. During episodic memory retrieval, bilateral increases in neural activations were observed in the precuneus, the lateral parietal, and the right dorsolateral and polar prefrontal cortex (23).

Taken together, these two single case studies provided evidence for a functional disturbance of the neural network known to be involved in episodic memory retrieval (22).

BRAIN AREAS IMPLICATED IN HYSTERIA BY FUNCTIONAL IMAGING

Table 26.1 summarizes the areas implicated in hysteria (and related disorders) by functional imaging. Clearly, the areas implicated are far from homogeneous. Furthermore,

TABLE 26.1

SUMMARY OF THE MAIN FINDINGS OF THE FUNCTIONAL IMAGING STUDIES WHICH INVESTIGATED HYSTERICAL SYMPTOMS (OR RELATED NONORGANIC DISORDERS)

Structure Implicated	Side	Change	Authors	N	Method	Comment
A. Hysterical paresthesia/anesthesia, hypnotically induced pain						
Prefrontal cortex	Contra	↑	Tiihonen et al., 1995 (6)	1	SPECT	Studied during sensorimotor loss and after recovery
Parietal cortex	Contra	↓				
SI	Contra	↓	Mailis-Gagnon et al., 2003 (7)	4	fMRI	Chronic pain with hysterical anesthesia
SII	Contra	↓				
Posterior parietal cortex	Contra	↓				
Prefrontal cortex	Contra	↓				
Rostral ACC	Contra	↓				
Thalamus	Bilateral	↑	Derbyshire et al., 2004 (20)	8	fMRI	Hypnotically induced pain is related to imagined as well as physically induced pain; hypnotically induced pain activates the areas also activated by physically induced pain; areas listed in this table are implicated when comparing hypnotically induced pain with imagined pain
Midanterior ACC	Contra	↑				
SII	Contra	↑				
Prefrontal cortex	Contra + ipsi	↑				
Parietal cortex	Ipsi	↑				
Thalamus	Contra	↓	Vuilleumier et al., 2001 (10)	7	SPECT	Studied during sensorimotor loss and after recovery; passive vibratory stimulation
Basal ganglia	Contra	↓				
B. Hysterical paralysis, hypnotically induced paralysis, and feigning						
ACC/orbitofrontal	Contra	↑	Marshall et al., 1997 (11)	1	PET	Within-subject comparison to good side, motor test
ACC and orbitofrontal	Contra	↑	Halligan et al., 2000 (18)	1	PET	Hypnotically induced paresis
Orbitofrontal/ventrolateral prefrontal	Right/left	↑	Ward et al., 2003 (19)	12	PET	Hypnosis induced within-subject design with (i) subjectively experienced paralysis, and (ii) intentionally simulated paralysis
DLPFC	Left	↓	Spence et al., 2000 (13)	3	PET	Hysteria vs. "feigning," left DLPFC hypofunction irrespective of side of hysterical paralysis

(continued)

TABLE 26.1

(continued)

C. Astasia-abasia						
Temporal cortex	N/A	↓	Yazící and Kostakoglu, 1998 (14)	5	SPECT	Left temporal hypoperfusion (n = 4; 1 bilateral, 3 unilateral); left parietal hypoperfusion (n = 1)
Parietal cortex						
D. Psychogenic amnesia						
ACC/orbitofrontal cortex	N/A	↑	Markowitsch et al., 1997 (21)	1	PET	Psychogenic fugue, activations all left hemispheric; when compared to controls no right hemisphere activations
Temporal cortex	N/A	↑				
SMA	N/A	↑				

N/A, not applicable (i.e., nonlateralized deficit); SI, primary motor cortex; SII, secondary somatosensory cortex; ACC, anterior cingulate cortex; DLPFC, dorsolateral prefrontal cortex; SMA, supplementary motor area; Contra/ipsi, signal change contralateral/ipsilateral to the side of symptomatology; Left, signal change in the left hemisphere irrespective of the side of symptomatology.
Note: "↑" or "↓" indicate whether the signal obtained with the different methods increased or decreased.

the effects observed are also heterogeneous: While some studies reported signal increases [which were mostly interpreted as "activations," e.g., active inhibitory processes exerted upon other areas (11)], others reported signal decreases [which were also mostly interpreted as resulting from active inhibitory processes (6) but could equally well reflect primary dysfunction of those areas (13)]. Finally, while some studies observed signal changes in the hemisphere contralateral to the symptomatology, others observed signal changes in the left hemisphere irrespective of the side affected (see Table 26.1). Any critical review of the literature could plausibly stop here and ask for more data.

Nevertheless, three conclusions can be drawn from the data currently at hand: (i) functional imaging can be used appropriately to study the neural mechanisms underlying hysteria and related disorders; (ii) the functional imaging data available imply a dysfunction *within* the neural networks that support normal sensorimotor processing (or memory, respectively); and (iii) if hysterical sensorimotor and cognitive impairments are found to be reliably associated with a distinct pattern of brain activation, then this association may form the basis for a neurobiological explanation for the symptom, which in turn may constrain and inform competing neuropsychological accounts.

Charcot (15) was the first to conjecture that in patients without any apparent structural injury to the brain, who nonetheless exhibited manifest symptoms that mimicked organic paralysis, sensory loss, or cognitive deficits such as aphasia, there would be "dynamic" or functional lesions in the regions to which structural damage could give rise to the same symptomatology (24). The physiologic basis for these functional lesions was hypothesized to be localized anemia or hyperemia "of which no trace is found after death" (25). Sigmund Freud, a student of Charcot's at the

time, realised that this required a close similarity between the behavioral effects of both the conventional "organic" lesion and the "dynamic" lesion (25). Freud argued (25) against this account, claiming that "hysteria behaves as though anatomy did not exist or as though it had no knowledge of it," but not revealing where in the brain the processes underlying hysteria might take place. Another 100 years were to pass before such a neurophysiologic account of hysteria could be tested using functional neuroimaging in apt paradigms. All the data available at present clearly suggest that Charcot and Freud were right when hypothesizing that the "lesions" would be functional and that their correlates would be either hyperemia or anemia.

THE ANTERIOR CINGULATE CORTEX "VERSUS" THE DORSOLATERAL PREFRONTAL CORTEX

Hysteria is a protean disorder, and therefore one would not necessarily expect that our current neurobiological findings will generalize across such different pathologies as hysterical blindness, deafness, or somatosensory loss. Two brain regions have nevertheless been particularly implicated by imaging studies of hysteria and related disorders. Spence et al. have argued that dysfunction of the DLPFC, a structure previously implicated in supervisory attentional processes (26) and volition (27), could underlie hysteria (4). Though conceptually compelling, only some of the functional imaging data (Table 26.1) support such a notion, and both hypoactivation as well as hyperactivation have been reported for DLPFC. The nature of the involvement of DLPFC thus remains poorly understood. Furthermore, DLPFC dysfunction has also been reported in other neuropsychiatric conditions including depression (28), psychomotor poverty (29), or delusion (30), which raises the question of symptom or disease specificity.

Many, though not all (Table 26.1), functional imaging studies of hysteria and related disorders indicate that the ACC may play a critical role in hysteria. More consistently than in the case of DLPFC, hyperactivation of the ACC is found. Marshall et al. (11) hypothesized that activation of the anterior cingulate (and orbitofrontal cortex, in their case) reflected active inhibitory processes. If, as Vogt et al. (12) suggest, cognition and motivation interact in the anterior cingulate cortex to determine an appropriate motor response, that response could be no response in the patient with hysteria. Furthermore, a predominantly evaluative, feedback-integrating role has been assigned to the ACC in cognitive control. Its direct anatomic connections to both inferior frontal and parietal regions also make it an important relay station that could exert top-down control on other brain areas (9). Nevertheless, as is the case with the DLPFC, the imaging evidence for a contribution of the ACC to hysteria remains scarce, and further studies are needed to elucidate its precise role in hysteria.

FUNCTIONAL DISINTEGRATION

One should keep in mind that functional imaging can only be used in the study of hysteria in a meaningful way if relevant cognitive (or neurophysiologic) theories are available that can be tested. The current lack of such theories is perhaps understandable, but highlights the need for theoretic guidance in developing appropriate paradigms and, ultimately, explanations. Furthermore, all functional imaging studies performed on the topic thus far have only attempted to localize areas of dysfunction: They have refrained from trying to explore the neural circuits within which the pathophysiology underlying the functional disturbance is found. New functional imaging methods that allow measurements of the functional integration of different brain areas in terms of effective connectivity are likely to allow novel insights into the functional disturbances of the neural networks involved. As Friston (31) writes: "Functional specialization is only meaningful in the context of functional integration and vice versa." It is reasonable to assume that the functional disturbances underlying hysteria are reflected, if not indeed caused by, changes in the normal functional integration within the neural networks supporting action, perception, or memory. Accordingly, future investigations of hysteria using functional imaging should attempt to go beyond mere localization of "abnormal activation patterns" in two ways: (i) they should test specific hypotheses about the neuropsychological and psychosocial mechanisms involved in hysteria, and (ii) they should put more emphasis on assessing changes in functional connectivity within the neural networks that would normally support the brain functions which are disturbed in hysteria.

CONCLUSIONS

Surprisingly, there have been few attempts to investigate the neurophysiologic basis of hysterical symptoms and it is only in the last 10 years that empirical studies have begun to appear. Not only is the number of studies available small, but the results obtained in that small number are far from homogeneous. Nevertheless, the attempt to employ functional neuroimaging in the study of the neural mechanisms underlying hysteria is an important step forward in our attempts to understand hysteria and complements psychological studies: Functional imaging studies allow the direct testing of specific hypotheses regarding the functional and psychological disturbances underlying hysteria. The data available also suggest that important insights can also be gained from studying malingering, feigning, and other related disorders. In particular, the study of hypnosis-induced positive or negative symptoms may prove a valuable approach.

One should keep in mind, however, that the detection of functional disturbances using functional neuroimaging does not allow for a direct translation into the mechanisms *causing* hysteria. Furthermore, one cannot conclude from the detection of functional disturbances in the brain that hysterical symptoms have a solely "organic" origin; the distal cause of the disorder could be psychogenic (e.g., psychological stress), even if the proximal cause is pathophysiologic (e.g., overactivity of parts of the anterior cingulate cortex). Likewise, a psychogenic distal origin of the disorder does not mean that functionally disturbed neural processes cannot be detected. The little imaging data available strongly suggest that "psychogenic" and "neural" processes do not exclude each other (32).

One critical caveat, however, has to be considered when interpreting all functional imaging data of patients with hysterical symptoms: Weeks, months, or even years of protracted symptoms are themselves likely to result in changes in the central nervous system. All or some effects observed could thus simply reflect neural plasticity in response to the symptomatology [and recovery thereof, as in the cases of the study of Tiihonen et al. (6) and Vuilleumier et al. (10)]. The latter aspect also makes functional imaging a valuable tool in studying recovery from hysteria and evaluating therapeutic efforts. Crucially, larger numbers of patients need to be recruited if one really wants to make a large step forward in the neuroimaging of hysteria. A major shortcoming of all studies mentioned above is their limited number of patients.

In conclusion, the current literature on the neural mechanisms underlying hysteria remains preliminary. Nonetheless, the data consistently suggest that alterations in regional brain activity may accompany the expression of conversion symptoms. The mechanisms underlying these altered patterns of neural activations in hysteria remain to be further explored. New imaging techniques and new approaches to data analysis including the assessment of changes in effective connectivity, as well as studying larger numbers of patients, seem a prerequisite for making substantial progress toward a better understanding of the pathophysiology associated with hysteria. Most importantly, testable hypotheses about the neuropsychological and psychosocial mechanisms of hysteria are needed to constrain functional imaging experiments of impaired volition, sensorimotor control, and memory.

ACKNOWLEDGMENTS

J.C. Marshall was supported by the British Medical Research Council. G.R. Fink is supported by the Deutsche Forschungsgemeinschaft (KFO-112).

REFERENCES

1. Halligan PW, Bass C, Marshall JC, eds. *Contemporary approaches to the study of hysteria: clinical and theoretical perspectives.* Oxford: Oxford University Press, 2001.
2. Trimble MR. *Somatoform disorders. A medicolegal guide.* Cambridge, MA: Cambridge University Press, 2004.
3. Ron MA. Somatization and conversion disorders. In: Fogel BS, Schiffer RB, Rao SM, eds. *Neuropsychiatry.* Baltimore, MD: Williams & Wilkins, 1996.
4. Spence SA. Disorders of willed action. In: Halligan PW, Bass C, Marshall JC, eds. *Contemporary approaches to the study of hysteria.* Oxford: Oxford University Press, 2001.
5. Halligan PW, Bass C, Oakley DA. *Malingering and illness deception.* Oxford: Oxford University Press, 2003.
6. Tiihonen J, Kuikka J, Viinamäki H, et al. Altered cerebral blood flow during hysterical paresthesia. *Biol Psychiatry.* 1995;37:134–137.
7. Mailis-Gagnon A, Giannoylis I, Downar J, et al. Altered central somatosensory processing in chronic pain patients with "hysterical" anesthesia. *Neurology.* 2003;60:1501–1507.
8. Mailis A, Plalper P, Ashby P, et al. Effects of intravenous sodium amytal on cutaneous limb temperatures and sympathetic skin responses in normal subjects and pain patients with and without complex regional pain syndromes (type I and II). *Pain.* 1997;70:59–68.
9. Stephan KE, Marshall JC, Friston KJ, et al. Lateralized cognitive processes and lateralized task control in the human brain. *Science.* 2003;301:384–386.
10. Vuilleumier P, Chicherio C, Assal F, et al. Functional neuroanatomical correlates of hysterical sensorimotor loss. *Brain.* 2001;124:1077–1090.
11. Marshall JC, Halligan PW, Fink GR, et al. The functional anatomy of a hysterical paralysis. *Cognition.* 1997;64:B1–B8.
12. Vogt BA, Finch DM, Olson CR. Functional heterogeneity in cingulate cortex: the anterior executive and posterior evaluative regions. *Cereb Cortex.* 1992;2:435–443.
13. Spence SA, Crimlisk HL, Cope H, et al. Discrete neurophysiological correlates in prefrontal cortex during hysterical and feigned disorder of movement. *Lancet.* 2000;355:1243–1244.
14. Yazící K, Kostakoglu L. Cerebral blood flow changes in patients with conversion disorder. *Psychiatry Res Neuroimaging.* 1998;83:163–168.
15. Charcot JM. *Clinical lectures on diseases of the nervous system.* London: New Sydenham Society, 1889.
16. McConkey KM. Hysteria and hypnosis: cognitive and social influences. In: Halligan PW, Bass C, Marshall JC, eds. *Contemporary approaches to the study of hysteria.* Oxford: Oxford University Press, 2001.
17. Oakley DA. Hypnosis and conversion hysteria: a unifying model. *Cogn Neuropsychiatry.* 1999;4:243–265.
18. Halligan PW, Athwal BS, Oakley DA, et al. Imaging hypnotic paralysis: implications for conversion hysteria. *Lancet.* 2000;355:986–987.
19. Ward NS, Oakley DA, Frackowiak RSJ, et al. Differential brain activations during intentionally simulated and subjectively experienced paralysis. *Cogn Neuropsychiatry.* 2003;8:295–312.
20. Derbyshire SWG, Whalley MG, Stenger VA, et al. Cerebral activation during hypnotically induced and imagined pain. *Neuroimage.* 2004;23:392–401.
21. Markowitsch HJ, Fink GR, Thöne AIM, et al. Persistent psychogenic amnesia with a PET-proven organic basis. *Cogn Neuropsychiatry.* 1997;2:135–158.
22. Fink GR, Markowitsch HJ, Reinkemeier M, et al. Cerebral representation of one's own past: neural networks involved in autobiographical memory. *J Neurosci.* 1996;16:4275–4282.
23. Markowitsch HJ, Calabrese P, Fink GR, et al. Impaired episodic memory retrieval in a case of probable psychogenic amnesia. *Psychiatry Res Neuroimaging.* 1997;74:119–126.
24. Marshall JC, Fink GR. Cerebral localization, then and now. *Neuroimage.* 2003;20:S2–S7.
25. Freud S. Quelques considérations pour l'étude comparative des paralysies motrices organiques et hystériques. *Arch Neurol.* 1893;26:29–43.
26. Shallice T, Burgess P. The domain of supervisory processes and temporal organization of behaviour. *Philos Trans R Soc Lond B.* 1996;351:1404–1412.
27. Frith CD, Friston K, Liddle PF, et al. Willed action and the prefrontal cortex in man: a study with PET. *Proc R Soc Lond B.* 1991;244:241–246.
28. Dolan RJ, Bench CJ, Liddle PF. Dorsolateral prefrontal cortex dysfunction in the major psychoses; symptom or disease specificity? *J Neurol Neurosurg Psychiatry.* 1993;56:1290–1294.
29. Liddle PF, Friston KJ, Frith CD. Patterns of cerebral blood flow in schizophrenia. *Br J Psychiatry.* 1992;160:179–186.
30. Spence SA, Brooks DJ, Hirsch SR. A PET study of voluntary movement in schizophrenic patients experiencing passivity phenomena (delusions of alien control). *Brain.* 1997;120:1997–2011.
31. Friston KJ. Beyond phrenology: what can neuroimaging tell us about distributed circuitry? *Annu Rev Neurosci.* 2002;25:221–250.
32. Marshall JC, Gurd JM, Fink GR. Catatonia, motor neglect and hysterical paralysis: some similarities and differences. *Behav Brain Sci.* 2002;25:587–588.

Diagnostic Techniques

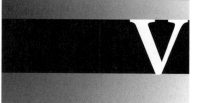

Hypnosis and Psychogenic Movement Disorders

27

John J. Barry

ABSTRACT

Many physicians have investigated hypnosis in the past for use in the diagnosis and treatment of movement disorders, especially those of psychogenic causation. The evolution of the use of hypnosis for this purpose is reviewed. The role of trauma and depression in the development of dissociative and, subsequently, movement disorders is reviewed. The physiologic basis of the hypnotic process is discussed. The use of hypnosis in the treatment of movement disorders is investigated. Probably the most researched use of hypnosis for the diagnosis and potential treatment of a movement disorder relates to its use in psychogenic nonepileptic seizures. The results of a study evaluating the use of hypnosis for this purpose are discussed as well. The unique advantages of this procedure over other suggestion techniques are examined.

INTRODUCTION

Hypnosis has had a long history, perhaps dating back to antiquity with Asclepian dream healing (1). In the modern era, the work of the 18th-century "healer" Franz Anton Mesmer represents the first introduction of a form of therapeutic intervention involving trance states. His work utilized the then current theory of an abnormal distribution of a "universal fluid." This fluid was believed to be redistributed by the use of magnetic energy. By the use of eye gaze and hand movements, Mesmer would re-equilibrate these fluids (2). Subjects eventually developed perceived involuntary behaviors that included convulsions, altered sensory and motor functioning, as well as other phenomena that were controlled by the magnetizer. Most of these patients were women and, interestingly, many of these behaviors developed before they were exposed to magnetism (1).

The Benjamin Franklin commission in 1784 discredited magnetism. In 1847, Braid developed a procedure called "monoideism." By the use of an induced trance state, the behavior of a receptive subject could be modulated. Braid attributed these phenomena to neural inhibition (3). Charcot continued this focus. He believed the hypnotic state contributed to neurophysiologic changes. In addition, he attributed susceptibility to the hypnotic state to mental dysfunction. This view was shared by Janet but opposed by Bernheim (4). Nevertheless, the association of hypnotic susceptibility with mental weakness has persisted to this day (1).

Behaviors that were originally attributed to possession and magnetism eventually began to be understood as manifestations of hysteria. In addition, the modern concepts of somatization and conversion were originally conceived of as expression of hysteria. It has been postulated that the development of the field of psychiatry as a new subdivision of medical specialties relied on the existence of hysteria as a unique disease entity (1).

In the middle of the 18th century, Pierre Briquet developed some of the fundamental concepts regarding conversion disorder. He conceptualized the components of this disorder as manifestations of a central nervous system dysfunction. In contrast, Russel Reynolds subsequently stressed the importance of psychological factors when considering conversion disorders (3).

In 1880, Freud and Breuer coined the term "conversion" to describe the clinical findings observed in their case of Anna O. The patient demonstrated a wide variety of somatic complaints including pseudocyesis. These symptoms were felt to be manifestations of unconscious conflicts (5). Hypnosis, learned through their work with Charcot, was pivotal in the treatment of Anna O. Furthermore, it was also a central concept in their published work, *Studies in Hysteria*, which appeared in 1895. Freud eventually abandoned hypnosis because of the "mysterious work behind hypnotism" and the possible problematic intensification of the transference process (4).

At this point in history, the hysteric was conceptualized as being ill rather than the victim of possession. Patients, most of whom were women, reported somatic illness consisting of convulsions, paralysis, and chronic pain. Their "illness" could also be explained in psychosocial terms with prominent primary (resolution of a psychic conflict) and secondary gain (accruing external benefits).

Charcot, along with Fredrick Myers and Gilles de la Tourette, introduced the concept of the fragmentation of psychic processes, so-called "dissociation." Janet emphasized the place of trauma in the development of memory fragmentation or dissociation. He also developed the concept of posttraumatic stress disorder (PTSD). Janet felt that the past experiences of a patient set up cognitive and emotional traces that predisposed to future dissociation of emotional experiences. He also noted that the trauma might be re-experienced in the form of flashbacks and behavioral re-enactments (6). This fragmentation of psychological experience could be understood as a manifestation of dissociation and is a critical component of the process of hypnosis. Additionally, such people as Simmel have utilized hypnosis to treat the psychological effects of trauma during World War II. It has also become a useful technique in the treatment of acute and chronic pain, anxiety disorders, weight control, smoking cessation, but most importantly, in the treatment of dissociative disorders in general and PTSD in particular (4). A further discussion of the history of hysteria has been documented elsewhere (7).

TRAUMA/POSTTRAUMATIC STRESS DISORDER

It appears that trauma and hysteria share a common etiology. Trauma appears to have a significant effect on the central nervous system. The pleomorphic physiologic effects of trauma on the nervous system suggest a possible neurobiologic phenomenon associated with hysteria. Van der Kolk (8) has reviewed the psychobiologic effects of trauma. These include psychophysiologic and neurohormonal fluctuations in levels of norepinephrine, glucocorticoid, serotonin, and endogenous opioids. In addition, trauma may induce neuroanatomic changes with its primary effects on hippocampal volume, amygdala activation, and right-hemispheric activation (8).

Trauma can also have profound effects on the motor system. This observation was noted in soldiers suffering the effects of continued stress. They were found to show evidence of tremors, hyperkinesis, excessive startle, and mutism (9). Patients, who have experienced trauma from any cause, especially in childhood, may be especially prone to the later development of abnormal motor movements under repeated stress. In addition, some authors (10) have emphasized the association of depression in the etiology of somatization. These proclivities may represent a fundamental biologic substrate and be particularly relevant to the phenomenon of nonepileptic seizures. However, others have questioned the validity of the causative link between trauma and PTSD. These issues have been discussed by Trimble (11).

HYPNOSIS: GENERAL COMMENTS

Hypnosis can be considered to consist of three primary components (4). The first, absorption, is the ability of participants to focus their attention while partially excluding awareness of peripheral events. The second, dissociation, is complementary to absorption and is that state of the participant that separates or fragments perceptions or consciousness from the surrounding world. Information is processed in a variety of systems. With dissociation, one of these systems appears to be acting separately from awareness and influences affect, cognition, or behavior. Finally, suggestibility is the ability to listen and respond to information from the hypnotist with a suspension of critical evaluation (4).

Hypnotic ability has been measured by a variety of psychometric tools. The Stanford Hypnotic Suggestibility Scale has excellent test-retest reliability, but is rather lengthy and more suitable for research purposes. Other, more clinically useful scales include the Stanford Hypnotic Clinical Scale, the Stanford Profile Scales of Hypnotic Ability, and the Hypnotic Induction Profile (HIP) (2). Spiegel et al. (12) standardized the HIP on a clinical population and attempted to measure all three components of the hypnotic process as well as the degree of involuntariness experienced by the subject. Hypnotic ability appears to be both a trait and state phenomena. Hypnotizability varies slightly over time with a peak in late childhood and declining somewhat into adulthood. However, individual hypnotic potential appears to be relatively stable over time (4). This observation was quantified in a study reviewing 50 subjects evaluated over a period of 25 years. A statistically significant stability coefficient of 0.71 was found with a non-significant change in mean scores (13).

HYPNOSIS/DISSOCIATION/ PSYCHOPATHOLOGY

It has been postulated that hypnotic ability can be used to differentiate varying psychopathologic states. As a corollary to this, those states characterized by high levels of dissociation, for example, PTSD, would be expected to display high levels of hypnotizability. In contrast, pathologic states like schizophrenia, where ability to focus and maintain attention is impaired, would be expected to have lower levels of hypnotizability (14). Frischholz et al. (15) evaluated this concept. They confirmed these expectations and found that higher hypnotic scores on the HIP and the Stanford Hypnotic Susceptability Scale Form C were found in those patients diagnosed with dissociative disorders and were lowest in those with schizophrenia. Patients with mood and anxiety disorders had intermediary scores (15). In a review of this issue, it was noted that controversy exists regarding the association of hypnotizability and psychopathology in general, but there appears to be agreement in respect to dissociative disorders (14).

An explanation of these findings focuses on the role of trauma, dissociation, and hypnotizability. It has been postulated that trauma, especially early in life, contributes to the persistent use of dissociation as a defense mechanism. The result of this method of processing experience is a fragmentation of the self to varying degrees. It would be expected that an individual who had a predilection to memory fragmentation would display a high level of dissociative ability. This, in fact, seems to be the case. Some researchers have even hypothesized a state of autohypnosis in those patients showing high levels of pathologic dissociation, that is, dissociative identity disorder (16).

As discussed earlier, Janet first discussed the interaction between trauma, both past and present, and dissociation. Recently, the roles of early childhood abuse and dissociation have been presented by several authors (17–19). In addition, trauma of other kinds has also been implicated, including those from combat (20), burn injury (21), and general acute stress (22). Causal links between self-reported trauma have been critically reviewed and questioned by others (23,24). It does appear, however, that people who have a premorbidly higher level of dissociability have a greater likelihood to develop PTSD with severe trauma (21,25).

HYPNOSIS AS A NEUROPHYSIOLOGIC PROCESS

The neurologic basis of hypnosis has been the subject of many studies. Hypnosis has no physiologic similarities to somnolence or sleep, despite the fact that *hypnos* in Greek refers to a sleep state. A particular electroencephalographic (EEG) signature for hypnosis has not been found (4), possibly because of contextual influences, that is, mood states (26). However, studies have suggested the presence of EEG changes in highly hypnotizable patients (27,28). In contrast to the EEG, event-related potentials (ERPs) may offer a more sensitive evaluation tool. ERPs may also be altered by the hypnotic state and appear to offer more characteristic physiologic changes. Patients who are highly hypnotizable have demonstrated specific psychophysiologic responses compared to those patients who have low hypnotizability (26,29,30). For example, more P300 alterations were seen in highly hypnotizable patients in response to positive obstructive and negative obliterating instructions than in poorly hypnotizable patients (26). These findings appear to lend credence to the trait conceptualization of hypnosis.

Finally, positron emission tomography (PET) has also been used to evaluate the physiologic basis of hypnosis. Two modes of investigation have been pursued. The first involves evaluating hypnosis as it is being used to alter other somatic states. Secondly, it has been evaluated independently in highly hypnotizable individuals.

Recent case studies lend credence to the concept of a common physiologic mechanism between hypnosis and hysteria, implicating the prefrontal region, dorsolateral, orbitofrontal, and anterior cingulate gyri (31,32).

In a study by Halligan et al. (31), the authors noted prior investigations implicating the frontal-limbic inhibitory areas as being involved in hysteria. The authors hypothesized that hypnotically activated paralysis would activate similar areas as those seen in a patient with a hysterical movement dysfunction. The right orbitofrontal and anterior cingulate regions were activated in both clinical situations.

Pain can also be modulated by hypnosis. PET studies performed during unpleasant stimuli ameliorated by hypnosis again show the same primacy of activity in the anterior cingulate (33,34). Auditory hallucinations induced in highly hypnotizable subjects also showed activation of the right anterior cingulate (35).

Two studies by Rainville et al. (36) evaluated the physiologic effects of PET in differing stages of the hypnotic process, that is, relaxation, absorption, and suggestion. The hypnotic state appeared to be characterized by activation in the anterior cingulate, and the intralaminar and mediodorsal nuclei of the thalamus. Furthermore, the right inferior frontal gyrus and the right inferior parietal lobe were activated in the state of absorption. The authors postulated an "executive attentional network" that was important in the development of the hypnotic state. In addition, hypnosis coupled with suggestion resulted in increased activity of the frontal cortices, especially on the left side, with medial and lateral posterior parietal cortical augmentations of regional cerebral blood flow (37). The prominent role of the anterior cingulate in hypnosis is not surprising, given its apparent role as a gating mechanism in both affect and cognition (38). The cingulate appears to be connected to other important anatomic regions including the amygdala, ventral striatum, orbitofrontal and anterior insular cortices, and periaqueductal grey that appear to be critical in the development of motivation, assessing stimuli, and in the regulation of behavior (39). A recent review (40) of functional imaging in the evaluation of conversion hysteria appears to confirm the apparent importance of the cingulate as well as the prefrontal cortex. The hypothesis that there may be corticofugal inhibition of somatosensory processing in patients with hysterical somatic symptoms was offered as one explanation of the findings. Other investigators have pointed to a biologic disconnection between somatic symptoms and awareness in these patients (40).

HYPNOSIS AND MOVEMENT DISORDERS

Hypnosis has been utilized to treat both physiologically and psychologically mediated movement disorders. Hypnotherapy has had documented efficacy in a therapeutic intervention for Gilles de la Tourette syndrome. A case study described a situation where tics and vocalizations were greatly ameliorated after 6 months of progressive relaxation induced via hypnosis (41). Similar case histories have been presented for patients with parkinsonian tremor (42) and for the physical and psychological effects of Hunington disease (43). Hypnosis has also been used effectively as an auxillary treatment in 14 hemiparetic patients with significant motor improvement (44). In addition, Rosenberg (45) reported a case of hypnosis induced elimination of a rhythmic movement sleep disorder and reviewed other sleep disorders where hypnosis resulted in a successful outcome. Hypnosis has been utilized in the treatment of movement disorders where psychological features may play an important role. Spasmodic torticollis is an example of such a movement disorder (46) and five case reports have documented the utility of hypnosis for desensitization and the eventual retraining of affected muscles (37,47,48).

USE OF HYPNOSIS IN PATIENTS WITH PSYCHOGENIC NONEPILEPTIC SEIZURES

Hypnosis has been most extensively studied in the diagnosis and possible treatment of psychogenic movement disorders. Andries Hoek used hypnotherapy in 1838 to treat one of his patients with "madness" consisting of amnesia, hallucinations, depression, and "pseudoepileptic seizures" (49).

Charcot used the term "hysteroepilepsy" to describe patients with psychogenic nonepileptic seizures (PNES). He also developed a technique of ovarian compression to treat these patients (50). It is interesting to note that many of these individuals, mostly women, had been traumatized in their lifetimes. The following figure is from Charcot's text, *Lectures on the Diseases of the Nervous System* (51). The depiction is of a woman with attacks in which she "is a prey to delirium, and raves evidently of the events which seem to have determined her first seizures. She hurls furious invectives against imaginary individuals, crying out, 'villains! robbers! brigands! fire! fire! O, the dogs! I'm bitten!'—reminiscences, doubtless, of the emotions experienced in her youth. . . . Compression of the ovary, in this case, is almost void of effect upon the convulsion." (51). It is also interesting to note that many of these women demonstrated their "illness" for visiting dignitaries and were often taken off the street and supported for extended periods of time. Certainly, significant elements of secondary gain were likely (Fig. 27.1).

PNES can be defined as episodic behaviors or sensations that resemble epileptic events but that are not associated with the abnormal electrical central nervous system discharges seen in people with epilepsy (52). The incidence of this disorder has been estimated at 2–33 per 100,000, but may be higher in select populations with 5% to 20% of patients referred to outpatient epilepsy clinics and diagnosed with PNES (53). Patients with epilepsy may also display features of PNES in from 3.6% to 58.8% when evaluated in comprehensive epilepsy centers with methodological differences possibly explaining the wide range (53). In addition, not only is the diagnosis of PNES often missed, but the misuse of antiepileptic drugs, episodes of pseudostatus epilepticus and the assumption of a chronically ill identity increase the morbidity and possible mortality from the disorder (54,55). The need for a sensitive and specific diagnostic technique is compelling.

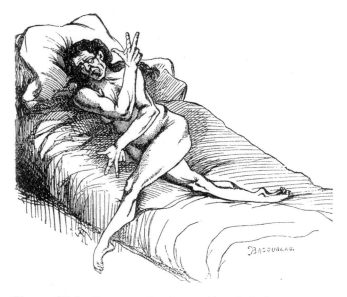

Figure 27.1 Hystero-epileptic attack; period of contortions. (Drawn by M. Richer from a sketch made by M. Charcot.)

Patients with PNES have been divided into five groups. First are those patients who exhibit convulsive symptoms because of inadequate coping strategies. These patients use PNES to galvanize attention to themselves and their distress. Secondly, there are those patients that embellish their physiologic symptoms with psychogenic ones. This group may also have physiologic epilepsy. The third group consists of those patients who are psychotic, and the forth those whose physical symptoms are misinterpreted. Finally, the fifth and most common subset consists of the emotional conflict group in whom unconscious psychological issues are manifested as physical dysfunction (56). It is this final category that is the topic of this discussion.

The utility of hypnosis in this population is not surprising, given the historical and clinical signs that are suggestive of the disorder. A history of physical or sexual abuse and induction by suggestion has been noted by Rowan (55) as characteristic. In addition, Bowman et al (57) in their evaluation of 45 patients with PNES have presented associated psychiatric diagnosis using the *Diagnostic and Statistical Manual of Mental Disorders*, Third Edition, Revised (DSM-III-R), criteria. They found affective illness past or present in 98% with most of these being a Major Depressive Disorder (80%). A lifetime history of PTSD was seen in 58% with a history of trauma seen in 84%. Finally, dissociative disorders were currently present in 91%. Given the incidence of trauma and dissociation, plus the level of suggestibility of this patient population, hypnosis would be expected to be a useful intervention.

There are primarily three suggestion techniques that have been reported to be useful for the diagnosis of PNES. Walczak et al. (58) evaluated 68 patients using the saline placebo infusion method. There were 40 patients with PNES in the study and 82% of them had one of their typical events induced by the procedure while being monitored under video-EEG. In two of the patients with epilepsy, physiologic seizures were induced. The sensitivity of the procedure was 82% and the specificity was 92%. In another study by Lancman et al. (59), the alcohol patch technique was utilized. In this procedure, the patient is informed that the application of the alcohol patch to the patient's neck may stimulate an event. In this study, 93 patients with PNES and 20 with epileptic events (EE) were evaluated. A sensitivity of 77.4% and a specificity of 100% were obtained.

Stagno et al. (60) and Devinsky and Fisher (61) have discussed the ethical considerations of both of these procedures. Although Walczak et al. (62) reported no long-term negative effects in their study, psychogenic status epilepticus has been induced by a provocative procedure, that is, saline infusion (63). With hypnosis, the technique and its purpose are completely explained to the patient.

Peterson et al. (64) first investigated the use of hypnosis in the diagnosis of patients with PNES in 1950. The authors postulated that patients with PNES would remember the specifics of their seizures in contrast to those patients with EE. There were 35 patients with PNES and 30 with EE who were hypnotized. In only those patients with PNES could specific details of their "seizures" be recalled. Schwartz (65) followed this investigation in 1955 by utilizing hypnosis to induce typical "seizures" under EEG monitoring. There were 26 patients who were entered into the study and only the ten patients diagnosed with PNES had a successful induction of a typical event.

Given the frequency of PNES and the need for a reliable and valid diagnostic intervention, plus the apparent utility both theoretically and in preliminary studies, a re-evaluation of hypnosis for this purpose was undertaken. The Hypnotic Induction Profile (HIP) was utilized because of its ease of administration and clinical utility (12). A description of the test itself is listed in Table 27.1 and was originally developed by Spiegel H and Spiegel D (12). The eye roll is a hypothesized measure of the biologic capacity of the patient to experience hypnosis. As noted previously, HIP scores have been shown in other studies to correlate well with levels of dissociability and differing psychopathologic states.

After the HIP score is obtained, the patient is then hypnotized again and a split screen technique is utilized as outlined in Table 27.2.

TABLE 27.1
HYPNOTIC INDUCTION PROFILE

Measure of hypnotizability.
Combines a measure of the patient's innate ability to be hypnotized, as measured by the eye-roll sign, with a measure of hypnotic expression, the induction score.
Scores range from 0 (no hypnotizability) to a maximum of 10.
A profile score is obtained which shows the patient's response pattern to the induction and represents the relationship between the patient's innate ability to be hypnotized and the actual level of hypnosis achieved by the test.

Adapted from Barry JJ, Atzmon O. Use of hypnosis to differentiate epileptic from nonepileptic events. In: Gates JR, Rowan JA, eds. *Nonepileptic seizures*. Boston, MA: Butterworth-Heineman, 2000:285–304.

TABLE 27.2
HYPNOSIS AND SEIZURE INDUCTION

Patient is hypnotized and taught self-relaxation.

Split-screen technique is used (visualize the word "relax" on the left side of the screen and "seizure" on the right).

Patients begin by focusing on the left side of the screen and imagining a relaxed and safe scene that is special for them.

The patient is then asked to shift to the other side of the screen and to recall their last seizure, and the extent of memory for that event is determined.

They are then asked to imagine themselves merging with the image on the screen and idiosyncratic, characteristic aspects of their events are suggested to them, if necessary.

Seizure induction ensues.

Patients are taught the technique and can often self-induce and terminate their PNES.

PNES, psychogenic nonepileptic seizures.
Adapted from Barry JJ, Atzmon O. Use of hypnosis to differentiate epileptic from nonepileptic events. In: Gates JR, Rowan JA, eds. *Nonepileptic seizures.* Boston, MA: Butterworth-Heineman, 2000:285–304.

Eighty-two patients seen in the Stanford Comprehensive Epilepsy center were evaluated with 69 patients meeting criteria for the study. Twenty-two patients had localization-related epilepsy (67). Thirty-six patients had PNES alone, while 11 patients had both PNES and NES. The results of the study are listed in Table 27.3.

It should be noted that there was one patient in this study who had an event during the hypnosis exercise. However, the patient was not hypnotizable, had several seizures the day the test was done, and repeat attempts at induction were not successful. In addition, she presented with a decrement profile indicative of the potential for hypnosis but without successful induction. Since a seizure occurred during the hypnosis exercise, induction could not be ruled out, thus, the specificity of the procedure was calculated at 95%.

HIP scores themselves were statistically different between those patients with EE and PNES only when all of the PNES patients were grouped together. The sensitivity of 77% with a specificity of at least 95% confirms the utility of hypnosis as a valid diagnostic technique. Additionally, hypnosis can also be used as a treatment modality, as well (68). Thus, hypnosis offers a viable alternative to other interventions like the alcohol patch and saline infusion techniques which employ suggestion in the diagnosis of PNES. It also offers distinct advantages, as well. Patients can be taught the procedure and can use the technique to occasionally resolve or more frequently modulate their disorder. It also fosters the therapeutic alliance so pivotal in establishing the groundwork for the psychotherapeutic process.

TABLE 27.3
HIP AND DIAGNOSIS BY SEIZURE INDUCTION

| Group | No. | Hypnotic Induction Profile scores | | Sensitivity | Specificity |
		Mean	SD		
EE	22	5.18[a,b]	3.31	—	—
NEE	36	6.80[a]	3.14	—	—
EE/NEE	11	6.92[a]	1.99	—	—
NEE + EE/NEE	47	6.83[b]	2.87	—	—
All patients	69	—	—	77%	95%

EE, epileptic events; NEE, nonepileptic events.
[a]Means are not different statistically ($p = 0.117$).
[b]Means are statistically significant ($p = 0.038$).

CONCLUSIONS

The purpose of this review was to explore the utility of hypnosis to diagnose and treat movement disorders, especially those with a psychogenic basis. The history of hypnosis starting with Mesmer, Charcot, Freud, and Janet have been discussed. The evolution of the concept of hysteria from possession/exorcism and magnetism was reviewed. In addition, the role of PTSD in the development of psychogenic movement disorders and perhaps the pathophysiologic basis of the disorder was also presented. The physiologic basis of hypnosis was reviewed as well, especially related to recent literature using PET scans. Hypnosis, as it is used currently, was defined. Differing hypnotic processes were reviewed generally, with one of the most clinically useful, the HIP, discussed in detail.

Finally the use of hypnosis for movement disorders was explored. Probably the most well-documented use of suggestion techniques in the diagnosis of movement disorders has been in the evaluation of PNES. The HIP and the use of a split-screen technique under hypnosis were evaluated and reviewed. With a sensitivity of 77% and a specificity of 95%, hypnosis can be a useful diagnostic technique in the investigation of patients with movement disorders that suggest an epileptic versus a psychogenic cause.

REFERENCES

1. Spanos NP, Chaves JF. History and historiography of hypnosis. In: Lynn SJ, Rhue JW, eds. *Theories of hypnosis—current models and perspectives.* New York: The Guilford Press, 1991:43–78.
2. Raz A, Shapiro T. Hypnosis and neuroscience: a cross talk between clinical and cognitive research. *Arch Gen Psychiatry* 2002;59(1): 85–90.
3. Guggenheim FG. Somatoform disorders. In: Sadock BJ, Sadock VA, eds. *Comprehensive textbook of psychiatry.* New York: Lippincott Williams & Wilkins, 2000:1504–1532.
4. Spiegel H, Greenleaf M, Spiegel D. Hypnosis. In: Sadock BJ, Sadock VA, eds. *Comprehensive textbook of psychiatry.* New York: Lippincott Williams & Wilkins, 2000:2128–2145.
5. Gabbard GO. Psychoanalysis. In: Sadock BJ, Sadock VA, eds. *Comprehensive textbook of psychiatry.* New York: Lippincott Williams & Wilkins, 2000:563–607.
6. van der Kolk BA, van der Hart O, Marmar CR. Dissociation and information processing in posttraumatic stress disorder. In: van der Kolk BA, McFarlane AC, Weisaeth L, eds. *Traumatic stress—the effects of overwhelming experience on mind, body, and society.* New York: The Guilford Press, 1996:303–327.
7. Trimble M. *Historical overview. Somatoform disorders a medicolegal guide.* Cambridge, MA: Cambridge University Press, 2004:1–20.
8. van der Kolk BA. The body keeps the score: approaches to the psychobiology of posttraumatic stress disorder. In: van der Kolk BA, McFarlane AC, Weisaeth L, eds. *Traumatic stress—the effects of overwhelming experience on mind, body, and society.* New York: The Guilford Press, 1996:242–278.
9. Kardiner A, Spiegel H. *War stress and neurotic illness.* New York: Paul B. Hoeber, Inc, 1947:428.
10. Katon W, Kleinman A, Rosen G. Depression and somatization: a review—Part 1. *Am J Med.* 1982;72:127–135.
11. Trimble M. Mechanisms. *Somatoform disorders a medicolegal guide.* Cambridge: Cambridge University Press, 2004:197–219.
12. Spiegel H, Spiegel D. *Trance and treatment.* New York: Basic Books Inc, 1978.
13. Piccione C, Hilgard ER, Zimbardo PG. On the degree of stability of measured hypnotizability over a 25-year period. *J Pers Soc Psychol.* 1989;56(2):289–295.
14. Nash MR. Hypnosis, psychopathology, and psychological regression. In: Fromm E, Nash MR, eds. *Contemporary hypnosis research.* New York: The Guilford Press, 1992:149–172.
15. Frischholz EJ, Lipman LS, Braun BG, et al. Psychopathology, hypnotizability, and dissociation. *Am J Psychiatry.* 1992;149(11): 1521–1525.
16. Butler LD, Duran REF, Jasiukaitis P, et al. Hypnotizability and traumatic experience: a diathesis-stress model of dissociative symptomatology. *Am J Psychiatry.* 1996;153(7):42–63.
17. Ganaway GK. Hypnosis, childhood trauma, and dissociative identity disorder. *Int J Clin Exp Hypn.* 1995;53(2):127–144.
18. Chu JA, Ganzel BL, Matthews JA. Memories of childhood abuse: dissociation, amnesia, and corroboration. *Am J Psychiatry.* 1999; 156(5):749–755.
19. Roelofs K, Keijsers GPF, Hoogduin KAL, et al. Childhood abuse in patients with conversion disorder. *Am J Psychiatry.* 2002; 159(11):1908–1913.
20. Brown P, van der Hart O, Graafland M. Trauma-induced dissociative amnesia in World War I combat soldiers. II. Treatment dimensions. *Aust N Z J Psychiatry.* 1999;33:392–398.
21. DuHamel KN, Difede J, Foley F, et al. Hypnotizability and trauma symptoms after burn injury. *Int J Clin Exp Hypn.* 2002; 50(1):33–50.
22. Bryant RA, Guthrie RM, Moulds ML. Hypnotizability in acute stress disorder. *Am J Psychiatry.* 2001;158:600–604.
23. Merckelbach H, Muris P. The causal link between self-reported trauma and dissociation: a critical review. *Behav Res Ther.* 2001; 39:245–254.
24. Frankel FH. Dissociation: the clinical realities. *Am J Psychiatry.* 1996;153(7):64–70.
25. Spiegel D, Cardena E. New uses of hypnosis in the treatment of posttraumatic stress disorder. *J Clin Psychiatry.* 1990;51(10): 39–46.
26. Jensen SM, Barabasz A, Barabasz M, et al. EEG P300 event-related markers of hypnosis. *Am J Clin Hypn.* 2001;44(2): 127–139.
27. Sabourin ME, Cutcomb SD, Crawford HJ, et al. EEG correlates of hypnotic susceptibility and hypnotic trance: spectral analysis and coherence. *Int J Psychophysiol.* 1990;10(2):125–142.
28. Williams JD, Gruzelier JH. Differentiation of hypnosis and relaxation by analysis of narrow band theta and alpha frequencies. *Int J Clin Exp Hypn.* 2001;49(3):185–206.
29. De Pascalis V, Carboni G. P300 event-related-potential amplitudes and evoked cardiac reponses during hypnotic alteration of somatosensory perception. *Int J Neurosci.* 1997;92(3–4):187–208.
30. Barabasz A, Barabasz M, Jensen S, et al. Cortical event-related potentials show the structure of hypnotic suggestions is crucial. *Int J Clin Exp Hypn.* 1999;47(1):5–22.
31. Halligan PW, Athwal BS, Oakley DA, et al. Imagining hypnotic paralysis: implications for conversion hysteria. *Lancet.* 2000;355: 986–987.
32. Marshall JC, Halligan PW, Fink GR, et al. The functional anatomy of a hysterical paralysis. *Cognition.* 1997;64:B1–B8.
33. Faymonville ME, Laureys S, Degueldre C, et al. Neural mechanisms of antinociceptive effects of hypnosis. *Anesthesiology.* 2000;92: 1257–1267.
34. Rainville P, Duncan GH, Price DD, et al. Pain affect encoded in human anterior cingulat but not somatosenory cortex. *Science.* 1997;277:968–971.
35. Szechtman H, Woody E, Bowers KS, et al. Where the imaginal appears real: a positron emission tomography study of auditory hallucinations. *Proc Natl Acad Sci.* 1998;95:1956–1960.
36. Rainville P, Bushnell MC. Hypnosis modulates activity in brain structures involved in the regulation of consciousness. *J Cogn Neurosci.* 2002;14:887–901.
37. Rainville P, Hofbauer RK, Paus T, et al. Cerebral mechanisms of hypnotic induction and suggestion. *J Cogn Neurosci.* 1999;11: 110–125.
38. Mayberg HS. Limbic-cortical dysregulation: a proposed model of depression. *J Neuropsychiatry Clin Neurosci.* 1997;9:471–481.

39. Devinsky O, Morrell MJ, Vogt BA. Contributions of anterior cingulate cortex to behavior. *Brain.* 1995;118:279–306.

40. Black DN, Taber KH, Hurley RA. Conversion hysteria: lessions from functional imaging. *J Neuropsychiatry Clin Neurosci.* 2004; 16(3):246–251.

41. Culbertson FM. A four-step hypnotherapy model for Gilles de la Tourette's syndrome. *Am J Clin Hypn.* 1989;31(4):252–256.

42. Wain HJ, Amen D, Jabbari B. The effects of hypnosis on a parkinsonian tremor: case report with polygraph/EEG recordings. *Am J Clin Hypn.* 1990;33(2):94–98.

43. Witz M, Kahn S. Hypnosis and the treatment of Huntington's disease. *Am J Clin Hypn.* 1991;34(2):79–90.

44. Radil T, Snydrova L, Hacik L, et al. Attempts to influence movement disorders in hemiparetics. *Scand Rehabil Med Suppl.* 1988; 17:157–161.

45. Rosenberg C. Elimination of a rhythmic movement disorder with hypnosis-a case report. *Sleep.* 1995;18(7):608–609.

46. Smith DL, DeMario MC. Spasmodic torticollis: a case report and review of therapies. *J Am Board Fam Pract.* 1996;9(6):435–441.

47. Schneiderman MJ, Leu RH, Glazeski RC. Use of hypnosis in spasmotic torticollis: a case report. *Am J Clin Hypn.* 1987;29(4): 260–263.

48. De Benedittis G. Hypnosis and spasmotic torticollis-report of four cases: a brief communication. *Int J Clin Exp Hypn.* 1996; 44(4):292–306.

49. van der Hart O, van der Velden K. The hypnotherapy of Dr. Andries Hoek: uncovering hypnotherapy before Janet, Breuer, and Freud. *Am J Clin Hypn.* 1987;4:264–271.

50. Ramani V. Review of psychiatric treatment strategies in nonepileptic seizures. In: Gates JR, Rowan AJ, eds. *Nonepileptic seizures.* Boston, MA: Butterworth-Heineman, 2000:259–267.

51. Charcot JM. *Lectures on the diseases of the nervous system.* Vol. 1. London: The Classics of Medicine Library, 1877:281.

52. Krumholz A. Nonepileptic seizures: diagnosis and management. *Neurology.* 1999;53:S76–S83.

53. Gates JR. Epidemiology and classification of nonepileptic events. In: Gates JR, Rowan JA, eds. *Nonepileptic seizures.* Boston, MA: Butterworth-Heineman, 2000.

54. King DW, Gallagher BB, Murvin AJ, et al. Pseudoseizures: diagnostic evaluation. *Neurology.* 1982;32:749–752.

55. Rowan AJ. Diagnosis of nonepileptic seizures. In: Gates JR, Rowan AJ, eds. *Nonepileptic seizures.* Boston, MA: Butterworth-Heineman, 2000:15–30.

56. Gates JR, Erdahl P. Classification of nonepileptic seizures. In: Rowan JA, Gates JR, eds. *Nonepileptic seizures.* Boston, MA: Butterworth-Heineman, 1993:21–30.

57. Bowman ES, Markland ON. Psychodynamics and psychiatric diagnoses of pseudoseizure subjects. *Am J Psychiatry.* 1996;153: 57–63.

58. Walczak TS, Williams DT, Berten W. Utility and reliability of placebo infusion in the evaluation of patients with seizures. *Neurology.* 1994;44:394–399.

59. Lancman ME, Asconape JJ, Craven WJ, et al. Predictive value of induction of psychogenic seizures by suggestion. *Ann Neurol.* 1994;35:359–361.

60. Stagno SJ, Smith ML. The use of placebo in diagnosing psychogenic seizures: who is being deceived. *Semin Neurol.* 1997; 17(3):213–218.

61. Devinsky O, Fisher R. Ethical use of placebos and provocative testing in diagnosing nonepileptic seizures. *Neurology.* 1996;47: 866–870.

62. Walczak TS, Papacostas S, Williams DT, et al. Outcome after diagnosis of psychogenic nonepileptic seizures. *Epilepsia.* 1995; 36:1131–1137.

63. Ney GC, Zimmerman C, Schaul N. Psychogenic status epilepticus induced by a provocative technique. *Neurology.* 1996;46: 546–547.

64. Peterson DB, Sumner JW, Jones GA. Role of hypnosis in differentiation of epileptic from convulsive like seizures. *Am J Psychiatry.* 1950;107:428–432.

65. Schwartz BE, Bickford RG, Rasmussen WC. Hypnotic phenomena, including hypnotic activated seizures, studied with electroencephalogram. *J Nerv Ment Dis.* 1955;122:564–574.

66. Barry JJ, Atzmon O. Use of hypnosis to differentiate epileptic from nonepileptic events. In: Gates JR, Rowan JA, eds. *Nonepileptic seizures.* Boston, MA: Butterworth-Heineman, 2000:285–304.

67. Barry JJ, Atzmon O, Morrell MJ. Discriminating between epileptic and nonepileptic events: the utility of hypnotic seizure induction. *Epilepsia.* 2000;41(1):81–84.

68. Bush E, Barry JJ, Spiegel D, et al. The successful treatment of pseudoseizures with hypnosis. *Epilepsia.* 1992;33:135.

The Sodium Amytal and Benzodiazepine Interview and Its Possible Application in Psychogenic Movement Disorders

28

Susanne A. Schneider   *Kailash P. Bhatia*

ABSTRACT

Sodium amytal, a medium-acting barbiturate, was first described in 1861. Since then it has been popular for its effectiveness in facilitating diagnostic and therapeutic interviewing, and we have reviewed its use here. Early studies that found particular utility in catatonia mainly focused on the responses of psychiatric patients. Amytal has also been found to be useful in conversion reactions, including those manifesting as movement disorders. Beneficial effects in posttraumatic torticollis and amelioration of posture and pain have been demonstrated. Furthermore, sodium amytal can help to differentiate conversion disorder from malingering and factitious behavior.

Combining the amytal interview with the use of video feedback was reported to lead to full recovery and a restoration of lost body function, and may be a useful tool in movement disorder patients.

Overall, sodium amytal is a relatively safe and useful drug facilitating diagnostic and therapeutic interviewing. However, there is a relative paucity of studies for the use in psychogenic movement disorders. Further studies including controlled investigations are needed. The amytal or benzodiazepine interview may also be a useful tool to increase our understanding of the pathophysiology of psychogenic movement disorders.

INTRODUCTION

As far back as 1861, Griesinger had described notable improvements in psychotic states after narcotic- or anesthetic-induced sleep (1,2). The synthesis of sodium amytal, a medium-acting barbiturate, by Schonle and Moment in 1923 led to the facilitation of diagnostic and therapeutic interviewing (2,3).

In 1930, Bleckwenn first reported the use of sodium amytal to produce "sleep and physical rest in psychotic patients" (4,5). In order to "break down the stubborn insomnia of the more severe psychoses" and to "simplify the management and materially shorten the course of the illness," he administered repeated injections of sodium amytal by means of general anesthesia to the patients (6,7). He noticed "a lucid interval for 1 to 2 minutes before the patient fell asleep" during which the patient "was rational and had complete insight into his condition" (2). Barbiturates have a sedating effect, and sodium amytal became the drug of choice to assist interviewing due to its rapid induction time and the elicited effect of released speech. These initial observations led to the practice of the use of sodium amytal for both diagnostic and therapeutic interviewing for over 75 years.

In the early 1960s, the recognition of barbiturate dependency and the introduction of alternative drugs like benzodiazepines, however, led to a decline in the use of amytal. In recent years, there has been fresh interest in amytal interviewing as a tool in clinical practice. Beneficial diagnostic use and successful treatment of conversion disorders, especially those with movement disorders like abnormal or fixed postures, have been described. Videotaping of amytal interviews has become possible and, in fact, is recommended, as such videos can be used as feedback in following sessions. They give evidence to the patient of the ability to move fixed or paralyzed body parts and may help to improve such symptoms.

Thus, amytal-assisted interviews may have a role in the diagnosis and therapy of psychogenic movement disorders. In this review, we will look at the historical aspects, method of use, and suggested clinical indications for amytal/benzodiazepine-assisted interviews and also review the aspect of its potential use for psychogenic movement disorders.

HISTORICAL ASPECTS

Following Bleckwenn mentioned above (4,5), Lindemann used subanesthetic doses of amytal to promote self-disclosure in both normal and abnormal individuals (8). He was the first to demonstrate possible benefits of the interview in a nonpsychotic population, as well (8,9). In 1935, an influential study by Thorner described the beneficial effects of sodium amytal in catatonia (10). He studied 18 patients, ten of whom, previously mute, began talking.

Waxy flexibility (cerea flexibilitas) was successfully ameliorated in all five affected cases. Twelve of 14 patients with previously compromised eating and nourishment "requested food and ate ravenously."

The event of World War II led to a marked increase in the use of sodium amytal. Battle traumatized soldiers would develop a variety of neurotic symptoms to escape the rigors of trench warfare. At this time, Horsely (1936) introduced a new technique termed "narcoanalysis." This defined a popular seven-stage procedure used to treat acute, traumatic neuroses (7,11). Retrieval and reintegration of "repressed memories" were achieved. In 1945, Grinker and Spiegel carried the work further. They used "narcosynthesis" to encourage "abreaction"—the free expression and release of previously repressed emotion (2,12). They outlined the importance of an early beginning with treatment before symptoms became fixed (9). At the technique's peak in popularity in 1949, Tilkin enthusiastically described "the future of narcosynthesis [as] infinite and possibilities [being] endless" (2,13). Narcosuggestion (14) and narcocatharsis were other new terms to make their appearance at that time.

One dubious application included the use of sodium amytal as a so-called "truth serum" for interviewing suspected criminals and also for prediction of response to electroconvulsive therapy (ECT) in schizophrenia (15).

By the 1960s, however, the use of sodium amytal started to wane due to a number of reasons. First, the risk of barbiturate dependency was increasingly recognized. Second, the appearance of new drugs, specifically neuroleptics like chlorpromazine in 1952 to treat catatonic schizophrenia or psychosis had a major effect on the decline in the use of sodium amytal interviewing (2). In addition, tricyclic antidepressants became available. Concurrently, benzodiazepines as safer alternative drugs to sodium amytal were introduced in those cases that needed it. Benzodiazepines were suggested as the preferred agent due to their possible reversibility by the GABA antagonist flumazenil and their broader therapeutic index.

CHEMICAL AND PHARMACOLOGIC PROFILE

Sodium amytal is a medium-acting barbiturate. Other names are amobarbital and isoamylethylbarbiturate. Chemically, amytal is 5-ethyl-5-(3-methylbutyl) barbituric acid or 5-ethyl-5-(3-methylbutyl)-2,4,6(1H,3H,5H)-pyrimidinetrione (16) (Fig. 28.1). As a consequence of their lipophilic chemical structure, barbiturates reach the brain quickly and need to be titrated carefully. As a medium-acting agent, amytal sedates more gradually; on the other hand, narcosis is more persistent (17). It depresses the cerebral cortex leading to changes in social behavior and intellectual operations (17). Due to this suppression of

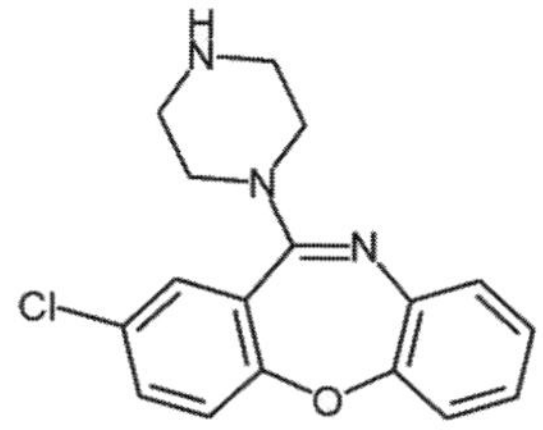

Figure 28.1 Amytal/Amobarbital

higher functions, the subject becomes less observant and more suggestible.

STUDIES AND SUGGESTED INDICATIONS FOR AMYTAL INTERVIEWS

Most of the early studies were either open-label or had relatively few cases, and there was a relative paucity of controlled studies focusing on sodium amytal interviewing. It was not until the 1960s that the first controlled studies to evaluate the usefulness of sodium amytal were attempted. Kavirajan, in a detailed review, analyzed the literature on the therapeutic and diagnostic studies using sodium amytal (15), and we will document some of the main findings below. In 1954, Weinstein and Malitz asserted the expediency of sodium amytal to identify organic brain injury, where it would cause disorientation and denial of illness, which would not occur in healthy subjects (15,18).

Around the same time, in a placebo-controlled trial, Shagass studied and outlined the usefulness of sodium amytal interviewing to differentiate between neurotic and psychotic depression, anxiety, schizophrenia, organic psychosis, and hysteria (19). He based his conclusions on the observation of the "sedation threshold" which defined the dose at which an individual manifested speech changes and specific EEG abnormalities (15,19).

Also, several controlled studies for catatonia were attempted, some of which had a favorable conclusion (20,21). Elkes observed increased accessibility, mobilization, and speech in catatonic patients who were given sodium amytal (20). Elkes also noted that saline in controls did not lead to a response. In contrast, Dysken published a more sceptical study in 1979 regarding the effects and utility of the amytal interview (22,23). In a placebo-controlled clinical trial, where subjects acted as their own controls, he investigated the diagnostic role in acute psychotic patients. Dysken perceived both the drug and the placebo to be clinically useful. He found no significant superiority of amytal over placebo in promoting disclosure of diagnostically useful information (23). Dysken was uncertain to what extent the benefit was a specific pharmacologic effect of sodium amytal or the result of the patient's expectation that a special drug would facilitate talking. In

conclusion, his findings would argue against widespread use of sodium amytal as a diagnostic tool in psychiatric illness (15). On the whole, various studies regarding catatonia were attempted over the years (24,25), but no unambiguous result was achieved. Kavirajan outlined a consensus from his review. He cited a study by Tollefson, who found that catatonic patients with primary psychiatric illness would at least transiently show an increased verbal expression. In contrast, those with "organic" catatonia would worsen or remain unchanged (15,26).

Similar results were found in patients with confusion (15,27,28). Amytal helped clear the sensorium in patients with functional confusion, while organic confusion was increased (27).

Subsequently, a "general rule" was described claiming that organic and nonorganic patients would show different reactions to administration of sodium amytal (15). However, it was pointed out that not all the cases of hysteria might improve (15,27).

Studies also aimed at evaluating the efficacy of sodium amytal compared to other agents and saline. Again, some studies were more favorable than others.

Hain, who used amobarbital, methamphetamine, hydroxydione, or saline for interviewing in psychoneurosis, found no significant differences among the different agents in promoting emotional expression or recall (15, 29). However, he noted that amytal was associated with less emotional change than was the placebo. Smith reanalysed the same data in a follow-up paper. He found that abreaction during the interview did not correlate with subsequent clinical change (30). In a later paper, he stressed that interviewer effects reached significance in measures of interview quality and outcome (31).

Thus, over the years, the main interest of the first attempted trials was the response to sodium amytal in patients with various psychiatric diseases, and its use, particularly for catatonia and functional confusion, was recognized. Studies also highlighted the usefulness for distinction between organic and nonorganic etiology. However, there was no clear consensus about the effectiveness of sodium amytal and its possible advantages above other drugs.

Given the confusion, Perry and Jacobs did a service by naming several indications for the use of sodium amytal, reviewing the conclusions of the different studies (9). Further, it was suggested that diagnostic versus therapeutic interviewing should be distinguished (9). The suggested indications were as follows: Amytal interviewing can be used as an aid to diagnose the mute or stuporous patient. Thus, it is indicated in catatonia symptoms and hysterical stupor. Sodium amytal also is useful to differentiate between depressive, schizophrenic, and organic stupors, and to elucidate unexplained muteness.

Therapeutic usefulness was shown in disorders of repression and dissociation. Posttraumatic stress disorders can be improved by abreaction induced by the amytal

TABLE 28.1
VALID INDICATIONS FOR SODIUM AMYTAL INTERVIEWS

A. Diagnostic aid
   1. Catatonia
   2. Hysterical stupor
   3. Depressive, schizophrenic, and organic dissociation
   4. Muteness
B. Therapeutic usefulness
   1. Abreaction of posttraumatic stress disorder
   2. Recovery of memory in psychogenic amnesia and fugue
   3. Recovery of function in conversion disorder

[Perry JC, Jacobs D. Overview: clinical applications of the amytal interview in psychiatric emergency settings. *Am J Psychiatry.* 1982;139(5):552–559.]

interview. Patients with psychogenic amnesia and fugue may achieve recovery of memory. Finally, amytal interviewing can ameliorate conversion disorders with a subsequent partial or full recovery of lost function. Valid indications are summarized in Table 28.1. The suggested procedure of an amytal interview (9), contraindications, and cautions are mentioned below.

ADMINISTRATION OF SODIUM AMYTAL AND PROCEDURE OF AMYTAL INTERVIEW

Before the infusion is given, its effects—that it will cause relaxation and the willingness to talk—should be explained to the patient.

An intravenous infusion of sodium amytal diluted to a concentration of 5% (500 mg per 10 mL of sterile water) is administered in 50-mg doses. It should not be given faster than 1 mL per minute (50 mg per minute) to prevent sleep or sudden respiratory depression (7,32). Overall, 200 to 1,000 mg are required for the whole procedure.

Titration should be based on the individual response to the medication. Infusion should be slowed when the patient becomes drowsy; it should be stopped when nystagmus occurs, speech becomes slurred, pulse oximeter shows less than 95%, or sleep.

The sedation threshold lies between 150 and 350 mg (9). To maintain the level of narcosis, 0.5 to 1 mL of sodium amytal should be administered every 5 minutes.

Combination with other drugs such as ammonium carbonate (32), methylphenidate (33), methyl amphetamine (15,34), or caffeine (35) to avoid sleep can be considered, as sleep limits the interview and the results. Studies have shown that 25% of catatonia patients fall asleep during amytal interviewing without additional caffeine (15,35).

The interview should begin with orientation questions, which are affectively neutral. It should then progress to emotionally laden material covering historical information with special attention to conflictual data (7,15). A typical interview lasts 30 to 60 minutes.

Videotaping of the interview is recommended (32). It can be used for feedback in subsequent sessions. This is a key point in order to ameliorate the symptoms of psychogenic disorders and especially those presenting with movement disorders.

CONTRAINDICATIONS AND CAUTIONS

Overall, sodium amytal administration is safe. Hart reported one case of respiratory arrest in 500 interviews, which could be reversed by intravenous caffeine benzoate (9,36). Paradoxic excitement as a reaction to amytal is very rare (9). A suicide attempt following an amytal interview was reported in one instance after recovery of conversion paralysis (37). Kwentus and others have noted that patients who have used particular symptoms as a major defense may become acutely depressed upon being cured, as conversion symptoms were their source of nonverbal communication or a way to control or manipulate others (17,32). It has been accounted that 12% to 30% of conversion patients have a moderate to severe depression (7). Thus, depressive and suicidal features should be assessed carefully before the interview and an appropriate follow-up should be provided.

Certain other precautions should also be regarded when using amytal. Barbiturates must not be used in patients with porphyria or in those who are allergic to this class of medication or are intoxicated with other sedatives, including alcohol. Barbiturates should be used with caution in patients with chronic obstructive pulmonary disease or potential airway problems, congestive heart failure, hypotension, liver disease, and renal failure (7,9). A cardiopulmonary resuscitation cart should be available in the event of a cardiac arrest or respiratory failure.

THE ROLE OF AMYTAL IN CONVERSION AND PSYCHOGENIC DISORDERS

Conversion disorders are thought to be an intrapsychic response to conflict, threat, or need leading to the loss of body functions, such as blindness, deafness, paralysis, or apnea (33,38). Various other symptoms like movement disorders can occur. This loss of function cannot be directly attributed to a lesion or dysfunction of the nervous system, and derives in most cases from psychological or psychiatric causes (39).

Freud and Breuer stressed the role of amnesia in conversion disorders (9). Later, Janet pointed out the importance of "retraction in the field of consciousness" including unawareness of bodily areas (9). Perry cited an experiment by Hernandez-Peon, which showed reduced evoked potentials in a hysterical patient with a hemianesthetic leg (9,40). Regarding these findings, Ludwig defined a neurophysiologic theory claiming the dissociation to be due to an increased inhibition of sensory and allied motor function from corticofugal tracts (9,41). A relief of conversion symptoms and return to normal attention were shown to be achieved by barbiturates (9). Evoked potentials normalized in the affected leg after administration of barbiturates (9,40).

Thus, electrophysiologically and clinically, conversion disorders show a good response to sodium amytal and other barbiturates. Recovery of a variety of symptoms due to conversion has been reported (9,42). These effects and the achieved clinical benefits were an important finding and show possibilities to treat conversion disorders, particularly as the majority of psychogenic movement disorders are conversion reactions.

Sodium amytal can also be helpful in detecting malingering and factitious behavior. It has been noted that malingerers may not illustrate the expected reaction to sodium amytal administration. Perry referred to Morris's description of two cases of malingerers who showed an unusual response (9,43). He reported a patient who became resistant to amytal and untalkative after injection. A second malingering mute patient spontaneously began to talk when the nurse was told—within his earshot—to prepare a drug which would elicit important information about whether the patient's illness was fake or real. Both responses are not typical for conversion patients treated with sodium amytal.

Kwentus observed that symptoms might worsen or become bizarre during the interview if there is a conscious wish to defeat the intervention (17). Malingering patients may have such wishes in order to gain and keep certain attention.

Factitious disorder is characterized by the intentional feigning of physical or psychological signs and symptoms (44). Münchausen syndrome is the best-known type of factitious disorder. A case report by McDonald reported the efficacy of sodium amytal to elicit information from patients with factitious disorders and to gain relief of symptoms (15,45). Marriage studied patients with Münchausen syndrome and borderline personality disorders who were treated with amytal. He found that amytal promoted disclosure in his factitious disorder patients (46). Accordingly, the procedure was asserted helpful to obtain "more accurate" historical information in patients with factitious disorder (15). However, Kent warned that after the administration of sodium amytal, patients may report fantasy as fact, and that sodium amytal should not be abused as "truth serum" (15,17).

These findings confirm the value of sodium amytal as a diagnostic tool in nonorganic illness like malingering and factitious disorder. Studies showed an usual response in such patients, in contrast to those presenting with conversion. Psychogenic patients show good response, as mentioned above. However, Ward cautioned that psychogenic patients might also not improve or may show an unusual response to sodium amytal (15,27). Thus, a negative response does not exclude a psychogenic origin.

THE ROLE OF AMYTAL IN PSYCHOGENIC MOVEMENT DISORDERS

There have been very few studies focusing on the effect of the amytal interview on symptoms in patients with psychogenic disorders, particularly those presenting with movement disorders. We will discuss the main studies (7,9,15,35,42,47).

An early nonexperimental study from 1944 by Lambert and Rees compared the efficacy of amytal interviews with hypnosis and conventional treatment of conversion disorders (9,42). Even then, they found the barbiturate interview to be preferable in the treatment of motor conversions.

Hurwitz discussed the effects of amytal interviewing in combination with narcosuggestion in five conversion disorder patients and demonstrated the restoration of conscious control over their disabled limbs. Four of five improved; however, three experienced a relapse within the next few months (15,35).

More recently, Fackler et al. studied 21 cases with suspected conversion disorder, four presenting with movement disorders (7). One patient exhibited generalized choreiform movements of the upper and lower extremities, which decreased in intensity after amytal-assisted interviewing. Fackler et al. also noted that those with movement disorders did better than patients with other conversion symptoms like pseudoseizures or focal neurologic symptoms (7).

Recently, Sa et al. (2003) showed sodium amytal to be useful in patients with posttraumatic painful torticollis (47). They evaluated 16 patients who had developed an abnormal dystonic posturing of the neck or shoulder after local trauma like motor vehicle accidents or work-related injuries. Patients presented with painful, fixed head tilt and shoulder elevation. Fourteen patients also exhibited non-dermatomal sensory deficits. Occurrence was shortly after trauma (some within minutes) and with progression to maximum within 2 weeks. Sa et al. emphasized that all patients fulfilled the criteria of psychogenic dystonia including characteristic features like fixed, unremitting posture, distractibility, stereotypic course, and involvement of litigation or compensation. The researchers noted that litigation or compensation was present in all 16 patients. Accordingly, they concluded that there was an important role of psychological factors in the etiology and maintenance of abnormal posture. Sodium amytal interviewing was carried out in 13 of 16 patients and beneficial effects were achieved, in contrast to controls that had received normal saline. Posture, pain, or both improved in all 13 patients. Posture normalized in nine of 13, spontaneous pain was abolished in five. Sensory deficits normalized or improved in five patients. Sa et al. rightly proposed that this condition should not be characterised as a form of dystonia, but to name it "posttraumatic painful torticollis" in order not to confuse different etiologies of organic and nonorganic origin.

THE USE OF VIDEO FEEDBACK IN PSYCHOGENIC/CONVERSION REACTION PATIENTS

In 1995, Bradley demonstrated sodium amytal to be a successful method for the treatment of psychogenic disorders especially when combined with the use of videos. He reported a patient with psychogenic paralysis to whom excerpts of the video showing transient relief during the interview were demonstrated and to whom the emotional rather than the neurologic origin of her symptoms were elucidated. While watching herself moving her thought-to-be paralyzed leg, she consciously moved it for the first time. The patient showed daily improvement (32).

This is only one example of improvement of symptoms after the presentation of the recorded amytal interview. Such use of videotapes in the sodium amytal interview can be helpful for different reasons. First, it allows the therapist to revisit or review important parts of the interview to resolve unclear points (32). Second, and more important, the video can be used as feedback and for treatment during the next sessions under the supervision of the therapist. Videos will show the discrepancy between the patient's perceived disability and the tasks performed during the amytal interview. The video proves to the patient the ability to perform certain tasks and movements, even though there is no memory of this. This evidence helps the patient to achieve a better concept of self by eliminating "distortions

concerning their behavior" (32). It may also help to "reinforce" those activities (32).

Overall, we wish to emphasize that sodium amytal is a valuable tool in diagnosis and therapy of psychogenic movement disorders, and that the additional use of videos can successfully help to promote recovery.

OTHER DRUGS

Currently, benzodiazepines like lorazepam are more often used than sodium amytal to assist interviewing, particularly in catatonia. They are administered orally or intravenously and the normal dose ranges between 1 and 8 mg. Individuals may respond within minutes or not for several hours. In contrast, narcosis induced by sodium amytal is more persistent and begins gradually due to the pharmacologic characteristics of this medium-acting barbiturate. Compared to amytal, benzodiazepines do not have a risk of respiratory suppression and they are easily reversible with the GABA antagonists like flumazenil.

CONCLUSION AND OPEN ISSUES

Conversion disorders are thought to be an intrapsychic response to conflict leading to the loss of body functions. Symptoms like blindness, movement disorders, and paralysis can be exhibited (32,38). Diagnosis and therapy of conversion disorders are difficult, and the evidence in diagnostic and therapeutic applications is limited. Particularly, the therapy of psychogenic movement disorders is not well-established and can be challenging to the clinician (39). Overall, prognosis of psychogenic movement disorders, particularly after a year of onset of symptoms, remains very poor with regard to permanent remissions.

Our review shows that sodium amytal and similar drugs can be successfully used to diagnose and treat conversion disorders, particularly those with movement disorders. In this regard, the reports of Fackler et al. (7) and Sa et al. (47) are notable. The reported cases who had initially presented with abnormal postures showed notable improvement or full recovery after sodium amytal administration (7,47). We expect that good results can be achieved by combining drug-assisted interview with video feedback (32). Videos presented to the patient in one of the following sessions will prove the ability to perform certain tasks and movements. In any case, most movement disorder specialists are familiar with using video to record interesting patients. Ideally, a team consisting of a movement disorder specialist and a psychiatrist with an interest in psychogenic conditions and experience with the amytal interview, as well as ancillary staff including a dedicated nurse specialist, would be required to make this successful. There is still a relative paucity of studies focusing on the sodium amytal interview in the field of movement disorders. There are only a few studies comparing the effectiveness and the long-term benefit of sodium amytal with other drugs assisting interviewing or other methods like hypnosis, insight-oriented psychotherapy, and memory retrieval. Questions on the safety of these methods have not been answered yet.

It also remains unclear which endpoints should be considered regarding the differentiation of organic versus psychogenic disorders. Furthermore, ethical aspects must be considered. Improvements regarding the consent of the patient have to be made.

A careful reassessment of sodium amytal may enhance our understanding of the pathophysiology of psychogenic disorders and psychogenic movement disorders. For instance, a functional imaging paradigm (and other studies) could be considered in the symptomatic phase prior to, during, and after the amytal interview in the recovery phase to shed more light on the pathophysiologic mechanism.

REFERENCES

1. Griesinger W. In: Robertson CL, Rutherford J, eds. *Mental pathology and therapeutics*. London: The New Sydenham Society, 1861.
2. Patrick M, Howells R. Barbiturate-assisted interviews in modern clinical practice. *Psychol Med*. 1990;20(4):763–765.
3. Schonle HA, Moment A. Some new hypnotics of the barbituric acid series. *J Am Chem Soc*. 1923;45:243–249.
4. Bleckwenn WJ. Production of sleep and rest in psychotic cases. *Arch Neurol Psychiatry*. 1930;24:365–372.
5. Bleckwenn WJ. Narcosis as therapy in neuropsychiatric conditions. *JAMA*. 1930;95:1168–1171.
6. Bohn RW. Sodium amytal narcosis as a therapeutic aid in psychiatry. *Psychiatr Q*. 1932;6:301–309.
7. Fackler SM, Anfinson TJ, Rand JA. Serial sodium amytal interviews in the clinical setting. *Psychosomatics*. 1997;38(6):558–564.
8. Lindemann E. Psychological changes in normal and abnormal individuals under the influence of sodium amytal. *Am J Psychiatry*. 1932;88:1083–1091.
9. Perry JC, Jacobs D. Overview: clinical applications of the Amytal interview in psychiatric emergency settings. *Am J Psychiatry*. 1982;139(5):552–559.
10. Thorner MW. The psycho-pharmacology of sodium amytal in catatonia. *J Nerv Ment Dis*. 1935;82:299–303.
11. Horsley JS. Narco-analysis. *J Ment Sci*. 1936;82:417–422.
12. Grinker RR. Treatment of war neuroses. *JAMA*. 1944;126:142–145.
13. Tilkin L. The present status of narcosynthesis using sodium pentothal and sodium amytal. *Dis Nerv Syst*. 1949;10:215–218.
14. Hoch PH. The present status of narco-diagnosis and therapy. *J Nerv Ment Dis*. 1946;103:248–259.
15. Kavirajan H. The amobarbital interview revisited: a review of the literature since 1966. *Harv Rev Psychiatry*. 1999;7(3):153–165.
16. Soine WH, Graham RM, Soine PJ. Identification of 5-ethyl-5-5(2-methylbutyl) barbituric acid as an impurity of manufacture in amobarbital. *J Pharm Sci*. 1992;81(4):362–364.
17. Kwentus JA. Interviewing with intravenous drugs. *J Clin Psychiatry*. 1981;42(11):432–436.
18. Weinstein EA, Malitz S. Changes in symbolic expression with amytal sodium. *Am J Psychiatry*. 1954;111:198–206.
19. Shagass C, Naiman J, Mihalik J. An objective test which differentiates between neurotic and psychotic depression. *Arch Neurol Psychiatry*. 1956;75:461–471.
20. Elkes J. Effects of psychsomimetic drugs in animals and man. In: Abramson HA, ed. *Neuropharmacology: transactions of the third conference*. New York: Josiah Macy, Jr. Foundation, 1957.
21. Stevens JM, Derbyshire AJ. Shifts along the alert-response continuum during remission of catatonic "stupor" with amobarbital. *Psychosom Med*. 1958;20:99–107.
22. Dysken MW, Chang SS, Casper RC, et al. Barbiturate-facilitated interviewing. *Biol Psychiatry*. 1979;14:421–432.
23. Dysken MW, Kooser JA, Haraszti JS, et al. Clinical usefulness of sodium amobarbital interviewing. *Arch Gen Psychiatry*. 1979;36:789–794.
24. Iserson KV. The emergency amobarbital interview. *Ann Emerg Med*. 1980;9:513–517.
25. Marcos LR, Goldberg E, Feazell D, et al. The use of sodium amytal interviews in a short-term community-oriented inpatient unit. *Dis Nerv Syst*. 1977;38:283–286.
26. Tollefson GD. The amobarbital interview in the differential diagnosis of catatonia. *Psychocomatics*. 1982;23:437–438.
27. Ward NG, Rowlett DB, Burke P. Sodium amylobarbitone in the differential diagnosis of confusion. *Am J Psychiatry*. 1978;135:75–78.
28. Shale JH, Gelenberg AJ. The amobarbital interview. *Mil Med*. 1980;145:825–828.
29. Hain JD, Smith BM, Stevenson I. Effectiveness and process of interviewing with drugs. *J Psychiatr Res*. 1966;4:95–106.
30. Smith BM, Hain JD, Stevenson I. Emotional expression, memory and feelings during and after interviews with drugs. *Behav Neuropsychiatry*. 1969;1(3):10–14.
31. Smith BM, Hain JD, Stevenson I. Controlled interviews using drugs. *Arch Gen Psychiatry*. 1970;22:2–10.
32. Bradley RH, Zonia CL, Caputo SJ. The amobarbital sodium interview in conversion disorders: use of video feedback in therapy. *J Am Osteopath Assoc*. 1995;95(2):122–125.
33. Hurwitz TA. Narcosuggestion in chronic conversion symptoms using combined intravenous amobarbital and methylphenidate. *Can J Psychiatry*. 1988;33(2):147–152.
34. Solomon GF, Zarcone VP Jr, Yoerg R, et al. Three psychiatric casualties from Vietnam. *Arch Gen Psychiatry*. 1971;25:522–524.
35. McCall WV. The addition of intravenous caffeine during an amobarbital interview. *J Psychiatry Neurosci*. 1992;17(5):195–197.
36. Hart WL, Ebaugh F, Morgan DC. The amytal interview. *Am J Med Sci*. 1945;210:125–131.
37. Menza MA. A suicide attempt following removal of conversion paralysis with amobarbital. *Gen Hosp Psychiatry*. 1989;11(2):137–138.
38. Kapfhammer HP, Dobmeier P, Mayer C, et al. Conversion syndromes in neurology. A psychopathological and psychodynamic differentiation of conversion disorder, somatization disorder and factitious disorder. *Psychothes Psychosom Med Psychol*. 1998;48:463–474.
39. Thomas M, Jankovic J. Psychogenic movement disorders: diagnosis and management. *CNS Drugs*. 2004;18(7):437–452.
40. Hernandez-Peon R, Chavez-Ibarra G, Aguilar-Figueroa E. Somatic evoked potentials in one case of hysterical anesthesia. *Electroencephalogr Clin Neurophysiol*. 1963;15:881–892.
41. Ludwig AM. Hysteria: a neurobiological theory. *Arch Gen Psychiatry*. 1972;27:771–777.
42. Lambert C, Rees WL. Intravenous barbiturates in the treatment of hysteria. *Br Med*. 1944;2:70–73.
43. Morris DP. Intravenous barbiturates: an aid in the diagnosis and the treatment of conversion hysteria and malingering. *Mil Surg*. 1945;96:509–513.
44. Bauer M, Boegner F. Neurological syndromes in factitious disorder. *Nerv Ment Dis*. 1996;184(5):281–285.
45. McDonald A, Kline SA, Billings RF. The limits of Munchausen's syndrome. *Can Psychiatr Assoc J*. 1979;24:323–328.
46. Marriage K, Govorchin M, Gerorge P, et al. Use of an amytal interview in the management of factitious deaf mutism. *Aust N Z J Psychiatry*. 1988;22:454–647.
47. Sa DS, Mailis-Gagnon A, Nicholson K, et al. Posttraumatic painful torticollis. *Mov Disord*. 2003;18(12):1482–1491.

Role of Anesthesia in the Diagnosis and Treatment of Psychogenic Movement Disorders

29

Stanley Fahn

ABSTRACT

When a patient presents with fixed postural deformities that do not yield to passive manipulation by the examiner, if those fixed postures persist in sleep, and if the physician suspects that the postural deformities may be due to a psychogenic movement disorder, then the possibility that those fixed postures are the result of contractures needs to be considered. The extent of the contractures will be the limiting factor in the degree of motor benefit that could be expected by treating the patient for a psychogenic movement disorder by the usual method of a combination of psychotherapy, physiotherapy, and medications for any psychiatric disorder. Therefore, it is important to know whether or not the fixed postures are the result of contractures, and to know the limitation of the range of motion possible because of those contractures. Examination of the fixed postures under deep anesthesia allows the physician to ascertain this knowledge, and to devise an effective plan of therapy. The essence of this chapter is that anesthesia provides information about the presence or absence of contractures, and if contractures are present, about the extent of benefit one might obtain by the routine psychotherapy–physiotherapy approach one utilizes for the treatment of psychogenic movement disorders.

An added benefit from the examination under anesthesia is the ascertainment of any fixed postures that failed to respond to passive manipulation or routine sleep *not* being due to contractures. This added lack of range of motion not due to contractures supports the notion that they were caused by a psychogenic movement disorder rather than an organic one. The acceptance by the patient that there was this noncontractured type of fixed posture, which can now be overcome by the patient voluntarily, adds greatly to the patient accepting the diagnosis of a psychogenic movement disorder and often leads to successful therapy of that condition. Informing the patient about the presence or absence of contractures, and about any noncontractured state of the fixed postures, aids in the patient often immediately eliminating the noncontractured component of the fixed postures. Fahn writes:

> An accurate diagnosis of psychogenic movement disorder as opposed to diagnosing an organic movement disorder is often one of the most difficult tasks in the movement disorder specialty. It is extremely important to be correct in the diagnosis, because only then can the appropriate therapy be initiated. The results of an incorrect diagnosis are detrimental. If a patient has a psychogenic disorder that is misdiagnosed, the patient will be given inappropriate and potentially harmful medication and is also denied the proper treatment to overcome the disabling symptoms. By postponing the appropriate psychiatric treatment, the cycle of disability is perpetuated. Untreated patients with psychogenic movement disorders are at risk for becoming career invalids with chronic disability (1).

INTRODUCTION

The first step in the diagnosis of a psychogenic disorder, like most medical conditions, is to be suspicious of the possibility of that diagnosis. In movement disorders, that suspicion rests on the phenomenology of the abnormal pattern of movements and on certain clues (1) in the history and examination. Fixed postures are sustained postures that resist passive movement, and such fixed postures are highly likely to be due to a psychogenic dystonia (2–4).

Once a psychogenic movement disorder is suspected, the next step is to establish the correct diagnosis, that is, document that the abnormal movements are indeed due to a psychogenic etiology. Just being suspicious that the signs and symptoms are psychogenic is insufficient for the diagnosis of documented psychogenic disorder. Fahn and Williams (2) categorized patients into four levels of certainty as to the likelihood of their having a psychogenic movement disorder. These four degrees of certainty are (i) documented psychogenic disorder, (ii) clinically established psychogenic disorder, (iii) probable psychogenic disorder, and (iv) possible psychogenic movement disorder. This classification has been used by subsequent authors (5–7). In order for the disorder to be documented as being psychogenic, the symptoms must be relieved by psychotherapy, by the clinician utilizing psychological suggestion including physiotherapy, by administration of placebos (again with suggestion being a part of this approach), or by the patient being witnessed as being free of symptoms when left alone, supposedly unobserved (1). Two special problems exist: (i) when the abnormal movements are paroxysmal, because getting better at times is part of a paroxysmal syndrome, so one cannot be certain if the improvement was due to the psychotherapeutic treatment

for psychogenicity; and (ii) if the abnormal movements had led to a fixed posture that resists passive movement possibly due to the development of contractures.

A contracture in a muscle is a shortened muscle that is resistant to passive stretch and is usually due to fibrosis of the muscle, ligaments, tendons, or the joints, preventing the muscle from stretching to its normal length. (An ankylosed joint due to bony growth would also result in a fixed posture and would be in the differential diagnoses of fixed postures along with contracture. X-rays would be able to detect such ankylotic joints, and we will not consider ankylosis any further.) The contracture thus presents as a fixed posture, that is, a posture that cannot be relieved by the examiner trying to straighten out the abnormally positioned body part. However, a fixed posture due to psychogenicity may be due to a contracture or may resemble a contracture, merely by resisting passive movement. How to distinguish between a contracture and a noncontracture fixed posture is the essence of this chapter. The ultimate, documented diagnosis of a psychogenic dystonia, as stated above, depends on getting the patient better; getting better, in terms of relieving fixed postures, depends on knowing if contractures are present and if noncontractured fixed postures are present.

The shortened muscle, if due entirely to a contracture, is electrically silent. Metabolic diseases, such as McArdle disease (8) due to muscle phosphorylase deficiency, can cause electrically silent contractions, thus technically physiologic contractures (9). But these disorders do not lead to persistent contractures. This type of physiologic contracture appears with protracted exercise, and is most readily seen in phosphorylase deficiency with anaerobic exercise, where the muscle's energy is derived from glycolysis and not

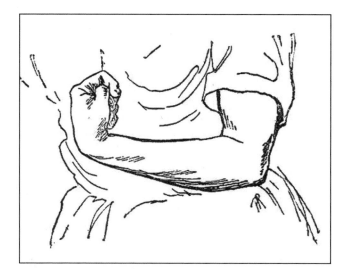

Figure 29.1 Drawing by Richer. "Hysterical contracture of the left arm." (From Oppenheim H. In: Bruce A, ed. *Text-book of nervous diseases*. Edinburgh: Otto Schulze and Co., 1911:1079, with permission.)

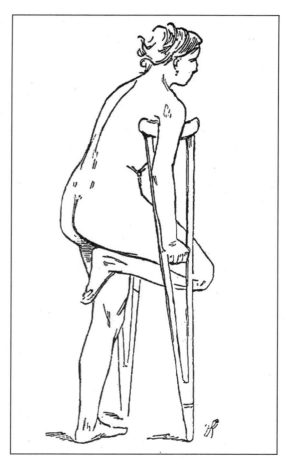

Figure 29.2 Drawing by Richer. "Hysterical flexion contracture of the right leg." (From Oppenheim H. In: Bruce A, ed. *Text-book of nervous diseases*. Edinburgh: Otto Schulze and Co., 1911:1079, with permission.)

mitochondria. Further discussion of physiologic contractures is not part of this chapter.

Contractures, as depicted in Figs 29.1 and 29.2 (10), more commonly result from fixed dystonias that persist during sleep. The dystonia can be due to an organic etiology or a psychogenic etiology. Organic dystonias usually disappear in deep sleep, whereas psychogenic dystonias may not, as depicted in Case Report 1 below. Important in the establishment of a psychogenic etiology is the observation that the abnormal posture can be improved with therapeutic techniques unique for psychogenic disorders. But, if a muscle contracture is present, whether due to psychogenicity or some other cause, the treating clinician is not able to restore that movement disorder to health by using the standard methods of treating a psychogenic movement disorder.

HOW DO CONTRACTURES OCCUR IN A PSYCHOGENIC MOVEMENT DISORDER?

In organic torsion dystonia, contractures can develop if the muscle remains in a fixed posture for a prolonged period of time, which usually includes during sleep. By the muscle not stretching out for such extended durations, fibrosis of the tendons can develop. The same mechanism occurs if the abnormal dystonic posture were due to psychogenicity. This means that the psychogenic dystonia needed to persist during sleep. Although most, but not all, movement disorders lessen or disappear during sleep, the fact that contractured psychogenic dystonic muscles can develop indicates that in those patients the abnormal postures persisted in sleep. This is most likely to occur in somatoform disorders where the subconscious psyche persists during sleep. Case 1 below illustrates that a psychogenic abnormal posture can persist during sleep, implying that the psychic mechanism inducing the posture remains in subconscious control during this period.

Gowers (11) may have been the first to mention that some spasmodic contractions persist in sleep. In his textbook, in the section on hysteria, Gowers mentioned that some spasmodic contractures persist in sleep and can relax only with chloroform narcosis, and if continued over years, can lead to permanent contractures that are no longer responsive to chloroform.

PATIENTS PRESENTING WITH FIXED POSTURES THAT DO NOT DISAPPEAR WHILE ASLEEP

Patients who present with fixed postures that persist while awake and also during sleep present a problem not only in establishing the diagnosis, as mentioned above, but also in determining the course of treatment. Fixed postures can arise from organic as well as psychogenic dystonia, and also from orthopaedic and arthritic conditions. If the treating physician suspects that the posture is due originally to a psychogenic basis, how should the physician proceed? Apply psychotherapy to see if the patient can improve; as mentioned in the introduction, a necessary step to document a psychogenic movement disorder may fail to show improvement in the fixed posture if it is entirely due to a contracture although psychogenic in origin. It is critical to determine with certainty that the fixed posture was psychogenic in origin so that a proper treatment regimen for such an etiology can be initiated. It is also important to determine how much of the fixed posture seen is the result of a contracture and how much is not due to contracture but an assumed fixed posture, possibly due to psychogenicity. Moreover, a fixed posture due to organic dystonia that disappears with deep sleep or anesthesia is potentially remedial because contractures are not present, and even brain stereotactic surgical therapy becomes an available choice. The two case reports below illustrate how deep sleep or anesthesia can lead to a treatment strategy. Case 1 turned out not to have contractures as the cause of her fixed postures; Case 2 turned out to have fixed postures partly due to contractures. These observations led to appropriate treatment in each case and at the same time reinforced the clinical diagnosis of psychogenic dystonia because the patients remained improved following the experience.

Thus, one of the first steps is to determine if contractures are present. Only then can one expect to know if there would be any relief of the fixed postures by simply treating the underlying psychogenic cause of the disorder. We thus have a vicious cycle. The diagnosis of a psychogenic movement disorder is established and documented by getting the patient better with appropriate therapy for such patients, but if the patient cannot physically improve because of contractures, then the diagnosis cannot be established.

The first step when confronted with a patient with fixed postures is to observe the patient when he or she is asleep. It is important that the patient be in deep sleep, which may require EEG electrodes. But even if the postures persist in Stage IV sleep, one cannot be absolutely certain whether contractures are present or if the subconscious psyche is maintaining that posture. Utilizing EMG electrodes on the affected muscle may not be helpful. Observing actual contractions would be an indication that the muscle has assumed the abnormal posture, at least in part, because of either voluntary or subconscious contractions. But an electrically silent muscle can also maintain the abnormal posture, and there still is no help in determining if fixed contractures due to tendon and ligament fibrosis are present. The simplest method is to place the patient under deep anesthesia and observe if the shortened muscle can be stretched. If contractures are found during deep anesthesia, then intensive physiotherapy or tendon-releasing surgery to relieve the contractures would need to be included in the treatment plan.

Knowing that contractures are not present may aid in the diagnosis of a psychogenic movement disorder. Very few patients with organic dystonia have abnormal postures that persist during sleep, although this can occur. Therefore, in a patient with a fixed posture even during sleep, the cause of the fixed posture may be organic or psychogenic if a contracture is present. If deep anesthesia reveals that there is no contracture, this finding may support a diagnosis of a psychogenic movement disorder, as seen in Case 1 below. If the fixed posture melts away with anesthesia, this is good news for the patient, and this information can be provided to the patient. This direct approach allows the patient to recognize that the fixed posture may not be organic, and may be an important first step for the patient to start the healing process toward recovery from the movement disorder. Then, if the fixed posture no longer recurs when the patient is awake, the patient may make a speedier recovery by accepting a diagnosis of a psychogenic cause of the previous fixed posture.

APPLYING ANESTHESIA TO DETERMINE IF CONTRACTURES ARE RESPONSIBLE FOR THE FIXED POSTURES

Anesthesia needs to be arranged with the anesthesiology department. The actual anesthesia procedure will usually be carried out after all the surgical cases for the day have been completed. It is safest to arrange for the patient to be admitted to the hospital for this testing. The neurologist should be present to examine the fixed postures to determine if contractures are present. It is also helpful to videotape the examination under anesthesia. The videotape serves as a medical record, but might also be useful to show to the patient should he or she have doubts about the findings under anesthesia. The anesthesiologist must apply the general anesthetic so that the patient is fully and deeply asleep. Then, the neurologist will attempt to open up closed joints and stretch out the muscles. If the muscle can be fully relaxed and stretched, and the closed joint can be fully extended, no contracture is present. If the muscle cannot be stretched or only partially stretched, with the joint not being extended, then a contracture is present.

If the contracture is less extensive than the severity of the "fixed" muscle that could not be stretched when the patient was awake, this indicates that some voluntary or subconscious muscle contraction was present to increase the degree of the fixed posture. Such failure to relax the muscle with the patient awake above and beyond any component of underlying contracture indicates that the fixed posture is psychogenic in origin.

If there is no contracture in a muscle that was resistant to passive stretch when the patient was awake, the diagnosis of a psychogenic fixed posture is likely. The differential diagnoses to be considered are (i) a voluntary contraction because of malingering or a factitious disorder, (ii) "involuntary" contraction due to a subconscious conversion posturing, or (iii) a very longstanding organic dystonia.

THERAPY IF CONTRACTURES ARE PRESENT

The presence and extent of a fixed contracture sets the limit as to the ultimate improvement one can anticipate from psychotherapy, standard physiotherapy, and medications (i.e., the standard therapeutic approach to treating psychogenic movement disorders). The presence of a fixed contracture indicates that orthopaedic procedures or special physiotherapy applications would be necessary to treat the contractures. Psychotherapy must therefore be coupled with intensive physiotherapy and often the addition of tendon-releasing surgery. Knowing the range of motion available to the involved joint, therefore, allows the neurologist to establish the best therapeutic strategy. It is important to improve the motor disability as well as the abnormal psyche that led to the deformity in psychogenic movement disorders.

In my experience in treating patients with psychogenic contractures, by informing the patient of the presence of the contracture immediately upon awakening from general anesthesia, the patient becomes convinced of the physical problem and also becomes more accepting of the diagnosis of a psychogenic movement disorder. This makes it easier to institute psychotherapy, along with physiotherapy.

CASE REPORTS

Two cases have been published that illustrate the value of anesthesia in patients with fixed postures, which are suspected of being caused by psychogenic dystonia (2). These two cases are reproduced here with the permission of the authors.

Case 1

Patient 8 of Fahn and Williams (2): Nurse with chronic equinovarus feet, which persisted during natural sleep but were supple under amobarbital sleep.

At age 19 (in 1966), while a nursing student, this woman twisted and fractured her right ankle, which was placed in a cast. She continued to have pain, and the foot was operated upon but without relief. Diazepam and phenobarbital had little effect. She continued in nursing school, and the right leg was braced. At age 23, the right foot turned in and remained that way despite casting; the pain had subsided. She was able to work as a nurse with a twisted right foot. Hypnotism, physiotherapy, hydrotherapy, psychotherapy, and various psychotropic medications were without benefit. A diagnosis of dystonia was made in 1971 (age 24). She had intermittent painful spasms.

In 1979 the right foot went into a severe painful spasm. Trials of clonazepam, trihexyphenidyl, and baclofen were without benefit. She became unable to straighten the foot and walked with a foot brace, which increased the pain. In the fall of 1979 the left foot began to turn in and eventually remained that way.

Examination in 1980 (age 33) revealed an overweight woman in obvious distress and almost tearful. The right arm showed postural and handwriting tremor, and also give-way weakness and drift without pronation. There was also limited facial contractions and slowness of rapid succession movements of the right hand. She could not wiggle her toes, yet they were of normal flaccid tone on passive movement. She was able to straighten the left foot but not past midline. It was turned in, but it became straight when the arms were being examined. She was referred back to the referring neurologist with the diagnosis of a psychogenic dystonia and with advice to have the patient see a psychiatrist for psychotherapy.

Within 18 months, and despite psychotherapy, the left foot became permanently turned in, and she returned for another consultation. Both feet were in an equinovarus posture that resisted passive movement. However, the toes remained flaccid, but she was unable to wiggle them on her own. Weak grips were found bilaterally. The remainder of the examination was unchanged from the previous year. She was admitted to the hospital in November 1982. EMG of the legs revealed that when the leg muscles were at rest, the ankle remained in a state of inversion, suggesting that fixed contractures may be present. The nurses reported that the feet remained turned in at night when the patient was asleep. Rigorous physiotherapy was given to attempt to straighten the feet, but this resulted in severe pain, so little was accomplished.

In addition to physiotherapy, she received placebo medication. Psychotherapy sessions including hypnosis yielded no initial symptomatic improvement but did point to features of dependence on parents and retreat from competitive vocational and social arenas in a manner strongly suggestive of a somatoform disorder. The psychiatrist detected depression and began her on phenelzine, increasing the dose gradually to 90 mg per day. After 4 weeks of hospitalization, an amobarbital interview was attempted, but the infusion put her to sleep. While she was asleep, her ankles became loose and the feet could be straightened but not everted. As she awakened, the ankles became tight again. The patient was informed of this finding and encouraged to continue with physiotherapy. She wanted to leave the hospital to attend Christmas church services and was told that she could not go home for Christmas on a pass unless she made progress. Two days before Christmas, the feet straightened and she was able to walk. All signs of dystonia disappeared. Phenelzine was tapered and discontinued approximately 6 months after discharge in the course of supportive outpatient psychotherapy. She lost weight, subsequently married, and is now raising a family. There has been no relapse since the 5 years after discharge.

Case 2

Patient 21 of Fahn and Williams (2): Fixed contractures of the legs and right hand because of continuous twisted posturing.

At age 31, this woman had complete loss of color vision for 1.5 hours. In 1973 (at age 50), she had a 15- to 30-minute distortion of the left visual field. In 1977 (age 54), she developed pain in the right thigh; an orthopaedist found no pathology. At age 58, the right foot became twisted. Tenotomies were not helpful. At age 59, the left foot twisted, and 3 months later (September 1982) she awakened with her legs crossed and locked together. This fixed posture persisted. Many medications were tried, all without benefit. In May 1983, a cervical spinal stimulator was tried without effect. In May 1984, intrathecal infusion of baclofen was tried without any lasting benefit.

The right hand became clenched, but she could still write. In 1985, the left arm developed decreased grip and mobility. She had not been able to walk but could manipulate from bed to wheelchair and the reverse.

She was admitted to hospital in January 1986, at which time we first saw her. Examination revealed the right leg wrapped around the left at the level of the knees, and the feet and toes were plantar flexed. The legs were fixed to any movement by the examiner. Yet she had no difficulty moving from the bed to the wheelchair or functioning on the toilet. The right hand was tightly fisted. We were unable to move the right thumb passively, yet she lifted it slightly to insert a pen under the thumb to allow her to write. She wrote normally despite abnormal posture of right arm and hand. There was give-way weakness of the left arm. The patient consented to be put to sleep under general anesthesia to allow us to determine the extent that the fixed postures were due to contractures or were free to be moved passively. She consented. Examination under general anesthesia revealed fixed contractures in the right knee and foot, but less severe than when she was awake, and the leg could be uncrossed. The fingers of the right hand also had contractures, but the hand could be partially opened. The right thumb was fully moveable.

After awakening from anesthesia and back in her room, the patient was informed of the results of the examination under anesthesia. She was told that the dystonia was due to subconscious emotional conflicts, which had generated real and disabling physical symptoms, but that she could improve with physiotherapy and psychotherapy. She was receptive to this plan. Psychiatric assessment disclosed that this woman had a chronically extremely unhappy marriage to a man who was chauvinistic, domineering, verbally abusive, unfaithful, alcoholic, and in recent years, impotent. It was impressive that the patient described these phenomena with a tone of masochistic resignation, but adamantly denied having any angry feelings about them. It was postulated by the psychiatrist that the patient's clenched fist and crossed legs represented the patient's body-language expression of feelings of repressed rage, which she could not express verbally. Because of features of depression, imipramine was also recommended.

With encouragement, physiotherapy, and psychotherapy, she subsequently improved. She was able to walk with a walker by the time of discharge. She subsequently underwent orthopaedic surgery to break the contractions in the leg and currently continues in a physiotherapy program. She has become active with her local chapter of the Dystonia Medical Research Foundation and has been a successful fundraiser.

CONCLUSION

The neurologist who has full knowledge of the cause of fixed postures and the degree of limited joint mobility will be in a position to better help the patient. Examination under anesthesia is a necessary early step to obtain this full knowledge. Such an examination usually leads to the affirmation that the disorder is psychogenic when the abnormal posture is greater than the degree of posture caused by the contracture. Another advantage is that by being informed of the results of the examination under anesthesia, there is better acceptance by the patient of a psychogenic movement disorder so that psychotherapy can more readily achieve a successful outcome.

REFERENCES

1. Fahn S. Psychogenic movement disorders. In: Marsden CD, Fahn S, eds. *Movement disorders 3.* Oxford: Butterworth-Heineman, 1994:359–372.
2. Fahn S, Williams DT. Psychogenic dystonia. *Adv Neurol.* 1988; 50:431–455.
3. Lang A, Fahn S. Movement disorder of RSD. *Neurology.* 1990;40: 1476–1477.
4. Schrag A, Trimble M, Quinn N, et al. The syndrome of fixed dystonia: an evaluation of 103 patients. *Brain.* 2004;127:2360–2372.
5. Koller W, Lang A, Vetere-Overfield B, et al. Psychogenic tremors. *Neurology.* 1989;39:1094–1099.
6. Ranawaya R, Riley D, Lang A. Psychogenic dyskinesias in patients with organic movement disorders. *Mov Disord.* 1990;5:127–133.
7. Lang AE. Psychogenic dystonia: a review of 18 cases. *Can J Neurol Sci.* 1995;22:136–143.
8. McArdle B. Myopathy due to a defect in muscle glycogen breakdown. *Clin Sci.* 1951;10:13–35.
9. Gasser HS. Contractures of skeletal muscle. *Physiol Rev.* 1930; 10:35–109.
10. Oppenheim H. In: Bruce A, ed. *Text-book of nervous diseases.* Edinburgh: Otto Schulze and Co., 1911:1079.
11. Gowers WR. *A manual of diseases of the nervous system,* 2nd ed. Vol. 2. Philadelphia, PA: Blakiston, 1893:998.

Clinical Neurophysiology of Myoclonus

30

Peter Brown

ABSTRACT

Few tests are available that help in the positive diagnosis of psychogenic movement disorders. The presence of a readiness potential prior to muscle jerks is good evidence in favor of a psychogenic etiology, although its absence is only moderately suggestive of an organic process. The remaining electrophysiologic assessments used in the evaluation of psychogenic myoclonus, like burst duration and latency, are mostly aimed at excluding organic etiologies.

INTRODUCTION

It has been estimated that around 20% of myoclonus cases in specialist movement disorder clinics have a psychogenic etiology and that this accounts for around 10% of all psychogenic movement disorders evaluated (1). The separation of psychogenic jerks from tics and myoclonus can be a particularly difficult clinical problem. Neurophysiologic investigation can be helpful in this regard, but should be interpreted in the setting of the clinical assessment.

ELECTROPHYSIOLOGIC FINDINGS INDICATIVE OF ORGANIC MYOCLONUS

There are several good electrophysiologic clues that jerks may have an organic etiology. First, there are three general observations that are highly suggestive of organic myoclonus. These are (i) a mean duration of electromyographic (EMG) activity during the jerks of 70 ms or less, (ii) a mean latency of EMG responses of under 70 ms in reflex jerks elicited by sound or peripheral somaesthetic stimuli, and (iii) a recruitment of muscles within jerks that has a stereotyped order and little temporal variability across trials. This stereotyped pattern of muscle recruitment may be the orderly craniocaudal pattern of cortical myoclonus or the caudorostral and rostrocaudal patterns of brainstem jerks (including hyperekplexia) and propriospinal myoclonus, in which EMG activity is initially recorded in muscles innervated by the lower brainstem or a given spinal segment, respectively. Second, there are those electrophysiologic findings specific to cortical myoclonus, namely, the presence of a time-locked cortical correlate that precedes spontaneous and action-induced jerks with a short latency and the presence of a giant cortical evoked potential following peripheral stimulation (2).

ELECTROPHYSIOLOGIC FINDINGS SUGGESTIVE OF PSYCHOGENIC JERKS

Here it is useful to consider spontaneous and reflex jerks separately.

Spontaneous Jerks

Self-paced voluntary movements are preceded by a premovement potential—the readiness potential or Bereitschaftspotential. This is a slow negative potential beginning around one second prior to movement and maximal over the vertex (3). It is illustrated by the thin electroencephalographic (EEG) traces in Figure 30.1. In contrast, a slow premovement potential does not precede organic spontaneous myoclonus, although a very much briefer cortical spike discharge or sharp wave may precede the EMG discharges in cortical myoclonus by an interval of 20 to 40 ms, depending on whether the muscle under investigation is in the upper or lower limb (2). The bold EEG traces in Figure 30.1 show the absence of premovement potential prior to EMG bursts in a patient with abdominal flexion jerks due to tics.

The presence of a long premovement potential beginning more than 800 ms prior to jerks is very good evidence in favor of psychogenic myoclonus during the recording session (4), although it will not distinguish those patients with entirely psychogenic jerks from those with an organic movement disorder who elaborate with a preponderance of psychogenic jerks.

The presence of an abbreviated premovement potential, beginning less than 800 ms prior to the jerks is less helpful. Libet (5) showed that healthy subjects can have such shortened premovement potentials if they do not deliberately think about the timing of the movement, so it is likely that some psychogenic myoclonus may also be accompanied by abbreviated premovement potentials. On the other hand, some organic forms of jerks may also be accompanied by what effectively appear to be abbreviated premovement potentials. This may, for example, be true of the minority of patients with tics. Karp et al. found very brief premovement potentials (similar to the very late NS'

component of the normal premovement potential) in two out of their five patients with tics (6). However, Obeso et al. reported a complete absence of premovement potentials preceding tics in their cases (7), and Tijssen et al. reported three patients with an unusual late-onset posttraumatic tic disorder that was also not preceded by any premovement potential (8). Shibasaki et al. reported premovement potentials in the chorea of choreoacanthocytosis (9), but this is difficult to interpret, given that the chorea in Huntington disease involves no such EEG potential. There has also been a report of abbreviated premovement potentials prior to the jerks of myoclonus-dystonia, although this has not been replicated (10).

Conversely, absence of a premovement potential prior to a jerk is by no means incontrovertible evidence that jerks have an organic etiology. First, a premovement potential is absent or abbreviated when healthy subjects deliberately make movements in response to an external triggering stimulus (11). Thus, we must take care to avoid cues that might form the trigger for seemingly spontaneous jerks in psychogenic myoclonus and tics. Second, premovement potentials may be small or even absent in some healthy subjects (4). Thus, if at all possible, a premovement potential should be demonstrated to exist prior to voluntarily mimicked jerks in those patients with an absent premovement potential prior to symptomatic jerks. Third, and of most concern, are the old reports of attenuated or absent premovement potentials in healthy subjects who repeatedly practiced a voluntary movement, for as little as one hour (12,13). Further research is necessary here to establish whether attenuation or loss of premovement potentials occurs independently of changes in arousal state, but nevertheless, the implication is clear that the repetition of the same movement over hours to years may change the way that movement is organized, thereby compromising the usefulness of the absence of a premovement potential as an indicator of organic myoclonus. It is perhaps no surprise, then, that a premovement potential may be absent in some patients in whom other clinical considerations strongly point to a psychogenic etiology (4).

Finally, the technique of back-averaging employed to demonstrate a premovement potential has several methodological limitations. The poor signal-to-noise ratio of the EEG usually demands that the EEG preceding at least 40 jerks is averaged. Thus, the examination is time-consuming and, more importantly, prohibitive in those patients with very infrequent jerks. Paradoxically, the technique is also unhelpful when jerks occur more frequently than every 6 seconds or so, as any premovement potential may be contaminated by afference or movement artifact related to the last jerk. Finally, contamination of the EEG by artifacts such as EMG or the absence of a clear EMG trigger for back-averaging may limit the usefulness of this technique under any circumstances. It remains to be seen whether other approaches such as frequency analysis (14,15) or

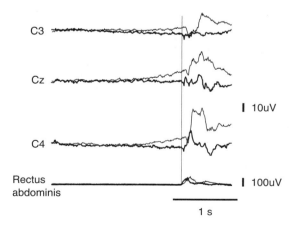

Figure 30.1 The bold traces are the averaged electroencephalographic (EEG) accompanying abdominal flexion jerks in a patient with tics. There is no premovement potential prior to the tics. The thin EEG traces are the averaged EEG accompanying voluntary abdominal flexion in the same patient, whereupon a normal premovement potential is seen to precede EMG activity.

examination of jerk-related EEG power decreases will be able to overcome some of these problems.

In conclusion, the finding of a long premovement potential beginning more than 800 ms prior to spontaneous jerks is very good evidence in favor of psychogenic myoclonus during the recording session. The presence of a shortened premovement potential (less than 800 ms in duration) also supports the diagnosis of psychogenic myoclonus, but cannot be taken as definite proof of the latter. The absence of a premovement potential prior to spontaneous jerks is suggestive, but again not diagnostic, of organic myoclonus.

Reflex Jerks

Unfortunately, there is no truly effective way of electrophysiologically demonstrating a psychogenic etiology in reflex jerks. As a general rule, a mean EMG response latency in excess of 100 ms does suggest a psychogenic process (16), but similarly long latencies may be seen in idiopathic hyperekplexia (17) and some cases of propriospinal myoclonus (18). The latter highlights that no single electrophysiologic criterion, such as reflex latency, is useful in distinguishing etiologies, and combinations of observations are far more useful. Thus, although the latency of reflex jerks may be long in some, but not all, cases of hyperekplexia and propriospinal myoclonus, these conditions can be distinguished from psychogenic myoclonus by their stereotypic patterns of caudorostral and rostrocaudal muscle recruitment from the brainstem (hyperekplexia) or a given spinal segment (propriospinal myoclonus).

In contrast, psychogenic myoclonus is characterized by a variable order of muscle recruitment and/or widely differing delays in the onset of EMG activity in different muscles between jerks (16), although no specific guidelines have been formulated. Finally, a mean duration of EMG activity in reflex jerks that is in excess of 70 ms is consistent with a psychogenic cause, but again may be true of the jerks in hyperekplexia (19) and some cases of spinal myoclonus (18).

CONCLUSION

Our present repertoire of electrophysiologic techniques largely serves to aid the exclusion of organic causes of myoclonus, but, with the exception of a long-duration premovement potential, provides little categoric support for the diagnosis of psychogenic myoclonus. Features such as long duration EMG bursts, long latencies in response to external stimuli, and variable patterns of muscle recruitment can be suggestive of psychogenic myoclonus, but are not diagnostic. Accordingly, electrophysiologic investigations should be interpreted in the light of other clinical assessments, rather than in isolation.

REFERENCES

1. Monday K, Jankovic J. Psychogenic myoclonus. *Neurology.* 1993; 43:349–352.
2. Shibasaki H, Kuroiwa Y. Electroencephalographic correlates of myoclonus. *Electroencephalogr Clin Neurophysiol.* 1975;39:455–463.
3. Kornhuber HH, Deecke L. Hirnpotentialänderungen bei Willkürbewegungen und passiven Bewegungen des Menschen: Bereitschaftspotential un reallerente Potentiale. *Pflügers Arch.* 1965;284:1–17.
4. Terada K, Ikeda A, Van Ness PC, et al. Presence of Bereitschaftspotential preceding psychogenic myoclonus: clinical application of jerk-locked averaging. *J Neurol Neurosurg Psychiatry.* 1995;58:745–747.
5. Libet B, Gleason CA, Wright EW, et al. Time of conscious intention to act in relation to onset of cerebral activity (readiness-potential). *Brain.* 1983;106:623–642.
6. Karp BI, Porter S, Toro C, et al. Simple motor tics may be preceded by a premotor potential. *J Neurol Neurosurg Psychiatry.* 1996;61:103–106.
7. Obeso JA, Rothwell JC, Marsden CD. Simple tics in Gilles de la Tourette's syndrome are not prefaced by a normal premovement EEG potential. *J Neurol Neurosurg Psychiatry.* 1981;44:735–738.
8. Tijssen MAJ, Brown P, Morris H, et al. Acquired startle-induced tics. *J Neurol Neurosurg Psychiatry.* 1999;67:782–784.
9. Shibasaki H, Sakai T, Nishimura H, et al. Involuntary movements in chorea-acanthocytosis: a comparison with Huntington's chorea. *Ann Neurol.* 1982;12:311–314.
10. Quinn NP, Rothwell JC, Thompson PD, et al. Hereditary myoclonic dystonia, hereditary torsion dystonia and hereditary essential myoclonus: an area of confusion. *Adv Neurol.* 1988;50: 391–401.
11. Papa SM, Artieda J, Obeso JA. Cortical activity preceding self-initiated and externally triggered voluntary movement. *Mov Disord.* 1991;6:217–224.
12. Kristeva R. Study of the motor potential during voluntary recurrent movement. *Electroencephalogr Clin Neurophysiol.* 1977;42:588.
13. Villa M, Barzi E, Beretta E, et al. The effect of distributed practice on the Bereitschaftspotential during skilled performance. *EPIC IX, International Conference on Event-Related Potentials of the Brain.* 2, Noordwijk, 1989;56–57.
14. Brown P, Farmer SF, Halliday DM, et al. Coherent cortical and muscle discharge in cortical myoclonus. *Brain.* 1999;122:461–472.
15. Grosse P, Guerrini R, Parmeggiani L, et al. Abnormal cortico-muscular and intermuscular coupling in high-frequency rhythmic myoclonus. *Brain.* 2003;126:326–342.
16. Thompson PD, Colebatch JG, Rothwell JC, et al. Voluntary stimulus-sensitive jerks and jumps mimicking myoclonus or pathological startle syndromes. *Mov Disord.* 1992;7:257–262.
17. Colebatch JG, Barrett G, Lees AJ. Exaggerated startle reflexes in an elderly woman. *Mov Disord.* 1990;5:167–169.
18. Brown P, Thompson PD, Rothwell JC, et al. Axial myoclonus of propriospinal origin. *Brain.* 1991;114:197–214.
19. Brown P, Rothwell JC, Thompson PD, et al. The hyperekplexias and their relationship to the normal startle reflex. *Brain.* 1991; 114:1903–1928.

The Diagnosis and Physiology of Psychogenic Tremor

31

Günther Deuschl   *Jan Raethjen*   *Florian Kopper*   *R.B. Govindan*

ABSTRACT

Psychogenic tremor is a common movement disorder. We interpret the diagnostic criteria that have been established in several previous papers in the context of two hypotheses of the pathophysiology of psychogenic tremor. One is a voluntarylike mechanism which should not be misinterpreted as a simulated tremor. In this case fatigue, entrainment test, cocontraction sign, and the coherence test between two trembling extremities are likely to be positive. Two is a clonuslike mechanism for which it is expected that the cocontraction sign would likely be positive, but fatigue and entrainment test may be negative. We propose that psychogenic tremor can be diagnosed based on clinical and neurophysiologic criteria alone.

INTRODUCTION

Psychogenic tremor may well be the most common psychogenic movement disorder. Prognosis is poor because the tremor persists despite treatment attempts in up to 90% of the patients on long-term follow-up (1) and more than 50% of the patients are unable to follow their professional careers (2,3). The epidemiology has never been formally investigated. There was an epidemic outbreak of psychogenic tremor during the First World War (4), but during more recent wars like the Vietnam War (5), tremor was found less frequently. The reasons for this peculiar difference have never been elucidated. Currently, the data from movement disorder referral centers show a prevalence of psychogenic tremor of about 2% to 5% of all referred patients with tremor (3,6).

The diagnosis requires careful neurologic assessment, but objective and more reliable tests are necessary. Some neurophysiologic tests have been proposed to confirm the diagnosis (3,7–15), but the sensitivity and specificity of these tests have not yet been sufficiently tested. The treatment of psychogenic tremor is not yet elaborated and only some small, uncontrolled cohort studies have been published.

The current paper summarizes the clinical diagnosis, electrophysiologic tools that may assist the diagnosis, and hypotheses on the pathophysiology of tremor.

THE CLINICAL FEATURES SEPARATING PSYCHOGENIC FROM OTHER TREMORS

Psychogenic tremor is not a diagnosis of exclusion, but can be separated on clinical grounds (see Table 31.1), and the diagnosis can be confirmed by additional electrophysiologic tests. Several studies have revealed very similar findings when assessing patients with psychogenic tremors clinically (3,6–8,16–19). We will summarize these findings here.

TABLE 31.1

CLINICAL CRITERIA FOR THE DIAGNOSIS OF PSYCHOGENIC TREMOR

Past medical history for conversion disorders
Sudden onset/remissions
Fatigue of tremor
Unusual combinations of rest, postural, and intention tremor
Variability of tremor frequency
Distractibility
Entrainment of tremor frequency
Cocontraction sign of psychogenic tremor
Absent finger tremor

Almost all of the papers refer to a past medical history for conversion disorders. However, this is not found in all the cases, and the patient's report may also be incomplete.

Most psychogenic tremors start suddenly and may have one or several spontaneous remissions and relapses. This is usually reported by the patients. Sometimes patients present in the emergency room with the first manifestation of their tremor. We saw this in 15% of our own series.

Another clinical feature which is only rarely mentioned is the fatigue of tremor (8). When patients are observed for extended time periods, the tremor may cease or at least diminish in amplitude. This fatigue can be clearly distinguished from the "waxing and waning" of many large-amplitude organic tremors.

All the descriptions mention that patients sometimes have unusual combinations of rest, postural, and action tremors. The detection of such special clinical features strongly depends on the experience of the investigating physician, and this is not an easily applicable clinical test. The important aspect is probably the reproducibility of tremor during various maneuvers: Organic tremors usually have a very similar movement performance when specific motor acts are repeatedly performed and the tremor always interferes mainly with specific parts of the movement. This may vary in psychogenic tremors very much. However, again, no data are available on the reliability of this criterion.

The variability of tremor frequency is usually easier to assess. Tremor frequencies can be separated clinically when they differ more than 1.5 to 2 Hz. In patients with psychogenic tremor, larger changes are sometimes observed that can then be regarded as a sign of psychogenic tremor. Organic tremors do not show such large variations (11,14,20).

An important part of the clinical investigation is the assessment of distractibility. Such distraction can be loading patients mentally (counting backwards) or asking them to perform complicated motor tasks. The expected result is then a loss of regularity of tremor, a change of frequency, a meaningful amplitude reduction, or even a cessation of tremor. A very elegant and easily applicable test is the entrainment test of tremor frequency, which is a formalized way to test distractibility clinically. The patient is asked to perform rhythmic voluntary movements with the less affected hand. The frequency of the imposed rhythmic movements should clearly differ from the tremor frequency and is usually chosen between 2.5 and 4 Hz. If patients cannot produce such a rhythm internally, the investigator can pace them externally. The observed parameter is the change of frequency in the contralateral extremity affected by tremor. It will be explained later why the entrainment test may be meaningfully explained in terms of pathophysiology.

The cocontraction sign is another important sign for the diagnosis of psychogenic tremor. The physician has to move the distal extremity around one joint (usually the wrist joint) while the tremor is present. It is the same testing procedure as for rigidity. The physician feels the resistance in both directions during tremor. This enhanced resistance persists as long as the tremor is present and ceases when the tremor stops. It is a kind of give-way relaxation when the tremor stops, and is one of the clinically reliable signs for the diagnosis of psychogenic tremor.

Finger tremor is mostly absent in psychogenic tremor. Finger tremor can be found when patients make a tremor by voluntary alternating movements, but not if they use the cocontraction mechanism for the production of the tremor.

ELECTROPHYSIOLOGIC TOOLS TO SEPARATE PSYCHOGENIC FROM OTHER TREMORS

The separation of tremors is based on various clinical features and can be assisted by electrophysiologic parameters like the frequency or amplitude of tremor, and more complex measures like the coherence between different muscles. Recently, these electrophysiologic techniques were applied to patients with psychogenic tremors. Some of these tests may even have a high specificity. The following summarizes the tests which have been reported to be helpful.

Electromyography

The electromyographic recording of two or three agonist–antagonist pairs has been recommended for assessing tremors of various origins (11,21–24). For psychogenic tremors, most of the authors did not find specific features, but recently Milanov et al. (13,25) described as typical features a tonic co-contraction superimposed on a reciprocal alternating bursting pattern of antagonists, and a variable frequency and amplitude. Prospective trials are necessary to confirm these observations.

Instantaneous Tremor Frequency Measurements

The measurement of tremor frequency can be done by hand or currently, more precisely, on the basis of accelerometer or electromyogram recordings which are subsequently analyzed with computer programs to determine the instantaneous frequency—the beat-to-beat frequency. Such recordings have shown that the spontaneous fluctuations of the frequency are much larger in patients with psychogenic tremor than in patients with essential tremor (ET) or Parkinson disease (PD) (14,20). A representative example is shown in Figure 31.1 (20). The investigators concluded that patients with psychogenic tremor have a higher spontaneous variation of tremor frequency than do patients with organic tremors. Due to the limited numbers of patients, the authors could not comment on the specificity of their tests.

Entrainment Test

The so-called entrainment test has now been used in several studies (8–10,12,14,15,20). The test requires the investigator to look at the trembling hand affected by presumed psychogenic tremor. The subject is then asked to perform a rhythmic movement with the other hand at a frequency clearly different from the tremor rhythm. The subject can do this self-paced or via an external signal (metronome, rhythmic clapping of the investigator). The test is to see if the trembling hand adopts the rhythm of the extremity performing voluntary rhythmic movements. The physiologic background of this test is that normal subjects cannot perform two different rhythms in two extremities over extended time periods. However, patients with organic tremors can perform, because of a pathologic oscillator which is presumed to function independently from the physiologic rhythmic movement generator.

Patients with various organic tremors have been tested. Figure 31.2 (20) shows the instantaneous frequencies from two patients with parkinsonian tremor and one with psychogenic tremor, before and after starting to perform rhythmic tapping with the contralateral hand. It is obvious that, in all patients, some change of the instantaneous tremor frequency occurs, but the most profound change toward the low contralateral tapping frequency is seen in psychogenic tremor. This is also confirmed by a larger study (14) demonstrating that the largest changes occur in psychogenic tremor, but that the frequency does not necessarily change toward the tapping frequency (Fig. 31.3).

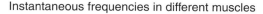

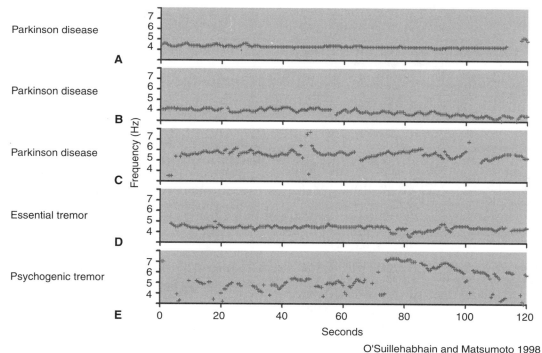

O'Suillehabhain and Matsumoto 1998

Figure 31.1 Variation of tremor frequency over time. **A:** Relatively stationary Parkinson disease rest tremor. **B:** Gradual slowing of Parkinson disease rest tremor. **C:** Small fluctuations of rest tremor in Parkinson disease. **D:** Small fluctuations of postural tremor in essential tremor patients. **E:** Very large fluctuations in psychogenic tremor. (From O'Suilleabhain PE, Matsumoto JY. Time-frequency analysis of tremors. *Brain.* 1998;121:2127–2134, with permission.)

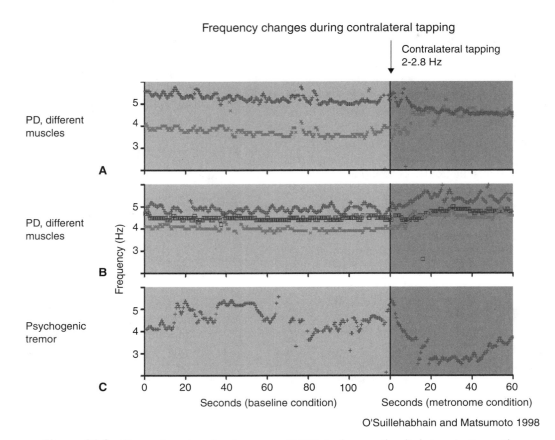

Frequency changes during contralateral tapping

Contralateral tapping
2-2.8 Hz

PD, different muscles

A

PD, different muscles

B

Psychogenic tremor

C

Frequency (Hz)

Seconds (baseline condition)   Seconds (metronome condition)

O'Suillehabhain and Matsumoto 1998

Figure 31.2   Change from baseline frequency (0–120 s) when another limb taps in time with a metronome. **A:** Parkinson disease: left biceps and left anterior tibial tremors both shift to 4.6 Hz from baseline modal frequencies of 5.2 and 3.8 Hz, respectively, when the right hand taps at 2 Hz. **B:** Parkinson disease: shift of modal frequency of masseter from 4.8 to 5.5, of right wrist flexor from 4.5 to 4.8, and of left anterior tibial muscles from 4.2 to 4.6 Hz when left hand taps at 2 Hz. **C:** Psychogenic tremor: Wide fluctuation of right thenar tremor, which shifts to the tapping frequency when the left hand taps at 2.8 Hz. PD, Parkinson Disease. (From O'Suilleabhain PE, Matsumoto JY. Time-frequency analysis of tremors. *Brain*. 1998;121:2127–2134, with permission.)

Coherence Analysis

Coherence analysis is a tool to analyze data from accelerometers or full wave rectified electromyographic data. Spectral analysis provides valid measures of the variance of amplitude and frequency of a time series (e.g., EMG or accelerometer data). Significant peaks in these spectra indicate rhythmic movements or rhythmic activity at the respective frequency, and mathematically sound statements can be made as to whether such a frequency peak is significant or not. Cross-spectral analysis is used to analyze the relation between two signals. Coherence between two such signals (two muscles or muscle and accelerometer) is analyzed according to established algorithms (24,26) and a significant coherency indicates correlated tremor activity in the two signals.

Coherence Analysis of Entrainment Tests

In a recent study of 25 patients with suspected psychogenic tremor, the EMG or accelerometer time series of two extremities was analyzed with coherence analysis when the patients were performing an entrainment test (15). The patients were asked to perform a voluntary rhythm with one extremity which was different from the tremor frequency. Patients with dystonic tremor and normal subjects served as controls. The pathologic tremors never showed coherence between the two different extremities, and 100% of the patients with psychogenic tremor had a significant coherence (Fig. 31.4). This is an encouraging result, but prospective studies in larger groups of patients are necessary.

Coherence Analysis of Bilateral Tremors

Coherence measurements have shown that in organic tremors, muscles within one arm show coherence very often, but almost never between muscles from different extremities (Fig. 31.5A) (27–30). The only exclusion from this rule is orthostatic tremor, which has a very high coherence in all the trembling muscles (31), but this condition cannot be misinterpreted as psychogenic tremor, because the tremor frequency in orthostatic tremor is much higher

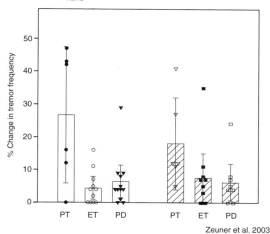

Change of tremor frequency during 3 Hz (open) or 4-5 Hz (hatched) tapping of the contralateral hand

Zeuner et al. 2003

Figure 31.3 The absolute percent change in tremor frequency is shown with 3-Hz tapping *(open columns)* and with 4- or 5-Hz tapping *(hatched columns)*. Patients with essential tremor (ET) and parkinsonian tremor (PD) could tap at 4 Hz only, whereas psychogenic tremor (PT) patients were asked to tap at 5 Hz. One patient with ET and three patients with PD were not able to tap at 4 Hz. The top of the column and error bars represent group mean and 95% CI; the symbols show the results of individual patients. For both tapping speeds, it is evident that the frequency change is largest in the psychogenic tremor patients. (From Zeuner KE, Shoge RO, Goldstein SR, et al. Accelerometry to distinguish psychogenic from essential or parkinsonian tremor. *Neurology.* 2003;61:548–550, with permission.)

than in any other tremor, including psychogenic tremor. In contrast, when normal subjects are mimicking tremor in two extremities, they have a high coherence between the muscle activities of both hands (Fig. 31.5B), indicating that normal subjects usually cannot maintain independent rhythms in their hands.

How can this be used to test for suspected psychogenic tremor? If patients have tremor in two extremities (preferentially in forearm muscles), the coherence between representative muscles from both arms can be measured. We found two types of coherence measures in a group of 15 patients with bilateral psychogenic tremor. One group (n = 7) had a high coherence between the arms, indicating that the motor system uses a similar mechanism as in the case of bilateral rhythmic movements of normal subjects. A representative example is shown in Figure 31.5C. The second group of eight patients had no coherence between the arms (Fig. 31.5D). This latter, noncoherent variant of psychogenic tremor has the same characteristics as tremor in a subject with an organic tremor. In this case, the tremor is most likely produced by cocontraction and using the mechanism of clonus to produce the tremor. These observations demonstrate that the entrainment test is very helpful, but does not fit all the cases with psychogenic tremor. Thus, if the entrainment test is negative, the possibility of a cocontraction tremor must be taken into account.

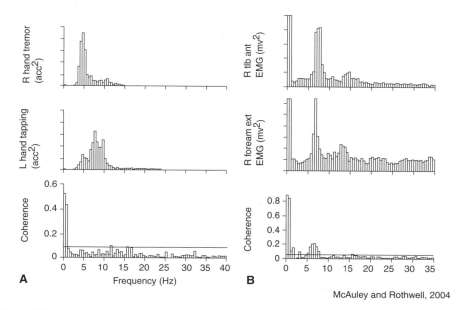

McAuley and Rothwell, 2004

Figure 31.4 Examples of the coherence entrainment test. The power spectra of two muscles from different limbs are displayed together with the coherence spectrum between these two muscles in the bottom row. **A:** Example of a patient with dystonic tremor with a 5-Hz tremor in the right hand. The patient taps as fast as possible with the left hand, leading to a broad range of frequencies covered by this movement. There is no significant coherence in the frequency band of the tremor and the tapping, indicating that the organic tremor rhythm can be maintained independently from the voluntarily produced tapping movement. **B:** Example of a psychogenic tremor present in the right lower leg and the right arm. The tremors from both limbs are clearly coherent. EMG, electromyograph. (From McAuley J, Rothwell J. Identification of psychogenic, dystonic, and other organic tremors by a coherence entrainment tremor. *Neurology.* 2003;61:548–550, with permission.)

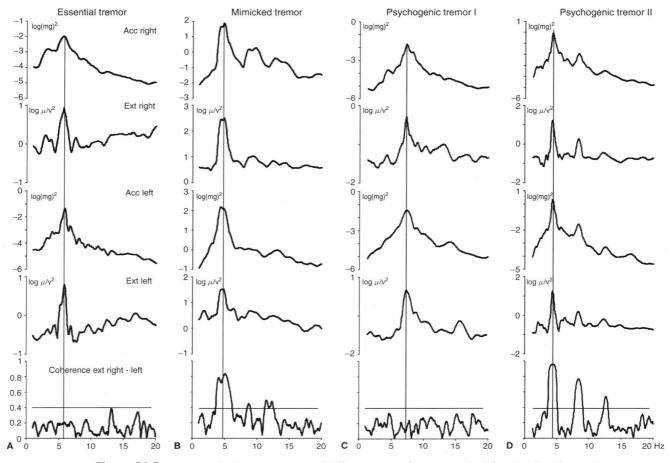

Figure 31.5 Power and coherence spectra of different types of tremor on the left and right sides. **A:** An example of accelerometric and forearm extensor electromyography power spectra for both hands of a patient with essential tremor. There is rhythmic activity at the same frequency on both sides, but these rhythms are not coherent as indicated by the coherency spectrum remaining below the 95% confidence limit *(straight line)*. **B:** A normal subject is mimicking hand tremor. The instruction was to move both hands repeatedly and independently up and down as quickly as possible. There is a significant coherence between the simulated tremor on the left and the right side. **C:** An example of a patient with psychogenic tremor. Similar to the essential tremor patient, there is no coherence between the tremors on both sides. **D:** Another patient with psychogenic tremor is displayed. In this case, there was a significant coherence between the tremors on both sides, resembling the spectra of bilaterally voluntarily mimicked tremor. (Modified after Raethjen J, Kopper F, Govindan RB, et al. Two different pathogenetic mechanisms in psychogenic tremor. *Neurology.* 2004;63:812–815, with permission.)

In summary, several electrophysiologic tests for the diagnosis of psychogenic tremor have been developed in the last 10 years. Specifically, the entrainment test and the coherence analysis seem to be good candidates for resolving the problem in the future. Prospective tests in large groups of patients are now necessary to assess the specificity and sensitivity of these tests.

THE PATHOPHYSIOLOGY OF PSYCHOGENIC TREMOR

Interestingly, the more recent literature does not comment on the pathophysiology of psychogenic tremor. However, the older neuropsychiatric literature discussed this issue summarizing the experience of the battlefield neuropsychiatry of the First World War, when psychogenic tremor was epidemic (4,21,32–37). Kretschmer commented in his 1918 article (32) "Gesetze der willkürlichen Reflexverstärkung und ihre Bedeutung für das Hysterie- und Simulationsproblem" ("The Laws of Voluntary Changes of Reflex Gain and Their Relevance for Hysteria and Simulation") that psychogenic tremor is closely related to a change of the gain of reflexes as the basis of psychogenic tremor. In modern terms, his interpretation of psychogenic tremor was that subjects change the gain of their tendon reflexes, and, therefore, "tremor" subsequently develops as a clonuslike rhythmic hyperkinesis. At that time, the neurologists were heavily discussing the question of whether this change of the reflex gain is voluntary or simulated. Then, the hypothesis was based on the observation of thousands of patients with psychogenic tremor, and specifically that some of them could tremble all day long, interrupted only when asleep; hypnosis was the treatment of first choice.

Today we may have a somewhat different view, but the discussion and research in this field is just beginning. Therefore, it may be justified to propose a schematic simple framework to further elaborate the pathophysiology of psychogenic tremor (Fig. 31.6): On the one hand, we assume that at the beginning, an (unconscious?) decision is made in the brain to develop a conversion symptom. There is a psychological or psychiatric background determining this, and we do not know much about it. Once the brain has made this decision, the next step is to select a movement disorder out of the wide range of different conversion symptoms (psychogenic tremor, sensory loss, psychogenic vertigo, etc.). We have no idea how this is determined and have not even begun to assess this question. Again, we must leave this question unanswered. Once the decision has been made to use psychogenic tremor as a conversion symptom, there may be several physiologic mechanisms which might serve to produce tremor. It is one of the assumptions of neurology—that the nervous system, and in particular, the motor system of patients with psychogenic tremor is intact. Therefore, we have to look for ways of how an intact and healthy nervous system can make rhythmic movements. The concept that we want to develop is therefore limited to this specific question within the much broader framework of questions related to psychogenic movement disorders in general.

We know next to nothing about how the brain decides to develop a psychogenic movement disorder. But it seems obvious that psychological/psychiatric factors play a role. How and why a specific movement disorder is selected by the brain is equally unknown. If it is tremor, there are at least two and probably more mechanisms by which the healthy brain can produce tremor. While we are currently beginning to understand the final step, we know little, if anything, about the first steps in this development, demonstrating that much remains to be done.

An important feature separating psychogenic tremor from other psychogenic disorders is that it is a positive symptom clearly differing from negative symptoms like hysterical blindness, deafness, or paresis. In the case of a negative psychogenic symptom like psychogenic paralysis, the subject has lost the ability to move the extremity selectively and consciously. In the case of positive symptoms like psychogenic tremor, a psychogenic gait disturbance, psychogenic parkinsonism, or psychogenic seizures, the motor activity can be positively investigated. We can compare it with normal movements, and thus can make comparisons with normal performance.

In the case of psychogenic tremor, the patient has an apparently normal motor system performing rhythmic movements. To the best of our knowledge, there are two ways to do this:

A. *Voluntary movementlike mechanism.* This can be done by just mimicking movement. Supporting such a mechanism is the observation that distraction and the entrainment test are positive in so many patients. To formulate it as cleanly as possible, this does not mean that the patient is voluntarily simulating tremor. The question of

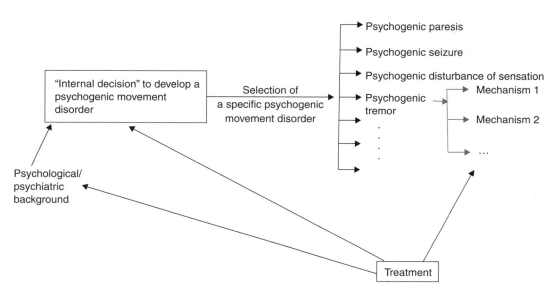

Figure 31.6 Schematic diagram of the putative steps for the development of psychogenic tremor.

why the patients use this mechanism is a different one and cannot yet be answered here. But we want to emphasize that the patient uses a normal capacity of the human nervous system. In this case, a few clinical and electrophysiologic features must be expected:

a. The subject should have a clear-cut fatigue. To perform rhythmic voluntary movements over long time periods is exhausting.
b. The cocontraction test should reveal voluntarylike rhythmic movements during tremor production.
c. The entrainment test should be positive because voluntary movements with one hand will entrain the trembling hand.
d. The coherence test should be positive, as bilateral voluntary movements cannot be performed unless with the same central movement program.

B. *Clonuslike mechanism.*   It is an everyday experience that normal individuals can produce a clonus of leg muscles after long and exhausting exercises with the legs (long-distance car-riding, etc.). This mechanism may operate to produce tremor also in the arms and in proximal joints. The subject must only maintain a steady cocontraction of antagonistic muscles to maintain this oscillation. It can be hypothesized from this mechanism that the frequency of this tremor may vary in different joints. This mechanism will be much more invariant to distracting maneuvers than the mimicked tremor, as only cocontraction is necessary to be maintained instead of the production of rhythmic movements. Thereby, even an otherwise normal nervous system can produce continuous tremor activity without too much of an effort. To some extent, any normal subject can produce such a tremor by cocontraction of arm muscles after some training.

There is an experiment reported in the literature that demonstrates the existence of this mechanism (38,39). Stimulation of Ia spindle afferents can cause a type of tremor in normal subjects. The excitation of Ia afferents was performed through continuous vibration of the triceps and biceps tendons. The tremor frequency was between 4 and 8 Hz, and it was maintained as long as the Ia excitation lasted. Different subjects had different preferred frequencies.

In this case, different clinical symptoms should be positive:

a. Fatigue should not be a major feature in these patients.
b. The subjects should have a clinical cocontraction sign. It should be easily discernible, as for this kind of movement disorder a continuous cocontraction is necessary.
c. The clinical entrainment test can be negative, as the cocontraction mechanism allows two independent oscillations in two different extremities.
d. Distractibility and frequency changes will be less obvious in this condition than in the voluntarylike mechanism.

e. The electrophysiologic coherence test can be negative because clonus can oscillate independently and noncoherently in two different extremities.

In summary, there are at least two different mechanisms, the voluntarylike and the clonus mechanism, that can produce psychogenic tremor. Assuming these two mechanisms, we can design a testable hypothesis for a prospective study of how each patient suffering from psychogenic tremor can be reliably diagnosed.

ACKNOWLEDGMENTS

This work was supported by the German Research Council (Deutsche Forschungsgemeinschaft, DFG).

REFERENCES

1. Feinstein A, Stergiopoulos V, Fine J, et al. Psychiatric outcome in patients with a psychogenic movement disorder: a prospective study. *Neuropsychiatry Neuropsychol Behav Neurol.* 2001;14: 169–176.
2. Scheidt CE, Köster B, Deuschl G. Diagnose, Symptomatik und Verlauf des psychogenen Tremors. *Nervenarzt.* 1996;67:198–204.
3. Deuschl G, Koster B, Lucking CH, et al. Diagnostic and pathophysiological aspects of psychogenic tremors. *Mov Disord.* 1998; 13:294–302.
4. Kentsmith DK. Principles of battlefield psychiatry. *Mil Med.* 1989;151:89–96.
5. Pary P, Lippmann SB, Turns DM, et al. Post-traumatic stress disorder in Vietnam veterans. *Am Fam Physician.* 1988;37:145–150.
6. Kim YJ, Pakiam AS, Lang AE. Historical and clinical features of psychogenic tremor: a review of 70 cases. *Can J Neurol Sci.* 1999; 26:190–195.
7. Marsden CD. Origins of normal and pathologic tremor. In: Findley LJ, Capildeo R, eds. *Movement disorders: tremor.* London: Macmillan, 1984:37–84.
8. Factor SA, Podskalny GD, Molho ES. Psychogenic movement disorders: frequency, clinical profile, and characteristics. *J Neurol Neurosurg Psychiatry.* 1995;59:406–412.
9. McAuley JH, Rothwell JC, Marsden CD, et al. Electrophysiological aids in distinguishing organic from psychogenic tremor. *Neurology.* 1998;50:1882–1884.
10. Spiegel J, Heiss C, Fruhauf E, et al. Polygraphic validation of distraction tasks in clinical differential tremor diagnosis. *Nervenarzt.* 1998;69:886–891.
11. Deuschl G. Differential diagnosis of tremor. *J Neural Transm Suppl.* 1999;56:211–220.
12. Brown P, Thompson PD. Electrophysiological aids to the diagnosis of psychogenic jerks, spasms, and tremor. *Mov Disord.* 2001;16:595–599.
13. Milanov I. Electromyographic differentiation of tremors. *Clin Neurophysiol.* 2001;112:1626–1632.
14. Zeuner KE, Shoge RO, Goldstein SR, et al. Accelerometry to distinguish psychogenic from essential or parkinsonian tremor. *Neurology.* 2003;61:548–550.
15. McAuley J, Rothwell J. Identification of psychogenic, dystonic, and other organic tremors by a coherence entrainment test. *Mov Disord.* 2004;19:253–267.
16. Tyrer PJ. Tremor in acute and chronic anxiety. *Arch Gen Psychiatry.* 1974;31:506–509.
17. Marsden CD. Hysteria—a neurologist's view. *Psychol Med.* 1986; 16:277–288.
18. Koller W, Lang A, Vetere-Overfield B, et al. Psychogenic tremors. *Neurology.* 1989;39:1094–1099.
19. Thomas M, Jankovic J. Psychogenic movement disorders: diagnosis and management. *CNS Drugs.* 2004;18:437–452.

20. O'Suilleabhain PE, Matsumoto JY. Time-frequency analysis of tremors. *Brain*. 1998;121:2127–2134.
21. Redfearn JWT. Frequency analysis of physiological and neurotic tremors. *J Neurol Neurosurg Psychiatry*. 1957;20:302–313.
22. Sabra AF, Hallett M. Action tremor with alternating activity in antagonist muscles. *Neurology*. 1984;34:151–156.
23. Hallett M. Differential diagnosis of tremor. In: Vinken PJ, Bruyn GW, Klawans HL, eds. *Handbook of clinical neurology*. Vol. 49. Amsterdam: Elsevier Science Publishers, BV, 1986:583–595.
24. Elble RJ, Koller WC. *Tremor*. Baltimore, MD, London: The Johns Hopkins University Press, 1990.
25. Milanov I. Clinical and electromyographic examinations of patients with psychogenic tremor. *Electromyogr Clin Neurophysiol*. 2002;42:387–392.
26. Lauk M, Timmer J, Lucking CH, et al. A software for recording and analysis of human tremor. *Comput Methods Programs Biomed*. 1999;60:65–77.
27. Raethjen J, Lindemann M, Schmaljohann H, et al. Multiple oscillators are causing parkinsonian and essential tremor. *Mov Disord*. 2000;15:84–94.
28. Hurtado JM, Lachaux JP, Beckley DJ, et al. Inter- and intralimb oscillator coupling in parkinsonian tremor. *Mov Disord*. 2000;15:683–691.
29. Ben-Paz H, Bergman H, Goldber JA, et al. Synchrony of rest tremor in multiple limbs in parkinson's disease: evidence for multiple oscillators. *J Neural Transm*. 2001;108:287–296.
30. Hellwig B, Haussler S, Schelter B, et al. Tremor-correlated cortical activity in essential tremor. *Lancet*. 2001;357:519–523.
31. Koster B, Lauk M, Timmer J, et al. Involvement of cranial muscles and high intermuscular coherence in orthostatic tremor. *Ann Neurol*. 1999;45:384–388.
32. Kretschmer E. Die Gesetze der willkürlichen Reflexverstärkung in ihrer Bedeutung für das Hysterie- und Simulationsproblem. *Zsch ges Neurol und Psychiat*. 1918;41:354–385.
33. Stern H. Die hysterischen Bewegungsstörungen als Massenerscheinung im Krieg, ihre Entstehung und Prognose. *Zsch ges Neurol und Psychiat*. 1918;39:246–281.
34. Wachholder K, Haas J. Untersuchungen über organischen und nichtorganischen Tremor. In: Siemerling E BO, ed. *Jahresversammlung der südostdeutschen psychiater*, 4th ed. Vol. 88. Berlin: Springer, 1929:470–477.
35. Altenburger H. Elektrodiagnostik. In: Bumke O FO, ed. *Handbuch der neurologie*. Vol. Band III. Berlin: Julius Springer, 1937:1036–1086.
36. Altenburger H. Zur Pathophysiologie psychogener Bewegungsstörungen. *Zsch ges Neurol und Psychiat*. 1937;158:133–135.
37. Jung R. Physiologische Untersuchungen über den Parkinsontremor und andere Zitterformen beim Menschen. *Zsch ges Neurol und Psychiat*. 1941;173:263–332.
38. Prochazka A, Trend PS. Instability in human forearm movements studied with feedback- controlled muscle vibration. *J Physiol*. 1988;402:421–442.
39. Jacks A, Prochazka A, Trend PS. Instability in human forearm movements studied with feedback-controlled electrical stimulation of muscles. *J Physiol*. 1988;402:443–461.

32

Natural History of Psychogenic Movement Disorders

Daniel T. Williams   *Blair Ford*   *Stanley Fahn*   *Marc Williams*

ABSTRACT

The term "psychogenic-neuropsychiatric movement disorders" (PNMDs) is advocated here for two reasons. The first reason is for precision of descriptive phenomenology, which will be explored below. The second reason is in the interest of facilitating acceptance of the diagnosis by patients and their families where it applies. This term is less likely than "psychogenic movement disorders" to be perceived as pejorative by these individuals, who often have long labored under the misimpression that the movement disorder symptoms were purely neurologic. Initial clarification of the formidable, and frequently primary, role of psychiatric contributants to these symptoms tends to come as a jarring shock to many such patients. Indeed, if conveyed too confrontationally by the evaluating clinician, this clarification may contribute to the patient's premature departure and associated refusal of crucial psychiatric intervention.

Psychogenic-neuropsychiatric movement disorders (PNMDs) are abnormal movements that cannot be considered to result directly from traditional "organic" diseases, but which rather derive primarily from psychological and psychiatric causes (1). The presumption inherent in the term "psychogenic movement disorders," as used over the past 20 years, was that they lacked either definable structural abnormality in the brain, or a definable physiologic abnormality, both of which are demonstrable in "organic" diseases (2,3). Yet we now are coming to appreciate that these distinctions between "organic" and "psychogenic" are arbitrary, representing relative points on a continuum, rather than categoric distinctions. We recognize that the psychomotor retardation that may accompany depression, the bizarre movements and postures of schizophrenia, and the stereotyped movements of autism all represent movement abnormalities characterizing psychiatric disorders where there is strong evidence of a pathologic-neurophysiologic underpinning. In this context, Vuilleumier et al. (4) documented a consistent decrease of regional blood flow in the thalamus and basal ganglia contralateral to the deficit in patients with "psychogenic" sensorimotor loss that were diagnosed as conversion disorders.

It is, therefore, not only to make diagnostic debriefing of patients more palatable, but also because it represents a more sophisticated contemporary understanding of the pathophysiology that the use of the term "psychogenic-neuropsychiatric movement disorders" is preferable. One can reasonably discern a qualitative difference between a relatively transient conversion disorder causing tremor that fully resolves with therapeutic suggestion and the relatively more fixed tremor of a Parkinson disease patient. Yet we know that the Parkinson patient's tremor can be exacerbated by emotional stress and that an untreated conversion disorder can become both physically and emotionally chronically incapacitating, such as by generating fixed contractures in extreme cases. This chapter will address the natural history of those neuropsychiatric movement disorders that have traditionally been viewed as "psychogenic," with a view to exploring relevant diagnostic and treatment considerations, as well as features of developmental course.

The first challenge faced by a clinician dealing with such a patient is to rule out the presence of an underlying "organic" neurologic condition. The second is to see that appropriate psychiatric evaluation and treatment are implemented. Having noted this, it must be added that the pathogenesis of the PNMD conditions discussed remains only partially understood, and the treatment, as in much of psychiatry, is largely empirical.

HISTORICAL CONSIDERATIONS

Most of the presentations at the symposium contributing to this volume that have dealt with the evolution of our understanding of PNMDs have focused on the seminal contributions of Briquet (5), Charcot (6), and Freud (7). It is worth adding that prior to these clinical formulations, the predominant historical perspective on these disorders derived from the variety of religious presumptions that viewed many forms of both physical and emotional illness as derivatives of adverse supernatural influences. As such, the contributions of William James (8) deserve mention in highlighting the role of dissociative phenomena in this domain. The role of dissociative mechanisms continues to be relevant, both regarding our understanding of symptom formation and in elucidating how the potentially powerful role of authoritatively sanctioned suggestion can sometimes be dramatically helpful in symptom alleviation (9), if appropriately applied.

A more contemporary influence of historical relevance is the clarification of the distinction between epileptic and nonepileptic seizures, facilitated greatly by the availability of electroencephalographic technology and its application in epilepsy monitoring units (10). This has provided a clear paradigm for the differentiation of neurologic from neuropsychiatric syndromes that might appear initially indistinguishable, and which may, in fact, coexist within the same patient. The tendency of epileptologists to avoid the pejorative use of such terms as "pseudoseizures" in favor of "nonepileptic seizures" constitutes a useful terminological model for movement disorder clinicians. While epileptologists indeed use the term "psychogenic nonepileptic seizures" in communicating with other clinicians, the tendency in communicating with patients and their families

is to use a more neutral term, such as "stress-induced nonepileptic seizures," a precedent worth considering by movement disorder neurologists.

There was not unanimity of opinion on this issue at the conference that generated this volume, and further evolution of terminology will likely ensue. Most significant clinically in working with a given patient is conveying one's findings sensitively and supportively so as to facilitate appropriate treatment intervention. This will inevitably involve a shift in linguistic nuance, depending on the intellectual capacity and level of psychological sophistication of a given patient.

EPIDEMIOLOGY

Neuropsychiatric symptoms have been estimated to account for between 1% and 9% of all neurologic diagnoses (11, 12). No specific epidemiologic data exists with regard to the incidence of psychogenic-neuropsychiatric movement disorders in population studies. In specialized movement disorder clinics, which tend to be at tertiary care centers, the rate of PNMDs tends to be around 3% of the total number of movement disorder patients (13,14). It is estimated, based on sampling similar patient populations, that 10% to 15% of patients with PNMDs have an underlying organic movement disorder, as well (1).

NEUROLOGIC DIAGNOSIS

Since most patients with PNMDs present to neurologists before they get to see a psychiatrist, the burden of initial diagnosis generally falls to the neurologist. In this regard, it is best to conceptualize the diagnostic process in these disorders as a two-stage process. The first stage is that of ruling out or circumscribing the role of definable neurologic illness, thus clarifying the necessary presence of a psychiatric disorder as an essential component of understanding some or all of the presenting symptoms. It is generally best for the neurologist to then facilitate the obtaining of a psychiatric evaluation so that a full psychiatric diagnostic assessment can inform treatment planning. It is important to note that delays in correct neurologic diagnosis and associated psychiatric treatment referral are likely to prolong a patient's pattern of disability (15). Further, some patients with undiagnosed PNMDs are subjected to inappropriate and sometimes aversive testing or potentially dangerous treatment, including unwarranted stereotactic neurosurgery (3).

It should also be re-emphasized that the role of the neurologist is primary in the establishment of the diagnosis of a neuropsychiatric movement disorder. No mental health professional should embark on treatment of such patients without a clear understanding as to the level of confidence with which the neurologic diagnosis has been either established or ruled out. The role of the mental health professional is to clarify the extent and potential relevance of discernable psychopathology as part of a collaborative assessment. If this appears relevant and a positive rapport has been established with the patient, ideally the psychiatrist will then take the lead in treatment, with appropriate collaborative support from the neurologist. This maintenance of a "team approach" is crucial to enhance acceptance of treatment to which the patient and family are often initially quite resistant.

The issues of movement disorder phenomenology and the differential diagnosis of neurologic versus psychogenic-neuropsychiatric movement disorders have been addressed earlier in this volume as well as elsewhere (1). Since it is our contention that the natural history of PNMDs is generally a byproduct of the patient's psychopathology and clinical management, rather than a byproduct of the presenting movement disorder phenomenology, we will address this issue with a primary emphasis on considerations of psychiatric referral, psychiatric diagnosis, and psychiatric treatment.

To our knowledge, there is no published prospective data on the natural history of PNMDs. We will review here the modest retrospective literature that is available, with some clinical observations drawn from our experience with these disorders over the past 20 years at the Columbia University Medical Center.

PSYCHIATRIC REFERRAL

As noted above, the issue of facilitating psychiatric referral is crucial with this group of disorders. Despite a close and longstanding collaborative relationship that our movement disorder group has with a psychiatrist experienced in treating patients with neuropsychiatric movement disorders, well over half the patients who are referred for outpatient psychiatric consultation fail to implement this recommendation.

Our initial response to this pattern of noncompliance with psychiatric referral by the neurologist was to preferentially admit all such patients that we could to the inpatient neurology service, once a strong probability of the diagnosis of a neuropsychiatric disorder was ascertained. Under the rubric of a "multidisciplinary diagnostic and treatment approach," the patient would be seen intensively by the admitting neurologist, the consulting psychiatrist, and a physical therapist. This hospitalization served several functions. It removed the patient from those environmental influences that were frequently contributory to the symptom formation and perpetuation, while it also allowed us to evaluate the patient more thoroughly in a more controlled environment. Further, the introduction of the psychiatrist as a routine member of the evaluation and treatment team made it more difficult for the patient to reject this intervention and allowed for the development of a therapeutic alliance while

multiple diagnostic and treatment strategies were ongoing simultaneously, assuring the patient that no organic contributions to symptoms were being overlooked.

Within a few days of admission, with our initial diagnostic impressions usually further clarified, we arranged for a conjoint debriefing session with both the neurologist and psychiatrist present to supportively present to the patient our diagnostic impressions and treatment recommendations. If neurologic workup was negative, this was supportively reviewed, together with the more favorable prognosis for recovery than would be the case with a degenerative neurologic disorder. We observed further that stress of various origins can contribute to physiologic aberrations that generate clear physical symptoms despite the absence of discernable structural lesions on the various diagnostic tests currently available. Commonly encountered clinical examples of how stress can activate the symptoms of hypertension, peptic ulcer disease, and asthma, among others, would often facilitate patient recognition of the plausibility and relevance of this conceptual model. A treatment plan was then outlined, tailored to the needs of the individual patient. Elements of this treatment plan, often including psychotherapy, pharmacotherapy, and physical therapy, would generally be started in the hospital in an effort to achieve as much symptomatic improvement as possible in the available duration of stay, to be continued on an outpatient basis as individually needed. There was always a follow-up appointment with both the neurologist as well as the psychiatrist to assure the patient and family that both spheres were being appropriately monitored in an effort to achieve full symptom resolution.

Over the past 20 years, however, it has become increasingly difficult to admit patients with suspected PNMDs to the inpatient neurology service because of the restrictions of rigid "managed care" guidelines. This is sometimes a short-sighted obstruction of effective treatment for patients who are otherwise resistant to appropriate psychiatric care and consequently suffer prolongation of an otherwise treatable disability. On the other hand, we have been pleasantly surprised by a significant number of positive responders to our revised format of requiring a routine outpatient psychiatric consultation *before* the full formulation of treatment recommendations by the neurologist, based on the clinically indicated *possibility* that stress may be contributing significantly to the presenting symptoms. Many of these patients, who were sufficiently insightful, motivated, and emotionally capable of responding to a combined neurologic and psychiatric outpatient treatment program, demonstrated resilience in their capacity to respond to such therapeutic intervention much beyond our initial expectations.

Case Study

Emily, a 30-year-old married attorney, was referred for psychiatric consultation when our senior movement disorder neurologist doubted, based on office consultation, that Emily's 10-year history of "myoclonus" was neurologically based. This syndrome had first presented during college, when Emily was academically as well as emotionally stressed and developed an episode of apparent viral encephalitis. This illness further compromised her academic functioning for a while, and left her with residual symptoms of episodic "myoclonic jerks," particularly at times of stress. Although she graduated both college and law school and married, she continued to be troubled by these persistent symptoms, which were not alleviated by a variety of anticonvulsant and antitremor medications. There was partial benefit from clonazepam, which was used in doses up to 4 mg per day.

Emily had previously participated in supportive–exploratory psychotherapy, albeit irregularly, over many years, without any discernable impact on the myoclonic symptoms. The therapy clarified clear traumatic emotional residua of the divorce of Emily's parents when she was an adolescent, resulting in Emily being thrust into the role of caretaker for her learning-disabled younger sibling. Emily had considerable residual ambivalence toward both parents, stress associated with her professional obligations as an attorney; and ambivalence regarding the prospect of motherhood. Emily sought consultation at our medical center because of a desire to discontinue medication in the face of her wish to become pregnant.

In psychiatric consultation, prompted by an atypical history for myoclonus and nonphysiologic findings on neurologic and electrophysiologic examination, the above history was reviewed supportively and the plausibility of a neuropsychiatric basis for the myoclonic symptoms was explained, expanding on its initial presentation by the consulting neurologist. There were indications of possible secondary gains associated with added solicitude and support from Emily's parents, spouse, and her supervisor at work when her myoclonic symptoms were activated by stress. Yet the patient's maintenance of a relatively high level of functioning, despite her longstanding symptoms, plus her active wish to eliminate medication as she planned her pregnancy, appeared to constitute favorable prognostic and motivational factors. Two additional psychiatric visits were scheduled. In the first, a supportive formulation of the dynamics of conversion disorder was articulated, including the neurophysiologic capacity of dissociative mechanisms to unconsciously transform emotional conflicts into physical symptoms. This was followed by the assessment of the patient's hypnotizability and the teaching of a self-hypnosis exercise to facilitate emotional–cognitive reorientation geared to facilitating symptom relinquishment. The premise was that, in light of the new incentive of a medication-free pregnancy, Emily might mobilize the resources to face ongoing conflicts in a more direct and healthy manner with the aid of this new perspective and psychotherapeutically reformulated strategies of adaptation. In the third session,

which was a conjoint session with her husband, the overall treatment strategy was further supportively reviewed, with initial observations of symptomatic improvement already evident. A plan for monitoring further symptom attenuation, together with tapering of clonazepam, was outlined. Emily cancelled her next appointment, however, and declined to schedule another.

Follow-up came three years later, when Emily set another appointment with the psychiatrist. She reported having become fully free of myoclonic symptoms in the wake of the prior three office visits, allowing tapering and discontinuation of clonazepam. A subsequent pregnancy was carried successfully to term, with the ensuing birth of a normal infant. Emily continued symptom-free for another one and a half years, when a resurgence of work and family pressures was associated with the recurrence of myoclonic symptoms. She initially returned to the neurologist who had previously maintained her on clonazepam and he chose to restart it. Emily returned to us after a year on clonazepam, which was clearly ineffective in symptom control, when she decided to become pregnant again. A similar course of multimodal psychotherapeutic intervention was commenced, with recommendation for more sustained treatment, in the hope of establishing a more sustained clinical improvement. This was indeed achieved within the course of several weeks. With the re-establishment of a symptom-free state, however, Emily again abruptly discontinued treatment and declined to schedule follow-up visits.

In contrast to Emily's impressive resilience (albeit resistance to appropriate follow-up treatment), many patients, based on initial outpatient psychiatric consultation, appear clearly unlikely to be responsive to outpatient treatment. Such a clinical assessment may be based on limitations of insight and receptivity to entertaining a neuropsychiatric hypothesis, inadequately supportive or conflicted family situations, and/or severe coexisting psychopathology. In such cases, the detailed report of the initial outpatient psychiatric consultation, coupled with the detailed report of the movement disorder neurologist's consultation, is frequently sufficient to persuade the relevant insurance carrier of the merits of an elective hospital admission, if the patient is receptive to this recommendation. This recommendation is predicated on the logical clinical and fiduciary premise that it is in the best interest of all concerned, including that of the insurance carrier, to give the patient an opportunity for comprehensive evaluation and treatment in an inpatient setting as an alternative to what otherwise frequently becomes a course of chronic disability, with an associated course of further expensive and unhelpful diagnostic and treatment interventions.

Quite apart from the bureaucratic and administrative constraints that need to be navigated in seeking to establish the most effective possible treatment plan, based on the diagnostic considerations of the individual patient, the attitude and tenor of the referring neurologist is crucial in influencing the prospects of the patient's accepting a psychiatric referral. If the psychiatric referral is perceived by the patient as a rejection and devaluation by the neurologist, because the symptoms are "not real" or "all in my mind," obviously the likelihood of successful referral are poor. Conversely, if the psychiatrist is a valued collaborator in a diagnostic and treatment endeavor which is presented as having a more favorable prognosis than would otherwise pertain, chances for successful referral markedly improve.

PSYCHIATRIC DIAGNOSIS

In our clinical experience, one of the most frequent impediments to the establishment of an accurate psychiatric diagnosis is the reluctance of many mental health professionals to adequately assess psychopathology when they are intimidated by the often dramatically impressive nature of the patient's obvious physical symptoms, coupled with the patient's strong conviction that the symptoms are of organic etiology. Faced with this formidable combination, and frequently not being fully informed regarding previous neurologic evaluations, the mental health professional may be reluctant even to consider a psychiatric diagnosis in light of the potentially embarrassing and problematic medical and legal consequences if a "psychiatric label" is mistakenly applied to a patient who actually has an undiagnosed primary neurologic disorder. Many patients consequently present to our group with the contention that they have been given "a clean bill of health" by a previously evaluating mental health practitioner, thereby reinforcing their reluctance to consider further exploration of potentially relevant psychopathology.

The best antidote to this quandary is to have a psychiatrist or psychologist with significant clinical experience in the complexities of the neurology–psychiatry interface who can undertake the process of evaluating potentially relevant psychopathology in such patients. This diminishes the prospects of a premature presumption that documented psychopathology, some of which will inevitably be found in every patient, is necessarily causative of the presenting physical symptoms (16). It should also allow flexibility to consider the possibility that significant psychopathology, when encountered, may be relevant and contributory to presenting neuropsychiatric symptoms. It is crucial to avoid a "rush to judgment," insofar as an adequate neuropsychiatric evaluation of these complex patients frequently requires several visits and communications between the neurologist and evaluating mental health professional.

Having noted the above, it is advisable that, after completion of the initial neuropsychiatric evaluation, a full multiaxial delineation of relevant psychopathology be organized in accordance with the nomenclature of the most current edition of the *Diagnostic and Statistical Manual of Mental Disorders* (DSM) of the American Psychiatric Association (17). This substantially facilitates appropriate differential diagnosis and associated treatment recommendations. The three most relevant diagnostic categories for describing the primary psychopathology associated with PNMDs include: somatoform disorders, factitious disorders, and malingering.

Somatoform Disorders

In accordance with current DSM definition, a somatoform disorder is one in which physical symptoms that cannot be explained by a diagnosable medical condition appear, after careful clinical assessment, to derive from psychological factors that are not under the patient's voluntary control (17). This implies that the symptom formation is not intentionally (consciously) produced by the patient. The two most commonly encountered forms of somatoform disorder, in our experience with patients having neuropsychiatric movement disorders, are conversion disorder and somatization disorder. The latter is also known as hysteria or Briquet syndrome. Other somatoform disorder subtypes that can be encountered as coexisting conditions in these patients include hypochondriasis, pain disorder, body dysmorphic disorder, and undifferentiated somatoform disorder.

In conversion disorder, the patient has one or more symptoms affecting voluntary motor or sensory function that suggest a neurologic or other medical condition. Psychological factors may be discerned to play the primary etiologic role in a variety of ways. There may be a temporal relationship between the onset or worsening of the symptoms and the presence of an environmental influence that activates a psychological conflict or need. Alternatively, the symptom may be observed to liberate the patient from an unwanted activity or encounter. As in all somatoform disorders, the symptom is not intentionally produced or feigned. (This is in contrast to factitious disorder or malingering.) The symptom cannot, after appropriate clinical investigation, be fully explained by a general medical condition, by the direct effects of a substance, or as a culturally sanctioned experience (17).

Case Study

Alan, an 18-year-old college student, was referred to our group after evaluation by neurologists, psychologists, and psychiatrists at three other medical centers for a 6-month history of uncontrolled, jerky movements, involving all four extremities. The first episode occurred after his first sexual experience with a girlfriend that he had courted avidly, but toward whom he had ambivalence related to her fending off his initial dating overtures. These initial symptoms subsided spontaneously, but recurred several months later, the night before a major paper was due and as college final exams were looming. Initial neurologic evaluation was unrevealing of any organic substrate and Alan was referred for psychotherapy. However, the symptoms worsened and persisted, precluding the taking of exams and prompting a sequence of numerous neurologic and psychiatric consultations in several disparate cities. Extensive blood studies, EEG, MRI of brain and spine, and a PET scan were all normal. One neurologic consultant recommended a brain biopsy to rule out a progressive viral encephalopathy. There were several nonphysiologic findings upon neurologic examination by our group. These findings, coupled with the persistence of disabling symptoms and the family's confusion about appropriate diagnosis and treatment, led to Alan's being admitted to our neurology inpatient service with a plan for more extensive neuropsychiatric assessment.

The extensive negative neurologic workup, coupled with the nonphysiologic findings pointing to a psychogenic etiology, allowed for a reassuring communication to the family of a favorable prognosis in this previously highly functional young man with no prior psychiatric or neurologic history. Activation of the patient's paroxysmal movements was noted by an exaggerated startle response. On the inpatient service, a combination of psychodynamically oriented individual and family psychotherapy helped to clarify conflictual issues regarding Alan's family life, his sexual identity, and his capacity for assertiveness that appeared together to have contributed to precipitating conversion symptoms under stressful circumstances. Treatment included supportive psychotherapeutic restructuring, utilizing a combination of hypnosis, antidepressant medication, and behavioral desensitization in conjunction with "reconditioning" by the physical therapy department. Alan's symptoms cleared progressively during his 2-week hospital stay. He was discharged to outpatient psychiatric treatment and was able to successfully re-enroll at college, maintaining his symptom-free state, with the benefit of follow-up psychiatric treatment.

Somatization disorder involves recurrent, multiple physical complaints of several years' duration for which medical care has been sought, but which cannot be fully explained by any known medical disorder or the direct effects of a substance (e.g., a drug of abuse or a medication). The symptoms are not intentionally produced or feigned, connoting psychodynamics analogous to those of conversion disorder. There are indications that somatization disorder may emerge from chronic, recurrent, untreated conversion disorder (18). Diagnostic criteria require four pain symptoms, two gastrointestinal symptoms, one sexual symptom, and one "pseudoneurologic" symptom. Other diagnostic requirements are that the symptoms commence before age 30, and result in treatment being sought or significant impairment in social, occupational, or other significant areas of functioning. The coexisting presence of factitious or malingering symptoms, together with unintentional symptoms, is not uncommon (17).

The term "undifferentiated somatoform disorder" applies when one or more physical symptoms persists for at least 6 months and shares the above somatoform characteristics, but does not meet the full criteria of a somatization disorder (17).

Factitious Disorders

The essential feature of factitious disorders is the intentional production of physical or psychological signs or symptoms due to a pathologic, psychological need. The primary motivation is to assume the sick role. External incentives for the behavior, such as economic gain or avoiding legal responsibility (as in malingering) are absent. There are often not only numerous medical evaluations and treatments, but numerous hospitalizations and surgical interventions, often in many different sites to avoid clarification of the psychiatric components that might be more evident with continuity of care. A chronic pattern frequently emerges, to which iatrogenic errors of diagnosis and intervention may contribute, reinforcing chronicity and intractability, as in the case of Münchausen syndrome. The apparent yearning to be cared for by assuming the role of a patient is frequently associated with severe dependent, masochistic, borderline, and antisocial personality features. Consequently, treatment prognosis is generally less favorable than in cases of somatoform disorders (17).

Case Study

Sandra, a 19-year-old student, came to us with a 10-year history of multiple complaints, including uncontrolled seizures, ambloyopia, and dystonia. Her 10-year history of evaluation and treatment for these disorders included 14 hospitalizations and three major surgical interventions at prestigious university medical centers. The parents came for admission to our medical center from another state, but failed to meet with the psychiatrist during the patient's several weeks of hospitalization. The mother was a nurse.

At age nine, the first onset of the turning in of Sandra's left foot with abnormal gait was observed. This eventually led to the diagnosis of torsion dystonia, which was complicated by surgical intervention to insert a metal rod in the foot in an effort to straighten it. A few years later, the emergence of scoliosis led, eventually, to spinal surgery, with the insertion of a metal rod to straighten the spine. Over time, although treated with numerous anticonvulsants for uncontrolled seizures, there was no clear record of a documented, abnormal EEG. The ambloyopia, which resulted in the patient's being declared legally blind, was never explained medically with regard to a discernible etiology. Finally, the patient was transferred from an adolescent psychiatry inpatient service at another medical center to the neurosurgery unit, where a cryothalamotomy was performed for what was thought to be a progressive form of torsion dystonia.

Upon evaluation at our medical center, it became clear that the findings on neurologic examination were not compatible with those of a neurologically based torsion dystonia. The absence of EEG documentation of prior seizures led to the suspicion that they may well have been nonepileptic. The patient, when observed unobtrusively by the nursing staff, was noted to be watching television from a substantial distance and to be manifesting other behaviors incompatible with the contended level of ambloyopia. During an effort at neuro-ophthalmologic evaluation, involving a visual-evoked response test, the patient was noted to be volitionally crossing her eyes, rather than attending to the visual stimulus, documenting a purposeful effort to confound medical evaluation and treatment.

Although there was partial improvement during the course of the hospital stay with supportive conjoint debriefing by the psychiatrist and neurologist, and sustained efforts at insight-oriented psychotherapy with this adolescent of at least average intellectual capacity, symptomatic improvement was modest. The patient returned to her home state and failed to respond to our recommendation for systematic follow-up with us.

Malingering

Malingering refers to the voluntary production of physical and/or psychological symptoms in the pursuit of a recognizably pragmatic goal. Examples of such goals would include financial compensation, avoidance of school or work, evasion of criminal prosecution, or acquisition of drugs. Frequent associated characteristics include a medical–legal context (e.g., pending litigation), a notable lack of cooperation during diagnostic evaluation and/or treatment, and the presence of an antisocial personality disorder. Malingering is not considered to be a mental disorder, though there may be substantial coexisting psychopathology (17).

PSYCHIATRIC DIFFERENTIAL DIAGNOSIS

The challenges here can be formidable. When faced with a patient having a neuropsychiatric movement disorder, it is often impossible, especially initially, to distinguish with confidence among somatoform disorders, factitious disorders, and malingering. A patient's volitional intentions are often impossible to ascertain, especially early in the course of assessment. Clarification may emerge however, in the course of further evaluation and treatment endeavors, as manifested by the patient's level of candor, responsiveness, and cooperation. The most important pitfall to avoid is that of becoming prematurely confrontational with the patient, or of assuming that the patient's difficulty in absorbing the subtleties of the concept of somatization necessarily connotes purposeful obstructionism that is associated with factitious disorders or malingering. Protracted efforts should be made, hopefully facilitated with participation by the evaluating neurologist, to enable the patient and relevant family members, if appropriate, to grasp the complexities of unconsciously based symptom formation. It is much better for the clinician to eventually come to the conclusion that he or she has been duped by a feigning patient than to make the more serious error of inappropriately alienating a potentially treatable patient by premature erroneous attribution of purposeful noncooperation.

COEXISTING PSYCHIATRIC CONDITIONS

A primary task of psychiatric differential diagnosis is indeed that of distinguishing between somatoform disorders, factitious disorders, and malingering. Yet most patients with neuropsychiatric movement disorders have other coexisting psychiatric diagnoses, as well (19). It is desirable to delineate these as fully as possible in accordance with the most recently available edition of the DSM of the American Psychiatric Association (17), insofar as this will inform treatment recommendations. Common examples of relevant psychopathology on axis I would include affective disorders, anxiety disorders, dissociative disorders, or psychotic disorders. Also common are axis II diagnoses, such as developmental disorders and personality disorders. One must, of course, be cognizant of the possibility of coexisting, undiagnosed organic illness (axis III). The identification of specific psychosocial stressors, such as school, work, family, or other environmental adversities should also be considered (axis IV). In this regard, due consideration should be given to the possibility of symptom modeling and secondary gain issues (pragmatic benefits of the symptoms). Specific inquiries should be made with regard to a possible history of physical, sexual, or emotional abuse, which may contribute to a coexisting dissociative disorder. A global assessment of the function (axis V) should be designated to signify the estimated extent of functional impairment. Some neuropsychiatric movement disorder symptoms may develop in vulnerable individuals who are incapable of directly negotiating the everyday demands of life, but these symptoms may also develop in relatively highly functioning individuals who are overwhelmed by either cumulative and/or unusually stressful life events.

A review of clinical experience with 24 patients with neuropsychiatric movement disorders who underwent a full psychiatric evaluation disclosed a range of characteristics (19). The demographic profile of a typical patient included a wide variation in age (from 11 to 60 years; mean age 36 years), predominantly women (79%), of average to above-average intelligence (96% combined), with a wide duration of symptoms (range less than 1 month to 23 years; mean duration of 5 years). The majority of adults were unable to work and were on disability (70%). The primary axis I psychiatric diagnoses were conversion disorder (75%), somatization disorder (13%), factitious disorder (8%), and malingering (4%). Dysthymia, as an associated psychiatric diagnosis, was present in 67% of patients. Additional associated diagnoses included major depressive disorder, adjustment disorder, organic mood disorder, psychotic disorder, obsessive–compulsive disorder, panic attacks, bipolar disorder, and others.

It should be emphasized that effectively treating coexisting psychiatric conditions can be crucial in enhancing the prospects of effectively alleviating the presenting neuropsychiatric movement disorder.

TREATMENT

In the absence of controlled clinical trials specifically for patients with psychogenic-neuropsychiatric movement disorders, empirical treatment has generally been focused on those features of psychopathology that can be identified in these patients (20). As such, a comprehensive psychiatric assessment is a crucial prerequisite to effective treatment. Those considerations which would ordinarily pertain to treating each category of relevant psychopathology would naturally pertain as well when dealing with a neuropsychiatric movement disorder. Associated considerations of relevance to the treatment of PNMDs will be addressed here.

Traditional treatment strategies for conversion disorders include considerations of predisposition, precipitating factors, and perpetuating factors (21).

Predisposition includes personality factors and past experiences that predispose to somatization; limitations of communicative ability due to intellectual, emotional, or social constraints; and underlying psychiatric or neurologic disorders.

Precipitating stressors may involve activation of psychological conflicts, for example, regarding sexual, aggressive, or dependency issues; or traumatic events, for example, those threatening one's physical integrity or self-esteem.

Perpetuating factors include both the extent to which the symptom resolves the conflict that gave rise to the symptom (primary gain) and associated pragmatic benefits of the symptom (secondary gain).

The goal of effective treatment involves not merely symptom relief in the short term, which can often be achieved by the use of suggestion or placebos, but consideration of the factors that produced the symptom and assessment of the possibilities of their sustained remediation. Implicitly, this involves evaluating the possibility of an underlying psychiatric or neurologic disorder, of which the patient may be unaware (22). This may also pertain regarding situations of past or present physical, emotional, or sexual abuse that may be either consciously suppressed or unconsciously repressed by the patient (23). Often a combination of both psychotherapy to deal with psychological conflicts, as well as active advice regarding redress of environmental stressors or abusers, is required for sustained symptom alleviation. Similarly, treatment must address those secondary gains of the symptom that may contribute to resistance to its relinquishment.

One may conceptualize a conversion symptom as a "dissociative disconnect," whereby the patient is overwhelmed with adversity beyond capacity for conscious processing or expression, leading to a more primitive communication of a "body language expression of distress" (24,40). The presenting conversion symptom thereby serves a partially protective function, albeit in a regressive and often maladaptive way. If the conversion symptom abates spontaneously after the resolution of a short-term precipitating conflict, no formal treatment may be needed and supportive reassurance or suggestion may suffice. Symptom persistence or exacerbation, however, clearly mandates therapeutic intervention to avoid potential chronicity that makes subsequent treatment intervention more difficult.

Psychotherapeutic interventions need to be mindful of the patient's self esteem and help to generate a more effective adaptive strategy for dealing with pre-existing conflicts by a process of emotional and cognitive "restructuring" that allows for more effective coping without need for the maladaptive symptom. Such treatment should ideally take into account as many relevant etiologic variables as possible and address them with a systems theory perspective that includes biologic, psychological, and social influences. This intervention is more palatable to the patient if presented supportively, with the therapist taking a collaborative stance in helping the patient to improve "stress management" strategies (21).

Hypnosis provides the advantage of providing the patient with a direct experience of dissociation under the protective rubric of the therapy setting (26,27). The current tendency to assess hypnotizability with standard scales allows the patient to experience a structured "mind-body" dissociative experience of a benign nature. This becomes a paradigm to then understand this capacity for dissociation to be both a vulnerability to symptom formation, but also a potential conduit for symptom relinquishment, when restructured under the guidance of the therapist. Thus, the therapist can first use the trance experience as an opportunity for transmitting a more sophisticated understanding of the dynamics of symptom formation (28). Having achieved this in a supportive therapeutic relationship, hypnosis can then be utilized as a vehicle for positive suggestions to improve coping strategies and thereby achieve symptom attenuation (29).

One recent randomized controlled trial attempted to evaluate the additional effect of hypnosis in a comprehensive treatment program for inpatients with persistent conversion disorder of the motor type. Moene et al. (30) treated 45 inpatients between 18 and 65 years of age with these symptoms, using symptom-oriented and insight-oriented techniques. A randomly selected subsample was also treated with hypnosis to ascertain whether this would yield additional therapeutic benefits. The comprehensive treatment program, either with or without hypnosis, resulted in significant clinical improvement on all clinical outcome measures. The addition of hypnosis had no additional effect on treatment outcome and hypnotizability was not predictive of patient outcome. Further systematic studies of this type would clearly be of interest.

Behavior therapy has significant advantages in addressing those contingencies of reinforcement that appear to have contributed to symptom formation and perpetuation. This is true regarding considerations of both primary and secondary gain of the symptom.

Speed (31) has advocated that this approach be used to the exclusion of insight-oriented psychotherapy of the type advocated above. Our preference has been to use it in a complementary manner. In this regard, we have found it important to adapt to the cultural or ideological preferences of the patient in using those interventions that are most palatable to the patient's conceptual style and level of sophistication. Some patients are accessible to introspective exploration and need a framework to understand the puzzling dynamics of unconsciously based mind–body interaction. Others find such an issue troublingly beyond their capacity and prefer a structured approach built on a purely neurophysiologic model, with supportive reassurance regarding the "biologic" components of their treatment, as a preferable and more palatable route to recovery.

Physical therapy can be extremely valuable in situations of symptomatic weakness, fixed postures, or gait abnormalities. This is so because it responds directly and supportively to the patient's physical symptom, while allowing psychotherapy to be more readily tolerated at the same time. The physical therapist provides encouragement, reassurance, hands-on intervention, and reinforcement for improvement. For patients who have difficulty grasping or accepting psychodynamic formulations, physical therapy can provide a face-saving mechanism of recovery, provided that other relevant treatment considerations of primary and secondary gain have been diplomatically dealt with effectively. Physical therapy may also be essential in treating or preventing disuse atrophy or contractures that may develop with more persistent conversion symptoms, as may occur in somatization disorders or undifferentiated somatoform disorders (32).

Pharmacotherapy can serve two valuable functions in treating patients with PNMDs. Clearly, pharmacotherapy is indicated for coexisting and often contributory psychiatric conditions, such as depression, anxiety, or psychosis. In addition, the coexistence of identifiable life stressors can often legitimately enable the neurologist and psychiatrist to delineate how stress-induced neurophysiologic alterations in the central nervous system can contribute to physical symptoms via perturbations of neurotransmitter balance in the brain. It can then be supportively explained that these neuropsychiatric medications have often been able to correct such perturbations and contribute to recovery. In this

regard, may not only pharmacologic treatment relieve an underlying psychiatric contributant to the conversion disorder, but it can also provide a conceptual bridge to facilitate the acceptance of a biologic rationale for recovery in a patient who is not receptive to postulated psychodynamic formulations.

A variety of other treatment interventions may each play a valuable role in selected patients with conversion-based neuropsychiatric movement disorders. These include: family therapy (to deal with contributory conflicts, abuse, dependency, or enabling issues); intravenous amobarbital infusions (particularly to evaluate the possible presence of contractures in cases of fixed, dystonic posturing); electro-convulsive therapy (for coexisting, treatment-resistant depression or mania); speech therapy (for aphonia, dysarthria, or other neuropsychiatric speech problems); or direct environmental intervention (to deal with contributory stressors or secondary gain influences).

Difficult challenges of treating patients with somatization disorder and undifferentiated somatoform disorder include the chronicity of the course and the proliferation of symptoms. These features frequently generate greater treatment resistance than a more time-limited conversion disorder. Since relevant psychodynamics in these disorders appear to include intensive help-seeking behavior directed to physicians, one recommendation for general management of these patients has included the scheduling of regular visits with a designated primary physician who can judiciously and supportively monitor presenting symptoms, provide appropriate reassurance, and avoid either ordering unnecessary tests, or harshly rebuffing the patient's exaggerated concerns. The merits of continuity with a consistent primary care physician, preferably supplemented by regular psychological and/or psychiatric care, increase the opportunity for the supportive measures that diminish anxiety-driven searching for additional medical evaluations (32).

The literature is sparse regarding specific treatment for these disorders. One randomized controlled trial studied primary care patients with medically unexplained symptoms, which presumably included some patients having these chronic disorders, though the psychiatric diagnoses are not specifically delineated (33). A larger number of patients treated with cognitive-behavioral therapy had a decrease in the intensity and number of symptoms, an improvement in functioning, and a decrease in illness behavior. The treatment was delivered in the primary care setting, involving 12 sessions over 8 weeks.

Kashner et al. (34) conducted a randomized controlled trial involving short-term, cognitive–behavioral group therapy (eight sessions) for patients with somatization disorder. This treatment reportedly yielded better physical and mental health status than that of the group not receiving the group therapy.

As with conversion disorders, there is a need to evaluate and treat comorbid psychiatric conditions, as well as other coexisting medical conditions. Similarly, the treating clinician should evaluate relevant family dynamics (past and present), ongoing stressors, dependency, and disability issues, as well as other secondary gain considerations that may pertain. A stance of therapeutic positivism regarding the feasibility of clinical improvement is advisable, recognizing that the extent of improvement is highly variable in this group of disorders.

Even more challenging is the group of factitious disorders, where the patient is aware of his or her purposeful fabrication of physical signs and symptoms, but is by definition not fully aware of the underlying pathologic motivation to engage in this self-defeating behavior pattern. In contrast to malingering patients, external pragmatic incentives, if present, play only a secondary role in symptom genesis.

Perhaps the first task of treating factitious disorder patients is the need to deal with the physician's anger at realizing the deliberate deception by a patient who has often consumed much time and other expensive medical resources with a self-inflicted illness (35). To combat the temptation to launch into a "triumphant unmasking confrontation," it is wise to recall that the patient is at least in part a victim of prior life traumas and deprivations, as well as of intrinsic, severe psychopathology, that led to the presenting, "sick," attention-seeking behavior. Therefore, humiliating and dismissing the patient will only reinforce the patient's already existing assumption that honest exploration of psychological components of the patient's illness is likely to be traumatic and unhelpful. This will counterproductively lead to persistence in the patient's duplicitous and self-defeating illness behavior.

Furthermore, there is an understandable pessimism associated with the most severe form of factitious disorder, the Münchausen syndrome, where the patient relentlessly pursues a lifestyle of unceasing patienthood. However, Reich and Gottfried (36) and Kapfhammer (37) have reported that up to 90% of factitious disorder patients do not have the Münchausen syndrome variant. This suggests the potential merits of supportively presenting a potentially efficacious treatment plan with judicious regard for the patient's self-esteem, so that the prospects of effective therapeutic engagement are enhanced.

When the diagnosis is clarified during a medical hospitalization, the merits of a nonconfrontational conjoint debriefing by both the neurologist and psychiatrist in the supportive manner described earlier in this chapter can be helpful. If the patient is insufficiently insightful, capable and/or motivated to respond to an individually oriented clarification of the diagnosis and related treatment recommendations, then inclusion of relevant family members with the patient's consent may be more helpful in addressing relevant dependency issues and other behavioral contingencies that require more leverage for effective implementation than the patient alone can provide. In all such discussions, efforts should be made to emphasize those contributants

to the patient's illness that were outside of the patient's awareness and/or control, in the interest of preserving the patient's self-esteem and, hopefully, a nascent therapeutic alliance. As with somatoform disorders, effective treatment of coexisting depression, anxiety, psychosis, and/or other coexisting psychopathology substantially increases one's prospects of effectively alleviating the presenting PNMD symptoms. Also, as with somatoform disorders, a variety of the same types of reorienting techniques geared to replace regressive somatization with more appropriate coping strategies is available. However, in some treatment-resistant patients who present a serious danger to themselves, initial transfer to a closed psychiatric unit may be essential for the patient's protection.

With regard to malingering, it is more appropriate to address management, rather than treatment, insofar as malingering is not considered to be a psychiatric disorder (35). We have already addressed the need to approach the diagnosis of malingering only after thoroughly exploring and excluding other treatable causes of presenting PNMD symptoms. Dealing with the malingering patient still presents significant challenges. First, it should be reiterated that angry confrontation of the patient is unlikely to help anyone and may be harmful to the physician in a variety of ways. If the patient presents at the outset with a clear pending litigation issue, it is advisable to formally request in writing all prior medical information of relevance and to have written permission to speak with the patient's attorney, as well as to have written permission to prepare a written report, before actually doing so. Although it is advisable to make a tactful but forthright statement to the patient about one's findings, it may be judicious to do so in the presence of a supportive independent observer, in the event of an unanticipated angry reaction by the patient. Having access to the patient's attorney can have the added potential benefit of another route of influence to the patient, since malingering patients are unlikely to relinquish their symptoms until their pragmatic goal is either achieved or recognized by the patient as not realistically attainable. The patient's attorney can be potentially helpful in the latter regard.

PROGNOSIS

Implicit in the above discussion is the expectation that the prognosis for any particular patient with a neuropsychiatric movement disorder would be influenced by a variety of factors. These would include the nature, chronicity, and severity of the underlying psychopathology; the nature, chronicity, and severity of contributory external stressors; the intrinsic strengths and resilience of the patient; as well as the effectiveness of the patient's support system, including the appropriateness and effectiveness of treatment. There is no indication, either in published reports to our knowledge, or in our clinical experience, that the particular movement disorder phenomenology manifested by the patient has prognostic predictive value.

It appears from follow-up studies of patients with untreated somatoform disorder, that the general outcome is poor and that spontaneous resolution of symptoms is uncommon. One recent study of 73 patients with "unexplained medical symptoms" who were admitted to the hospital, with a presumed substantial representation of neuropsychiatric somatoform symptoms found that the index symptom was unimproved or worse in over half the patients after a 6-year follow-up interval (38). A comparable outcome was reported in a 4-year follow-up study of 70 patients with conversion disorder and somatization disorder (39). Indeed, the pattern of recurrent, undiagnosed and/or untreated conversion disorder in childhood and adolescence has been postulated, based on follow-up studies, to lead developmentally to the more chronic and treatment-resistant features of somatization disorder (18).

Relatively speaking, a better prognosis is associated with conversion disorder in patients who have been hospitalized if they are aged less than 40, with a short duration of symptoms, who have had a recent change in marital status, and who experience expeditious symptom remission by the end of the hospital admission (40). Several studies suggest that the presence of an underlying treatable psychiatric disorder, such as depressive disorder or anxiety disorder, connotes a more favorable prognosis (19,38,40). Contrawise, poorer prognosis is associated with the presence of a personality disorder, pending litigation, and current or prospective secondary gain in the form of financial compensation (41). Furthermore, simply being in medical treatment *per se* does not predict a better outcome. A 10-year follow-up study of 73 patients with conversion disorder found that the patients with the most primary physician contact had the least likelihood of symptom remission (41). Thus, the data currently available suggests that benign neglect of these patients with regard to psychiatric treatment is unwise.

A somewhat more sanguine prognosis is suggested for patients with psychogenic neuropsychiatric somatoform disorder, when treated with the type of integrated and relatively intensive treatment strategy advocated in this chapter. In the series of 24 patients reported by our group (42), all treatment responders were those with conversion disorder or somatization disorder. None of those with factitious disorder or malingering improved. It must be conceded, however, that this was not a controlled, prospective study and the diagnoses of some patients changed to a more pathologic variant during the course of evaluation and treatment, as signs of uncooperativeness, purposeful dissimulation, and personality disorder emerged over time. For patients with somatoform disorder, there was no correlation between favorable outcome and such variables as age at onset, gender, intelligence level, or specific movement

disorder phenomenology. In this retrospective review, the integrated treatment strategy outlined here resulted in sustained improvement (longer than 1 year) in 54% of patients. Complete symptom resolution was achieved in 25%, considerable improvement in 21%, and moderate improvement in 8% by the end of active treatment. Patients considered not significantly improved included 22% with modest improvement and 12% with no improvement. Some relapse after initial improvement was observed in about 20% of patients over time, as determined when contacted at follow-up. Of those who were functioning actively before the onset of their neuropsychiatric symptoms, 25% were re-employed full-time at the conclusion of treatment, 10% were employed part-time, and 15% were normally functional as homemakers or students. While chronicity of neuropsychiatric symptoms has been associated with less favorable prognosis in other series of these patients (40,43), we encountered several patients who, with effective diagnostic clarification and active treatment, were able to achieve complete and sustained symptom resolution. This is noted in an effort to dispel a self-fulfilling therapeutic nihilism in approaching such patients.

A recent follow-up report of PNMD patients by the Baylor Movement Disorder Group (44) located 39 responders of a sample of 113 identified patients. At follow-up, 56% of the contacted patients had improved, 8% did not change, and 36% had worsened. Psychiatric diagnoses and psychiatric treatment, if any, are not specified in this abstract, nor was it clear what proportion had received psychiatric intervention. Interestingly, however, the most frequent reason cited by patients for their improvement was effective treatment by the physician. While it is not clear in this abstract whether a neurologist or psychiatrist or both are being credited, the potentially therapeutic benefit of a positive attitude by the physician in facilitating symptomatic improvement in the patient is noteworthy.

CONCLUSIONS

In the absence of prospective data on the evolutionary course of psychogenic-neuropsychiatric movement disorders, we are limited in describing the natural history of these disorders by the data available in retrospective and follow-up reports of clinicians working actively with these patients. What does appear clear by consensus of those working in this area, is that this diverse group of patients represents a fascinating challenge to clinicians at the neurology-psychiatry interface. It is clearly the primary task of the neurologist to carefully diagnose movement disorder symptoms phenomenologically, with a view to either ruling out or defining the extent of any identifiable organic substrate. The next task is that of facilitating referral to a mental health professional capable of diagnosing relevant psychopathology and collaborating in the formulation of a treatment plan that is both acceptable to the patient and realistically likely to be effective. A supportive explanation of the diagnosis that is sensitive to the patient's intellectual capacity, prior conception of the illness, and self-esteem appears to be a crucial determinant influencing the patient's capacity to be engaged effectively in treatment. While there are many factors influencing response to treatment, those of particular significance include the effectiveness of communication among the neurologist, the mental health professional, and the patient; the nature, severity, and chronicity of relevant psychopathology in the patient; the nature, severity, and chronicity of stressors affecting the patient; and the level of resilience and environmental support available to the patient, including the availability and effectiveness of treatment.

Based on the data currently available, it appears advisable to individualize treatment, utilizing as many relevant interventions as appear likely to be helpful in treating relevant psychopathology, modifying environmental stressors, and strengthening the patient's coping capacities with a view to symptom abatement. Further study is needed to assess the specific efficacy of particular treatment approaches and to clarify those prognostic factors that influence long-term response to treatment.

REFERENCES

1. Fahn S, Williams DT, Ford B. Psychogenic movement disorders. In: Noseworthy JH, ed. *Neurological therapeutics: principles and practice.* Vol. 2. London: Martin Dunitz, 2003:2677–2687.
2. Fahn S, Williams DT, Reches A, et al. Hysterical dystonia, a rare disorder: report of five documented cases. *Neurology.* 1983;33 (Suppl. 2):161.
3. Fahn S, Williams DT. Psychogenic dystonia. *Adv Neurol.* 1988; 50:431–455.
4. Vuilleumier P, Chicerio C, Assal F, et al. Functional neuroanatomical correlates of hysterical sensorimotor loss. *Brain.* 2001;124:1077–1090.
5. Trimble MR. Somatization disorder. In: Hallett M, Fahn S, Jankovic J et al., eds. *Psychogenic movement disorders: psychobiology and therapy of a functional disorder.* Advances in neurology. Philadelphia, PA: Lippincott Williams & Wilkins, 2004.
6. Goetz CG. Charcot and psychogenic movement disorders. In: Hallett M, Fahn S, Jankovic J et al., eds. *Psychogenic movement disorders: psychobiology and therapy of a functional disorder.* Advances in neurology. Philadelphia, PA: Lippincott Williams & Wilkins, 2004.
7. Tomlinson WC. Freud and psychogenic movement disorders. In: Hallett M, Fahn S, Jankovic J et al., eds. *Psychogenic movement disorders: psychobiology and therapy of a functional disorder.* Advances in neurology. Philadelphia, PA: Lippincott Williams & Wilkins, 2004.
8. James W. *The varieties of religious experience.* New York: Modern Library, 1994.
9. Brown RJ. Dissociation and conversion in psychogenic illness. In: Hallett M, Fahn S, Jankovic J et al., eds. *Psychogenic movement disorders: psychobiology and therapy of a functional disorder.* Advances in neurology. Philadelphia, PA: Lippincott Williams & Wilkins, 2004.
10. Lesser R. Treatment and outcome of psychogenic non-epileptic seizures. In: Hallett M, Fahn S, Jankovic J et al., eds. *Psychogenic movement disorders: psychobiology and therapy of a functional disorder.* Advances in neurology. Philadelphia, PA: Lippincott Williams & Wilkins, 2004.
11. Marsden CD. Hysteria: a neurologist's view. *Psychol Med.* 1986; 16:277–288.
12. Lempert T, Dietrich M, Huppert D, et al. Psychogenic disorders in neurology: frequency and clinical spectrum. *Acta Neurol Scand.* 1990;82:335–340.
13. Factor S. Psychogenic movement disorders: frequency and type in a movement disorder center. In: Hallett M, Fahn S, Jankovic J et al., eds. *Psychogenic movement disorders: psychobiology and therapy of a functional disorder.* Advances in neurology. Philadelphia, PA: Lippincott Williams & Wilkins, 2004.
14. Thomas M. Psychogenic tremor: characteristics and longitudinal follow-up. In: Hallett M, Fahn S, Jankovic J et al., eds. *Psychogenic movement disorders: psychobiology and therapy of a functional disorder.* Advances in neurology. Philadelphia, PA: Lippincott Williams & Wilkins, 2004.
15. Crimlisk HL, Bhatia KP, Cope H, et al. Patterns of referral in patients with unexplained medical symptoms. *J Psychosom Res.* 2000;49:217–219.
16. Moene FC, Landberg EH, Hoogduin KA, et al. Organic syndromes diagnosed as conversion disorder: identification and frequency in a study of 85 patients. *J Psychosom Reesearch.* 2000;49:7–12.
17. American Psychiatric Association. *Diagnostic and statistical manual of mental disorders,* 4th ed., text revision. Washington, DC: American Psychiatric Press, 2000.
18. Williams DT. Somatoform disorders, factitious disorders and malingering. In: Noshpitz J, ed. *Handbook of child and adolescent psychiatry.* Vol. 2. New York: James Wiley & Sons, 1997:563–578.
19. Williams DT, Ford B, Fahn S. Phenomenology and psychopathology related to psychogenic movement disorders. *Adv Neurol.* 1995;65:231–257.
20. Ford B, Williams DT, Fahn S. Treatment of psychogenic movement disorders. In: Kurlan R, ed. *The treatment of movement disorders.* Vol. 2. Philadelphia, PA: JB Lippincott Co, 1994:475–485.
21. Ford CV. Conversion disorder and somatoform disorder not otherwise specified. In: Gabbard GO, ed. *Treatment of psychiatric disorders,* 3rd ed. Washington, DC: American Psychiatric Press, 2001: 1755–1776.
22. Bowman ES. Pseudoseizures. *Psychiatr Clin North Am.* 1998;21: 649–657.
23. Roelofs K, Keijsers GP, Hoogduin KA, et al. Child abuse in patients with conversion disorder. *Am J Psychiatry.* 2002a;159:1908–1913.
24. Spitzer C, Spelsberg B, Grabe HJ, et al. Dissociative experiences and psychopathology in conversion disorders. *J Psychosom Res.* 1999;46:291–294.
25. Hallett M. Voluntary and involuntary movements in humans. In: Hallett M, Fahn S, Jankovic J et al., eds. *Psychogenic movement disorders: psychobiology and therapy of a functional disorder.* Advances in neurology. Philadelphia, PA: Lippincott Williams & Wilkins, 2004.
26. Spiegel D, Maldonado J. Hypnosis. In: Hales R, Yudofsky S, Talbott J, eds. *The american psychiatric press textbook of psychiatry,* 3rd ed. Washington, DC: American Psychiatric Press, 1999:1243–1274.
27. Raz A, Shapiro T. Hypnosis and neuroscience: a cross talk between clinical and cognitive research. *Arch Gen Psychiatry.* 2002;59:85–90.
28. Roelofs K, Hoogduin KA, Keijsers GP, et al. Hypnotic susceptibility in patients with conversion disorder. *J Abnorm Psychol.* 2002;111:390–395.
29. Williams DT. Hypnosis. In: Weiner J, Duncan M, eds. *Textbook of child and adolescent psychiatry,* 3rd ed. Washington, DC: American Psychiatric Press, 2003:1043–1054.
30. Moene FC, Spinhoven P, Hoodguin KA, et al. A randomized clinical trial on the additional effect of hypnosis in a comprehensive treatment program for inpatienys with conversion disorder of the motor type. *Psychother Psychosom.* 2002;71:66–76.
31. Speed J. Behavioral management of conversion disorder: retrospective study. *Arch Phys Med Rehabil.* 1996;77:147–154.
32. Smith GR. Somatization disorder and undifferentiated somatoform disorder. In: Gabbard GO, ed. *Treatment of psychiatric disorders,* 3rd ed. Vol. 2. Washington, DC: American Psychiatric Press, 2001:1735–1753.

33. Speckens AE, van Hembert AM, Spinhoven P, et al. Cognitive behavioral therapy for medically unexplained physical symptoms: a randomized controlled trial. *Br Med J.* 1995;311:1328–1332.

34. Kashner TM, Rost K, Cohen B, et al. Enhancing the health of somatization disorder patients: effectiveness of short-term group therapy. *Psychosomatics.* 1995;36:462–470.

35. Eisendrath SJ. Factitious disorders and malingering. In: Gabbard GO, ed. *Treatment of psychiatric disorders*, 3rd ed. Vol. 2. Washington, DC: American Psychiatric Press, 2001:1825–1842.

36. Reich P, Gottfried LA. Factitious disorders in a teaching hospital. *Ann Intern Med.* 1983;99:240–247.

37. Kapfhammer HP, Rothenheausler HB, Dietrich E, et al. Artifactual disorders—between deception and self-mutilation: experiences in consultation psychiatry at a university clinic. *Nevenarzt.* 1998;69:401–409.

38. Crimlisk HL, Bhatia K, Cope H, et al. 6 year follow-up study of patients with medically unexplained symptoms. *Br Med J.* 1998; 316:582–586.

39. Kent DA, Tomasson K, Corvell W. Course and outcome of conversion and somatization disorders: a four-year follow-up. *Psychosomatics.* 1995;36:138–144.

40. Couprie W, Wijdicks EF, Rooijmans HG, et al. Outcome in conversion disorder: a follow-up study. *J Neurol Neurosrg Psychiatry.* 1995;58:750–752.

41. Mace CJ, Trimble MR. Ten year prognosis of conversion disorder. *Br J Psychiatry.* 1996;169:282–288.

42. Williams DT, Ford B, Fahn S. Phenomenology and psychopathology related to psychogenic movement disorders. In: Wiener WJ, Lang AE, eds. *Behavioral neurology of movement disorders.* Advances in neurology. New York: Raven Press, 1995:231–257.

43. Factor SA, Podskalny GD, Molho ES. Psychogenic movement disorders: frequency, clinical profile, and characteristics. *J Neurol Neurosurg Psychiatry.* 1995;59:406–412.

44. Thomas M, Vuong KD, Jankovic J. Long term prognosis of psychogenic movement disorders, 2003.

Treatment

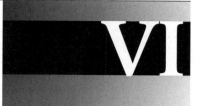

Treatment of

Conversion Disorder

33

P. Rosebush   *Michael F. Mazurek*

ABSTRACT

Over the course of 12 years, we have assessed and treated 45 patients with conversion disorder and have found that this extremely disabling condition is very responsive to treatment. It is, unfortunately, underdiagnosed, and often poorly managed. Our summary of the demographic and clinical characteristics of our sample is followed by detailed descriptions of five representative cases. Based on our experience to date, we identify the barriers to diagnosis and treatment followed by the essential elements of successful treatment which usually involve hospitalization.

INTRODUCTION

The condition we call "conversion disorder" (CD) was known to physicians at least as far back as the 16th century, and perhaps even earlier (1). By the late 19th century, it had become one of the first neurologic or psychiatric illnesses for which an effective treatment was available. An early breakthrough in this regard was the discovery by the Parisian neurologist Charcot that the symptoms of CD could be dramatically reversed with hypnosis. Soon afterward, the Viennese neurologist and neuroscientist Breuer recognized, through his successful treatment of the patient Anna O, that psychotherapeutic intervention could be even more effective than hypnosis, producing not merely an amelioration of symptoms, but an actual cure. This striking ability of psychotherapy to treat CD persuaded Breuer's younger Viennese colleague, Freud, to break from neurology and establish psychiatry as an independent discipline.

By the late 1800s, CD had become one of the few neuropsychiatric conditions that was amenable to treatment. It is, therefore, ironic that CD has become an underrecognized and poorly treated cause of chronic disability. In our experience, there are two major reasons for this state of affairs: (i) the failure of physicians to make the diagnosis, and (ii) uncertainty about how the problem should be treated once a diagnosis has been made.

CURRENT STUDY

Over a 12-year period from 1992 to 2004, we have diagnosed CD in 45 patients, according to the *Diagnostic and Statistical Manual of Mental Diseases*, Fourth Edition (DSM-IV), which requires that the following diagnostic criteria be met:

- A patient must have one or more symptoms or deficits affecting voluntary motor or sensory function that suggest a neurologic or other general medical condition.
- Psychological factors are judged to be associated with the symptoms or deficit because the initiation or exacerbation of the symptoms or deficit is preceded by conflicts or other stressors.
- The symptom or deficit is not intentionally produced or feigned.
- The symptom or deficit cannot, after appropriate investigation, be fully explained by a general medical condition or by the direct effects of a substance, or as a culturally sanctioned behavior or experience.
- The symptom or deficit causes clinically significant distress or impairment in social, occupational, or other important areas of functioning, or warrants medical evaluation.

This series did not include any individuals who were involved in litigation. The majority of patients were referred with a tentative diagnosis of conversion disorder, after extensive investigations failed to yield another condition that might account for their presentation, or when the course of a presumed condition, such as multiple sclerosis, was atypical. In a number of instances, we made the diagnosis after being asked to consider whether a rare metabolic or degenerative neuropsychiatric disorder might explain the clinical picture.

Nature of the Conversion Disorder

The frequency of CD type in the 45 patients was as follows:

- Limb paralysis or immobility in 23 (50%); for 19, this was the predominant feature.
- Seizurelike activity in 15 (37%); for 13, this was predominant.
- Bizarre excessive movements such as dystonic posturing, choreoathetosis, or coarse tremulousness in 17 (38%); this was the primary manifestation in eight.
- Speech disturbances in seven (15%); the main conversion feature in two.
- Ataxia in five (11%); predominant in two.

In total, 20 patients (44%) manifested more than one type of neurologic abnormality and of these, almost half displayed more than two types of disturbance. Seventeen patients (38%) complained of sensory symptoms such as pain, shocklike sensations, vibrations, or paresthesias, and six (13%) endorsed cognitive problems in the form of poor concentration, "confusion," disorientation, and memory impairment.

Burden of Illness

All patients were severely affected by their illness, as reflected in the following:

- A period of complete inability to work, attend school, or care for children or family as before (40/45; 100%).
- Being bedridden (13/45; 29%) or regularly using assistive devises such as a cane, walker, or wheelchair (13/45; 29%).
- Daily dependence upon caregivers for feeding, dressing, mobilization, hygiene, toileting, or safety (22/45; 50%).
- Long duration of symptoms: this was more than two years in 27 patients (60%).
- A mean Global Assessment of Function (GAF) score of 35. This represents a score of 50 or less in all but one case, and 30 or less in 16 (35%). A score of 50 reflects serious impairment in social, occupational, or school functioning, and a score of 30, an inability to function in almost all areas.

Psychiatric Comorbidity

Psychiatric

Twenty-seven patients (60%) met DSM-IV criteria for at least one other psychiatric illness in their lifetime. These disorders included: personality (n = 16; 35%); affective (n = 10; 22%); anxiety (n = 6; 13%); somatization (n = 9; 20%); posttraumatic stress (n = 2; 4%), and anorexia nervosa or bulimia (n = 3; 6%). Seventeen patients (38%) had received psychiatric treatment in the past for one of the aforementioned diagnoses. The identified comorbid conditions were active at the time of our assessments in 11 (24%). It is noteworthy that none of the patients had experienced psychotic symptoms or been diagnosed with schizophrenia, and over 75% had no history of any type of substance abuse.

Response to Treatment

Of the 45 patients assessed, 32 engaged in treatment, four were beginning treatment at the time of this report, and nine others had refused involvement in our program. Of those who refused treatment, only one enjoyed spontaneous improvement, and another, a 22-year-old woman, died from the complications of prolonged immobility secondary to leg paralysis. She had been bedridden for 4 years and developed contractures and recurrent infections, eventually succumbing to a pulmonary embolus. Efforts to engage her in psychiatric treatment were angrily rejected.

Twenty-six (81%) of the 32 patients who engaged in treatment had complete resolution of all conversion signs and symptoms, and no longer required care or use of assistive devices. The six other patients had partial, but functionally significant, improvement. They no longer required care from others and were able to return to work or school, but continued to experience symptoms or "episodes" intermittently.

All but two of the patients treated were hospitalized with an average length of stay of 8 weeks (range: 1 week to 6 months).

CASE STUDIES

Our approach in this article will be to describe in detail a number of these cases, with attention to the issues that helped give rise to the conversion symptoms and pointed the way to a successful therapeutic plan. This will be followed by a discussion of the barriers to diagnosis and treatment of this condition. We conclude with an attempt to summarize the principles of treatment that have proven effective in our patients.

Case 1: Conversion Disorder Presenting as Multiple Sclerosis

This 33-year-old married mother of two, BT, was well until the age of 30, when she began to experience leg weakness, urinary retention, paresthesiae, and easy fatigability and muscle pain. She was referred to a neurologist, who recorded a number of abnormal findings including clonus, increased muscle tone, and absence of abdominal reflexes. She was diagnosed as having probable multiple sclerosis, and for the next three years was followed in the MS clinic of a teaching hospital. Over the first year of her illness, she deteriorated rapidly and lost control of her legs and bladder. Numerous investigations were undertaken, including magnetic resonance imaging (MRI) of the brain and spinal cord, electromyography (EMG), electroencephalography (EEG), evoked potentials (EVP), lumbar puncture, myelogram, cystoscopy, and cystometrogram. She was eventually referred to us for a second opinion because the severity of her disability seemed to be out of keeping with the persistent absence of lesions on repeat MRI scans.

When we initially assessed BT at age 33, she had been confined to a wheelchair for two years and was treating her "neurogenic bladder" with regular self-catheterization. She was taking 16 different medications for treatment of depression, muscle spasms, pain, constipation, and bladder dysfunction. We were not able to find any convincing abnormalities on neurologic examination.

Medical History

Prior to the age of 30, BT had no history of neurologic or psychiatric illness. There was no history of substance abuse. She did, however, have childhood asthma, for which she was reportedly hospitalized on multiple occasions before the age of 10.

Relevant Personal History

BT was raised in poverty by an abusive, alcoholic father and a mother who was "always sick" with "leg problems." She had to assume care for her younger siblings and remembered feeling overwhelmed by their demands. During hospitalizations for asthma she enjoyed a respite from her responsibilities and the strife at home. BT fondly recalled the attention she received from nurses.

Following completion of high school, she married a man from a different ethnic background with a large extended family. There were culturally endorsed expectations that BT would care for her husband's ill mother and grandmother, as well as help out with the family business. At the same time, she was expected to work full-time, care for their own children, and manage the household. BT attempted to keep up with these multiple demands for a number of years, but felt trapped, deprived, and inadequate. She particularly felt that she was neglecting her own children just as she had been neglected. Shortly before the development of her CD, BT was involved in a minor motor vehicle accident for which she was found to be at fault. While neither she nor anyone else was hurt, a young child was in the other vehicle and BT recalled hearing him cry. In the months that followed, she became "obsessed" with the cry of this child. It was over this period of time that she began to experience the leg weakness, paresthesiae, and bladder symptoms.

In trying to understand BT, why she developed CD when she did, and what issues would have to be addressed and resolved in psychotherapeutic treatment, we considered the factors below.

Predisposing Factors

- Parental neglect and abuse which resulted in low self-esteem and chronically unmet needs.
- Identification with a sick mother for whom she was prematurely responsible.
- Repeated hospitalizations for asthma during which she was exposed to the only nurturing environment she knew as a child, and provided with relief from an abusive, neglectful home situation.

Precipitating Factors

- Extreme fatigue secondary to overwork.
- An increasing sense of being trapped, neglected, and taken advantage of in her marital and social situation.
- A sense of inadequacy and failure as she took on more responsibilities and yet felt she did nothing very well.
- A minor motor vehicle accident in which she heard a child crying. This seemed to personify her own needs as well as those of her own children, whom she thought she was neglecting.

Perpetuating Factors

- Being cared for when she was ill, but not when she was well.
- Being released from overwhelming responsibilities as a result of being disabled.
- Not wanting to acknowledge her intense anger and other conflicted feelings about her family of origin as well as her marital situation.
- Failure of physicians to accurately diagnose her condition earlier.

Approach to Treatment

At the time of our initial assessment, we asked BT to consider that "stress" and "pent-up emotions" might be playing at least some role in her condition. We presented her inability to walk in terms of a simple analogy, comparing her motor system to the engine of a car. If the car will not run, one possible explanation might be a breakdown of some vital engine part. Alternatively, there might be a disconnection between the ignition and an otherwise normal motor. In this case, the car can function if an appropriate starter signal can be restored. BT responded to this notion of a "mind-body disconnection" as an explanatory model for her inability to move her legs. We indicated to her that, in our opinion, her central nervous system "motor" was fundamentally sound, and that she therefore had the potential for a complete recovery. We emphasized the importance of trying to understand what was causing the "disconnection" at the same time as she received physiotherapy for her motor dysfunction.

BT was hospitalized in our neuropsychiatry inpatient service for 6 months. During this time, all medications were tapered and discontinued. We discouraged self-catheterization and initiated physiotherapy three times a week with a focus upon learning to walk and regaining control over her motor function. Daily psychotherapy sessions were carried out. Much time was spent inquiring about her past life, earlier development, and why she had become who she was. She was also encouraged to talk about her life prior to her illness. Interventions typically involved helping her to correctly identify the feelings that had been aroused in different situations, both in her early life and later in her marriage. We acknowledged her ability to put her own needs aside and her strong sense of responsibility and compassion for others. At the same time, we pointed out the absence of an appropriate sense of entitlement to have her own needs met. Her self-esteem was low and she clearly harbored a deep sense of deprivation. She was also angered by others' expectations of her. She felt intense, yet unexpressed, anger toward her husband for his role in creating and allowing a situation that recapitulated important aspects of her early life. BT saw herself as a victim and without any control. These unconscious feelings of anger had resulted in significant problems with intimacy as she distanced herself from others, including her husband and her own children, in order to avoid overt expression of her rage. The intensity of her rage—a word she began to use—often frightened her and, although she had no history of aggression, she was concerned that she might hurt someone. Feelings of rage eventually gave way to sadness and she developed a clinical depression, which was treated with antidepressant medication. Efforts to engage her husband in marital therapy were unsuccessful.

Outcome and Follow-up

Six months after admission, BT was no longer using the wheelchair. She walked with a cane and required assistance in going up and down stairs. At this point she was discharged and seen in twice-weekly psychotherapy by one of us (PR) for the next 2 years. Antidepressant medication was continued during this time. Eight months after discharge, she was walking normally, and within a year she had returned to her factory job. She soon assumed full-time hours and began to coach baseball in her spare time. She initiated a separation from her husband and maintained full custody of her children. At 5-year follow-up, she had remarried, and at 10-year follow-up, continued to work full-time with no relapses of her CD or hospitalizations for other reasons.

Case 2: CD Presenting as a Neurometabolic Disorder

This 13-year-old girl, HN, was healthy and developing normally until the age of 9, when she began to complain of a range of medical symptoms, including excessive fatigability, headache, gastrointestinal disturbances, and weakness. She was hospitalized for investigations, initially at her local hospital and later for a full year on the pediatric service of a major out-of-province teaching hospital. At times she required tube feeding. Extensive testing failed to yield a diagnosis. Meanwhile, she continued to clinically deteriorate to the point where she was confined to a wheelchair. She was eventually referred to us with the provisional diagnosis of an inherited neurometabolic disorder, with the hope that we might be able to provide biochemical and genetic characterization of her problem.

When we initially assessed her at the age of 13, HN was completely unable to walk. She had been confined to a wheelchair for one year, and had not attended school for two. She was reluctant to go outside, claiming that it made her feel "nervous." Despite the fact that she had not been diagnosed with any specific psychiatric disorder, several selective serotonin reuptake inhibitor antidepressant medications had been prescribed over the previous 3 years. She had no response and repeatedly developed akathisia with use of these agents.

We observed HN interacting with hospital staff prior to our initial formal assessment. When not in her wheelchair, she was in bed, requiring assistance with toileting, feeding, and turning. With any effort to move her legs, she displayed striking "overflow" choreoathetotic movements of her head, arms, and torso. Otherwise, her neurologic examination showed no convincing abnormalities. There were striking inconsistencies between what she could do when distracted and what she was purportedly able to do in response to specific requests.

Investigations

In view of the clinical history, we undertook fairly extensive investigations, including a cranial MRI, EMG, muscle biopsy, EEG, evoked potentials, ophthalmologic assessment, cognitive testing, and various enzyme analyses, all of which yielded normal results.

Relevant Personal History

HN came from a stable, well-adjusted family and had a normal upbringing. By temperament she was shy, anxious, and easily frightened. At age 9, six months prior to her first bout of illness, she had witnessed the unprovoked and repeated stabbing of a classmate by another classmate's mother. She and the child who was assaulted were alone in the school cloakroom at the time. HN did not reveal this history herself and when asked about it replied, "It didn't really bother me because I was busy tying up my shoes." Shortly after this horrific event, her dog, which had always provided her with a sense of protection, died. Despite these events, she denied experiencing any stress other than that caused by her illness.

In arriving at a formulation we considered the following:

Predisposing Factors
- An anxious temperament.

Precipitating Factors
- Witnessing a life-threatening assault.
- Death of a pet.

Perpetuating Factors
- Failure to consider a diagnosis of CD.
- Ongoing secondary gain of being able to avoid almost all social situations, including the added social and interpersonal expectations that would naturally have begun to occur around this age.

Approach to Treatment

While comfortable having a neurologic assessment, HN was initially very upset about seeing a psychiatrist and voiced her concern that our involvement meant she was "crazy" and "imagining everything." Despite this, she did not resist hospitalization and listened intently to our explanation that she was suffering from a stress-related illness that had caused her to lose control of her legs. We emphasized that investigations had indicated that the "hard-wiring" required for walking was intact, but that her brain was having difficulty "cueing up" the motor program that would normally allow her to walk and use her legs normally. We likened this to a CD player having problems "reading" the information on a particular compact disc, making it impossible to play the recorded music. We explained that stress can be present and affect the body without any real *emotional* awareness. We put it in terms of stress disturbing the "cueing" function in the brain, with the result that some of the motor "programs" may not get "played" properly. An important, explicitly stated goal of psychotherapy was that she would become more conscious of how life events made her feel so that the "short-circuiting" to her body might be interrupted.

An obvious concern in this case was the possibility of Münchausen-by-proxy. We found no evidence for this. In fact, HN's mother was able to leave her daughter in the hospital for treatment while she returned home to another province.

Treatment and Outcome

HN met DSM-IV diagnostic criteria for major depression, somatization disorder, and social phobia, as well as CD. She was treated with Nortriptyline, low-dose alprazolam, and a program of desensitization to being outside. Physiotherapy began at the outset, for 2 hours three times a week. Many sessions were videotaped and later reviewed with her. This allowed her to see the abnormalities in her gait and have a keener sense of what needed to be corrected.

Daily psychotherapy focused upon her sense of vulnerability and fear of being harmed. She acknowledged that her worst fears about the world being a dangerous place had come true when she witnessed the assault on her classmate. The relationship between this traumatic incident and the development of her CD came into relief when she spontaneously said, "But, I don't feel afraid because I don't think anyone would hurt a sick little girl in a wheelchair," starkly drawing attention to the defensive function her paralysis had served.

Six months after admission, HN was walking normally without any assistance. She was discharged at this time and returned to school 2 months later without experiencing any relapse. She remained on the regimen of Nortriptyline and alprazolam for one year after discharge. At 3-year follow-up she was socializing in an age-appropriate manner and engaging in competitive dancing. At 6-year follow-up she had experienced no further conversion symptoms.

Case 3: CD Presenting as Dystonia

This 30-year-old married woman, KL, was the mother of three children, ages 12, 9, and 6, when she was admitted for assessment and treatment of a severe movement disorder of 4 years duration. She had been either bedridden or wheelchair-bound for the previous year. Family members and medical specialists referred to "attacks" of muscle spasms which could last up to 10 hours a day and which involved opisthotonus, extensor posturing of her limbs, and choreoathetotic movements. KL also suffered intermittently from a severe stutter with bizarre, incomprehensible speech patterns. She had been admitted on multiple occasions to the neurology service at several different hospitals and had twice been admitted to the ICU of her local hospital because of acute shortness of breath and an inability to swallow. She had been treated symptomatically for muscle spasms and pain, with a provisional diagnosis of multiple sclerosis, later switched, without supporting evidence, to a diagnosis of heterozygous adrenaleukodystrophy. Although the diagnosis of a conversion disorder had been suggested by one of us (MM) several years before when she presented to the emergency room of our own hospital, the patient, her husband, and her parents vehemently and litigiously rejected any suggestion of a psychiatric component to her illness. KL eventually agreed to see us at the behest of her family, who were overwhelmed by her needs and saw that the medical approach was failing. By that time, she had been unable to work for 3 years and was unable to care for her children. Her husband had left his job and had unsuccessfully tried to establish a business in their home because of his wife's condition. An agency provided daily home care.

At the time of admission, KL described her husband as well as her children as "very understanding" and denied any family or marital problems. She did not think her illness had had a negative impact on the children. On the second day of hospitalization, her husband informed the staff that he was leaving the marriage and emphasized that we needed to understand his wife's early life in order to understand the current problem.

Medical History

A review of KL's medical records supported a diagnosis of somatization disorder for 10 years prior to the development of CD. She had a history of migraine headaches dating from adolescence, episodes of "fainting," and many gynecologic problems. Her medications at the time of admission included the following: morphine sulphate, 60 mg every 4 to 6 hours, administered subcutaneously by her husband; Gravol, 50 mg four times per day; Artane, 32 mg per day, and clonazepam, 6 mg per day.

Relevant Personal History

KL's CD began shortly after she learned about her husband's infidelity. While they remained together, she became pathologically jealous and preoccupied with the possibility that he might leave her for another woman. This situation, in turn, triggered memories of a similar experience when she was 9, at which time she discovered her father's infidelity and informed her mother. It was KL's understanding that this revelation, for which she was responsible, precipitated the family breakdown, which followed soon after. Her parents separated and she lived with her mother, who became physically and emotionally unwell. She rarely saw her father, and with her mother, moved repeatedly to new schools and new neighborhoods. KL assumed considerable responsibility for taking care of her mother and often accompanied her to hospital emergency rooms when she was sick.

Family History

This was positive for various types of movement disorders on her father's side. She had an aunt with "dystonia" and a first cousin with cerebral palsy. Numerous other paternal relatives were reported to have "tics," "shakes," and "stuttering." Her mother seemed to have had a somatoform disorder and was treated for depression.

Investigations

KL had undergone many investigations in the several years prior to her admission. These included two EMG studies; EEG on two occasions; cranial and spinal MRIs; visual, auditory, and brain stem evoked potentials; and a lumbar puncture. These were all normal. Neurologic examination did not show any convincing abnormalities, but was limited by KL's severe movement disorder. Blood work on admission revealed an elevated creatine phosphokinase level of over 3,000. Her urine was negative for myoglobin.

Treatment Approach

KL displayed striking la belle indifférence. She smiled constantly and frequently laughed. Early on in her hospitalization, she was intermittently inattentive, impaired in her short-term memory, and disorganized in her thought processes. These cognitive features were judged to be secondary to the many centrally acting medications she was receiving, and resolved after they were withdrawn. Amitriptyline, 75 mg at bedtime, was prescribed to treat her initial insomnia as well as her complaints of headache, which predated withdrawal of her opiate medication.

Physiotherapy began immediately and involved breathing, relaxation exercises, and a gradual increase in normal motor activities with hierarchic expectations of control over her movements. She was reassured about her potential for full recovery and of our understanding of the stresses she had been under and that we felt had been affecting her physical health. In psychotherapy the following issues that emerged as significant were as follows:

- Anger about her husband's infidelity, complicated by her fear that he would abandon her.
- Longstanding feelings of guilt about revealing her father's infidelity when she was 9 and the role this had played in precipitating her parents' separation as well as her mother's illnesses.
- Her identification with her mother, who provided a role model for physical illness as an indicator of distress.
- Her unconscious feelings of abandonment by both parents at the time of their separation which, in turn, had engendered low self-esteem, chronic anxiety, and anger.
- Guilt about her inability to care for her own children during her years of disability and the fact that she had exposed them to the same situation that she had found so troubling in her youth.

Despite years of resistance to psychiatric intervention, KL was very responsive to the support that was offered in the hospital and easily engaged in psychotherapy. Her denial and la belle indifférence gave way to the expression of sadness, grief, guilt, and anger. She came to understand and accept that when she felt physically unwell, it often signaled psychological and emotional distress. We discussed her family history of movement disorders and the role of inheritance in lowering her threshold for developing motor problems in response to stress.

Outcome

KL's conversion disorder resolved completely over a 3-month hospitalization and her mood was euthymic at the time of discharge. Her husband did indeed leave the marriage. Six months after leaving the hospital, KL resumed driving and was caring for her children full-time. At 3-year follow-up she was well, with no recurrence of any somatic or psychiatric symptoms, and was involved in a new relationship. Her only medication has been amitriptyline 25 to 50 mg at bedtime, lowered over time from 75 mg.

Case 4: CD Presenting as a Tourette-like Syndrome

This 50-year-old, thrice-married woman, KD, with two grown children had, at the time she was referred to us, been on disability for 10 years because of treatment-resistant depression, chronic fatigue, and fibromyalgia. She was referred by a neurologist because of a 4-year history of muscle spasms and tics involving her face arms, legs, and torso, as well as intermittent leg "paralysis" and periods of stuttering and screaming. She would often hit and bite her husband during her "spells."

Relevant Personal History

KD was one of five children who grew up in a poverty-stricken family. She felt very close to her father but said he was often absent. She described her mother as "irritable," unaffectionate, withdrawn, and critical, and thought that her manner had driven KD's father away. Despite excelling academically, KD's self-esteem was always low and she felt lonely and neglected. With respect to personality style, she described herself as a "control freak" who "never showed emotion."

Her first two marriages were with emotionally and physically abusive men, and she terminated both relationships. One of her children had died of sudden infant death syndrome at 6 months of age while in the care of her mother. They never spoke about this event and KD could not recall grieving except on one occasion, 3 years later, when she became overwhelmed by sadness after a clergyman at her church expressed sympathy for her experience.

Several months after her father's death, when KD was 40 years old, she developed irritable bowel syndrome, fibromyalgia, and chronic fatigue. Prior to this she had been medically well and functioning, in her words, as a "super-woman," managing home, family, and work responsibilities. She had also just met her third husband who was not only *not* abusive but exceptionally attentive, kind, and solicitous. Following her father's death, she and her husband moved into her mother's home in order to provide her with support and company. She felt that her mother always "competed" with her for medical attention. Whenever KD was unwell, she said her mother would come down with something even more severe. In fact, KD accused her mother of making up, or exaggerating, her physical complaints.

KD experienced her first "spasm" at a family dinner after a brother suggested that she was taking financial advantage of their mother by living in her home. She felt "overwhelmed with rage" and perceived her mother as inadequately defending her against her brother's charges. She and her mother became increasingly estranged to the point of having no verbal communication, even though they continued to live in the same house. Over a period of 2 years in this situation, KD developed more and more symptoms and became increasingly dysfunctional to the point that her husband was caring for her 24 hours a day.

Prior to admission KD had been tried on a host of different psychotropic medications without any beneficial effect upon her symptoms. She remained dysphoric, and yet had gained 100 pounds, which resulted in elevation of her blood pressure and the development of obstructive sleep apnea. At the time of admission, she was taking the following drugs: lorazepam, 4 mg per day; clonazepam, 2 mg per day; Imovane, 7.5 mg per day; valproic acid, 1,000 mg per day; chlorpromazine, 25 mg at bedtime; and sertraline, 150 mg per day.

Investigations

The following investigations had been carried out prior to presentation to us: two cranial MRIs, 24-hour EEG telemetry, three neurologic consultations, and extensive blood work. All were normal. A sleep study confirmed sleep apnea and continuous positive airway pressure (CPAP) was recommended.

Treatment Approach

KD was hospitalized for 4 months. Her medications were withdrawn and replaced with alprazolam, 3 mg per day. She was instructed in relaxation exercises and advised to use them in order to abort the spasms, which she could anticipate. Insight-oriented psychotherapy was directed to identification and expression of emotion and understanding the sources of her anger and sadness. She was most consciously aware of intense anger toward her mother because of her neglect and repeated failures of empathy, as well as the fact that one of her own children had died while in her care. She began to feel deep regret that she had never been able to spend time with her father, and that his death had ended any possibility of rectifying this. KD herself first articulated the connection between her bodily pain, diagnosed soon after his death as fibromyalgia, and her unacknowledged grief. As she reflected upon early experiences, gave expression to her emotions, and came to understand what she was feeling, her conversion symptoms resolved.

Outcome

At the time of discharge, KD had recovered completely from her conversion disorder, and at 3-year follow-up was euthymic and without conversion symptoms. Her marriage remained stable, and she started several entrepreneurial ventures including a dog-breeding business. She also became an active member and volunteer of her local church committee.

Case 5: CD Presenting as a Dyskinetic Movement Disorder

BG is a 40-year-old, single woman living with her elderly parents, who was referred to us with probable CD after prolonged and extensive investigations at a movement disorder center failed to yield a neurologic diagnosis. Her presenting problem was the development, over 24 hours, of dysphagia, an inability to walk or speak, and writhing, dyskinetic movements of her pelvis and lower torso. All of her symptoms worsened and were accompanied by anxiety if she was outside her home.

Relevant History

BG had not been well for 3 years prior to presentation, beginning with the development of chronic low back pain after she sustained a very minor muscle strain from bending forward. She had been investigated extensively for this and no explanation could be found for her persistent complaint and disability. For 3 years she used a cane and gradually reduced her hours of work from 14 a day to none, 6 months prior to the development of the movement disorder described above. For one of the 3 years, she took high doses of Percocet and Tylenol #3, from which she eventually weaned herself. Shortly after she had developed back pain, her mother suffered a cerebral vascular accident, her father was diagnosed with cancer, and her only sibling, a younger sister, left home for the first time to live independently.

One afternoon, 6 months prior to presentation, while her father was at a doctor's appointment, his "favorite cat" escaped from the house into the backyard and was savagely attacked by a neighboring pit bull. BG, the only one at home at the time, helplessly witnessed the cat's prolonged dismemberment. Several days later, she found herself "flooded" with memories from the ages of 5 to 7, when she was repeatedly sodomized in the backyard of her grandmother's house by the man who lived next door. These were not new memories, but ones she thought she had "put aside" years ago. She had never told anyone about this experience, but had an enduring sense of being "guilty" and "dirty." She was very aware that her avoidance of intimacy or any relationships outside the home was related to this early, abusive experience.

BG had no personal or family history of psychiatric illness and had been medically well prior to the development of back pain 3 years before her presentation.

Personal and family psychiatric history was entirely negative and the patient had no medical problems other than chronic low back pain.

Predisposing Factors
- Sexual abuse as a child.

Precipitating Factors
- A minor back injury which led to a type of discomfort that unconsciously "reminded" her of her experience of being sodomized as a child.
- Loss of her sister and the threat of loss of her parents.
- Witnessing a lethal attack on the family cat in the backyard and feeling helpless to do anything. The setting of this trauma in the backyard reminded her of her own frightening experience of abuse by a neighbor at her grandmother's home as a child.

Perpetuating Factors

In this case, BG's movement disorder was appropriately investigated and then quickly identified as CD, which led to an appropriate referral for treatment. We believe she would have benefited from attention to the role of psychological factors in the development of chronic low back pain and the degree of dysfunction it caused. It became clear, during psychotherapy sessions with BG, that the minor muscle strain she experienced 3 years before had provoked somatic memories of the discomfort she experienced while being sodomized as a child.

Treatment Approach and Outcome

We saw BG in the outpatient department for several months prior to her admission to the hospital because she was very reluctant to be separated from her family. During this time, her clinical presentation remained unchanged and she became increasingly depressed. Although she was actively involved in physiotherapy, none of her improvements in the clinical setting were being transferred into her day-to-day life. At the behest of her family she eventually agreed to come into the hospital. By this time she had been unable to walk and had had abnormal excessive movements for 6 months.

In the hospital we instituted hierarchic expectations of motor independence even before the abnormal movements had resolved. At the same time, BG was instructed in breathing techniques, relaxation exercises, and yoga. A program of desensitization to her fear of being in public spaces was instituted and her depression was treated with an antidepressant agent. Daily psychotherapy sessions focused upon the early experience of abuse, her longstanding avoidance of relationships outside of her family, her fear of losing her parents, and her guilt about not being able to save her father's cat, just as she felt chronically guilty about not being able to prevent the sexual abuse she experienced as a child.

BG was easily engaged in psychotherapy and at one point said, "I think it's good that I had a problem with my movements, because it told people something was wrong." As she became able to express her feelings, and address distorted cognitions about her experiences as a child, she became more and more mobile and her abnormal movements resolved.

After one month of hospitalization, BG was no longer depressed and was walking independently and making plans to return to work. During one particular excursion outdoors during which she walked independently for the first time, BG became tearful and said, "I feel so free."

BARRIERS TO THE DIAGNOSIS OF CONVERSION DISORDER

In almost every case we treated, the patient had been followed for many years by one or more neurologists, and had had multiple medical and neurologic consultations. Many of these patients were regarded as having an intractable neurodegenerative or demyelinating disorder, with no consideration of a diagnosis of CD. In our experience, failure to make the diagnosis typically occurs either because CD was never considered in the differential or because the treating physicians were concerned about missing an "organic" diagnosis.

Failure to Consider the Diagnosis of CD

Many of our patients were followed for years by experienced clinicians, with diagnoses such as multiple sclerosis, epilepsy, dystonia, or Tourette syndrome. The patient would typically present with neurologic symptoms and signs that were suggestive of the early phases of a known neurologic disorder. The initial diagnosis, in other words, was usually a reasonable one. Over time, however, the initial provisional diagnosis tended to become entrenched, even in the absence of the expected supportive evidence from neurologic investigations. The difficulty in recognizing CD is magnified in a patient who has a coexistent neurologic disorder, such as multiple sclerosis or epilepsy. In these cases, there are, typically, clear-cut abnormalities on the EEG or MRI scan. The problem arises when, for unidentified psychological reasons, the patient experiences so-called symptom amplification. A natural tendency for the treating physician is to ascribe all clinical deterioration to the identified neurologic illness. This can result in a failure to consider the possibility that at least some of the patient's clinical dysfunction might be due to conversion symptoms. Elements that might help alert one to the possibility of CD include the following: atypical or inconsistent clinical features; functional deterioration that is out of keeping with the degree of abnormality evident on neurologic examination and investigations; an inappropriate lack of emotional response to the deteriorating clinical situation; and plausible evidence of "secondary gain."

Fear of Missing an "Organic" Diagnosis

For most of the past 100 years, there has been a strong tendency to regard neuropsychiatric problems in general, and movement disorders in particular, as being *either* "organic" *or* "functional." This dichotomous approach persists today, despite a wealth of neuroscientific evidence that life experiences and state of mind (the "psychological") can have powerful effects on the structure and function of the brain (the "biologic"). The problem is exacerbated by a tendency among neurologists, in particular, to equate the "organic" with the "real." Torsion dystonia, for example, is often regarded as being more "real" than psychogenic dystonia, despite the fact that we still have a poor understanding of the pathophysiology of dystonia or why it affects specific body parts in particular individuals. This mindset influences clinical practice. The single-minded search for an "organic" neurologic diagnosis can result in blindness to blatant evidence of CD. It is noteworthy that ignoring or missing a diagnosis of CD does not carry the same weight of embarrassment as missing a diagnosis of, for example, multiple sclerosis, even though CD is potentially curable, whereas the functional disabilities arising from multiple sclerosis are generally not responsive to therapeutic interventions.

This relative lack of concern among physicians about missing a "functional" problem such as CD, as opposed to an "organic" illness, is reflective of the general stigma attached to psychiatric illness. It is as if the overriding and even exclusive priority of the physician is to identify an "organic" diagnosis in order to spare the patient from a "less acceptable" psychiatric one, even if the latter is treatable and the former is not. Even within the field of psychiatry there has developed a tendency to regard CD as less "biologic" than other categories of psychiatric illness such as obsessive–compulsive or mood disorders.

BARRIERS TO TREATMENT
Failure of the Patient to Engage in Therapy

The psychodynamic understanding of CD posits that the patient's neurologic dysfunction is a defense against conflicts or unbearable thoughts or feelings. Because these psychological defenses are the very core of CD, it is understandable that there will be resistance on the part of the patient to anything that threatens to weaken or remove them. At the same time, many patients feel there is a stigma associated with being given a psychiatric, as apposed to a medical or neurologic, diagnosis, and will vociferously deny any emotional or psychological problems. If a psychiatric diagnosis is proffered, patients and their families may predict that it will be proven wrong and may even threaten legal action. In part, this reaction reflects the stigma of psychiatric illness, and in part, it emerges from the understandable concern that when attention is turned to psychological issues, any physical problems the patient may be experiencing will no longer be seriously investigated. For all of these reasons, patients with CD are not easily engaged in treatment and this interferes with the initiation of appropriate treatment. Most physicians do not have the time, nor do they wish to expend the effort, convincing patients of their diagnosis, especially when it involves finding a language and an explanatory model that encompasses both the psychological and physical and makes sense to the individual. Being able to formulate an understanding of why the condition developed is challenging. Hesitancy to make a diagnosis of CD is thus compounded by uncertainty about the best way to engage the patient in accepting the diagnosis.

Tendency to Associate CD with Malingering

Physicians are often ambivalent about CD because of its problematic association with malingering and factitious disorder. This sense that the CD patient is in some way "faking" illness can lead to a withholding or punitive attitude in which the patient is regarded as being "undeserving" of sympathy or even care. In our experience, some families readily adopt this attitude. In two of the cases we have described, (BT and KL), the patient's spouse, after years of providing solicitous and hyperattentive care while the patient was bedridden and wheelchair-bound, abandoned the family soon after the diagnosis of CD was made. Recovery for such patients means more than the overcoming of physical disability; it can also mean the loss of an emotional support system. This can pose an added barrier to recovery.

Failure to Recognize an Underlying Neurologic Illness

We noted earlier that CD can be difficult to recognize in patients with a coexistent neurologic disorder. The reverse is also true. Once the treating physician identifies conversion symptoms, there is a tendency to attribute all complaints to the CD. This can, in some cases, result in the overlooking of a treatable condition, as happened with one of our patients whose severe bilateral carpal tunnel syndrome had for years gone untreated because her paresthesias and tendency to drop things were assumed to be related to her CD. Even if the underlying neurologic problem is not amenable to therapy, a failure to make the diagnosis can undermine the trust that is essential if the patient is to engage with treatment of the CD. We treated an 11-year-old boy who developed CD following a sport-related concussion. In addition to his inability to walk, he also complained of headaches, sensitivity to lights, reduced stamina, and easy fatigability. All of these were understood as a tendency to somatize and to avoid treatment. When we first saw him, he clearly felt that no one understood how he was feeling. As part of our diagnostic workup, we ordered visual evoked potentials. They were grossly abnormal and certainly confirmed his sense that something was wrong with his brain. Once we informed him and his parents of the results, advised them that this was most likely secondary to a persistent postconcussive syndrome, and acknowledged that this might indeed affect his stamina, he became easily engaged in a program to treat his inability to walk, which we stated clearly was a manifestation of CD. Eight months following his concussion, he was able to ambulate after 2 weeks of intensive treatment.

The Shift Away from "Psychodynamic" Psychiatry

Over the past 40 years, psychiatric illnesses have been diagnosed according to criteria outlined in various editions of the *Diagnostic and Statistical Manual of Mental Disorders* (DSM) (2). This has involved defining psychiatric syndromes in terms of clinical features and natural history, without presumptions of causality or underlying pathology. The widespread adoption of DSM-based diagnosis has meant a shift away from trying to understand psychiatric illness in terms of psychodynamic processes. This has resulted in a withering of the conceptual tools for understanding and treating CD, which is, after all, the paradigmatic condition for demonstrating the efficacy of psychodynamic psychotherapy. It has also resulted in a de-emphasis of the role of psychological processes in mental health, and a concomitant loss of psychotherapeutic skills among psychiatrists. As a consequence, CD, which was once the most treatable, and even curable, of neuropsychiatric disorders, is arguably diagnosed and treated less effectively today that 100 years ago.

The Contemporary Health Care Environment

There has been, in recent years, a massive shift away from hospital-based treatment, indeed, from any form of long-term psychotherapeutic intervention. This has a particularly negative impact upon the treatment of CD, which, in our experience, can require months for a full response. This is unfortunate, since CD is a curable disorder that, left untreated, makes significant and ongoing demands on the health care system.

ELEMENTS OF THE TREATMENT PROCESS

Our treatment program rests upon a very close working relationship between neurology and psychiatry, and the active, ongoing involvement of both disciplines in the treatment process. Essential steps are as follows:

Step 1: *Creating a supportive, nonjudgmental environment that will allow an in-depth inquiry and exploration of the person's life.* We believe this is most effectively undertaken if both the neurologist and the psychiatrist are present. It has long been observed that people respond positively when someone listens to them with interest, compassion, and empathy. That said, these patients do not readily identify the events in their lives that are highly relevant to the development of their condition; indeed, they will typically deny any significant occurrences initially. If one conceptualizes CD as a somatic defense against psychological problems, this makes sense. These patients are working hard to protect themselves from psychological insight and awareness of the underlying problems while the psychiatrist is doing the opposite. The initial inquiry involves close attention to fluctuations in the physical manifestations in response to what is being discussed. At points of exacerbation, the physician should encourage further exploration of the particular situation as well as the expression of emotion. There should be attention to both the primary (unconscious) and secondary (more conscious) gains that appear to be afforded by the disability.

Step 2: *Identifying the psychosocial setting in which conversion symptoms first appeared.* It is important to identify any perceived or remembered trauma including injury, illness, neglect, abuse, deprivation, or loss. Determine whether the patient has ever been seriously ill or had a relationship with someone suffering from a serious or prolonged medical or neurologic illness. If so, what was the patient's role or involvement? In doing so, one is searching for whether the patient had a role model for illness behavior and whether there had been premature or overwhelming caretaking expectations of the patient which compromised his or her own care.

Step 3: *Finding a language and an explanatory model that engages the patient and offers a framework within which to understand the disorder.* This is the most critical step because, unless it is done successfully, patients will not become involved in treatment. While the specifics will differ from patient to patient, the model must acknowledge the reality of the motor dysfunction and the patient's conscious wish to recover. We have found a number of images that have proven useful in this regard. One involves the example of an athlete in a "slump." In this scenario, an admired sports hero is unable to do something he or she had previously mastered. "Stress" and its ability to affect physical health is another concept that many patients accept and seem to intuitively understand.

To some extent, the success of a stress model would appear to depend upon the individual acknowledging stressful events prior to the onset of the CD, which is typically *not* the case. We have found, however, that patients can accept the notion of *unconscious* feelings and the possibility that while they may be emotionally stoic—to the point of ignoring their feelings—their bodies may have absorbed the impact of certain stressful life events. Another explanatory image is that of being petrified, scared stiff, or frozen with fear. The example of trembling as an abnormal, excessive movement that accompanies fear or more striking examples from the animal world, when intense fear "paralyzes" movement, can be effective.

Step 4: *Deciding whether to hospitalize.* While some CD patients can be treated on an outpatient basis, we have found hospitalization to be the most effective and efficient setting for those most severely affected by the disorder. As treatment is time- and labor-intensive, it requires a team of health professionals. Hospitalization allows consistent, intensive, and integrated interventions, which emphasize progress and prevent regression. By being in the hospital, patients are removed from the environment in which their disorder developed and to which it may have become conditioned. This encompasses the physical setting as well as aspects of interpersonal and family life that might be enabling or perpetuating the disorder. That said, we have carried out successful treatment on an outpatient basis with highly motivated patients whose families are supportive of our understanding and our interventions.

Step 5: *Ensuring that appropriate medical and neurologic investigations are carried out and maintaining an open mind to the need for further tests even after treatment has started.* Mai (3) has said that after an adequate diagnostic workup has been completed, the physician should refrain from further re-examinations and additional investigations, on the grounds that this will only encourage patient denial of the psychological nature of the disorder and result in ongoing and unnecessary tests. Our experience has been different. We have found that patients can be given a diagnosis of CD with "confidence and authority" at the same time as a spirit of open-mindedness and ongoing inquiry is imparted. As with any illness, we feel that the diagnosis of CD should be reconsidered over the course of treatment if the patient is not recovering, and further investigations should be based upon consideration of the individual situation. In fact, we advise patients at the outset that we believe it is important to maintain an open mind with respect to the primary diagnosis as well as emergent or concurrent conditions. This not only reassures the patient but takes pressure off physicians who often feel that, once a diagnosis of CD is made, the door to reformulation is closed. While there are many examples of "gross overinvestigation" in patients with CD—with the attendant risk of iatrogenic illness and delays in instituting appropriate treatment (4)—we disagree with a rigid directive to stop all medical investigations at a certain point. This approach seems especially prudent given that "organic" illnesses often coexist with CD. It also allows one to begin treatment of the CD when the diagnosis is strongly suspected and yet investigations are incomplete.

Step 6: *Treating concurrent psychiatric and medical conditions.* In our experience these most frequently include depression, anxiety, social phobia, and headache. Complaints of pain and/or insomnia often respond to low-dose amitriptyline. Benzodiazepines can help with symptoms of anxiety and muscle tension.

Step 7: *Stating explicitly, at the outset, that the patient has the potential to recover fully,* although there may be periods of relapse as well as shifts in the nature of the dysfunction. We have found that anticipating relapses and shifting symptomatology can abort their occurrence, or at least shorten their duration.

Step 8: *Setting forth a timetable of achievable milestones,* with explicit statements to the patient about what will be accomplished, in terms of motor control recovery, by the end of each upcoming block of time.

Step 9: *Involving a physiotherapist and/or speech therapies, from the beginning* in developing individually tailored programs of graduate activity. This aspect of treatment serves to validate the physical dimension of the disorder and is an important face-saving device for both family and patients who are prone to regarding success from purely psychological intervention as evidence that the illness was not "real." Patients should be instructed early on in deep breathing and relaxation techniques. Activities that emphasize control over one's mind and body, such as yoga, are very helpful for patients with abnormal excessive movements. The allied health care professionals involved in these aspects of the treatment can encourage and compliment patients on their progress in a much more explicit manner than the person who is doing psychotherapy. In coordinating the physical and psychotherapeutic parts of treatment, Leslie (5) has commented upon the importance of moving from the "physical" to the "psychological" at a pace with which the patient and family can cope. Continued involvement of physiotherapy should be reconsidered if the patient is not responding or is not transferring improved motor skills to other settings. We have had patients who "recover" in physiotherapy but remain unchanged in all other settings. Physical and functional goals for a particular block of time, whether it be in days or weeks, should include the

expectations that these are consolidated in and out of the formal treatment hours.

Step 10: *Allowing frank discussion about the fact that others have accused the patient of "faking" illness.* Unfortunately, many of our patients have been previously treated in a dismissive, mocking, hostile, or belittling way by physicians. For example, one young woman was asked, "So what's your next story going to be?" In another instance, a 12-year-old boy recalled being terrified when the neurologist pulled away his walker and said, "I know you can walk." During a hospital fire, a 14-year-old girl who had been bedridden and unable to walk for 3 months was told that staff had no way of taking her out of the building, mistakenly predicting that in an emergency situation she would be able to move. Patients have been humiliated by being told they will have to wear diapers if they "insist" on needing help with toileting. In the same spirit, referral to psychiatry is presented as a threat or punishment if the patient stubbornly persists in failing to recover.

Step 11: *Meeting regularly with patients in order to understand and, in turn, have them understand what the conversion disorder means, what functions it serves, and why it developed when it did.* In every case we have encountered to date, there is a rich and compelling narrative that ties together aspects of the patient's past and present life and makes sense of the illness. This is, of course, the aim of the "formulation" in psychiatry. The therapeutic power of being understood by another and understanding oneself cannot be underestimated in any illness, but perhaps especially in CD.

Step 12: *Teaching patients about the role of the brain in physical/medical illness.* This would include the ways in which the brain controls many aspects of physical health; the effects of stress on both mental and physical functioning; the concept of mind-emotion-body disconnection; the interrelationship of mood and movement; and unconscious versus conscious experiences. The exact nature of the information transfer will, of course, depend upon the educational and knowledge level of the patient.

Step 13: *Using videotapes* for feedback and correction of deficits or abnormalities as well as for assessment of progress.

SUMMARY

CD is an important and underdiagnosed cause of major neurologic disability. It is essential to recognize signs and symptoms (6) when they arise, since they are potentially treatable and curable (7). Even patients with severe and profound dysfunction can enjoy an excellent clinical outcome with an appropriate multidisciplinary approach.

Individuals with CD are initially reluctant to accept this diagnosis. Recovery typically takes place over the course of many months and requires patience and persistence on the part of the treatment team.

REFERENCES

1. King H. Once upon a text: hysteria from Hippocrates. In: Gilman LS, King H, Porter R, eds. *Hysteria beyond Freud.* Berkeley, CA: University of California Press, 1993:3–90.
2. American Psychiatric Association. *Diagnostic and statistical manual of mental disorders,* 4th ed. Washington, DC: American Psychiatric Association, 1994.
3. Mai FM. Hysteria in clinical neurology. *Can J Neurol Sci.* 1995;22:101–110.
4. Leary PM. Conversion disorder in childhood-diagnosed too late, investigated too much? *J R Soc Med.* 2003;96:436–438.
5. Leslie SA. Diagnosis and treatment of hysterical conversion reactions. *Arch Dis Child.* 1988;63:506–511.
6. Speed J. Behavioral management of conversion disorder: retrospective study. *Arch Phys Med Rehabil.* 1996;77:147–154.
7. Stone J, Zeman A, Sharpe M. Functional weakness and sensory disturbance. *J Neurol Neurosurg Psychiatr.* 2002;73:241–245.

34

Treatment of Psychogenic Movement Disorder: Psychotropic Medications

Valerie Voon

ABSTRACT

Psychogenic movement disorder (PMD) is a subtype of conversion disorder (CD) characterized by symptoms of tremor, dystonia, myoclonus, and gait disorders.

The treatment literature is sparse with multiple methodological flaws. There are no psychotropic treatment studies specific to PMD. The limited literature on psychotropic treatment studies (dopamine receptor antagonists and antidepressants) in CD and other functional disorders is reviewed, focusing on potential pathophysiologic mechanisms. A hypothesis on the mechanism of action of antidepressants on psychogenic movement symptoms is proposed. General recommendations for psychotropic treatments are suggested and common patient questions raised in the prescribing of psychotropic medications in this population are addressed. Finally, recommendations for treatment studies in PMD are discussed. Our observations suggest that the efficacy of antidepressants on psychogenic movement symptoms can be dissociated from cross-sectional psychiatric diagnoses and measurements of depression or anxiety, consistent with the literature on antidepressants and other functional disorders. The presence of any depressive or anxiety symptoms, regardless of severity, should be actively treated, given the otherwise poor prognosis of the chronic PMD population. There may also be a rationale for a trial of antidepressants in PMD patients without overt comorbid psychiatric diagnoses, although further studies are necessary to support this observation. The preliminary evidence suggests that active intervention with antidepressants can alter the prognosis of patients with chronic PMD.

INTRODUCTION

Psychogenic movement disorder (PMD) is a subtype of conversion disorder (CD) characterized by symptoms of tremor, dystonia, myoclonus, and gait disorders. CD, a broader term focusing on unexplained neurologic symptoms, is classified in the *Diagnostic and Statistical Manual of Mental Disorders*, Fourth Edition (DSM-IV) (1), as a somatoform disorder—a type of disorder with unexplained physical symptoms related to underlying psychological factors.

The community point prevalence of CD is reported at 50 per 100,000 with the prevalence over a period of a year at approximately twice this rate (2). PMD itself is diagnosed in approximately 2% to 3% of patients in subspecialized movement disorder clinics (3). The differences between prognostic outcomes in acute versus chronic CD patients are profound, with recovery rates of 90% versus 45%, respectively (4). Yet, despite the high rates of disability, the financial burden, and the poor prognosis in patients with chronic symptoms, these patients are often underrecognized and undertreated (5).

The literature on the treatment of CD mirrors this clinical reality. The treatment literature is sparse and focuses on behavior therapy, rehabilitation, hypnosis, and psychotherapeutic techniques (6). Existing studies have multiple methodological flaws including small sample sizes, lack of controls, and heterogeneous populations (6). The mix of acute and chronic patients and the presence of different conversion subtypes in study populations confound the results of most studies.

The limited literature on psychotropic treatment studies (dopamine receptor antagonists and antidepressants) will be reviewed, focusing on potential pathophysiologic mechanisms. There are no psychotropic treatment studies specific to PMD; as such, this chapter focuses on psychotropic studies of CD and other specific somatoform disorders. A hypothesis on the mechanism of action of antidepressants on psychogenic movement symptoms will be proposed. General recommendations for psychotropic treatments will be suggested according to published guidelines and literature on the treatment of the comorbid psychiatric disorders. Common patient questions raised in the prescribing of psychotropic medications in this population will also be addressed. Finally, recommendations for treatment studies in PMD and issues in design and implementation will be discussed.

DOPAMINE RECEPTOR ANTAGONISTS

Rampello et al. (7) report on a two-month open-label trial in 18 patients with mixed CD symptoms of paralysis, anesthesia, and pseudoseizures, comparing haloperidol, 6 mg (n = 6), and sulpiride, 800 mg (n = 12). The sulpiride 800 mg group had a statistically significant improvement ($p < 0.002$) in comparison to the haloperidol group on the Middlesex Health Questionnaire (hysterical traits and symptoms). The sulpiride arm was extended a further 2 months at a lower dose of 400 mg with a subsequent loss in the improvement of symptoms. The authors conclude that a hyperdopaminergic state may play a pathophysiologic role in the CD symptoms.

The study can be further reinterpreted in light of recent PET imaging studies by Kapur and Seeman (8). Antipsychotic occupancy of the D2 receptor between 65% and 80% has been demonstrated to correlate with efficacy on the psychotic symptoms of schizophrenia, whereas occupancy of greater than 80% correlates with the emergence of extrapyramidal symptoms (EPS).

Haloperidol is a D2 receptor antagonist with a slow dissociation constant, which at 6 mg occupies greater than 80% of D2 receptors. The results for the haloperidol arm in the study by Rampello et al. may thus be confounded by EPS side effects, which were not reported. Sulpiride, an atypical antipsychotic, is a D2 and D3 receptor antagonist with a rapid dissociation constant. At a dose of 800 mg, sulpiride occupies less than 80% of D2 receptors. In the study by Rampello et al., sulpiride 800 mg was effective on CD symptoms; at 400 mg, the efficacy was lost. In this light, Rampello et al. suggest that antipsychotic agents targeting CD symptoms may be efficacious at doses similar to those required for antipsychotic effects, and that higher doses that may result in EPS symptoms should be avoided. Functional neuroimaging studies focusing on dopaminergic activity may be potentially useful, and the role of the D3 receptor remains to be clarified.

In addition to the small sample size, the open-label nature of the study, and the need for replication of findings, significant design issues limit the generalizability of the Rampello et al. study to the PMD population. The study population was a heterogeneous group of patients experiencing a range of CD symptoms which did not include PMDs. Different pathophysiologic mechanisms may mediate the production of these differing symptoms. The duration of symptoms was also not reported, creating potential confounders given the differences in prognoses between acute and chronic symptoms. Finally, the outcome measure of the study focused only on the CD symptoms, whereas clinically relevant outcome measures should focus more broadly on functional status, quality of life, and psychiatric symptoms in addition to the motor symptoms.

ANTIDEPRESSANTS

The evidence for the efficacy of antidepressants in PMD comes from the literature on overlapping functional disorders demonstrated to respond to antidepressants and our own clinical experience with the PMD population. In a cohort of 24 PMD patients reviewed by Williams et al. (9), 70% of these patients either had been treated or were currently being treated with antidepressants.

Antidepressants and Functional Disorders

A range of functional disorders including functional somatic syndromes, somatization disorder and globus hystericus have been demonstrated to respond to antidepressants. These functional disorders may have overlaps with PMD, thus indirectly supporting the role for antidepressants in PMD.

Functional somatic syndromes, previously recognized in the medical literature as discrete clinical entities, have recently been theorized to have a common underlying pathophysiology, and similar responses to treatment (10, 11). The most common of these medically unexplained syndromes include chronic pain, irritable bowel syndrome, chronic fatigue syndrome, and fibromyalgia. The functional somatic syndromes notably do not include CD, although there may indeed be some degree of pathophysiologic overlap. A metaanalysis of 94 randomized controlled trial (RCT) studies of a variety of functional somatic syndromes demonstrated that these syndromes can respond to antidepressants (12). The response was dissociated from the presence of depression although the exact relationship between these syndromes and depression and anxiety remains to be clarified. The concept of the "affective spectrum disorders" with disorders of similar comorbidities, heritability, and response to treatment has also been proposed. Such a scheme classifies the functional somatic syndromes as a form of an affective disorder (13).

An overlapping relationship may also exist between somatization disorder and CD. In one longitudinal study, 65% of patients initially diagnosed with CD were subsequently rediagnosed with somatization disorder in a 10-year follow-up (14). Similarly, in one cross-sectional study, 20% of patients admitted to a conversion disorder ward had diagnoses of somatization disorder (15).

An 8-week open-label trial of nefazodone in patients with somatization disorder (n = 15) resulted in a 75% improvement in global outcome (Clinical Global Improvement), functioning (Medical Outcome Study Short Form—36), and somatic symptoms (visual analog scale) (16). Notably, neither depression (Hamilton Depression Rating Scale) nor anxiety (Hamilton Anxiety Rating Scale) measures were predictive of outcome, suggesting that the improvement of somatization disorder with antidepressants was independent of comorbid depressive or anxiety symptoms.

Globus hystericus, a CD symptom also known as functional dysphonia, has been reported in case reports to respond to antidepressants and to ECT prompting a suggestion of this symptom to be a manifestation of depression (17).

Antidepressants and Psychogenic Movement Disorder: Clinical Experience

A review of the clinical psychiatric experience of the Movement Disorders Centre at the Toronto Western Hospital (TWH) supports the utility of antidepressants in the treatment of PMD.

From January 2003 to July 2004, 23 patients with diagnoses of PMD underwent psychiatric assessment. Fifteen patients were treated with antidepressants and followed in a nonblinded prospective manner. Eight patients were not followed due to distance (n = 2), follow-up with the patient's psychiatrist (n = 2), and patient refusal (n = 4). The diagnosis was made by a movement disorders neurologist utilizing Fahn and Williams's definite and probable criteria for the diagnosis of PMD (9). Patients in whom the diagnosis of factitious symptoms, or malingering, could not be definitively made were included within the cohort. Four patients with suspected neurologic disorders at the time of assessment were not included in the analysis. The symptoms were of chronic duration (longer than 3 months). Treatment visits occurred on average every 2 weeks, ranging from weekly to monthly.

The patients were assessed for psychiatric diagnoses with the Mini International Neuropsychiatric Inventory (MINI) (18), a shortened version of the Structured Clinical Interview for the Diagnosis of DSM-IV disorders. The diagnoses of panic attacks, chronic pain, somatization disorder, hypochondriasis, factitious symptoms, or malingering are not coded in the MINI and were made using DSM-IV criteria. The previous and current use of antidepressants (type, dose, and duration) was reviewed through patient interview, collateral information, and pharmacy record review.

A history of physical and sexual abuse was ascertained using the following questions: Have you ever experienced physical or sexual abuse? Has anyone ever touched you in a way that made you uncomfortable? Were you disciplined excessively as a child?

The severity of depressive symptoms was assessed using the clinician-rated Montgomery-Asberg Depression Rating Scale (MADRS) (19), and the patient-rated Beck Depression Inventory (20). Anxiety symptoms were assessed using the patient-rated Beck Anxiety Inventory (21). The Clinical Global Impression of Severity and Change of overall (nonmotor symptoms and function) and motor symptoms was documented.

The outcomes are summarized here and reported in greater detail elsewhere (22). The characteristics of the group were as follows: 18 women and five men; 16 married; mean age 43.5 (standard deviation 13.5); mean duration illness 73.0 (standard deviation 65.1); and 40% previously on antidepressants. Somatization disorder was identified in three (13%); stressors at onset in 12 (52%); previous models in eight (35%); abuse history in two (9%); and "la belle indifférence" in five (22%). There were no significant differences between the treated and untreated groups.

The group's MADRS improved following antidepressant treatment ($p < 0.01$) assessed at a mean of 3 months. Supportive psychotherapy was provided concurrently for three and family intervention in one. Ten of the 15 patients treated with antidepressants maintained a PMD diagnosis, with five diagnosed with primary hypochondriasis, somatization disorder, or likely factitious symptoms or malingering. Eight of the ten PMD patients had marked improvements, with one having mild improvement. Seven patients attained complete resolution of motor symptoms. Three of these patients did not have a current depression or anxiety diagnosis and had low baseline depression and anxiety scores, with one patient having anxiety disorder diagnoses but low measurement scores. The patient who did not improve did not have a current psychiatric diagnosis and had low measurement scores. The other PMD patients had diagnoses of major depression, generalized anxiety, panic disorder, and/or agoraphobia.

The five patients with alternate primary diagnoses did not improve with antidepressant treatment alone.

Antidepressants and Psychogenic Movement Disorders: Discussion of Clinical Experience

The patient population was a group with psychogenic movement symptoms of chronic duration, although the final diagnoses revealed greater diagnostic heterogeneity. The patients with likely factitious symptoms or malingering did not improve; given the inherent difficulties in the diagnosis of these patients, inclusion of these patients represents a potentially significant confounder. Somatization disorder was likely underdiagnosed as extensive collateral or medical records were not obtained.

Nine percent of patients had a history of physical or sexual abuse. The evaluation was limited in that only three screening questions were asked, and that emotional abuse or neglect was not screened. However, the results stand in contrast to that of the literature on pseudoseizures demonstrating a high association with a history of trauma (23,24). Although trauma has been suggested as a potential precursor for the mechanism of dissociation in pseudoseizures (23,25), it appears not to be as relevant in the PMD population. Furthermore, this difference also suggests that the populations may have differing underlying personality traits and prognoses.

Forty percent of patients were either previously or currently on antidepressants, keeping with the known literature (9). However, closer review of the antidepressant history reveals that only 17% of the patients had an adequate trial (an adequate dose for at least 6 weeks' duration) of antidepressants, and that only 13% of these patients were currently using antidepressants of an adequate dose. Optimal doses were thus likely not achieved during any of these previous trials. Despite the high association of PMD with antidepressant use, the patients were still undertreated.

The range of antidepressants utilized in our treatment trials included the specific serotonin reuptake inhibitors (SSRI), paroxetine and citalopram, and venlafaxine, a dual serotonin and norepinephrine reuptake inhibitor (SNRI). The dose ranges were in the upper range of normal.

Forty percent of patients with clinician-rated and patient-rated depression and anxiety scores of normal severity had marked improvements on antidepressants. Detailed psychiatric assessment of these three patients revealed diagnoses ranging from *previous* major depression (likely in partial remission), *previous* posttraumatic stress disorder (likely in partial remission), and generalized anxiety disorder, panic attacks, and agoraphobia. These results suggest that the efficacy of antidepressants on global and motor outcomes may be dissociated from current cross-sectional psychiatric diagnoses and measurements of depression or anxiety.

Alternative explanations for the results include the placebo effect, or the effects of supportive psychotherapy. However, the results remained sustained over months, arguing against a placebo effect. The psychotherapy was performed on an as-needed basis. The lack of a consistent weekly psychotherapeutic intervention argues against a significant contribution from the psychotherapy. However, given the known high short-term placebo response in this population, further RCT studies would be necessary to control for the effects of placebo or psychotherapy.

The results suggest that 80% of PMD patients with chronic symptoms of moderate severity can have marked improvements in global and motor outcomes when treated with antidepressants. Seventy percent of the patients had a complete resolution of their motor symptoms. These outcomes are in marked contrast to the outcomes reported in the literature on chronic untreated PMD symptoms, and suggest that active intervention may indeed shift prognosis. The subgroup with primary diagnoses of other somatoform disorders, factitious symptoms, or malingering, representing one-third of the treated group, had poor outcomes. The outcome of the patients who were not followed was not known. Notably, the study population was seen in a tertiary movement disorder clinic and was influenced by the method of referral (outpatients on a one-year waiting list). This data represents a very small series of patients treated in an open-label fashion. Further studies will be required to support these observations.

WHY ARE ANTIDEPRESSANTS EFFECTIVE IN PSYCHOGENIC MOVEMENT DISORDER?

The high prevalence of comorbid mood and anxiety disorders in the PMD population has been well-established (26). However, the data reviewed suggest that antidepressants may be effective for both the global and motor outcomes of PMD dissociated from a cross-sectional diagnosis of a mood or anxiety disorder. The rationale for efficacy can be understood as follows: Firstly, antidepressants may be treating an unrecognized comorbid depression or anxiety. Specific deficits associated with depression or anxiety may thus still mediate the expression of these symptoms. However, this explanation may be insufficient on its own, as only a small proportion of patients with depression or anxiety develop PMD symptoms. Secondly, depression or anxiety may indeed not be present in a subsection of the PMD population, suggesting then that antidepressants, or medications with serotonergic or noradrenergic activity, may have a direct effect on PMD symptoms.

Treatment of an Underrecognized Depression or Anxiety

In addition to the overt diagnosis of major depression, antidepressants may be treating an underrecognized comorbid depression or anxiety. In clinical practice, disorders such as dysthymia and generalized anxiety disorder are commonly underrecognized (27,28).

Dysthymia is a chronic, low-grade depression associated with vegetative and cognitive symptoms. The prevalence of dysthymia in the general population is 3.1%; however, the prevalence of dysthymia in primary care populations has been documented at 8%, suggesting a clustering in medical settings (27). Dysthymia is a disabling psychiatric state associated with somatic, social, and occupational dysfunction. Seventy-five percent of the patients with dysthymia progress to a major depressive episode. Despite the associated morbidity, the majority of patients with dysthymia are not diagnosed until their first major depressive episode (27). Dysthymia is a potentially treatable condition and has been demonstrated to respond in RCT studies to a range of antidepressants (29,30). Recent literature reviews suggest that antidepressants may be more effective than psychotherapy in the treatment of dysthymia (29,30).

The concept of a subsyndromal symptomatic depression (SSD) further extends this hypothesis of underrecognition of the underlying psychiatric disorders (31–33). The clinical assessment of patients and the subsequent decision for treatment is frequently cross-sectional (i.e., does this patient currently fulfill the criteria for a mood disorder?) rather than made in consideration of the longitudinal course of mood disorders. This tendency is based in part on the evolution of the DSM-IV as a categoric entity. SSD is a term utilized to describe patients who do not meet criteria for a depression or dysthymia, as they do not have a depressed mood or anhedonia. However, the endorsed symptoms such as fatigue or suicidal ideation are qualitatively similar to that of a major depression. SSD has been suggested to represent either the active premorbid or active residual state of major depression. Patients fulfilling the criteria for SSD have a significantly elevated risk of psychosocial dysfunction, suicide, and future depression (31–33). PMD patients with a comorbid SSD, despite its associated morbidity, may thus not be clinically recognized or adequately treated.

In addition to the mood disorders, anxiety disorders such as generalized anxiety disorder (GAD), an entity characterized by excessive generalized worries, is also poorly recognized and diagnosed in medical practices (28). The community prevalence is 5.1% and the primary care prevalence, similar to that of dysthymia, is higher at 8% (28,34). There is a high comorbidity of GAD with functional somatic syndromes and the disorder is associated with significant somatic, occupational, and social dysfunction (28,34). GAD is a potentially treatable condition and has been demonstrated to respond in RCT trials to paroxetine, venlafaxine and imipramine (35).

Antidepressants may thus treat psychogenic movement symptoms indirectly by treating the comorbid state of depression or anxiety, which may not necessarily be clinically recognized.

The Effect of Antidepressants on PMD Symptoms

Our clinical observations suggest that antidepressants may be efficacious in the treatment of PMD symptoms. The following hypothesis on the mechanism of antidepressant action on PMD symptoms, albeit speculative, is presented to spur further discussion on the pathophysiology of PMD.

Deficits in motor initiation and the inhibition of translation of motor initiation to motor command have been suggested as potential mechanisms in the pathophysiology of psychogenic paralysis (36,37). However, the deficits associated with the hyperkinetic movements of PMD remain to be determined. It can be hypothesized that abnormalities in the inhibitory control of motor programs may underlie the pathophysiology of hyperkinetic PMD symptoms. Indirect support for this hypothesis comes from the observation of the response of PMD symptoms to SSRIs. The animal literature implicates serotonin in the pathophysiology of behavioral inhibition (38). Serotonin acts to restrict the behavioral response to external arousing stimuli; the behavioral response is potentiated in the absence of serotonin. Reduced serotonin function is reported to increase pain sensitivity, startle behavior, exploratory behavior or locomotor activity, and aggressive and sexual behavior (38). Similarly, the literature on serotonin and human behavior implicates low serotonin levels in the mechanisms underlying behavioral impulsivity (39). From this literature on serotonin and behavioral inhibition, one could speculate that serotonin may also be implicated in inhibitory control mechanisms of motor programs. Hence, the improvement of PMD symptoms with antidepressants may be related more specifically to the treatment of the impaired motor inhibitory control rather than to the general treatment of depression or anxiety. The study of the pathophysiology of PMD would need to consider the high comorbidity with depression as a study confounder and the role of state- or trait-specific deficits of depression as mediators of the PMD symptoms. Notably, in addition to the presence of impaired motor inhibition, a second factor is also necessary to explain the reason a specific motor symptom predominates.

Alternatively, serotonin itself may have a more direct effect on PMD symptoms. Animal studies have implicated serotonin discharge patterns in the suppression of irrelevant sensory processing and the facilitation of motor activity (40, 41). Aberrant serotonin discharge patterns could be hypothesized to result in the impaired processing of irrelevant sensory information and impaired modulation of motor function. This may explain the association of psychogenic motor symptoms with the subjective sensations of pain or other somatic symptoms, and further explain the potential overlap of functional somatic syndromes with PMD.

RECOMMENDATIONS FOR PSYCHOTROPIC TREATMENT: EVIDENCE-BASED STRATEGIES

In the absence of medication studies in PMD, the selection of antidepressants should be guided by the literature on the comorbid psychiatric diagnoses. A review is not within the scope of this paper; relevant points will be discussed. Practice guidelines on the treatment of specific psychiatric disorders can be found online (42).

Comorbid depression or dysthymia should be actively treated. It can be suggested that the presence of any depressive or anxiety symptoms, regardless of severity, should be aggressively treated, given the otherwise poor prognosis in the chronic PMD population.

In the treatment of major depression or dysthymia, SSRIs are considered first-line agents, given the wealth of evidence from Level I data and their relatively innocuous side-effect profile. SNRIs (venlafaxine) can be considered when an SSRI trial has failed from lack of efficacy or due to side effects. SNRIs can be considered first-line in the context of a moderate to severe depression, given the evidence for relatively greater efficacy for moderate to severe depression and for hospitalized inpatients. SNRIs can also be considered first-line in the context of comorbid symptoms of chronic pain, given evidence for efficacy on these symptoms (43). Mirtazapine (an α-2 antagonist and serotonin 2A, 2C, and 3 receptor antagonist) can be considered where there are significant sleep difficulties, and/or significant anxiety features. Mirtazapine may have a more rapid onset of action, but sedation and weight gain can present difficulties for long-term compliance (44,45). The SSRI fluoxetine or bupropion [a norepinephrine and dopamine reuptake inhibitor (NDRI)] can be considered in cases of significant fatigue or apathy, but should be avoided with comorbid anxiety. The management of depression should include optimization of doses, augmentation, combination treatments, and the use of electroconvulsive therapy as necessary.

Generalized anxiety disorder has been demonstrated in RCT trials to respond to venlafaxine, paroxetine, and imipramine, although there is likely a range of antidepressants with efficacy (35).

Atypical antipsychotics have most recently been demonstrated to be efficacious as augmentation agents to antidepressants for the treatment of depression and may be considered in this context (46). There is insufficient evidence to support the use of antipsychotics as a single agent in the treatment of depression or PMD. The use of typical antipsychotics is likely not indicated, given their known side-effect profile.

In treatment trials of chronic depression and dysthymia, recent literature reviews suggest that psychotherapy alone may not be sufficient treatment. In particular, medication has been demonstrated to be superior to psychotherapy in the treatment of dysthymia (29,30). In the treatment of chronic depression, RCT evidence demonstrates that combined medication and psychotherapy is significantly more efficacious than either treatment alone (29,30). The evidence supporting a greater advantage of combined therapy for dysthymia is more limited.

The use of an adjunctive long-acting benzodiazepine such as clonazepam may be especially useful for anxiety symptoms, particularly in the short term. Benzodiazepines may improve symptoms in the short term but do not treat the underlying psychiatric illness and should be utilized only in conjunction with antidepressants or for symptomatic relief. Benzodiazepines are not recommended as a single agent in the long-term treatment of mood or anxiety disorders.

The use of mood stabilizers should be limited to the treatment of the underlying mood disorder.

There is insufficient evidence at present to make recommendations on the use of antidepressants for PMD in the absence of comorbid psychiatric disorders. However, in the context of a known poor prognosis without intervention, the possibility of underrecognition of psychiatric diagnoses, indirect evidence, and case reports (as reviewed) suggesting the potential efficacy of antidepressants and the relative safety of antidepressants, the risk-benefit ratio supports a clinical trial of antidepressants in this subset of patients.

COMMON PATIENT QUESTIONS SPECIFIC TO PSYCHOTROPIC MEDICATIONS

The following section reviews practical issues and psychoeducation related to antidepressant treatment and PMD. The discussion is in question-and-answer format and is informed by both clinical experience and evidence from the literature.

1. *I've already tried antidepressants.* Let me look at your previous antidepressant use. It's very common for people to have inadequate trials because of low doses or medications being stopped early because of side effects. There is a wide range of antidepressants and combinations with different types of actions that you've likely not tried.

2. *The depression isn't causing the symptoms. I'm depressed because of the symptoms.* It's very common to hear that. On a clinical level, we treat the depression the same

way. We used to have a concept of endogenous (primary and biologic) and reactive (secondary and psychological) depression from which psychiatry has since moved away. We know now that clinical depression that occurs as a result of stressors can still be mediated by chemical changes and that the people who develop clinical depression regardless of the cause may have an underlying vulnerability to depression.

3. *I don't want to become addicted.* That's a very common worry. There is absolutely no risk of addiction to antidepressants. There is a withdrawal syndrome that you may experience if you stop the medications suddenly (47,48). It's more common with venlafaxine or paroxetine and might last a few days to weeks. There is no harm associated with the symptoms, although they can be uncomfortable. We can easily avoid this by making sure that you don't run out of your medications and if we need to stop them, we'll do it slowly.

4. *I want to do this myself. I don't want to depend on a pill.* It would seem to me you've already been trying to do this yourself for the last X years. The symptoms and suffering you're experiencing are no different from those of someone who's had a heart attack or has diabetes. Depression is a very real illness that shouldn't be treated any differently. However, the antidepressant is only one part of the answer. We'll need to work on some of the avoidance behaviors that have built up over the years because of your illness. Aerobic exercise has also been shown to be useful in the treatment of mild depression and prevention of depression (45). Rehabilitation can also be very useful for deconditioning from lack of use. The therapy and exercise will also give you some sense of control over the symptoms.

5. *Do I have to be on this forever?* No. I can't say specifically about the movement symptoms, but I can tell you about the depression. For one episode of depression, the antidepressants should be continued for at least one year after you've become well (45). There is evidence to show that this significantly decreases the risk of relapse. Then we can consider gradually decreasing the dose and we'll follow you closely for any relapse. If the depression is more complicated or if there has been more than one episode, at least two years is the current recommendation (45).

6. *Will it change my personality?* No. That's always a good question. This is not a "happy pill." There are a few interesting studies of antidepressants on healthy volunteers or people who don't have psychiatric diagnoses. They found that in the short term, it improved negative mood, and made them more social, but didn't make their mood more positive (49). There's a suggestion that antidepressants might cause a shift away from focusing on material with a negative emotional tone, similar to how certain forms of psychotherapy might work (50). "Personality" is a broader idea and is affected by how you grew up, your past experiences, and your relationships which shape who you are as a person—antidepressants can't change that.

7. *I'm very sensitive to medications.* We'll start very low and go slowly to try to avoid side effects. The side effects also tend to improve after a week or so.

8. *What if you're missing something? I don't want the antidepressants to just mask the symptoms.* I work very closely with the movement disorders team. We'll send you off for lab tests to rule out any medical issues contributing to your depression or anxiety (complete blood count, thyroid stimulating hormone, Vitamin B12, red blood cell folate). If the treatment doesn't work, or even if it's only partly effective, we will readdress the issue to see if there may be something hidden that can't be detected as well because the effects of the depression or anxiety are obscuring it. The antidepressants cannot mask any of the other diseases.

9. *You mean I'm also depressed?* Oddly enough, it's actually very good news from my perspective that you're (anxious, depressed, etc.) because I know I can help you.

RECOMMENDATIONS FOR PSYCHOTROPIC TREATMENT TRIALS

The following recommendations for psychotropic treatment trials are based on the literature and clinical experience.

Given the potential differences in prognoses, pathophysiology, and associated comorbidities, the inclusion criteria should be restricted to focus on psychogenic movement symptoms. Group comparisons with different diagnoses, particularly paralysis and pseudoseizures, may be particularly instructive. As the duration of conversion symptoms has been shown to correlate with prognosis, acute symptoms (less than 3 months) should be excluded and the minimum duration for chronicity defined. The diagnosis of definite factitious symptoms and malingering are clinically difficult to make and overlaps can occur within the same individual with conversion disorder. A working definition to exclude probable malingering or, alternatively, randomization on the basis of probable conversion disorder versus probable factitious symptoms or malingering may be of utility.

Multicenter trials may be necessary to obtain sufficient power, given the relatively small numbers at each site. Randomized controlled trials of adequate duration with longitudinal follow-up should be performed, given the high short-term placebo response in this population.

Relevant clinical outcomes such as quality of life, functioning, and subjective impairment should be measured. In addition, structured psychiatric diagnostic interviews, clinician- and patient-rated depression and anxiety rating scales, and validated PMD measurement scales should also be considered.

The selection of antidepressant to be studied depends on the study objective. Citalopram, a highly specific serotonin reuptake inhibitor or reboxetine, a specific norepinephrine reuptake inhibitor, may be useful in correlating pathophysiology. However, clinical efficacy may be more likely with agents with dual mechanisms. Comparison of normal and high doses may be useful given the clinical observation of efficacy at higher doses. Based on the studies of the response of chronic depression to combination antidepressants and psychotherapy, consideration should be made to the design of a trial to include an arm with such a combination.

CONCLUSION

PMD is a complex neuropsychiatric disorder expressed through poorly understood neurobiologic and neuropsychological correlates and influenced by psychological stressors, personality traits, and sociocultural context. PMD, as a representative disorder for the study of functional and conversion symptoms, holds promise given the observable (and hence, measurable) nature of the symptoms in contrast to the less observable states of anesthesia, pain, or fatigue. The positive nature of the symptoms versus that of conversion paralysis, for instance, may signify underlying differences in pathophysiology. Furthermore, our observation of the lack of an association of PMD with a history of abuse, in contrast to pseudoseizures, suggests potentially differing pathophysiology underlying personality traits and prognoses.

We have observed that the efficacy of antidepressants on psychogenic motor symptoms can be dissociated from cross-sectional psychiatric diagnoses and measurements of depression or anxiety. This finding is consistent with the literature on antidepressants and functional somatic syndromes and somatization disorder. The exact relationship with depression and anxiety remains to be determined. Understanding the effect of psychotropic agents on PMD symptoms may further elucidate underlying pathophysiologic mechanisms of PMD.

The presence of any depressive or anxiety symptoms regardless of severity should be actively treated given the otherwise poor prognosis, significant rate of disability, financial burden, and subjective suffering in the chronic PMD population. Recent reviews have suggested that in the treatment of dysthymia, medication may be superior to psychotherapy. The evidence further suggests that the treatment of chronic depression, combined medication, and psychotherapy is superior to either medication or psychotherapy alone; the evidence is less strong for dysthymia. Given the lack of medication trials in PMD, the general psychiatric literature is useful to guide in the choice of antidepressants, psychotherapy, or a combination of both. In the assessment of the risk–benefit ratio, there may

also be a rationale for a trial of antidepressants in PMD patients without overt comorbid psychiatric diagnoses. The preliminary evidence suggests that active intervention with antidepressants can alter the prognosis of patients with chronic PMD, although further studies are required to support this observation.

It should be emphasized that psychotropic medications represent only one treatment modality. Given the learned dysfunctional behavioral adaptations and changes in interpersonal relationships in PMD patients, which often perpetuate the symptoms, and the impact of chronic symptoms on the functioning of PMD patients, treatment will likely be multimodal, including psychotropics, psychotherapy, and rehabilitation.

REFERENCES

1. American Psychiatric Association. *Diagnostic and statistical manual of mental disorders*, 4th ed. Washington, DC: American Psychiatric Association, 1994.
2. Akagi H, House A. The epidemiology of hysterical conversion. In: Halligan PW, Bass C, Marshall JC, eds. *Contemporary approaches to the study of hysteria: clinical and theoretical perspectives*. New York: Oxford University Press, 2001.
3. Factor SA, Podskalny GD, Molho ES. Psychogenic movement disorders: frequency, clinical profile and characteristics. *J Neurol Neurosurg Psychiatry.* 1995;59:406–412.
4. Ron MA. The prognosis of hysteria/somatization disorder. In: Halligan PW, Bass C, Marshall JC, eds. *Contemporary approaches to the study of hysteria: clinical and theoretical perspectives*. New York: Oxford University Press, 2001.
5. Bass C, Peveler R, House A. Somatoform disorders: severe psychiatric illnesses neglected by psychiatrists. *Br J Psychiatry.* 2001; 179:11–14.
6. Wade DT. Rehabilitation for hysterical conversion states: a critical review and conceptual reconstruction. In: Halligan PW, Bass C, Marshall JC, eds. *Contemporary approaches to the study of hysteria: clinical and theoretical perspectives*. New York: Oxford University Press, 2001.
7. Rampello L, Raffaele R, Nicoletti G, et al. Hysterical neurosis of the conversion type: therapeutic activity of neuroleptics with different hyperprolactinermic potency. *Neuropsychobiology.* 1996;33: 186–188.
8. Kapur S, Seeman P. Does fast dissociation from the dopamine D2 receptor explain the action of atypical antipsychotics?: A new hypothesis. *Am J Psychiatry.* 2001;158:360–369.
9. Williams DT, Ford B, Fahn S. Phenomenology and psychopathology related to psychogenic movement disorders. In: Weiner WJ, Lang AE, eds. *Behavioral neurology of movement disorders. Advances in neurology.* New York: Raven Press, 1995.
10. Wessely S, Nimnuan C, Sharpe M. Functional somatic syndromes: one or many? *Lancet.* 1999;354:936–939.
11. Aaron LA, Buchwald D. A review of the evidence for overlap among unexplained clinical conditions. *Ann Intern Med.* 2001; 134:868–881.
12. O'Malley PG, Jackson JL, Santoro J, et al. Antidepressant therapy for unexplained symptoms and symptom syndromes. *J Fam Pract.* 1999;48:980–990.
13. Hudson JI, Mangweth B, Pope HG, et al. Family study of affective spectrum disorder. *Arch Gen Psychiatry.* 2003;60:170–177.
14. Mace CJ, Trimble MR. Ten-year prognosis of conversion disorder. *Br J Psychiatry.* 1996;169:282–288.
15. Marsden CD. Hysteria—a neurologist's view. *Psychol Med.* 1986; 16:277–288.
16. Menza M, Lauritano M, Allen L. Treatment of somatization disorder with nefazodone: a prospective, open-label study. *Ann Clin Psychiatry.* 2001;13:153–158.

17. Cybulska EM. Globus hystericus or depressivus? *Hosp Med.* 1998;59:640–641.
18. Sheehan DV, Lecrubier Y, Sheehan KH, et al. The Mini-International Neuropsychiatric Interview (MINI): the development and validation of a structured diagnostic psychiatric interview for DSM-IV and ICD-10. *J Clin Psychiatry.* 1998;59 (Suppl 20):22–33.
19. Davidson J, Turnbull CD, Strickland R, et al. The Montgomery-Asberg depression scale: reliability and validity. *Acta Psychiatr Scand.* 1986;73:544–548.
20. Beck AT, Steer RA, Garbin MG. Psychometric properties of the beck depression inventory: twenty-five years of evaluation. *Clin Psychol Rev.* 1988;8:77–100.
21. Beck AT, Epstein N, Brown G, et al. An inventory for measuring clinical anxiety: psychometric properties. *J Consult Clin Psychol.* 1988;56:893–897.
22. Voon V, Lang AE. Antidepressant outcomes in psychogenic movement disorders. *J Clin Psychiatry* (in press).
23. Bowman ES, Markand ON. Psychodynamics and psychiatric diagnoses of pseudoseizure subjects. *Am J Psychiatry.* 1996;153:57–63.
24. Prueter C, Schultz-Venrath U, Rimpau W. Dissociative and associated psychopathological symptoms in patients with epilepsy, pseudoseizures and both seizure forms. *Epilepsia.* 2002;43:188–192.
25. Harden CL. Pseudoseizures and dissociative disorders: a common mechanism involving traumatic experiences. *Seizure.* 1997;6:151–152.
26. Feinstein A, Stergiopoulos V, Fine J, et al. Psychiatric outcome in patients with psychogenic movement disorder: a prospective study. *Neuropsychiatry Neuropsychol Behav Neurol.* 2001;14:169–176.
27. Klein DN, Santiago NJ. Dysthymia and chronic depression: introduction, classification, risk factors and course. *J Clin Psychol.* 2003;59:807–816.
28. Culpepper L. Generalized anxiety disorder in primary care: emerging issues in management and treatment. *J Clin Psychiatry.* 2002;63(Suppl 8):35–42.
29. Arnow BA, Constantino MJ. Effectiveness of psychotherapy and combination therapy for chronic depression. *J Clin Psychol.* 2003;59:893–905.
30. Michalak EE, Lam RW. Breaking the myths: new treatment approaches for chronic depression. *Can J Psychiatry.* 2002;47:635–643.
31. Sadek N, Bona J. Subsyndromal symptomatic depression: a new concept. *Depress Anxiety.* 2000;12:30–39.
32. Pincus HA, Davis WW, McQueen LE. 'Subthreshold' mental disorders. A review and synthesis of studies on minor depression and other "brand names." *Br J Psychiatry.* 1999;174:288–296.
33. Judd LL, Akiskal HS, Maser JD, et al. A prospective 12-year study of subsyndromal and syndromal depressive symptoms in unipolar major depressive disorders. *Arch Gen Psychiatry.* 1999;56:764–765.
34. Kessler RC, Wittchen HU. Patterns and correlates of generalized anxiety disorder in community samples. *J Clin Psychiatry.* 2002; 63:4–10.
35. Kapczinski F, Lima MS, Souza JS, et al. Antidepressants for generalized anxiety disorder. *Cochrane Database Syst Rev.* 2003;2: CD003592.
36. Spence SA, Crimlisk HL, Cope H, et al. Discrete neurophysiological correlates in prefrontal cortex during hysterical and feigned disorder of movement. *Lancet.* 2000;356:162–163.
37. Marshall JC, Halligan PW, Fink GR, et al. The functional anatomy of a hysterical paralysis. *Cognition.* 1997;64:B1–B8.
38. Lucki I. The spectrum of behaviors influenced by serotonin. *Biol Psychiatry.* 1998;44:151–162.
39. Hollander E, Rosen J. Impulsivity. *J Psychopharmacol.* 2000;14 (Suppl 1):S39–S44.
40. Jacobs BL, Fornal CA. Serotonin and motor activity. *Curr Opin Neurobiol.* 1997;7:820–825.
41. Jacobs BL, Fornal CA. Activity of serotonergic neurons in behaving animals. *Neuropsychopharmacology.* 1999;21:9–15.
42. American Psychiatric Association. Psychiatric guidelines, American Psychiatric Association online. http://www.psych.org/psych_pract/treatg/pg/prac_guide.cfm. Accessed October 30, 2003.
43. Fishbain D. Evidence-based data on pain relief with antidepressants. *Ann Med.* 2000;32:305–316.
44. Nutt DJ. Care of depressed patients with anxiety symptoms. *J Clin Psychiatry.* 1999;60(Suppl 17):23–27.
45. Thompson C. Mirtazapine versus selective serotonin reuptake inhibitors. *J Clin Psychiatry.* 1999;60(Suppl 17):18–22.
46. Thase ME. What role do atypical antipsychotic drugs have in treatment-resistant depression? *J Clin Psychiatry.* 2002;63:95–103.
47. Black K, Shea C, Dursun S, et al. Selective serotonin reuptake inhibitor discontinuation syndrome: proposed diagnostic criteria. *J Psychiatry Neurosci.* 2001;26:152.
48. Haddad PM. Antidepressant discontinuation syndromes. *Drug Saf.* 2001;24:183–197.
49. Harmer CJ, Hill SA, Taylor MJ, et al. Toward a neuropsychological theory of antidepressant drug action: increase in positive emotional bias after potentiation of norephinephrine activity. *Am J Psychiatry.* 2003;160:990–992.
50. Knutson B, Wolkowitz OM, Cole SW, et al. Selective alteration of personality and social behavior by serotonergic intervention. *Am J Psychiatry.* 1999;155:373–379.

Rehabilitation in Patients with Psychogenic Movement Disorders

35

Christopher Bass

ABSTRACT

Psychogenic movement disorders (PMDs) are a heterogeneous group of clinical conditions that are unlikely to have a single cause. They bear a similarity to somatoform disorders, in particular, to conversion disorders of the motor type. Evidence from a number of recent follow-up studies suggests that without treatment these patients have a poor prognosis, and over 80% continue to exhibit abnormal movements. These disorders will have a range of initiating psychosocial and/or physical causes, and maintaining factors are also likely to be diverse. A key component of management and rehabilitation will involve the detailed assessment of not only the physical symptoms and psychosocial state, but also functional impairments. The World Health Organization (WHO) model of disability as formulated in the *International Classification of Impairments, Disabilities and Handicaps* (ICIDH) will be adopted to illustrate the complex relationship among the various influences on disability. It is unwise to commence treatment before a sound psychosocial formulation has been established, with special emphasis on relevant maintaining factors.

Management will also depend, to a large extent, on the resources available to the diagnosing neurologist, for example, inpatient beds with mental health and medically trained nurses, local neuropsychiatry and clinical psychology services, and rehabilitation or physiotherapy services.

No systematic, randomized controlled trials of treatment in patients with PMDs have been published to date, only case series. Evidence from research into the management of somatoform disorders suggests that a rehabilitation approach based on (but not exclusively) cognitive–behavioral therapy (CBT) is likely to be the most effective method of managing these patients. Some of the present methods of rehabilitation will be described, with emphasis on the strengths and weaknesses of various approaches. To be effective, however, rehabilitation approaches have to address all the health domains that may be affected, including not only the patient's illness beliefs and perceived disabilities, but also satisfaction with their social role functioning associated with the illness; family; occupational factors; and potential adverse effect (in terms of rehabilitation) of the benefits available from the social and welfare institutions.

INTRODUCTION

The management of patients with psychogenic movement disorders (PMDs) is beset with difficulties. First, the diagnosis has to be established by a neurologist after relevant organic disease has been excluded. Second, the neurologist has not only to explain to the patient that there is no serious underlying organic disease, but also provide an explanation for the symptoms that is comprehensible to the patient. Third, unless the neurologist has the requisite qualifications, he or she invariably has to refer the patient to a mental health care worker (in practice either a clinical psychologist or a psychiatrist) in order for the patient to receive treatment. This is a skilled process requiring the neurologist to provide a rationale for the referral without alienating the patient

In this chapter, I will briefly discuss the clinical characteristics and longitudinal course of patients with PMDs and point out the features that these patients have in common with those with motor conversion disorder. I will also briefly describe the principles used in traditional rehabilitation programs. I will also review the current evidence for the efficacy of treatment of these disorders, and will introduce the World Health Organization (WHO) model of illness published as the *International Classification of Functioning, Disability and Health* (WHO ICF) (1). This provides a unified and standard language and framework for the assessment of health and some health-related components of well-being. Finally, because cognitive–behavioral therapy (CBT) has been shown to be the most effective treatment to date in patients with medically unexplained or "functional" syndromes, this approach to management will be briefly described.

How Should These Disorders Be Classified?

It is likely that PMDs bear a strong clinical resemblance to what psychiatrists call somatoform disorders [*Diagnositc and Statistical Manual of Mental Disorders*, Fourth Edition (DSM-IV)]. These illnesses have attracted a number of different terms such as "functional somatic syndromes" (2) or

"functional" disorders (3). It is becoming increasingly apparent that the multitude of functional syndromes such as IBS, chronic fatigue syndrome, and fibromyalgia share more similarities than differences (4).

It has also been suggested that some patients with PMDs are deliberately feigning or simulating their symptoms. It is extremely difficult, however, for physicians to infer levels of conscious awareness, the degree of consciously mediated intention, and the motivations that accompany the symptoms presented by patients (5). As pointed out by Miller (6), the distinction between hysteria and malingering "depends on nothing more infallible than one man's assessment of what is going on in another man's mind."

CLINICAL CHARACTERISTICS OF PATIENTS WITH PSYCHOGENIC MOVEMENT DISORDERS

Patients with PMDs have characteristics in common with those of motor conversion disorder (see Chapter 13). Without treatment, the prognosis in patients who present to tertiary care clinics is very poor (see Table 35.1). Early diagnosis and treatment is likely, therefore, to have a beneficial effect on prognosis, and those factors which have been shown to be associated with a good prognosis in motor conversion disorders are also likely to apply in patients with PMDs, that is, young age; short duration of symptoms, and sudden onset. Conversely, older patients with fixed dystonic postures of long duration who are involved in litigation are likely to be more resistant to the effects of any intervention (7).

TREATMENT STUDIES: PRACTICAL ISSUES

Before any discussion of treatment, it is important to consider the resources available to the neurologist to manage these patients. Some neurologists may have no access whatever to mental health resources, whereas others may have close collaborative links with either clinical psychology or

TABLE 35.1

RECENT FOLLOW-UP STUDIES OF PATIENTS WITH UNEXPLAINED MOTOR SYMPTOMS WHO PRESENT TO SECONDARY/TERTIARY CARE

Study	No. of Points	Mean Follow-up (years)	Mean Age at Follow-up	Axis I Disorder	Axis II Disorder	Outcome (Same or Worse)
Crimlisk et al., 1998 (8)	88	3.3	49	71%	45%	>90%
Feinstein et al., 2001 (9)	72	6.0	43	75%	53%	52%
Stone et al., 2003 (10)	60	12.5	48	—	—	83%

psychiatry services. There is no doubt that the successful management of patients with PMDs requires the cooperation of a number of clinical specialties, including psychologists, nurses, physiotherapists, and occupational therapists (OTs). Some patients may be so disturbed or disabled (or both) that they may require inpatient admission to a specialized unit with access to both mental health and medical nurses, as well as physiotherapists and OTs. In the opinion of this writer, every neurology service should have access to a specialist liaison psychiatry service (11).

Assessment

Before treatment begins, however, a comprehensive psychosocial formulation must be established. It goes without saying that the assessment should be multidimensional, that is, involve an assessment of symptoms and signs, but also emotional distress, illness beliefs, and functional impairments.

A number of instruments are helpful in assessing these various health domains. They include the Symptom Checklist-12 (SCL-12) to measure somatic symptoms (12); the Hospital Anxiety and Depression Scale to measure anxiety and depression (13) (the Depression and Anxiety scales devised by Beck are also useful); and the Illness Beliefs Questionnaire, which provides a rating of illness attitudes and concerns (14). There are several measures of functional impairment, including the Dartmouth COOP (15) and the Barthel Index (16).

It is also essential to have working knowledge of the initiating factors and of the maintaining factors, as the latter will often be the focus for any intervention (see description of WHO ICF model below).

PRINCIPLES OF REHABILITATION

Traditional behavioral approaches to rehabilitation are based on the premise that the symptoms reported by the patient are interpreted as physical but are amenable to recovery. Treatment aims to bring about a gradual increase in function through a combination of physical and occupational therapies. The patient receives rewards and praise for improvement of function, and withdrawal of reinforcement for continuing signs of disability. Avoiding direct confrontation of psychological problems and providing "face-saving" techniques are also regarded as key components (17). Rehabilitation has recently seen many practical innovations, but the major advances in rehabilitation are conceptual rather than practical (18). First, the approach to patients has moved from a predominantly medical one to one in which psychological and sociocultural aspects are equally important. Second, the need for organized specialist rehabilitation services involving a multidisciplinary team is recognized as essential.

What is the Evidence?

There are no large, randomized controlled studies of rehabilitation in patients with psychogenic movement disorders. Neither is there any good evidence to support the use of one specific intervention for patients with either conversion disorders or PMDs. A variety of different physical and psychological treatments have been used to treat motor conversion disorders, and these are shown in Table 35.2. Unfortunately, most of the available evidence consists of single cases or case series that have recently been reviewed by Wade (19). The shortcomings of these various "unimodal" therapies are that they tend to act on only one health domain. For example, functional electrical stimulation (FES) is directed toward movement; behavioral treatment at behavior, and so on. Although it is conceivable that one particular intervention may well have an effect on several areas, for example, FES may alter beliefs by showing that movement is possible and might reduce perceived disability (by allowing the patient to walk), it is unlikely to change the "disease label" used by the patient.

One recent exception is a randomized controlled trial in outpatients with motor conversion disorder (20). The study included 45 patients and the setting was a general psychiatric inpatient unit. The treatment involved group-based activities using cognitive and behavioral techniques as well as problem-solving and physiotherapy. Primary outcome measures were the Video Rating Scale for motor conversion symptoms (VRMC), the D (disabilities) code items from the *International Classification of Impairments, Disabilities and Handicaps* (ICIDH), and the Symptom Checklist-90 (SCL-90). The "experimental" condition consisted of eight weekly sessions of 1-hour hypnosis.

Patients tended to have chronic conditions (mean duration of symptoms for 3.9 years), with the majority having paresis or paralysis and one quarter having had their houses adapted considerably for their impairments.

TABLE 35.2

TREATMENTS USED IN REHABILITATION

Physical
Functional electrical stimulation (FES)
Biofeedback
Psychotherapy
Strategic-behavioral
Medication, e.g., amytal interview

Psychological
Hypnosis
Psychotherapy
Behavioral intervention
CBT (cognitive–behavioral therapy)

Other
Symptomatic treatment
Further investigation

According to the VRMC, 65% of the patients were substantially to very much improved at posttreatment assessment and 84% at the 6-month follow-up. The additional use of hypnosis did *not*, however, affect treatment outcome.

It is difficult to interpret the findings of this study, because the treatment was complex and involved a number of different components. In its favor, however, it adopted a randomized design; used a multidisciplinary team which employed a variety of behavioral, cognitive, and other rehabilitation approaches; and used standardized outcome measures.

A FRAMEWORK FOR FUTURE RESEARCH: THE WHO ICF MODEL

In the absence of good experimental evidence, a possible framework for future research can be developed. This draws on published evidence, and in this chapter I will use a model based on the WHO ICIDH, which is particularly useful for patients in whom there is a disability which is out of proportion to known disease and signs. The model provides opportunities for intervention, and is well-suited to the kind of multidisciplinary approach that is likely to be successful in these patients.

The original classification system used identifies four levels of change and three contextual domains that interact with these four levels. It makes the assumption that any illness may lead to or arise from changes at the level of *pathology* (the person's organ), *impairment* (the person's body), *disability/activity* (the person's goal-directed behavior), or *handicap/participation* (the person's social position as perceived by self and others). Important contextual factors may impact on the specific features any illness: The three contextual domains include the person's *own context* (attitudes, beliefs, expectations, past experience),

the person's *physical context* (objects and people acting as caregivers), and the person's *social context* (legal and cultural setting, laws, etc.). There is no reason to believe that all illness is initiated by or follows from primary pathology, and a systems analytic approach would predict the opposite—that some illness would arise at other levels, for example, abnormal illness beliefs. The model is shown diagrammatically in Figure 35.1.

The ICIDH was developed under the auspices of the WHO and was first published in 1980 (21). The ICIDH has recently been revised and updated, and the new WHO ICF represents another important advance (1), although it does not take account of temporal factors in illness, or have any method for handling the question of free will or patient choice (22). This is an important consideration in rehabilitation (and in most areas of health care), because much impairment and limitation of activities cannot be adequately explained by known pathology. Finally, it does not consider personal values or quality of life. The revised model proposed by Wade and Halligan (22) is summarized in the two tables that cover both the classification of the person and the classification of his or her context in contextual terms (Tables 35.3 and 35.4).

The revised model can be interpreted as a systems analytic approach to illness: Each level and each context is a separate system that is largely self-contained but may interact with each other system to a greater or lesser extent. The model emphasizes that whatever the primary cause of an illness, many factors will have an influence on its manifestations. Although it represents an advance, the model has been criticized as reflecting the determinism of the medical model. Wade and Halligan (22) point out that patients experience a sense of control and influence over their behavior by choosing (wherever possible) between different courses of action. The notion of free will and personal

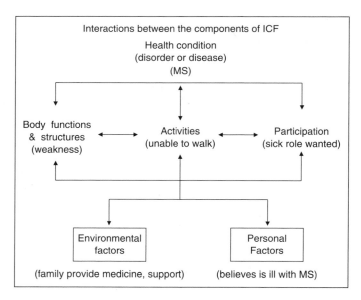

Figure 35.1 Interactions between the components of the *International Classification of Functioning.*

TABLE 35.3

EXPANDED WHO ICF MODEL OF HEALTH AND ILLNESS: THE PERSON

Level		Classification in Illness	
In Health	In Illness	Subjective/Internal	Objective/External
Person's Organ Structure/anatomy Function/physiology	**Pathology** Refers to abnormalities or changes in the structure and/or function of an organ or organ system.	**Disease** Label attached by the patient on the basis of information gained from others including health care staff.	**Diagnosis** Label attached by others, usually on beliefs, and basis of assessment and investigation of structure and physiology.
Person's Body Structure/anatomy Function/capacity	**Impairments** Refers to abnormalities or changes in the structure and/or function of the whole body set in personal context.	**Symptoms** Somatic sensations, experienced moods, thoughts, etc.	**Signs** Observable abnormalities (absence of or change in capacity or structure), explicit or implicit.
Free will	*Free will*	*Free will*	*Free Will*
Person in Environment Behavior	**Activity limitation** Refers to abnormalities, changes, or restrictions in the interaction between patients and their environment or physical context (i.e., changes in the quality or quantity of behavior).	**Perceived Ability** What patients feel they can do, and feelings about the quality of performance.	**Disability/Activities** What others observe that a patient does do, with quantification of that performance.
Person in Society Roles	**Participation Restriction** Refers to changes, limitations, or "abnormalities" in the position of patients in their social context.	**Role Satisfaction** Patients' judgment (valuation) of their own role performance (what and how well).	**Handicap/Participation** Judgment (valuation of important others (local culture) on role performance (what and how well).
Totality			
Quality of Life Refer to patients' own evaluation or summation of their capacities and performance at all levels, taking into account also some contextual matters and based on their expectations and values. No difference between quality of life whether ill or not, although some people refer to "health-related quality of life," which usually covers disease-specific changes in impairment and activities, with a greater or lesser focus on emotion.		**Happiness** Patients' assessment of and reaction to achievement or failure of important goals *and* sense of being a worthwhile person.	**Status** Society's judgment on success in life made on the basis of closeness to judged "normality" in terms of activities, roles, and material possessions, making allowance for disease and impairment.

responsibility remains a core belief for most democratic and legal conceptions of human nature, and it may help explain illness not produced by disease, injury, psychopathology, or psychosocial factors.

The model is shown in more detail in Figure 35.2 in a patient with a fixed dystonia, which has led her to retire to a wheelchair. This state has been reinforced by the family and medical services, which provide sick notes and disability aids. The model shown in the figure would suggest that intervention could be targeted at one or more of many sites, with the most obvious being "personal context," which includes beliefs and expectations. However, it is also important to address wider issues such as the attitudes and responses of family members and of health care professionals (22).

A number of predictions arise from the WHO ICF model:

A. Some illnesses will not have any specific underlying pathology. The prime cause might be within one level, or might be at other levels, or even arise from the contextual factors.

B. The model emphasizes that whatever the prime cause of an illness, many factors will have an influence on its manifestation. That is to say, disability may follow from a mixture of pathological, structural abnormalities within cells or organs, causing functional abnormalities, and psychological abnormalities that are best considered as abnormal functioning of the whole person in the absence of any specific structural abnormality. PMDs arise primarily from *psychological* malfunction.

TABLE 35.4

EXPANDED WHO ICF MODEL OF HEALTH AND ILLNESS: THE CONTEXT

Context		Classification	
Type	*Comment*	*Subjective/Internal*	*Objective/External*
Personal Context	Primarily refers to attitudes, beliefs, and expectations often arising from previous experience of illness in self or others, but also refers to personal characteristics and to the values of the individual.	**"Personality"** Patients' beliefs, attitudes, expectations, goals, etc.	**"Past History"** Observed/recorded behavior prior to and early on in this illness.
Temporal Context	Primarily refers to patients' position both in their own lifespan and in the course of their own illness. Also covers time and type of onset and prognosis.	**Memories and Expectations** Reflection on a different past. Expectation of a different future. Degree of certainty/uncertainty.	**Past abilities and Prognosis** Documented or known past abilities, likely future abilities (+/− intervention), predictable changes.
Social Context	Primarily refers to legal and local cultural setting, including expectations of important others, but also includes wider national cultural (including religious) setting.	**Local Culture** The people and organizations important to patients, and their culture; especially family, close friends, and people in the same accommodation.	**Society** The society lived in and the laws, duties, and responsibilities expected from and the rights of members of that society.

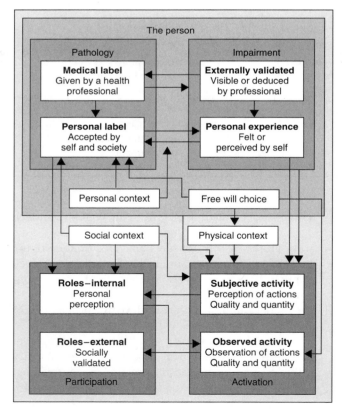

Figure 35.2 Proposed model of illness.

C. The model predicts that patients with similar presentations, for example, tremor or dystonia, may have different underlying causes and mechanisms that contribute to their disability, that is, patients will have varying proportions of their disability (or handicap) explained by their pathology. For example, a patient may be in a wheelchair but without any pathology (23). In such a patient, it may be important to fulfill the role as a chair of the local dystonia society, to avoid the need to leave home and work, and to be cared for by an important other person.

D. It is unlikely that a single intervention will be successful, even in a group of apparently homogeneous patients.

Using the WHO ICF model, it is clear that intervention in one domain may have an effect in another. For example, improving the functioning in a limb by physiotherapy may alter or modify the patient's beliefs, but also perceived disability as well as family expectations, and so on.

Wade has pointed out, however, that none of the accepted treatment regimes pay much attention to patients' satisfaction with their social role functioning associated with the illness or to the adverse effect of the patients receiving welfare benefits (24). This is an important omission, especially as the impact of financial incentives on disability, symptoms, and objective findings has been convincingly shown in several recent studies. For example, there has been a systematic review of 13 cohort studies of whiplash injuries (25), a metaanalysis of 18 studies after closed head injuries (26), and another metaanalysis of 32 studies of patients receiving compensation for chronic pain (27). A recent longitudinal study of 200 chronic back pain patients also adds support to this position (28). In this study litigants scored higher on all measures of pain and disability in comparison with a matched nonlitigating group. Moreover, litigants' scores on all measures dropped following settlement of litigation. Finally, a well-designed study of 2002 of unselected people involved in rear-end car collisions in Lithuania, where few drivers had personal injury insurance, showed clearly that the absence of a compensation infrastructure resulted in no significant difference between accident victims and uninjured controls with regard to head and neck symptoms (29).

PSYCHOLOGICAL TREATMENTS

I have suggested in this chapter that patients with PMDs share similarities with those with conversion disorders and that these disorders are likely to have similar etiologic mechanisms to other somatoform disorders, such as chronic fatigue syndrome, noncardiac chest pain, and chronic widespread pain (fibromyalgia). In all these disorders, the primary initiating factor may be at any level in the WHO ICF model, and the initiation and maintenance of the illness will often depend on or be potentiated by other factors. Treatments need to be directed at either the initiating factor (if that can be identified, which is not always possible) or at one or more of the other maintaining factors. It is unlikely that any one specific treatment will be effective in all cases.

Most of the evidence-based treatments in this field involve CBT or interpersonal therapy (IPT). These usually have to be undertaken by trained clinical psychologists or other clinicians. However, increasing numbers of specialist nurses are being trained to deliver these treatments, so they should become more widely available.

Cognitive–Behavioral Therapy

CBT is widely advocated for patients with medically unexplained symptoms. This form of usually brief psychotherapy is concerned mainly with helping the patients overcome identified problems and ascertain specified goals. It encourages self-help techniques such as relaxation and self-management of stress and anxiety. It discourages "maintaining factors" such as repeated body self-checking, and challenges patients' negative or false beliefs about symptoms. A cognitive–behavioral approach may also help with the formulation. An example is given in Figure 35.3.

In a recent German study, CBT (summarized in a treatment manual) was effective in treating patients with somatoform disorders in a tertiary care setting. Patients received individual and group treatment, and the main therapeutic focus was on identifying and modifying

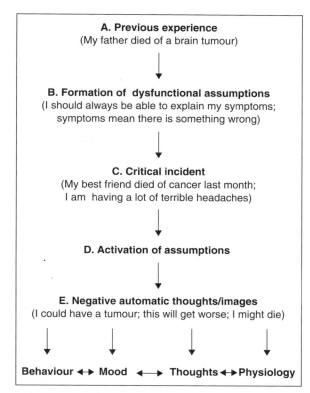

Figure 35.3 Cognitive–behavioral formulation of a patient with functional symptoms.

dysfunctional perceptions and thoughts. Dysfunctional assumptions and misinterpretations were identified and patients were encouraged to undertake behavioral experiments. The patients with somatoform disorders improved significantly compared to the control group with respect to physical symptoms, health anxieties, dysfunctional beliefs about the body and health, and psychosocial functioning. Furthermore, 2 years after treatment there was a treatment-related cost-offset for both outpatient and inpatient care (30).

A systematic review of 31 controlled trials (29 of which were randomized) compared the effectiveness of CBT with controlled therapy for unexplained symptoms. In 71% of the studies, physical symptoms improved to a greater extent in patients treated with CBT than in the controls (31). Group CBT also helps patients with medically unexplained symptoms.

Interpersonal Therapy

There are four large studies of IPT (or a related from of dynamic therapy) in patients with functional syndromes (32). All have been conducted on patients with chronic functional complaints. Three of the four studies showed that physical symptoms improved to a greater extent following psychotherapy, compared with control interventions. Two showed an improvement in health status and quality of life for IPT compared with a controlled intervention.

The most recent trial, involving 257 participants, demonstrated that patients who received psychotherapy in comparison with usual care show significant reductions in health service utilization in the year following treatment; IPT is thus a cost-effective treatment. The results of the trial also suggested that patients with a history of sexual abuse respond particularly well to IPT.

PHARMACOLOGIC TREATMENTS

There is evidence from randomized controlled trials (RCTs) and systematic reviews that antidepressants (both tricyclics and selective serotonin reuptake inhibitors (SSRIs) can be useful in the treatment of patients with medically unexplained symptoms (such as poor sleep and pain), whether or not depression is present (33).

CONCLUSION

Rehabilitation is a problem-solving process with multiple interventions at different levels and in different places, and it is based on an analysis of a person's illness using the ICF model or some other model of illness. In psychogenic movement disorder the treatment will need to be focused more on the subjective aspects of the illness and less on the external aspects. Treatments aimed at altering beliefs are already part of rehabilitation interventions for patients disabled secondary to definite pathology, for example, stroke and cardiovascular disease, and psychological therapies that are directed towards modifying illness beliefs have been shown to be effective in these disorders (14,34). Randomized controlled trials using evidence-based treatments as part of a multifaceted rehabilitation approach appear to hold promise in patients with psychogenic movement disorders.

REFERENCES

1. WHO. International clarification of functioning, disability and health. Geneva: World Health Organization, 2001 (http://www.who.int/en).
2. Barsky AJ, Borus JF. Functional somatic syndromes. *Ann Intern Med.* 1999;130:910–921.
3. Stone J, Wojcik W, Durrance D, et al. What should we say to patients with symptoms unexplained by disease? The number needed to offend. *Br Med J.* 2002;325:1449–1450.
4. Wessely S, Nimnuan C, Sharpe M. Functional somatic syndromes: one or many? *Lancet.* 1999;354:936–939.
5. Halligan P, Bass C, Oakley D. Willful deception as illness behavior. In: Halligan P, Bass C, Oakley D, eds. *Malingering and illness deception.* Oxford: Oxford University Press, 2003:3–28.
6. Miller H. Accident neurosis. *Br Med J* 1961;1:919–925.
7. Ron M. The prognosis of hysteria/somatisation disorder. In: Halligan P, Bass C, Marshall J, eds. *Contemporary approaches to the study of hysteria.* Oxford: Oxford University Press, 2001:271–283.
8. Crimlisk HL, Bhatia K, Cope H, et al. Slater revisited: 6-year follow up study of patients with medically unexplained motor symptoms. *Br Med J* 1998;316:582–586.
9. Feinstein A, Stergiopoulos V, Fine J, et al. Psychiatric outcome in patients with a psychogenic movement disorder: a prospective study. *Neuropsychol Behav Neurol* 2001;14(3):169–176.
10. Stone J, Sharpe M, Rothwell PM, et al. The 12-year prognosis of unilateral functional weakness and sensory disturbance. *J Neurol Neurosurg Psychiatry* 2003;74(5):591–596.
11. Gotz M, House A. Prognosis of symptoms that are medically unexplained. *Br Med J.* 1998;317:536.
12. Derogatis L, Melisartaros N. The brief symptom inventory: an introductory report. *Psychol Med.* 1983;13:505–605.
13. Zigmond A, Snaith RP. The hospital anxiety and depression scale. *Acta Psychiatr Scand.* 1983;67:361–370.
14. Weinman J, Petrie K, Moss-Morris R, et al. The illness perception questionnaire: a new method for assessing the cognitive representation of illness. *Psychol Health.* 1996;11:431–445.
15. Jenkinson C, Mayou R, Day A, et al. Evaluation of the Dartmouth COOP charts in a large scale community survey in the United Kingdom. *J Public Health Med.* 2002;24:106–111.
16. Wade D, Collin C. The Barthel ADL Index: a standard measure of physical disability? *Int Disabil Stud.* 1988;10:64–67.
17. Teasell R, Shapiro A. Rehabilitation of chronic motor conversion disorders. *Crit Rev Phys Rehab Med.* 1993;5:1–13.
18. Wade DT, de Jong BA. Recent advances in rehabilitation. *Br Med J.* 2000;320:1385–1388.
19. Wade DT. Rehabilitation for hysterical conversion states. In: Halligan P, Bass C, Marshall J, eds. *Contemporary approaches to the study of hysteria.* Oxford: Oxford University Press, 2001:330–346.
20. Moene F, Spinhoven P, Hoogduin K, et al. A randomised controlled clinical trial on the additional effect of hypnosis in a comprehensive treatment programme for inpatients with conversion disorder of the motor type. *Psychother Psychosom.* 2002;71:66–76.
21. Wood P. *International classification of impairments, disabilities and handicaps: a manual of classification relating to the consequences of disease.* Geneva: World Health Organization, 1980.
22. Wade DT, Halligan P. New wine in old bottles: the WHO ICF as an explanatory model of human behavior. *Clin Rehabil.* 2003;17:349–354.
23. Davison P, Sharpe M, Wade D, et al. "Wheelchair" patients with non-organic disease: a psychological enquiry. *J Psychosom Res.* 1999;47:93–103.
24. Wade DT. Medically unexplained disability—a misnomer, and an opportunity for rehabilitation. *Clin Rehabil.* 2001;15:343–347.
25. Cote P, Cassidy JD, Carroll L, et al. A systematic review of the prognosis of acute whiplash and a new conceptual framework to review the literature. *Spine.* 2001;26:445–458.
26. Binder L, Rohling M. Money matters: a meta-analytic review of the effects of financial incentives on recovery after closed head injury. *Am J Psychiatry.* 1996;153:7–10.
27. Rohling M, Binder L, Langhinrichsen-Rohling J. Money matters: a meta-analytic review of the association between financial compensation and the experience and treatment of chronic pain. *Health Psychol.* 1995;14:537–547.
28. Bryan Suter P. Employment and litigation: improved by work, assisted by a verdict. *Pain.* 2002;100:249–257.
29. Schrader H, Obelieniene D, Bovin G, et al. Natural evolution of late whiplash syndrome outside the medicolegal context. *Lancet.* 1996;347:1207–1211.
30. Hiller W, Fichter M, Rief W. A controlled treatment study of somatoform disorders including analysis of healthcare utilisation and cost-effectiveness. *J Psychosom Res.* 2003;54:369–380.
31. Kroenke K, Swindle R. Cognitive behavioral therapy for somatisation and symptom syndromes: a critical review of controlled clinical trials. *Psychother Psychosom.* 2000;69:205–215.
32. Guthrie E. Psychodynamic interpersonal therapy. *Adv Psychiat Treat.* 1999;5:135–145.
33. O'Malley P, Jackson J, Santoro J, et al. Antidepressant therapy for unexplained symptoms and symptom syndromes. *Fam Pract.* 1999;48:980–990.
34. Petrie K, Cameron L, Ellis C, et al. Changing illness perceptions after myocardial infarction: an early intervention randomised controlled trial. *Psychosom Med.* 2002;64:580–586.

Psychogenic Injuries and the Law

36

Michael I. Weintraub

ABSTRACT

The successful prosecution of a tort claim or a workers' compensation claim requires proof that an *objectively confirmed* personal injury occurred. Relying on medical and expert opinions supporting the causal association, judges, juries, or administrative boards can make appropriate decisions regarding compensation. It is important to recognize that in the area of psychogenic illness, the courts have rejected compensation for obvious, conscious malingering (medical lying). However, on the other hand, the legal system has recognized that psychogenic symptoms and illness on a *subconscious* basis are indeed compensable. There is, however, a general skepticism and cynicism both by jurors and the judiciary as to the merits of the injury, and without detailed and convincing medical support, the injury will not achieve the same financial award status and success as an organic causation. This chapter will discuss various court decisions in many states which address this complex topic. It will also discuss physicians' liability to third parties for injuries caused by patients having psychogenic illness during symptomatic episodes.

INTRODUCTION

Unraveling the role of psychogenic illness in personal injury law and compensation is a formidable task. It is estimated that there are 18 million lawsuits per year in the United States, with individuals claiming compensation for both economic and noneconomic damages. Objective traumatic injury traditionally generates claims in state and federal courts and in the workers' compensation and Social Security system. However, claims for psychogenic injuries have become more numerous in the past two decades, and symptoms unsupported by documented physical trauma have become more common. In addition, there has been an increase in health care fraud problems. Ideally, the courtroom is the arena to determine justice and provide compensation. However, the reality is that there are different applications of the law with different scenarios. It cannot be disputed that there is a critical need for both physicians and attorneys to distinguish between psychogenesis and malingering, in order that medicine and law serve the best interest of the community. This article will review the climate and standards of admissibility of evidence.

Definitions: Scientific Admissibility of Evidence

To distinguish between compensable, psychogenic injury and malingering, juries (in court cases) and administrative judges (in workers' compensation and Social Security cases) must rely upon information and opinion provided in the testimony of expert witnesses. Accordingly, the standards for admissibility of expert opinion play an important role in the outcome of jury claims. In 1923, the federal courts concluded the Frye Rule (1) that specifically dealt with the admissibility of an expert's opinion based on data from a predecessor of the modern polygraph or lie detector test. It concluded that the underlying "principle or discovery . . . from which the deduction is made must be sufficiently established to have gained general acceptance in the particular field in which it belongs." Thus, the Frye General Acceptance Standards defined admissibility as "reliability" and then deferred to an undefined "scientific community" for its "general acceptance." This was essentially the law of the land until 1973.

On June 28, 1973, the Supreme Court held that sections, Federal Rules of Evidence (FRE) 702 (2), superseded the Frye Test because it found scientific admissibility too restrictive. Thus, the FRE ruling authorizes judges to admit medical or scientific testing if it will assist the judge or jury. Helpfulness is the touchstone of admissibility. A witness can be qualified as an expert "by knowledge, skill, experience, training, or education." This rule did not expressly address the reliability of expert testimony and the trial judge was afforded great latitude (3). The trial judge, a layperson, had to decide if potentially controversial or perhaps ambiguous scientific evidence should be admitted to assist in clarifying a scientific issue for the jury. In view of many of the trial judges' limitations of lack of scientific background, and so on, it is not surprising that many creative theories developed, leading critics of the legal system to claim that judges permitted "junk science" and thus "junk justice" (4).

Not unexpectedly, this came under the purview of the Supreme Court and led to the *Daubert* decision (5), in which it attempted to formulate standards for trial courts to apply in determining whether scientific testimony is sufficiently reliable to be allowed into evidence. According to *Daubert*, general acceptance of any technical or scientific method is linked to the peer-review literature and is based on scientific language, principles, and explicit scientific standards. Moreover, it also discussed statistical standards. Thus, speculation is unacceptable. Moreover, it mandated that the trial judge must be more vigilant and serve as "gatekeeper," assuring that "scientific tests or evidence admitted is not only relevant but reliable." It also encouraged FRE 706 permitting judges to appoint their own independent witnesses, especially resolving issues of scientific complexity (6). Rule 403 allows judges to exclude testimony if relevant expert opinions "will prejudice, confuse, or mislead the jury" (7). On December 1, 2000, Rule 706 of FRE was amended to include that testimony is the product of reliable principles and methods, based on specific facts or data, and has been applied reliably to the facts of the case (8).

While most state courts and laws conform with the Federal Rules of Procedure and Evidence, some do not, and therefore, the same testimony from a given expert witness might be admissible in some state courts but not in federal courts and vice versa. Over 40 states, however, have adopted these guidelines.

The workers' compensation system, and Social Security disability system use their own set of rules which are usually decided by a judge or a panel of judges. Eligibility claims require that an injury has occurred so as to safeguard against fraud, yet workers' compensation and Social Security disability systems have come to realize that physical trauma (alleged or perceived) may have an emotional consequence and, therefore, are more willing to permit recovery. In fact, the following cases (9–12) provide awards for psychological trauma in the absence of physical injury.

The four most common psychogenic complaints seen in both state and federal litigation as well as the worker's compensation system are (i) chronic pain, (ii) traumatic brain injury/cognitive encephalopathy, (iii) reflex sympathetic dystrophy (complex regional pain syndrome 1 and 2), and (iv) fibromyalgia.

Despite the fact that these symptoms are subjective and intangible and cannot be quantified, they may be responsible for a significant amount of the award (13).

Definition of Terms: Psychogenic Illness

Hysterical conversion reactions (HCR) is a 20th-century term based upon a late 19th-century idea proposed by Freud. It has been defined as a subconscious, nonverbal communication and symbolic representation reflecting the patient's knowledge of the body (real or presumed). These symptoms arise because the patients, usually women, wish to obtain some gain (financial or interpersonal). The diagnosis is *not* confirmed by exclusion or personality traits, but rather when the clinician demonstrates, on examination, that these symptoms do not conform to known anatomic and physiologic patterns of innervation. The dramatic HCR seen in the days of Charcot, that is, paralysis, blindness, deafness, convulsions, and so on, have been frequently replaced in order to conform to our present society. The four most common psychogenic illness claims are (i) chronic pain, (ii) traumatic brain injury/cognitive encephalopathy, (iii) reflex sympathetic dystrophy/chronic regional pain syndrome 1 and 2, and (iv) fibromyalgia.

Malingering

Malingering is the false and fraudulent imitation or exaggeration of physical disease or mental symptoms in order to obtain financial rewards, drugs, or avoid jail or military duty. It is a behavior pattern, usually in men, that is deliberate, under conscious control, and goal-directed for personal advantage.

Malingering and HCR can coexist and at this time, it is difficult to distinguish them. As noted in the video-EEG case presented by Dr. John Morris, when the patient was presented with good news that his "seizures" were not organic, he muttered to his wife, "What will this do to insurance?" The use of videotape has been extremely helpful in resolving claims and has been found to be admissible as evidence in litigation over the past 25 years. In 1993, the FRE amended the definition of "photographs" to explicitly include "videotape evidence" (14).

DETECTION OF MALINGERING AND DECEPTIVE BEHAVIOR

Any deficit can be faked in a civil claim for psychological damage. It is extremely difficult to calculate the degree of health care fraud, but purposeful misrepresentation of claims was found to be acceptable in 20% of those claimants surveyed by the Public Attitude Monitor (PAM) (15) survey, and alarmingly, acceptable in 46% of those surveyed in New York, Pennsylvania, and New Jersey (16).

Recently, a specific type of fraud was uncovered in a New Jersey undercover operation known as "Ghost Riders" (17). In this videotaped staged bus accident, it was noted that several outsiders jumped on the stopped vehicle, mingled, and claimed injury. Surprisingly, a large number of individuals also submitted claims despite the fact that they were not near the scene of the accident. Thus, if one of these individuals went to a physician for care, how could the physician determine the validity of his or her statements? Thus, debunking claims for "injury and chronic pain and suffering" is extremely difficult without a videotape. If this problem confronts the scientific community, how valid is it that juries can easily reach a verdict. The emotions and sympathy of jurors can be fraudulently manipulated as demonstrated in the Lennahan case (18). This was a retired police officer who was married to an insurance claims adjustor. He left New York and settled in Florida with complaints of low back pain that were felt to be compensation-related. He ultimately required a laminectomy and alleged disability, receiving over $400,000 from the compensation system. He also secondarily sued his neurosurgeon for complications of the above surgery that left him with dementia, cognitive disability, and inability to function. A prominent neurologist provided a letter of causality despite the fact that it was alleged that he never examined the patient. The jury found for the plaintiff and awarded over $2 million. The involved neurosurgeon and the malpractice carrier agreed to provide surveillance videotape, and after the patient received compensation, he was noted to be performing executive tasks, sophisticated contractual agreements, purchasing a large boat, and also dancing a victory jig. This was demonstrated and shown on *20/20*. It was also demonstrated to the attorney general and to the judge, and the verdict was reversed. Money was returned except for the legal fees which the Florida Supreme Court felt were justified for the attorneys since they were "fooled" just like the jury.

STATE AND FEDERAL CASES

The benchmark and threshold is that a physical injury has occurred, usually verified by others. The claim is supported by a medical witness as to causality. If accepted, compensation is rendered. Emotional injury or psychological trauma indicates that individuals are not required to demonstrate a physical injury but only that they were exposed to an event that could have produced bodily injury or damage leading to disability. A specific "zone of danger or injury" has been used by the courts to establish for family members to recover from emotional trauma (shock, sorrow, fear) of seeing at close hand the infliction of serious physical injury upon a loved one.

Examples of psychogenic illness (PI) and litigation are described in *Hagen v Coca-Cola Bottling Company* (19), and *Rotundo v Kennedy* (20).

WORKERS' COMPENSATION, SOCIAL SECURITY, AND VETERANS ADMINISTRATION DISABILITY PROGRAM

In the United States, the worker's compensation system was developed as an alternative to tort litigation. The system was based on a no-fault principle and was designed to provide an efficient remedy to relieve the economic and social burden arising from work-related injury. The benefits include medical care, cash payments, and rehabilitation services. Claimant abuse is often a major problem. In a *New York Times* article (21), it was noted by Gorelick that a half dozen compensation attorneys sustained a flurry of minor accidents, that is, lifting a briefcase, inspecting a chair, and so on, that resulted in awards totaling $670,000. One attorney injured his back lifting his briefcase out of his car trunk, yet the injury did not cause him to miss any work or even his golf game. A worker's compensation judge awarded him $95,000. In defense of the award, the senior judge stated that the lawyers were not "thieves, cheats, or exploiters" but merely "aware of the worker's compensation laws." Thus, financial incentive and a knowledge of the system reward a significant group of claimants. However, it should not be inferred that the system is without merits for the majority of workers.

The following examples represent claims for psychogenic disability (22,23).

It remains to be established what happens to claimants after litigation has been settled. Despite the diversity of opinion, most neurologists in the United States perceive that a significant number return to their prelitigation status. However, until well-controlled outcome studies are available, one must be cautious in the final conclusion.

PHYSICIAN LIABILITY TO THIRD PARTIES

This is a creative type of litigation which allows patients to bring lawsuits against physicians who care for individuals involved in accidents that lead to subsequent injury or death to others. Thus, the duty to warn the public is at issue as well as the confidentiality of the doctor–patient relationship. Recently, the Health Insurance Portability and Accountability Act (HIPAA) rulings have indicated that physicians can be held liable for breaking this duty of confidentiality to third parties when the patient does not give consent (24).

Facts

Physicians are mandated in six states (California, Delaware, Nevada, New Jersey, Oregon, and Pennsylvania) to report individuals with epilepsy to the Department of Motor Vehicles (25). It is unclear as to whether they are mandated to report individuals with pseudoseizures. However, there has been a flurry of lawsuits for injuries caused by individuals who have diabetes, or have taken medication that may produce drowsiness, alcoholism, and so on. The following cases illustrate the above.

- *Crosby v Sultz*, 592 A. 2d 1337 (PA Ct. 1991). A noninsulin-dependent diabetic patient struck a mother and her three children who were pedestrians. They filed suit against the patient and a secondary action against her physician, asserting that the diabetes caused a temporary lapse of consciousness at the wheel and caused the accident. A trial court dismissed the complaint, indicating that diabetes was not a reportable disease to the Department of Motor Vehicles (26).
- Estate of *Wittloeft v Leiskaddon*, 733 A. 2d 623 (PA 1999). A patient with poor vision drove and struck and killed a bicyclist. Trial court did not find that the ophthalmologist had a duty to the bicyclist (27).

As a general rule, physicians are not liable to third persons harmed as a result of an auto accident caused by a patient's condition. The only major exception is the *Tarasoff v Regents of University of California* decision (28) in which psychologists and psychiatrists must warn the public if individuals have been singled out for potential harm by one of their patients. Several states besides California have also found that physicians have a duty to warn *identifiable* third parties of a risk of harm.

Dilemma

Recently, in 2003, an 86-year-old individual in Santa Monica, California, barreled through a farmer's market, killing at least ten individuals and injuring dozens. Preliminary tests indicated that the driver was not impaired by alcohol or drugs, but was elderly. This caused nationwide outrage directed toward elderly drivers and their increased incidence of accidents, especially in states like Florida. The American Medical Association sent a "Physician's Guide to Assessing and Counseling Older Drivers" to all physicians in the United States, emphasizing

that "*safe driving is a matter of function, not age*" (29). Thus, individuals with psychogenic illness who have impaired functions, that is, dystonia, tremor, pseudoseizures, severe tics, and so on, may be a potential danger to the public. Obviously, each case is individualized, but how do physicians defend themselves from third-party claims when the individuals have constant movement disorders of head, neck, arms, feet, or combinations thereof when they need to operate a vehicle with dexterity and safety so as to avoid an accident?

In conclusion, psychogenic illness and the law is an evolving concept and will continue to be a problem in the future.

REFERENCES

1. *Frye v US* 293 F. 1013 (D.C. Cir), 1923.
2. Federal Rules of Evidence § 702 PUB L #93-595, 88 STAT 1926, 1975.
3. Weinstein JB. Expert witness testimony: a trial judge's perspective in medical/legal issues facing neurologists. *Neurol Clin.* 1999;17: 355–362.
4. Huber P. *Galileo's revenge: junk science in the courtroom.* New York: Basic Books, 1991.
5. *Daubert v Merrill-Dow Pharmaceuticals,* 113 S Court 2786 1993.
6. Federal Rules of Evidence. Rule 706, 88 STAT 1926 1975.
7. Federal Rules of Evidence. Rule 403, 88 STAT 1975.
8. Kulick RJ, Driscoll J, Prescott JC, et al. The Daubert standard, a primer for pain specialists. *Pain Med.* 2003;4:75–80.
9. *American Smelting NREF. Co. v Industrial Commn.,* 59 Ariz. 87, 123 P. 2d 163 1942.
10. *Carter v General Motors,* 361 Mich. 577,106 N.W. 2d 105 1960.
11. *Bailey v American General Insurance Co.,* 154 Tex. 430, 279 S. W. 2d 315 1955.
12. *Allis Chalmers Mfg. Co. v Industrial Commn.,* 57 IL. 2d 257, 312 N. E. 2d 280 1974.
13. Weintraub MI. Chronic pain in litigation. What is the relationship? *Neurol Clin.* 1995;13:341–349.
14. Marcus RP. Admissibility and effects of videotape of medical procedures in litigation. *J Legal Med.* 2001;22:401–429.
15. Insurance Research Council. *Public attitude monitor.* Oak Brook, IL: Insurance Research Council, 1992, (Survey).
16. Insurance Research Council. *Public attitude monitor.* Oak Brook, IL: Insurance Research Council, 1993, (Survey).
17. Kerr P. Ghost riders are target of an insurance sting. *New York Times.* 1993, 8/18/93.
18. Lavin JH. Everyone believed the plaintiff except his doctor. *Med Econ.* 1991;68:34–41.
19. *Hagen v Coca-Cola Bottling Company,* 804 So. 2d 1234, (FLA) 2001.
20. Application of Rotundo, 36 Misc. 2d 332, 234 N.Y.S. 2d 859 (Sup. Ct.) 1962.
21. Margolick D. At the Bar. *New York Times,* April 30, Section B16, 1993.
22. *Greer v Coca-Cola Bottling Company,* 420 So. 2nd 540 (LA Ct. App.) 1982.
23. *Moccia v Eclipse Pioneer Division of Bendix Aviation,* 375 N.J. Super. 470 1959.
24. Health Insurance Portability and Accountability Act (HIPAA), of 8/21/96 Public Law 104-191, 1996.
25. Finucane AK. Legal Aspects of Epilepsy. In: Weintraub MI, ed. *Medical-Legal Issues Facing Neurologists; Neurol Clin.* 1999;17: 235–243.
26. *Crosby v Sultz,* 592 A 2d 1337 (PA Ct.), 1991.
27. *Estate of Witthoeft v Kiskaddon,* 733 A. 2d 623 (PA), 1999.
28. *Tarasoff v Regents of University of California,* 551 P. 2d 334 (Cal), 1976.
29. AMA News, August 4, 2003.

Therapeutic Approaches to Psychogenic Movement Disorders

37

Joseph Jankovic   *C. Robert Cloninger*   *Stanley Fahn*
Mark Hallett   *Anthony E. Lang*   *Daniel T. Williams*

ABSTRACT

This review summarizes a roundtable discussion among experts asked to address therapeutic approaches to psychogenic movement disorders. They were also asked to answer the following two questions: (i) How do you tell the patient the diagnosis? and (ii) What is the therapeutic plan? The summary is written in a didactic style and the word "we" is used when there was relative unanimity of opinion.

INTRODUCTION

Management of psychogenic movement disorders (PMD) has received little attention from either neurology or psychiatry communities. When primary care physicians suspect a somatoform disorder, either conversion or somatization (hysteria), or encounter patients with medically unexplained symptoms (1), they rarely initiate therapy. Because of their uncertainty about the diagnosis and because they regard such patients as difficult to manage, they usually refer these patients to specialists. Patients with PMD are usually referred to neurologists who may or may not refer the patients in turn to movement disorder specialists. As general neurologists are becoming more sophisticated in recognizing typical movement disorders, they tend to refer the unusual or atypical ones to specialists in

movement disorders. This is one reason why there is an exponential increase in the incidence of PMD in movement disorders centers (2). Because there is no definitive diagnostic test for PMD, the diagnosis must be made by a neurologist skilled in recognizing typical and atypical movement disorders. After the diagnosis is established, it is prudent for the neurologist to consult a psychiatrist, psychologist, psychotherapist, physical or occupational therapist, spiritual leader, or other mental health professional, preferably one experienced in the psychological management of such patients. It is often desirable for the mental health consultant to become involved not only with the patient but also with his or her spouse, companion, parent, or "significant other" to work toward the common goal of returning the patient into the mainstream of life. While a team approach to the management of PMD is essential for optimal results, the responsibilities of the treating physicians must be well-defined. It is imperative that the nonneurologic consultants adequately understand the neurologic diagnosis by detailed briefing from the referring neurologist in order to be able to effectively explicate and reinforce it with the patient and relevant family members. Effective briefing of the mental health consultant by the referring neurologist should avoid inappropriate transmission of perceptions of doubt that will undermine the patient's confidence in the diagnosis. They should avoid any perceptions of doubt and avoid challenging the diagnosis. There is nothing more disruptive to the care of patients with PMD than a pronouncement by the consulting psychiatrist or other mental health professional that "there is nothing psychologically wrong with you that can account for the symptoms."

THERAPEUTIC STRATEGIES

As there are no published controlled therapeutic trials of PMD, the management of such patients has engendered considerable uncertainty. There is no consensus even among the experts about the best therapeutic approach to patients with PMD. Therefore, the treatment strategies described here are largely based on empirical observations and cumulative personal experience of the authors. When relevant, differences of opinion among the authors will be pointed out.

The treatment of PMD starts with the diagnosis. Many patients with psychogenic disorders have a previous history of other medically unexplained symptoms, and confirmation of prior diagnosis of functional or somatoform disorder may help make the diagnosis of psychogenic disorder (3). The diagnosis, usually made by a neurologist knowledgeable about movement disorders, is based not only on exclusion of organic causes, but also on positive criteria. As described in earlier chapters in this book, these positive criteria include the presence of various clues such as abrupt onset, changing pattern and intensity of the movement, variable frequency, deliberate slowness of movement and speech, verbal gibberish, bizarre movement and gait, excessive startle, and movements that are incongruous with any recognized organic movement disorders. Other features include distractibility, spontaneous remissions, suggestibility, la belle indifférence, embellishment, and manifestations of exhaustion and fatigue (2). In addition, the patient may exhibit other medical or neurologic signs, such as false "give-way" weakness, unexplained paralysis or blindness, false sensory loss, pseudoseizures, and other neurologic symptoms typically associated with hysteria (4). The presence of contractures or the occurrence of the movement disorder during sleep does not exclude the diagnosis of PMD (5). Particularly challenging are those patients who manifest both PMD and an organic disorder (6). Coexistent "organic" neurologic disorder was present in 37% of patients with psychogenic tremor followed for over 3 years (7).

Before the diagnosis is disclosed to the patient, it is critical that the clinician is confident about the diagnosis based on personal evaluation of the patient, and after carefully reviewing all previous medical records, laboratory tests, imaging studies, and history of prior medications and other treatments. Such records may now be more difficult to access in the United States because of the recently enacted Health Insurance Portability and Accountability Act (HIPAA). It is also important to note that under this federal law, patients may now request their own records. Physicians, therefore, must have an open and honest relationship with their patients, and should be certain that their medical records accurately reflect their diagnosis, discussions, and recommendations.

If there is any uncertainty about the diagnosis, it is advisable to admit the patient to the hospital, preferably to the neurology service, to complete the evaluation. However, since insurance carriers and third-party payers often deny hospital admissions for psychiatric diagnoses, the evaluation may need to be completed in an outpatient setting (8). In the United States, using the CPT code 316 (*Psychologic factors in physical conditions classified elsewhere*) and additional codes to identify the associated condition (e.g., tremor, dystonia, myoclonus, tics, gait disorder) may legitimately facilitate approval for admission and insurance coverage. While it is not considered ideal to inform the patient about the diagnosis at the initial visit, this is sometimes unavoidable, particularly if the patient is allowed only one visit to the specialty clinic. In such cases, we always emphasize to patients that we will be working with their referring physicians to design the most appropriate treatment plan. An experienced clinician learns to read the patient's body language before making a decision to disclose the diagnosis at the initial visit. We strongly recommend videotaping patients (after signing an informed consent) before disclosing their diagnosis, because their attitude and the nature of the movement disorder may change after they are informed about our impression. Some patients even insist on revoking consent for previous videotape and request that the tape be destroyed.

At least one member of this panel recommends using the term "neuropsychiatric movement disorders" as a preferable term, rather than "psychogenic movement disorders" both for debriefing patients, as well as for general clinical description of this group of disorders. This is not only likely to be more palatable to patients with these disorders, but also effectively conveys a more sophisticated contemporary understanding of the pathophysiology of these disorders.

How the diagnosis is conveyed to the patient may be as important as the actual diagnosis. If presented in a compassionate, supportive, hopeful, nonconfrontational, and professional manner, it is more likely that the patient will react positively, and any potential anger directed against the physician can be diffused and neutralized. When informing the patient about the diagnosis, it is important to emphasize the positive aspects of the diagnosis, specifically that a favorable prognosis is likely, as there is no evidence of any structural neurologic damage or any neurodegenerative disease, such as Parkinson disease. Furthermore, since their disorder is not life-threatening and in fact is potentially completely reversible or resolvable, the patient and family should understand that we are actually conveying the "good news" that this is not a degenerative disease. It is important to indicate that we understand that they are not performing the movements on purpose and that they are not "crazy." We also emphasize that we recognize the obvious disability that their movements are causing. Many patients feel that the severity of the symptoms or the resulting disability is quite incompatible with a diagnosis of a psychological cause, and it is important to clarify this misconception.

In our discussion with the patient, we attempt to attribute some of the symptoms to "stress" as this tends to be a more acceptable explanation to patients than a psychiatric diagnosis. Although many patients initially deny any presence of stress, we explain that stress is not always recognized by the patient, but the brain can react to stress in this manner. Once a mutually trusting relationship is established, subsequent interviews with the patients and their family members or friends often identify major stress factors, such as emotional, sexual, or physical abuse, or other stresses at home or at work. To help patients accept the notion of stress-related symptoms, we usually point out that stress is a frequent cause of many physical ailments. Stress may, for example, cause high blood pressure, increased gastric acid production, bowel disturbances, dermatitis, and other physical signs including abnormal movements. We then emphasize that it is up to the patient, preferably with help from a knowledgeable mental health professional, to learn about potential stress factors and to adopt techniques that reduce the effects of stress on the body. At that point, we often recommend that the patient consult a mental health professional knowledgeable in both stress management and the general management of psychogenic movement disorders. In addition to muscle relaxation techniques, such as biofeedback, we often recommend yoga and meditation. We also explain that an active physiotherapy program is usually necessary to retrain the muscles to function normally again, or to desensitize the stress-induced reflexes that produce the abnormal muscle jerks. Also, point out that the patients need to participate in their own care and must work at physiotherapy to get their muscles retrained. These approaches encourage the patients to participate in their own care and empower them to help themselves.

It is also helpful to emphasize that the majority of patients are unaware of the relevance of stress to the development of their movement disorder symptoms. By definition, patients with somatoform disorders have an unconscious mechanism associated with symptom formation. This explanation further diminishes the prospects of unproductive confrontation that is inevitable if the patient feels unjustly accused of purposeful production of nonphysiologic symptoms.

The discussion of the exact term to use for the diagnosis generated particularly lively discussion. Some experts felt strongly that the term "psychogenic movement disorder" was accurate, used commonly, and hence, was the preferred term. Others thought that the implication that this was a psychiatric condition, even though accurate, would turn the patient away. Another popular term was "functional disorder," which was to be explained as a disorder of

the way the brain was working. This is the special element of the "good news"; since the brain is not damaged, recovery is particularly possible. Stone et al. (9) interviewed 102 general neurology outpatients to survey their attitudes toward specific labels for psychogenic seizures ("pseudoseizures") and found that "stress-related seizures" and "functional seizures" were significantly less offensive than "symptoms all in the mind," "hysterical seizures," and other labels. Another related approach is to tell patients that they have a specific movement problem, such as "tremor," but, opposed to situations like essential tremor or Parkinson disease, the etiology is stress.

We usually tell the patient that, based on our experience, we expect one of two types of reactions when we present a diagnosis of PMD: Some patients become angry and decide to seek another opinion, the vast majority, however, accept the diagnosis and express willingness to work with the neurologist, the psychiatrist, the physiotherapist, and other specialists, as well as with their referring or primary physicians. We then emphasize that long-term studies have found that patients who accept the diagnosis and follow our treatment plan generally have a much better prognosis than those who continue to seek other opinions through "doctor shopping" (7). Indeed, some patients in the latter group continue to consult other physicians, often undergo unnecessary, expensive, and risky procedures, and develop Münchausen syndrome (10).

There are very few studies of predictors of long-term outcome in patients with PMD. Williams et al. (11) noted a permanent benefit in 52% of their patients (n = 131), with complete, considerable, and moderate relief in 25%, 21%, and 8%, respectively. Of those who were previously employed, 25% were able to resume full-time work, 10% part-time work, and 15% functioning at home. These investigators utilized psychotherapy in all patients, along with supplemental approaches such as family sessions (58%), hypnosis (42%), and placebo therapy (13%). Antidepressants were utilized in 71% of their patients, and 8% underwent electroconvulsive therapy. Factor et al. (12) reported resolution of symptoms in 35% of their patients with PMD over a 6-year period. Feinstein et al. (13), however, reported persistence of abnormal movements in 90% of 88 patients followed up for an average of 3.2 years. In a longitudinal study of 127 patients with psychogenic tremor followed for at least 3 years, 55.1% reported improvement in tremor on a global rating scale at last follow-up (7). Based on a structured interview, this improvement was attributed by the patients to the physician's prescribed treatment (48.7%), elimination of stressor(s) (19.5%), specific medication (14.6%), stress management (9.8%), biofeedback (7.3%), and psychotherapy (4.9%) or a combination of these. Dissatisfaction with the physician was identified as the strongest prognostic risk factor of poor long-term outcome. Unwillingness to accept the physician's diagnosis and denial or lack of insight into possible stressors (i.e., personal, family, or social) are the main reasons why patients become disenchanted with their physicians. Therefore, gaining insight into underlying psychodynamic mechanisms is essential for effective treatment and favorable outcome.

While the neurologist usually focuses on establishing the neurologic diagnosis, the primary role of the psychiatrist is to explore the psychodynamic basis of the PMD and to develop a therapeutic plan for the primary psychopathology as well as for psychiatric comorbidities, such as associated personality disorder, depression, anxiety, and other psychiatric conditions. About half of patients with PMD have depression, although many deny any symptoms of sadness (7). The psychiatrist should help the patients to shift their focus from their symptoms and their disability to a goal-oriented therapy. Cognitive–behavioral therapy (CBT) has been used effectively by psychiatrists and psychotherapists to manage patients with somatoform disorders, hypochondriasis, and factitious and malingering disorders (14,15). One of the primary aims of CBT is to help patients identify their dysfunctional beliefs and to modify their maladaptive behavior that perpetuates the symptoms. This individually conducted or group therapy is designed to engage the patients in more productive activities and to dissuade them from seeking additional opinions and treatments. This is usually coupled with a program of graduated physical conditioning, relaxation techniques, and the teaching of coping skills that would allow the patient to function as normally as possible at home and at work. The psychodynamic underpinning may involve conflicts related to guilt, relieved by the physical suffering associated with the movement disorder. Many patients become dependent on their spouses, frequently requesting their assistance (even calling them at work and demanding that they come home to attend to their needs), transferring their usual responsibilities to them, and turning them into their personal caregivers. Typically, the patient, usually a young woman, is accompanied to the visit by an overly attentive and overprotective spouse. The psychiatrist and other therapists must use their skills to break this dependency. Avoidance of emotional conflict by displacing true feelings with physical symptoms may be another psychodynamic mechanism of PMD that has to be explored and addressed by the treating psychiatrist. Recognizing and facing the emotional conflicts and dealing with the avoidance may be an important stepping stone in the management of patients with PMD.

The use of placebos in the management of psychiatric disorders is controversial. The debate usually focuses on the ethics of using placebo as a diagnostic tool or as a treatment. Many physicians feel that placebos deceive the patient and thus violate the trusting doctor–patient relationship. On the other hand, placebos have been used effectively in diagnosing nonepileptic seizures (pseudoseizures) (16,17). Although they have not been systematically studied in PMD when used judiciously and with full disclosure to the patient, placebos may be useful in further defining the diagnosis of PMD. Furthermore, the response to a placebo may be used to support the reasons for the diagnosis during discussion with the patient. In addition to "curing" the abnormal movement, placebos may be used to better characterize the movement disorder. For example, when patient's symptoms are not present, or are very mild at the time of the visit ("today is a good day"), a double-blind injection of active or inactive drug (saline placebo), coupled with a powerful suggestion that the agent will trigger or transiently exacerbate the movement, may "reveal" the full symptom and thus allow for assessment of the nature of the movement disorder (18). If used in this instance, it is critical that the procedure is fully explained to the patient and an appropriate consent is obtained. When the physician's motives behind the use of placebo, namely, the need to appreciate the full spectrum of the movement disorder in order to understand the severity and to help establish the diagnosis with the ultimate aim to help the patient, are honestly discussed, placebos may not only help in defining the disorder, but may lead to more effective management. Provocative techniques without placebo, such as suggestion, hyperventilation, and photic stimulation, have been used successfully to induce psychogenic nonepileptic seizures (19). One of the authors (JJ) often applies a tuning fork to the affected area (e.g., tremulous limb) and uses a suggestion to make the movement disorder either better or worse. Such "placebo" techniques may be useful in better defining the phenomenology of the PMD and establishing the diagnosis. Although placebos have been used occasionally as a treatment, instead of potentially habit-forming or dangerous drugs, we generally do not condone or advocate such an approach.

In addition to insight-oriented psychotherapy, psychological support, stress management, and physical and occupational therapy, pharmacologic treatment of underlying depression and anxiety plays an important role in the management of patients with PMD. Although controlled trials are lacking, antidepressants and antianxiety drugs may be extraordinarily helpful as an adjunct to the CBT and other neurobehavioral therapies. The choice of antidepressants is often dependent on whether there is an associated anxiety, in which case the selective serotonin reuptake inhibitors (SSRI) are often beneficial; if insomnia is present, then the tricyclics may have some advantages. Mirtazapine—an antidepressant that enhances noradrenergic and serotonergic transmission and acts as a presynaptic α-2, 5HT2, and 5HT3 receptor antagonist—seems to have fewer side effects than do the typical SSRIs. Since patients often check the Internet or other sources for potential side effects, they may find it reassuring that the mirtazapine has been reported to improve tremor, at least in a small, open-label study (20). The drug, however, has not been found to be effective in essential tremor in a double-blind, placebo-controlled trial (21).

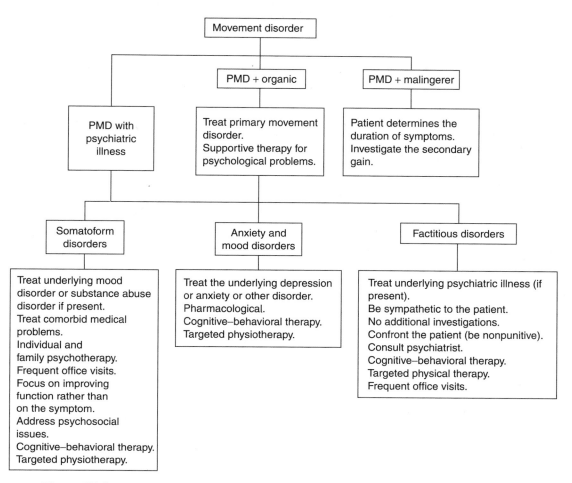

Figure 37.1 Guideline for management of psychogenic movement disorders. [From Jankovic J, Thomas M, Vuong KD. Long-term outcome of psychogenic tremor. *Neurology* 2004;62(Suppl 5): A501.]

Finally, it is important to individualize the therapy and customize it not only to the particular patient and his or her symptoms, but also to the specific disorder (Fig. 37.1). The treatment approach will be different depending on the patient's personality and psychopathology (22). Thus, in patients with somatization and conversion disorder, evidence of depression should be sought, and they should be encouraged to return to their previous function as soon as possible. Patients with hypochondriasis should be reassured that they do not have the disease they fear. They may also benefit from CBT (23). In this approach, the patients are instructed how to correct factors that cause them to amplify the somatic symptoms. Patients with factitious disorder should be confronted with evidence that they have manufactured their symptoms, and at the same time should be provided with appropriate emotional support.

Since predisposition to stress appears to be an important risk factor for PMD, identification of individuals who are at risk for developing psychogenic disorders in response to stress would represent an important advance in the treatment and prevention of this common disorder. Future genetic-epidemiologic studies may uncover genetic factors that would explain why some individuals react to stress by exhibiting physical signs and would provide evidence for a role of gene–environment relationship in psychogenic disorders (24).

REFERENCES

1. Sharpe M. Medically unexplained symptoms and syndromes. *Clin Med.* 2002;2:501–504.
2. Thomas M, Jankovic J. Psychogenic movement disorders: diagnosis and management. *CNS Drugs.* 2004;18:437–452.
3. Schrag A, Brown RJ, Trimble MR. Reliability of self-reported diagnoses in patients with neurologically unexplained symptoms. *J Neurol Neurosurg Psychiatry.* 2004;75:608–611.
4. Stone J, Zeman A, Sharpe M. Functional weakness and sensory disturbance. *J Neurol Neurosurg Psychiatry.* 2002;73:241–245.
5. Fahn S, Williams DT. Psychogenic dystonia. *Adv Neurol.* 1988; 50:431–455.
6. Ranawaya R, Riley D, Lang AE. Psychogenic dyskinesias in patients with organic movement disorders. *Mov Disord.* 1990;5:127–133.

7. Jankovic J, Thomas M, Vuong KD. Long-term outcome of psychogenic tremor. *Neurology.* 2004;62(Suppl. 5):A501.

8. Barsky AJ, Borus JF. Somatization and medicalization in the era of managed care. *JAMA.* 1995;274:1931–1934.

9. Stone J, Campbell K, Sharma N, et al. What should we call pseudoseizures? The patient's perspective. *Seizure.* 2003;12:568–572.

10. Turner J, Reid S. Munchausen's syndrome. *Lancet.* 2002;359: 346–349.

11. Williams DT, Ford B, Fahn S. Phenomenology and psychopathology related to psychogenic movement disorders. *Adv Neurol.* 1995;65:231–257.

12. Factor SA, Podskalny GD, Molho ES. Psychogenic movement disorders: frequency, clinical profile and characteristics. *J Neurol Neurosurg Psychiatry.* 1995;59:409–412.

13. Feinstein A, Stergiopoulos V, Lang AE. Psychiatric outcome in patients with a psychogenic movement disorder: a prospective study. *Neuropsychiatry Neuropsychol Behav Neurol.* 2001;14: 169–176.

14. Barsky AJ. The patient with hypochondriasis. *N Engl J Med.* 2001;345:1395–1399.

15. Krahn LE, Li H, O'Connor MK. Patients who strive to be ill: factitious disorder with physical symptoms. *Am J Psychiatry.* 2003; 160:1163–1168.

16. Devinsky O, Fisher R. Ethical use of placebos and provocative testing in diagnosing nonepileptic seizures. *Neurology.* 1996;47: 866–870.

17. Bhatia M, Sinha PK, Jain S, et al. Usefulness of short-term video EEG recording with saline induction in pseudoseizures. *Acta Neurol Scand.* 1997;95:363–366.

18. Levy RS, Jankovic J. Placebo-induced conversion reaction: a neurobehavioral and EEG study of hysterical aphasia, seizure, and coma. *J Abnorm Psychol.* 1983;92:243–249.

19. Benbadis SR, Johnson K, Anthony K, et al. Induction of psychogenic nonepileptic seizures without placebo. *Neurology.* 2000;55:1904–1905.

20. Pact V, Giduz T. Mirtazapine treats resting tremor, essential tremor, and levodopa-induced dyskinesia. *Neurology.* 1999;53:1154.

21. Pahwa R, Lyons KE. Mirtazapine in essential tremor: a double-blind, placebo-controlled pilot study. *Mov Disord.* 2003;18: 584–587.

22. Stone J, Carson A, Sharpe M. Functional symptoms in neurology: management. *J Neurol Neurosurg Psychiatry.* 2005;76(Suppl 1): 13–21.

23. Barsky AJ, Ahern DK. Cognitive behavior therapy for hypochondriasis: a randomized controlled trial. *JAMA.* 2004;291:1464–1470.

24. Caspi A, Sugden K, Moffitt TE, et al. Influence of life stress on depression: moderation by a polymorphism in the 5-HTT gene. *Science.* 2003;301:386–389.

Abstracts

ABSTRACT 1

Right Lateral Prefrontal Area May be Activated in Psychogenic Tremor

Michiko Kimura Bruno, Andrew Goldfine, Kenji Kansaku, Takashi Hanakawa, Zoltan Mari, Louis J. Ptacek, Mark Hallett

Objective: To identify areas of brain activation during psychogenic tremor.

Background: Tremor is one of the most common psychogenic movement disorders in clinical practice (1). As with other psychogenic movement disorders, tremor can be disabling and limit quality of life of patients. Secondary gain and psychiatric disturbances are not always identified, and the neuronal mechanism leading to psychogenic tremor remains unclear.

Methods

Subjects: We performed functional magnetic resonance imaging (fMRI) of two patients with psychogenic tremor. The study was approved by the Institutional Review Board, and both subjects gave written informed consent to participate in the MRI scanning according to institutional guidelines. The first patient was a 59-year-old right-handed woman, who started having right hand tremor at age 45 after antibiotic injection. The second patient was a 19-year-old man, who started having right hand tremor approximately 6 months prior to presentation, when he graduated high school and started college. Both patients had characteristic features of psychogenic tremor, such as distractibility, variability (in tremor frequency, intensity, and direction), and entrainment.

Task: Patients were given three different audio-instructed tasks: "rest," "hold," and "move," which were 25 seconds long. During "hold," they positioned their hands in a way that was most likely to produce their tremor. During "move," they were instructed to voluntarily mimic their tremor. "Hold" and "move" condition was always followed by rest, and this was repeated five times in one session. Both patients underwent three sessions. Their hand movements were monitored by videotape recording throughout the scanning.

Imaging and Data Analysis: BOLD contrast image volumes were acquired at 1.5 T (GE-Signa Horizon LX system, Milwaukee, WI) using gradient-echo, echo-planar imaging (TR/TE = 2,500 ms/ 25 ms, FA = 90°, slice thickness/gap = 5/1 mm, FOV = 22 × 22 cm^2, matrix size = 64 × 64). Statistical parametric mapping (SPM2, Wellcome Department of Cognitive Neurology, Institute of Neurology, University College London, London, UK) (2) was used to analyze the data. Significant hemodynamic changes for each contrast were assessed using *t*-statistics on a voxel-by-voxel basis. Correction for multiple comparisons across the whole brain volume examined was made, and areas of activity above a threshold corresponding to $p < 0.05$ corrected ($Z > 4.5$) are reported. Video recording of the tremor was reviewed to determine the timing of tremor (T) versus mimicking (M) versus rest (R). In addition to these three conditions, activation related to T–M, T–R, M–R, M–T were calculated.

Results: In both patients, analysis of T condition alone demonstrated generalized activation of the brain. Significant activation was observed in the right lateral prefrontal areas in the T–M (tremor–mimic) condition. In Case 1, there was also a robust activity in the right parietal lobe, in the supramarginal gyrus. The x, y, z coordinates of the first three significant areas of activation in T–M condition are shown in Table A1.1.

Discussion: Although both patients had tremor in their right hand, they demonstrated significant activation in their right side with T–M condition. Previous physiologic studies have shown involvement of prefrontal cortex in hysterical paresis patients (3,4). Prefrontal cortex, particularly the dorsal prefrontal cortex, is thought to be involved in "volition" (5). Our data suggest that right prefrontal cortex may have an important role in the generation of psychogenic tremor.

TABLE A1.1

X, Y, Z COORDINATES OF ACTIVATION IN T–M CONDITION

	Order	Z-value	*p*-value	x	y	z	Region
Case 1	1	9.30	0.000	48	−52	46	R Parietal
	2	8.86	0.000	34	40	28	R Lateral Prefrontal
	3	8.02	0.000	−36	38	24	L Lateral Prefrontal
Case 2	1	6.44	0.000	−6	−76	−46	L Cerebellar
	2	6.04	0.000	42	52	−18	R Prefrontal
	3	4.90	0.031	−16	64	4	L Prefrontal

1. Miyasaki JM, Sa DS, Galvez-Jimenez N, et al. Psychogenic movement disorders. *Can J Neurol Sci.* 2003;30(Suppl. 1):S94–100.
2. Friston KJ, Holmes AP. Statistical parametric maps in functional imaging: a general linear approach. *Hum Brain Map.* 1995;2:189–210.
3. Marshall JC, Halligan PW, Fink GR, et al. The functional anatomy of a hysterical paralysis. *Cognition.* 1997;64:B1–B8.
4. Spence SA, Crimlisk HL, Cope H, et al. Discrete neurophysiological correlates in prefrontal cortex during hysterical and feigned disorder of movement. *Lancet.* 2000;355:1243–1244.
5. Frith CD, Friston K, Liddle PF, et al. Willed action and the prefrontal cortex in man: a study with PET. *Proc R Soc Lond B Biol Sci.* 1991;244: 241–246.

ABSTRACT 2

Transcultural Comparison of Psychogenic Movement Disorders

Esther Cubo, Vanessa K. Hinson, Christopher G. Goetz, Pedro J. Garcia Ruiz, Justo Garcia de Yebenes, Maria J. Marti, Maria C. Rodriguez Oroz, Gurutz Linazasoro, José Chacón, Antonio Vázquez, Javier López del Val, Sue Leurgans, Joanne Wuu

Introduction: Psychogenic movement disorders (PMD) are generally defined as movement disorders that do not typify a known structurally or biochemically based disease, and appear to have associated significant psychological factors. Syndromes of psychogenic origin account for 1% to 9% of all neurologic diagnoses (1), and abnormal movements or motor disorders are among the most frequent presentations (2,3). Movement disorders described as psychogenic in origin include: dystonia, tremor, myoclonus, parkinsonism, tics, hemiballismus, chorea, and a host of bizarre gait and stance disturbances (1–5).

To date, there have been only a few reports from primarily single-center studies on PMD in the medical literature. Prompted by the lack of cross-cultural comparative data, we compared the phenomenology, anatomic distribution, and functional impairment of PMD in the United States (US) and Spain.

Methods

Patient Population: Consecutive patients from one US site (Rush Medical College, Chicago, Ill) and from eight Spanish university centers (Madrid, Barcelona, San Sebastián, Sevilla, Zaragoza, Pamplona), diagnosed with PMD by a movement disorder specialist were included. The diagnosis of PMD was based on the Fahn and Williams criteria (2), and the rating instrument used was the PMD scale (3).

Procedure: All patients were videotaped at rest and during speech and walking. The first author (EC) then reviewed videotapes and scored presence and severity of the ten PMD phenomena (action tremor, resting tremor, dystonia, myoclonus, bradykinesia, tic, chorea, cerebellar features, athetosis, and ballism). Gait and speech were rated for severity, duration, and incapacitation.

Statistical Analysis: Summary statistics were presented in mean, SD, frequency, and/or percentage. US and Spanish patients were compared across types and locations of PMD using chi-square or Fisher's exact test, as appropriate. Statistical significance was set at 0.05 (two-sided).

Results

Demography: The patient series was composed of 88 US patients and 48 Spanish patients. Women predominated (72% and 73%) in both groups. Spanish patients were older (mean 48.0 years, SD 16.6) than the US patients (mean 40.3 years, SD 13.5). All Spanish subjects were white, whereas the US group was more diverse: 84% white, 12% African American, 3% Asian, and 1% Hispanic.

PMD Phenomenology: The most frequently observed phenomenon in both countries was action tremor, seen in 48% of US and Spanish patients. Likewise, the other four most frequently observed phenomena in both countries were resting tremor, dystonia, myoclonus, and bradykinesia. Resting tremor was significantly more frequent among the US patients compared to the Spanish patients (40% vs. 21%, $p = 0.02$). Gait and speech disorders were similarly distributed in the two groups, with gait problems occurring in 47% (Unites States) and 50% (Spain), and speech dysfunction in 18% (United States) and 23% (Spain) (Table A2.1). There were no statistically significant differences between US and Spanish patients in the mean scores of duration, severity, and incapacity for any type of movements, gait, and speech.

Single vs. Multiple Phenomena: Whereas in Spain, most patients (64%) displayed a single movement type, the US patients more frequently showed multiple phenomena, with only 43% having a single movement type.

Location: The most frequently involved anatomic areas in both groups were upper extremities, followed by lower extremities for action tremor, resting tremor, and bradykinesia. Dystonia was more frequently located in face and neck. Shoulder involvement was significantly more frequent in US patients ($p = 0.01$).

Discussion: Despite possible cultural and referral bias, these two groups of university referral PMD subjects were remarkably similar in their movement types, anatomical distribution, and functional impairment. In accordance with prior studies,

TABLE A2.1

SUMMARY OF LOCALIZABLE MOVEMENT DISORDERS, BY PHENOMENA, AND GAIT AND SPEECH

	US (n = 88)	Spain (n = 48)	p-value
Action Tremor (AT)	42 (48%)	23 (48%)	0.98[a]
Resting Tremor (RT)	35 (40%)	10 (21%)	0.02[a]
Dystonia (D)	25 (28%)	14 (29%)	0.93[a]
Myoclonus (M)	11 (12%)	8 (17%)	0.51[a]
Bradykinesia (B)	12 (14%)	3 (6%)	0.17[a]
None of the above	16 (18%)	1 (2%)	0.002[a]
Tic (T)	6 (7%)	0	0.09[b,d]
Chorea (CH)	4 (5%)	1 (2%)	0.66[b,d]
Cerebellar features (CE)	4 (5%)	0	0.30[b,d]
Athetosis (ATH)	1 (1%)	0	N/A[d]
Ballism (B)	1 (1%)	0	N/A[d]
No abnormality	7 (8%)	5 (10%)	N/A[d]
Gait[c]	41 (47%)	24 (50%)	0.75[a]
Speech	16 (18%)	11 (23%)	0.51[a]

[a]Likelihood ratio chi-square test.
[b]Fisher's exact test.
[c]Gait evaluation not available for one Chicago subject (patient had cast on).
[d]Insufficient power to detect any significant difference. (Results listed here for documentation purpose.)

we found that PMDs were more prevalent in women than in men, and they were most common in upper and lower extremities. Gait and speech dysfunction were similarly distributed in both countries. Our findings from the two cultures are similar to other previously reported single-center samples, though some authors have reported myoclonus or dystonia as frequent forms of PMD (5). We have found action tremor to be the most frequent PMD in both countries. The primary difference between our cultural comparison was that PMD usually occurred as multiple movement disorders in the United States and more frequently as a single phenomenon in the Spanish population. Cultural differences or referral bias may account for the latter observation.

1. Lempert T, Dietrich M, Huppert D, et al. Psychogenic disorders in neurology; frequency and clinical spectrum. *Acta Neurol Scand.* 1990;82: 335–340.
2. Fahn S, Williams D. Psychogenic dystonia. *Adv Neurol.* 1988;50: 431–455.
3. Hinson V, Cubo E, Comella C, et al. *Neurology.* 2003;60(Suppl. 1): A212.
4. Cloninger CR, Maron RL, Cruze SB, et al. A prospective follow-up and family study of somatization in men and women. *Am J Psychiatry.* 1986;145:875–878.
5. Factor S, Podskalny GD, Molho ES. Psychogenic movement disorders: frequency, clinical profile, and characteristics. *J Neurol Neurosurg Psychiatry.* 1995;59:406–412.

ABSTRACT 3
Psychogenic Movement Disorders: Frequency and Type in a Movement Disorders Center

Stewart A. Factor, Eric S. Molho, Donald S. Higgins Jr., Anthony J. Santiago

Acknowledgments: This work was supported by the AMC Parkinson Research Fund and Riley Family Chair in Parkinson's Disease.

Background and Objective: Psychogenic movement disorders (PMD) are commonly seen by movement disorders specialists and represent a significant diagnostic and therapeutic challenge. The frequency of PMD in the general population has not been studied. It has been examined in a general neurology setting. In one report of 4,470 consecutive neurology patients, 9% (405 patients) were psychogenic with 3.9% of these (16 patients) having a movement disorder (1). Most of these were patients with tremor. In movement disorder clinics, few studies have examined the frequency of PMD. In the study of our clinic in 1995 (2), 3.3% (28) of 842 consecutive movement disorder patients seen over a 71-month period were diagnosed with PMD, and another study reported 2.1% of 3,700 patients (3). These estimates are low compared to the 10% to 20% incidence of pseudoseizures reported in epilepsy. The most common types of PMD seen in our study (2) and by others (3,4) were tremor and dystonia. The objective of this study was to evaluate the frequency of PMD in a movement disorders center and the types of movements that are most commonly seen. We also examined characteristic features of each type. This is an update of our prior experience.

Methods: This was a retrospective evaluation of PMD in a single movement disorder center. We performed a database search for the diagnosis of PMD in 3,826 consecutive movement disorder patients seen from July 1988 to July 2003. For those found with this diagnosis, the medical records were reviewed when available. Data was collected on age, gender, Fahn classification (5), type of movement disorder, other psychogenic features on examination, prior psychiatric diagnoses, the precipitating event, obvious secondary gain, mode of onset (abrupt or gradual), relief with distraction, presence of selective disabilities, stimulus sensitivity, a history of multiple somatizations and a prior history of psychogenic disorders.

Results: Of 3,826 movement disorder patients seen over 15 years, 135 (3.5%) had a diagnosis of PMD. Medical records were available for 127 (94%). Of these, 83 were definite, 39 probable, and five possible by Fahn classification. Mean age was 43, 69% were women, and mean duration of disease at time of initial evaluation was 41 months. With regard to type of psychogenic movement disorder, 60 (47%) had tremor, 30 (24%) dystonia, 17 (13%) myoclonus, 11 (9%) parkinsonism, and nine (7%) others. Of patients referred to our clinic for evaluation and management of a specific movement disorder (i.e., tremor, dystonia, etc.), the following percentages were psychogenic: 12% for tremor, 5% dystonia, 32% myoclonus; and 0.8% parkinsonism. The distribution of tremor, dystonia, and myoclonus are shown in Table A3.1. Key clinical features of psychogenic tremor included distractibility (87%), entrainment of tremor with other repetitive movements (27%), paroxysmal episodes (22%), stimulus sensitivity (17%), and changing location (7%). Dystonia and tremor occurred together in 7%. Key clinical features for dystonia included distractibility (47%), paroxysmal episodes (20%), and stimulus sensitivity (27%). For myoclonus, distractibility occurred in 47%, paroxysmal bouts in 24%, and stimulus sensitivity in 53%. In cases of psychogenic parkinsonism, 100% had tremor, 57% reported slowness, 14% had increased tone, and 86% had a gait disorder.

In the 127 PMD patients, other psychogenic features were seen on exam in 63%, including nonphysiologic weakness, sensory loss, slow movement, and gait disorders. Secondary gain was apparent in 57% (financial in 37%) and a precipitating event was described in 53%. A prior psychiatric diagnosis was reported in 50% (37% depression). The following additional clinical characteristics were noted: abrupt onset 55%, selective disability 54%, fatigue from the movements during the exam 26%, a history of somatizations 44%, and prior psychogenic disorder 22%.

Conclusion: PMD makes up about 3.5% of patients seen in a subspecialty movement disorders clinic. Similar figures are reported from Columbia University and Baylor College of Medicine (S. Fahn and J. Jankovic, *personal communication*, 2003). The majority of cases have tremor and dystonia, and approximately 70% have some kind of shaking (2–4). Previous reports indicated that psychogenic tremor and dystonia have characteristic locations and features (2,5–8), adult onset, unilateral lower limb or generalized paroxysmal dystonia, and bilateral upper extremity involvement for tremor, but this study demonstrates that the location is more varied. Of the clinical characteristics, distractibility seems to be more common with tremor, while stimulus sensitivity is more common with myoclonus. A substantial number of patients report a precipitating event,

TABLE A3.1
DISTRIBUTION AND CLINICAL CHARACTERISTICS OF PMD

Distribution	Tremor (n = 60)	Dystonia (n = 30)	Myoclonus (n = 11)
Head	5%	37%	—
Upper limbs			
Unilateral	30%	3%	—
Bilateral	12%	—	35%
Lower limbs			
Unilateral	—	20%	—
Bilateral	10%	—	12%
Segmental (neck & limb)	—	3%	—
Hemi	—	17%	—
Upper & lower limbs	13%	—	—
Generalized	28%	20%	53%
Clinical characteristics			
Distractibility	87%	47%	47%
Paroxysmal	22%	20%	24%
Stimulus sensitive	17%	27%	57%
Entrainment	27%	—	—

secondary gain, and prior psychiatric illness, as demonstrated in prior studies (2–9). By the time these patients reach a movement disorder specialist, the mean duration of illness is 41 months, indicating that PMD is a chronic disorder and represents an even greater therapeutic challenge, since prior studies have demonstrated that early intervention is an important ingredient for recovery (1,2).

1. Lempert T, Dietrich M, Huppert D, et al. Psychogenic disorders in neurology: frequency and clinical spectrum. *Acta Neurol Scand.* 1990;82: 335–340.
2. Factor SA, Podskalny GD, Molho ES. Psychogenic movement disorders: frequency, clinical profile and characteristics. *J Neurol Neurosurg Psychiatry.* 1995;59:406–412.
3. Fahn S. Psychogenic movement disorders. In: Marsden CD, Fahn S, eds. *Movement disorders 3.* Oxford: Butterworth-Heinemann, 1994:359–372.
4. Miyasaki JM, Sa DS, Galvez-Jimenez N, et al. Psychogenic movement disorders. *Can J Neurol Sci.* 2003;30:S94–S100.
5. Fahn S, Williams DT. Psychogenic dystonia. *Adv Neurol.* 1988;50:431–455.
6. Koller W, Lang A, Vetre-Overfield B, et al. Psychogenic tremors. *Neurology.* 1989;39:1094–1099.
7. Kim YJ, Pakian S-I, Lang AE. Historical and clinical features of psychogenic tremor: a review of 70 cases. *Can J Neurol Sci.* 1999;26: 190–195.
8. Lang AE. Psychogenic dystonia: review of 18 case. *Can J Neurol Sci.* 1995;22:136–143.
9. Feinstein A, Stergiopoulos V, Fine J, et al. Psychiatric outcome in patients with a psychogenic movement disorder: a prospective study. *Neuropsychiatry Neuropsychol Behav Neurol.* 2001;14:169–176.

ABSTRACT 4
Psychogenic Hemifacial Spasm (Psych-HFS); Incidence and Clinical Features

Néstor Gálvez-Jiménez, Melanie J. Hargreave

Hemifacial spasm (HFS) consisting of brief clonic jerking movements of the facial muscles innervated by the facial nerve has been classically described as resulting from vascular compression of the root exit zone of the VII cranial nerve (1–5). Reported HFS cases due to causes other than vascular compression are exceedingly rare (6). Similarly, psychogenic hemifacial spasm (Psych-HFS) is extremely rare. No exact figures are available on the true prevalence of this disorder in the medical literature. In a recent review of the topic (6), we found that psychogenic facial movements including psychogenic blepharospasm accounted for only 1.5% of 259 cases of psychogenic movement disorders seen at two large movement disorders centers. Tan et al. (7) recently reported psychogenic facial spasms in 2.4% of all patients referred for evaluation of HFS at the Baylor College of Medicine Movement Disorders Center. The aim of our study was to assess the incidence and clinical features of psychogenic hemifacial spasm in a tertiary referral center over a 7-year period. In order to be included, the patients had to fulfill the classical definition of HFS. Other forms of "facial spasms" deemed of psychogenic origin by the examiner such as psychogenic blepharospasm, psychogenic facial dystonic contractions, or other ill-described movements were not included.

Methods: All patients with movement disorders (MDS) were identified using the *International Classification of Diseases*, Ninth Revision, Clinical Modification (ICD-9-CM), coding system. These patients' medical records were reviewed and cross-referenced for the presence of HFS, other movement disorders, and psychogenicity as diagnosed by a movement disorders specialist (NGJ). The Cleveland Clinic Florida database is based on the ICD coding system, and patients diagnosed with HFS and psychogenic MDS are hence registered in these fashion. In addition, the files of the Movement Disorders Program with "interesting and unusual cases" (MJH) was queried and cross-referenced with the ICD code results. The great proportion of patients were identified after July 1996 when the Movement Disorders Program at the Cleveland Clinic Florida was initiated; therefore, only those patients seen during the last 7 years were included. No cases of Psych-HFS were diagnosed or recorded as such in the medical record database before July 1996.

TABLE A4.1

PATIENT DEMOGRAPHICS AND PHENOMENOLOGY

Patient	Gender	Onset	Age at Onset	Reason for Visit	Main Diagnosis	Other MDS
1	Female	Abrupt	37	Gait difficulties	Psychogenic gait (robotic)	Psychogenic limb and truncal (bizarre) dystonia (at rest and "action induced") Psychogenic hemifacial spasm (rt) (trigger or on action) Psychogenic tremor
2	Male	Unknown, progressive (?)	61	Dopa-resistant Parkinson disease	Psychogenic parkinsonism	Psychogenic hemifacial spasm (rt) (variably present during the examination) Psychogenic tremor
3	Female	Abrupt	32	Jerks and shakes	Psychogenic tremor	Psychogenic dystonia (right hand and torticollis) at rest and/or induced Psychogenic hemifacial spasm (rt) (trigger or on action during examination)
4	Female	Abrupt	26	Idiopathic torsion dystonia and tremor	Psychogenic dystonia	Psychogenic gait (ataxic) Psychogenic alternating hemifacial spasm (triggered during examination)
5	Female	Abrupt	42	Essential tremor	Psychogenic tremor Psychogenic disequilibrium/ gait	Psychogenic ataxia (gait & limb) Psychogenic hemifacial spasm (rt) (triggered)

MDS, movement disorders; rt, right.

Results: A total of 82 HFS patients were identified out of 1,757 MDS patients diagnosed and treated during the 7-year period. The total number of psychogenic MDS patients with Psych-HFS was five. The incidence of Psych-HFS, defined as the number of new cases with the disease in proportion to the total population, was 0.3% of all MDS in our series (five Psych-HFS/1,757 total MDS patients × 100). Psychogenic-HFS represented 6% of all cases with HFS (five Psych-HFS/82 HFS × 100). The incidence per year was 0.04%. (Incidence per year = Incidence/7 years. 0.3% incidence/7-year period). All five cases of psychogenic HFS had other accompanying, more prominent psychogenic movement disorders (Table A4.1) including psychogenic tremor in five patients, psychogenic dystonia in three, psychogenic gait disturbances, including ataxia (limb and gait) in three and psychogenic parkinsonism in one patient. All psychogenic HFS patients were women but one (4:1 women–men ratio) with an average age at onset of 30 years (32–61 yr). Surprisingly, all symptoms of HFS were localized to the right side, except in one patient (patient 4) who had alternating symptoms. In one patient, a "robotic" gait disturbance accompanied Psych-HFS. Routine blood testing and chemistry including copper studies when appropriate were normal. Magnetic resonance imaging (MRI) of the brain and MR angiography were normal. Past history of multiple somatizations in four patients and anxiety and depression in five were documented. The onset of HFS was abrupt in four, and progressive and unknown in one. The following clues suggested that the HFS and accompanying movement disorders were of psychogenic origin: abrupt onset in four patients, multiple somatizations in four, and secondary gain in three patients. Clinically (Table A4.2), the character of the movement was variable in all, with exacerbations and reduction with attention or distraction in all, tremor was entrainable in all, response to placebo in one (patient 4), and abrupt discontinuation of the abnormal movement in two after psychiatric intervention and reassurance (patients 3 and 5).

Discussion: In our experience, psychogenic hemifacial spasm is exceedingly rare, with a calculated incidence of 0.3% of all movement disorders, and 6% of all cases of hemifacial spasm evaluated at our program over a 7-year period. The yearly incidence is estimated at 0.04%. It is more common in women and was not the reason for initial neurologic consultation. In all instances, Psych-HFS was accompanied by other, more dramatic psychogenic movement disorders. Tremor, dystonia, psychogenic gait, and parkinsonism were the most common psychogenic movement disorders associated with Psych-HFS in our series. These abnormal movements may distract the examiner when categorizing all possible combinations of movement disorders observed in a given patient, perhaps resulting in a lower-than-expected reported incidence in the medical literature. Why most patients had symptoms localized to the right is intriguing but may relate to cerebral hemispheric brain dominance, as all patients in our series were right handed. When evaluating patients with facial spasms, Psych-HFS should only be considered if the patient's phenomenology fulfills the clinical definition for

TABLE A4.2
CLINICAL FEATURES/CLUES TO PSYCHOGENICITY

Patient	Response to "Trigger" Maneuvers (Tuning Fork, Touch, Command, Deep Pain)	Somatizations/Other Associated Diagnosis or Complaints	Secondary Gain	Psychiatric History
1	+ Tremor and HFS	Myofascial pain syndrome, generalized "aches and pains"	Requesting disability	Depression
2	+ Tremor and HFS		Disability	Depression
3	+ Dystonia, tremor and HFS	Pain to touch		Depression and anxiety
4	+ Tremor, dystonia and HFS	Myofascial pain syndrome, chronic tension-type headaches, irritable bowel syndrome	Divorce proceedings, attention from husband	Depression
5	+ Tremor and HFS	Lightheadedness (no true vertigo), irritable bowel syndrome, chronic daily headaches		Depression and anxiety

HFS, has evidence on exam of psychogenicity, and a thorough neurologic and medical examination fails to demonstrate a cause for the symptoms. In those HFS patients whose symptoms are indisputably psychogenic, there is no need for neuroimaging studies.

1. Gardner WT, Sava GA. Hemifacial spasm: a reversible pathophysiologic state. *J Neurosurg.* 1962;19:240–247.
2. Jannett PJ, Abbasy M, Maroon JC, et al. Etiology and definitive microsurgical treatment of hemifacial spasm: operative techniques and results in 47 patients. *J Neurosurg.* 1977;47:321–328.
3. Maroon JC. Hemifacial spasm: a vascular cause. *Arch Neurol.* 1978; 35:481–483.
4. Maroon JC, Lunsford LD, Deeb ZL. Hemifacial spasm due to aneurysmal compression of the facial nerve. *Arch Neurol.* 1978;35:545–546.
5. Calbucci F, Tognetti F, Bollini C, et al. Intracranial microvascular decompression for cryptogenic hemifacial spasm, trigeminal and glossopharyngeal neuralgia, paroxysmal vertigo and tinnitus: surgical techniques and results. *Ital J Neurol Sci.* 1986;7:359–366.
6. Galvez-Jimenez N, Hanson MR, Desai M. Unusual causes of hemifacial spasm. *Semin Neurol.* 2001;21:75–83.
7. Tan EK, Jankovic J. Psychogenic hemifacial spasm. *J Neuropsychiatry Clin Neurosci.* 2001;13:380–384.

ABSTRACT 5
Electrophysiologic Testing in Psychogenic Tremor: Does It Always Help?

Serena Wan-Si Hung, Gregory F. Molnar, Peter Ashby, Robert Chen, Valerie Voon, Anthony E. Lang

Objective: A case report to demonstrate that electrophysiologic studies may occasionally produce misleading results in psychogenic tremor.

Background: Electrophysiologic studies demonstrating entrainability, lack of frequency dissociation (frequency difference between two limbs), coactivation of antagonist muscles of the tremulous joint, and an increase in tremor amplitude with loading have been shown to be helpful in diagnosing psychogenic tremor.

Methods: We report a case of psychogenic tremor that was suspected clinically. Electrophysiologic studies were performed by an experienced investigator before and after cognitive behavior therapy and antidepressant treatment.

Case Report: A 21-year-old right-handed man presented with a 7-month history of arm tremor that started bilaterally. Left arm tremor resolved spontaneously. He had trouble with his handwriting or holding a glass of juice, but not with typing or lighting a cigarette. He had multiple somatic complaints and was diagnosed with anxiety disorder 1 year prior to the onset of the tremor. On examination, the tremor was present in his right wrist and fingers at rest, with posture, and action, with no significant change in amplitude or frequency. Little or no dampening between rest and posture was noted. The tremor seemed to abate completely for brief periods and appeared to diminish during distraction with finger-to-nose or complex arithmetic tasks. He was neurologically normal otherwise with a normal MRI. Due to strong clinical suspicion of psychogenicity, cognitive behavioral therapy and venlafaxine was started, after which his tremor diminished to involve only the right index finger and showed more obvious signs of psychogenic tremor including inconsistent frequencies, entrainment, and distractibility.

Electrophysiologic Studies (Prior to Treatment): Recordings were done from the forearm flexors and extensors bilaterally with accelerometer over the right wrist. At rest, tremor frequency was 6 Hz and driven by 7-ms, often synchronous bursts in the flexors and extensors of the right wrist. No entrainment to the left hand tapping frequency (3–5 Hz) was seen with the right wrist tremor remaining at 5.5 to 6 Hz (Fig. A5.1). Tremor frequency and amplitude were unaffected by 100-7 test and touching numbered fingers in various patterns with the left hand. These features supported an organic cause of the tremor.

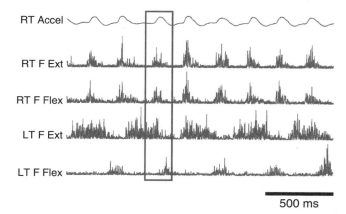

Figure A5.1 Before treatment, recording during tapping with left hand showed no entrainment. Accel, accelerometer; Ext, extensor; F, forearm; Flex, flexor.

Electrophysiologic Studies (after Treatment with Cognitive Behavior Therapy and Venlafaxine): After treatment, tremor improved to involve only the flexion and extension of the right index finger. Frequency of tremor varied with different positions of the right arm (4.6 Hz at rest, 5.1 Hz with only right arm outstretched, 5.5 Hz with both hands outstretched). Distraction with various tasks (2.7 Hz with voluntary flexion/extension of right wrist, 4 Hz with voluntary flexion/extension of left wrist, 0.9 Hz with finger-to-nose test performed with right upper extremity, 3.5 Hz with 100-7 test) was evident. Entrainment with tapping of the left index finger was seen (Fig. A5.2). With weighting of the right arm in the outstretched position, the peak tremor frequency changed to 6.1 Hz and the amplitude of the tremor increased compared to without weighting. These features supported the diagnosis of a psychogenic tremor.

Conclusion: Although electrophysiologic studies have been helpful in confirming the diagnosis of psychogenic tremor, the case above demonstrated the possibility of false negative tests. In some cases, a high index of suspicion and repeated careful clinical and electrophysiologic evaluations may be necessary to confirm the diagnosis.

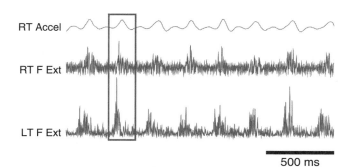

Figure A5.2 After treatment, recording during tapping with left hand showed entrainment. Accel, accelerometer; Ext, extensor; F, forearm.

ABSTRACT 6

The Relationship of Type of Dysphonia to Patient Report of Treatment Outcome

Christy L. Ludlow, Kimberly A. Finnegan, Steven Bielamowicz, Nazli Haq, Frank Putnam

Introduction: Spasmodic dysphonia (SD) begins in mid-life—the cause is unknown. It is classified as a focal dystonia and 50% of patients report onset after an upper respiratory infection and/or chronic stress. The disorder involves involuntary laryngeal muscle spasms producing voice breaks in vowels in adductor SD or breathy breaks in abductor SD. The treatment of choice for SD is botulinum toxin injection; it is 90% effective in adductor SD and 60% effective in abductor SD. Functional voice disorders (FVD) include muscular tension dysphonia and psychogenic voice disorders; both are considered secondary to stress or psychological factors. Currently, differentiation is dependent upon response to voice therapy, muscular tension dysphonia responds to manual circumlaryngeal massage, and psychogenic disorders respond to voice training and reassurance. The purpose was to identify what factors are predictive of patient response to treatment.

Methods: This was a prospective study of consecutive admissions that included a 3-day multidisciplinary team evaluation and consensus meeting of otolaryngology, speech pathology, neurology, psychiatry, and social work. The team reviewed neurologic findings; psychiatric diagnosis based on Standardized Clinical Interview for DSM, Personality Diagnostic Questionnaire-Revised, Schedule for Affective Disorders and Schizophrenia-Lifetime, and the Dissociative Experience Scale (Bernstein and Putnam, 1986); speech changes during sodium amytal IV; a psychosocial interview by a social worker; otolaryngologic examination; and speech symptom description by a speech-language pathologist. The team came to a consensus diagnosis and treatment recommendation of: SD and botulinum toxin injection; FVD and psychiatric referral and voice therapy; or both SD with FVD and botulinum toxin, counseling, and voice therapy. The team met with the participant and conveyed their decision and corresponding treatment regimen. A retrospective multiple regression determined which of the examination findings and blinded counts of speech symptoms differed among the diagnostic groups. The measures of speech symptoms were counts of the numbers of voice breaks and voice quality ratings of breathy, harshness, and tremor. Two years after the study, the participants were contacted to determine what treatment they had received and the outcome.

Results: Sixty-one participants with idiopathic voice disorder were diagnosed as having SD in 38 (15 adductor, 16 abductor, seven tremor), FVD in 16, and mixed (SD and FVD) in seven. Six (9.8%) were lost to follow-up. A stepwise logistic regression differentiated among SD, FVD, and mixed; the significant predictors were mean number of voice breaks in sentences and breathiness ratings. SD differed from FVD on number of breaks ($t = 3.325$, $p = 0.001$) and breathiness ($t = -2.036$, $p = 0.042$). Mixed differed from FVD on number of breaks ($t = 2.512$, $p = 0.012$) but not on breathiness ($t = -1.615$, $p = 0.106$). Comparisons among patient groups on benefit received from botulinum toxin injections were significant (chi square = 9.647, $p = 0.047$). A nonsignificant trend for a greater response to voice therapy occurred in the FVD group compared to SD (chi square = 7.867, p = 0.097).

Summary and Conclusions: The type of symptoms (voice breaks) was the best identifier for spasmodic dysphonia in comparison with functional voice disorders. Breathy voice quality without voice breaks was typical of functional voice disorders compared to SD. None of the other examinations—response to sodium amytal, neurologic, psychiatric, and psychosocial status—could accurately predict the group consensus diagnosis. A significant relationship was found between diagnosis and reported treatment outcome. A significantly larger number of patients with SD benefited from botulinum toxin than FVD, and a trend occurred for more FVD to benefit or recover from therapy alone. Only a few SD patients benefited from voice therapy. Voice breaks would be the most accurate measure for selecting patients who would benefit from botulinum toxin injection and not voice therapy.

ABSTRACT 7

The "Chair Test" to Aid in the Diagnosis of Psychogenic Astasia-Abasia

Michael S. Okun, Hubert H. Fernandez, Kelly D. Foote

Objective: To describe a new test to aid in the diagnosis of psychogenic astasia-abasia.

Background and Significance: The diagnosis of psychogenic gait disorders can often be difficult, particularly for the general practitioner, or general neurologist, due to its diverse clinical spectrum. Contained in Paul Blocq's original descriptions of hysterical gait disorders are 11 case descriptions of patients with astasia-abasia (meaning "unsteady gait, unsteady station"). One description, Case 3, was of a patient, Henri Gob, who had a hysterical gait disorder, but could propel a chair while seated normally. This observation by Blocq may be useful in the modern neurologic examination.

Methods: Paul Blocq's original 1888 paper on astasia-abasia was translated from French to English. Based on Case 3, Henri Gob, we developed a paradigm to aid in the identification of astasia-abasia. We describe the first nine consecutive patients who presented with astasia-abasia who underwent "chair testing." Each patient was seen by a movement disorders neurologist, and diagnosed with astasia-abasia. Each patient was then asked to walk 20 to 30 feet forward, turn around, and walk 30 feet back toward the examiner, twice. The patients were then asked to sit in a swivel chair with wheels and a back rest and to propel the chair forward and backward 20 to 30 feet in two trials. The qualitative results of the trials were recorded. This was then compared to the control group of 19 consecutive movement disorder patients with gait problems but without psychogenic gait disorders who performed the chair test.

Results: Nine consecutive patients with psychogenic gait disorders were examined (Table A7.1). Eight of the nine were women, with an average age of 47.6 (range 18–76). When applying characteristics described by Hayes of psychogenic gait disorders, our psychogenic group was found to have the following characteristics: 9/9 (100%) had exaggerated effort, 6/9 (66%) had extreme slowness, 9/9 (100%) had variability throughout the day, 2/9 (22%) had unusual postures, 7/9 (78%) had collapses, 6/9 (67%) had tremors, hyperkinetic, or ballistic movements, and 9/9 (100%) showed distractibility.

Compared to their walking, eight of the nine patients in the psychogenic group "performed well" on the chair test, showing improved ambulation when seated in the chair. One patient was frozen and would not attempt to walk or use the chair even with the assistance of the examiner. By contrast, all 19 control patients "performed equally" when walking or ambulating using the chair.

Conclusion: The "chair test" is a safe and efficient neurologic examination maneuver that can be used to aid in the differentiation of psychogenic from neurologic gait disorders. More studies are needed to determine the sensitivity and specificity of this test.

TABLE A7.1
CHARACTERISTICS OF THE PSYCHOGENIC GAIT PATIENTS AND RESPONSE TO THE CHAIR TEST

Patient	Age	Sex	Features of Gait	Neuro/ psych Diagnosis	Secondary Gain	Chair Test	Exag- gerated Effort	Extreme Slowness	Variability Through Day	Unusual Postures	Collapses	Tremors	Distractibility
1	18	F	Unsteady, high steps, shaking tendency to fall without injuring	Depressive symptoms; migraine	No	(+)	(+)	(−)	(+)	(−)	(+)	(+)	(+)
2	68	F	High steps, jumping, high amplitude dyskinesia "off"	Depressive symptoms; Parkinson disease	No	(+)	(+)	(+)	(+)	(+)	(−)	(+)	(+)
3	59	F	Unsteady, lurching, fainting	Depressive symptoms; craniofacial dystonia	Possible	(+)	(+)	(+)	(+)	(−)	(+)	(−)	(+)
4	36	F	Ataxia, unsteady, falling without injury	Depressive symptoms	No	(+)	(+)	(+)	(+)	(−)	(+)	(−)	(+)
5	76	F	Unsteady, unusual arm and leg movement, ballism	Bipolar disorder; depressive symptoms	No	(+)	(+)	(−)	(+)	(−)	(−)	(+)	(+)

(continued)

TABLE A7.1
(Continued)

Patient	Age	Sex	Features of Gait	Neuro/psych Diagnosis	Secondary Gain	Chair Test	Exaggerated Effort	Extreme Slowness	Variability Through Day	Unusual Postures	Collapses	Tremors	Distractibility
6	28	F	Unsteady, fainting, ballistic movements in arms/legs	Depressive symptoms	No	(+)	(+)	(+)	(+)	(+)	(+)	(+)	(+)
7	49	F	Twisting movements in trunk/legs, unsteady, fall without injury	"Fibro-myalgia;" depressive symptoms	Possible	(+)	(+)	(+)	(+)	(−)	(+)	(+)	(+)
8	52	F	Unsteady, fall without injury, zig-zag walking	Depressive symptoms	No	(+)	(+)	(−)	(+)	(−)	(+)	(−)	(+)
9	43	M	Akinetic, frozen, held upright by examiner	Depressive symptoms	Possible	(−)	(+)	(+)	(+)	(−)	(+)	(+)	(+)

ABSTRACT 8
Simultaneous Examination of Patients by Neurologist and Psychiatrist Provides Clues for the Diagnosis of Psychogenic Movement Disorders

Ghislaine Savard, Michel Panisset

Introduction: Psychogenic movement disorders (PMD) represent a most difficult challenge to the neurologist. Some clinical features are suggestive of the diagnosis, but no sign is pathognomonic (1). Referral to a psychiatrist without special expertise in PMD may not be of help (2). We report our experience with simultaneous examination of patients with PMD by neuropsychiatrist and neurologist with a view to delineate the strengths of this approach in diagnosis-making and in treatment initiation.

Methods: Consecutive patients with suspected PMD from two movement disorders clinics were interviewed and examined by the neurologist and by the neuropsychiatrist separately and then jointly. First, the neurologist established a diagnosis of PMD as "documented" or "clinically established" according to criteria by Fahn et al. (3). Second, the neuropsychiatrist formulated a diagnostic impression according to the *Diagnostic and Statistical Manual of Mental Disorders*, Fourth Edition, Text Revision (2000). Malingering was not retained as a medical illness. Third, the neurologist, in the presence of the neuropsychiatrist, disclosed the working diagnosis of PMD, provided opportunity for psychoeducation, and proposed joint follow-up and treatment. Neurologic and psychiatric diagnoses were then reviewed in the light of the third session. Any perception of deceit was addressed (4).

Results: Seven patients were evaluated. All were suspected by the neurologist to have "documented" or "clinically established" PMD occurring alone or superimposed on a movement disorder (MD). When interviewed by the neuropsychiatrist alone, the patients focused on the somatic symptoms and were often unable to discuss psychiatric issues. But during the joint interview, the patients, while attempting to establish a privileged therapeutic alliance with the neurologist, displayed psychological distress in various, often nonverbal, ways, which the neuropsychiatrist could witness. All patients agreed to joint follow-up (Table A8.1).

TABLE A8.1

Case	Patient's Presentation	MD Specialist Diagnosis	Neuropsychiatric Diagnosis	Joint Diagnosis of PMD Second to:
1 (GL) 55-year-old woman	1. Head tremor 2. Many complaints 3. Resistant to all medications	1. Atypical syndrome of gait/hand and head tremors	1. Chronic dysthymia 2. Substance abuse (BZD) 3. Dependant personality disorder	Factitious disorder
2 (DR) 52-year-old man	1. Progressive postural tremor 2. Incoordination 3. Concentration poor 4. Variable symptoms	1. Atypical gait/abnormal movement	1. Anxious disorder, NOS	Conversion disorder
3 (IH) 76-year-old man	1. PD 2. Anxiety 3. Intolerant to all medications	1. PD stage 2/5	1. Obsessive personality traits	Psychological symptoms affecting PD
4 (TNTT) 57-year-old woman	1. PD 2. Gastralgia NYD 3. Tremor disappeared with kung fu 4. Poor concentration 5. Intolerant to most medications	1. PD 2. Give-way weakness 3. Total gastrointestinal evaluation negative	1. Anxiety disorder, NOS 2. Stomach pain disappeared with mirtazapine	Psychological symptoms affecting PD
5 (DL) 44-year-old woman	1. Ataxia 2. Myoclonus 3. Variable symptoms 4. Suggestibility	1. Atypical ataxia	1. Substance abuse in remission	Factitious disorder
6 (RS) 44-year-old woman	1. Floppy head 2. MRI of C spine and EMG normal	1. No dystonia, no myopathy	1. Delusional state, somatic	Delusional state
7 (WB) 53-year-old woman	1. Torticollis 2. Botox toxin pre-MRI 3. Tic like movements 4. Whispers, barely vocal	1. Posttraumatic dystonia	1. Posttraumatic stress disorder	Factitious disorder

EMG, electromyographic; MRI, magnetic resonance imaging; NOS, not otherwise specified; PD, Parkinson disease.

Conclusions: Joint interviews pave the way to a better understanding of the psychopathology underlying PMD. Without them, psychiatric data is lost, diagnostic certainty is low, and follow-up is unproductive. Self-deceit likely hampers these patients' abilities to team up with the psychiatrist unless joint neurologic follow-up is secured.

1. Miyasaki JM, et al. Psychogenic Movement Disorders. *Can J Neurol Sci.* 2003;30(Suppl. 1):S94–S100.
2. Feinstein A, et al. Psychiatric outcome in patients with a psychogenic movement disorder: a prospective study. *Neuropsychiatry Neuropsychol Behav Neurol.* 2001;14:169–176.
3. Fahn S, Williams DT. Psychogenic dystonia. *Adv Neurol.* 1988;50: 431–455.
4. Ford CV. *The psychology of deceit.* Washington, DC: American Psychiatric Press, 1996:333.

ABSTRACT 9
The Syndrome of Fixed Dystonia— An Evaluation of 105 Patients
Anette Schrag, Michael Trimble, Niall P. Quinn, Kailash P. Bhatia

We describe the clinical features of 105 patients presenting with fixed dystonia, and report the prospective assessment and investigation of 41 such patients. Most patients were women (85%) and had a young age of onset (mean 30.1 years SD 13). A peripheral injury preceded onset in 64%, and spread of dystonia to other body regions occurred in 55%. After an average follow-up of 3.3 years (overall disease duration, 8.4 years), partial (19%) or complete (8%) remissions had occurred in a minority of patients. The fixed postures affected predominantly the limbs (90%) and rarely the neck/shoulder region (6%) or jaw (4%). Pain was present in most patients and was a major complaint in 41%. Features of complex regional pain syndrome (CRPS) were found in 41%, but these were mild in the majority. No consistent investigational abnormalities were found; no patient tested (n = 25) had a mutation in the DYT 1 gene, and only one patient had neurophysiologic features of stiff limb syndrome. Neuropsychiatric assessment in the prospective group revealed dissociative (42% vs. 0%, $p = 0.001$) and affective disorders (50% vs. 85%, $p = 0.01$) significantly more common in the fixed dystonia than in a control group. Thirty-six percent of patients fulfilled classification criteria for psychogenic dystonia; 29% fulfilled the *Diagnostic and Statistical Manual of Mental Disorders*, Fourth Edition, criteria for somatization disorder, which was only diagnosed after examination of the primary care records in many cases; and 24% fulfilled both sets of criteria. However, 10% of the prospectively and 47% of the retrospectively studied patients did not have any suggestion of psychogenic dystonia, and detailed investigation failed to reveal an alternate explanation for their clinical presentation.

Fixed dystonia is a heterogeneous condition, which overlaps with CRPS and somatoform disorder, a history of which should be sought from these patients. The syndrome of isolated fixed dystonia in the remaining subjects appears to differ from both of these disorders and from primary dystonia, and its etiology remains obscure.

ABSTRACT 10
Appraisal of Clinical Diagnostic Criteria for Psychogenic Movement Disorders
Paula Gerber, Holly A. Shill

Objective: To review clinical diagnostic criteria for psychogenic movement disorders, and to identify possible new criteria.

Background: Psychogenic movement disorders are a rare but difficult entity in clinical neurology. Previous work by Fahn and Williams (1) and Factor et al. (2) has shown that there are certain features suggestive of a psychogenic disorder (Table A10.1).

Methods: We retrospectively reviewed selected patients in a movement disorders specialty clinic who were deemed psychogenic. Out of 800 patients seen in a 10-month period, 15 met this criterion.

Results: Eighty-seven percent were women. Tremor was the most frequent complaint (67%), followed by myoclonus (47%), gait disorders (33%), and dystonia (13%). Common features in these patients included pain (73%), coexisting psychiatric disease (73%), other psychogenic features on exam (73%), and history of trauma (60%). The median number of positive systems on review of systems was 5 (range 2–10). Previously described clues to a psychogenic process including distractibility, selective disability, and abrupt onset were 47%, 27%, and 27% in our series, respectively. Fifty-three percent of patients had a clearly identifiable secondary gain; 73% had either an identifiable or a possible secondary gain. Forty percent of patients had a family history of a movement disorder, and 47% reported family history of a neurologic disorder. Also, 57% of patients reported a response to some form of medication.

Conclusion: These results are mostly consistent with those previously reported. Compared to Factor et al. (2), we report a lower frequency of distractibility (47% vs. 86%), abrupt onset (27% vs. 54%), and selective disability (27% vs. 39%). However, dystonia was comparatively rare in our series, while gait disorders were more frequent. Many of the features originally described by Fahn and Williams (1) were present in our patients, including pain, potential for secondary gain, and other psychogenic exam findings. In addition, we identified a positive family history as an additional clue to a psychogenic process, suggesting that modeling may be important.

1. Fahn S, Williams D. Psychogenic dystonia. *Adv Neurol.* 1988;50: 431–455.
2. Factor S, Podskalny G, Molho E. Psychogenic movement disorders: frequency, clinical profile, and characteristics. *J Neurol Neurosurg Psychiatry.* 1995;59:406–412.
3. Fahn S. Tremor, psychogenic, peripheral and paroxysmal movement disorders. In: *A comprehensive review of movement disorders for the clinical practitioner.* August 1–4, 2002, syllabus:1153–1181.

TABLE A10.1

SUMMARY OF CHARACTERISTICS OF PATIENTS WITH PSYCHOGENIC MOVEMENT DISORDERS

Patient	Age/sex	Presenting Complaint	Other Complaints	Suggestive Exam Findings
1	49/M	Gait disorder, falls, postural instability	Back pain	
2	59/F	R hand tremor	Pain, dizziness, ataxia, dysphagia, speech problems	Give-way weakness
3	52/F	Myoclonus	Essential tremor	Variable latency DTRs
4	61/F	Bilateral tremor, R >L	Insomnia, involuntary limb movements, cramps	
5	50/F	Pain, spasms of R side, dystonia		Tearful affect, deliberate slowness, distractible myoclonus
6	37/F	Gait disturbance	"Jerks," facial twitches, spasms, pain, migratory numbness	Exaggerated DTRs
7	60/F	Gait disturbance, "stiff legs"	Paresthesias, slow speech	Give-way weakness, gegenhalten
8	51/F	Tremor, "jerks"		Suggestible, whole-body jerking
9	48/F	Tremor	Balance disturbance, "fine motor" problems	Give-way weakness, activation rigidity
10	39/M	Tremor, night myoclonus	Back pain, memory problems, syncope, urinary retention	Give-way weakness, activation rigidity, distractible tremor
11	34/F	Dystonia, tremor		Fixed posture, distractible tremor
12	29/F	Tremor, spasms	Back pain	Deliberate slowness, depressed affect
13	50/F	Gait disturbance, tremor	Cramps, headache, speech and memory troubles, EDS	
14	56/F	Tremor, gait disturbance, stiffness	Chronic fatigue	Give-way weakness, gegenhalten, distractible
15	49/F	Tremor, myoclonus	Pain, tingling, cramps, scotomata	

ABSTRACT 11

Psychogenic Facial Spasm (the Smirk) Presenting as Hemifacial Spasm

Daniel Tarsy, Alexandra Dengenhardt, Cindy Zadikoff

Psychogenic Movement Disorders: Psychobiology and Therapy of a Functional Disorder

Abstract: Large surveys of PMD in movement disorder clinics have reported a low incidence of psychogenic facial spasm. We report three patients with psychogenic facial spasm seen in a single movement disorders clinic within one year. They were each referred for possible hemifacial spasm. All were women ranging in age from 28 to 53 who had acute onset of symptoms without progression 8 to 11 months prior to consultation. Facial movements were constant in two patients and fluctuated in the third. Two patients reported episodic motor symptoms in one upper extremity. There was a previous history of anxiety and other somatizations in two patients. Examination showed prominent unilateral elevation of one corner of the mouth in each patient which created a cartoon-like, smirking facial expression. Other unusual facial movements were present in all three patients. Other psychogenic signs were present in three patients and inconsistent and changing signs with distractibility in two patients. Two patients stopped working. There was litigation in one case. The diagnosis of psychogenic facial spasm was made in these patients based on several features. All had acute onset of symptoms with maximal severity, a static course, normal diagnostic studies, inconsistent symptoms over time, signs incongruent with hemifacial spasm, and a history of psychiatric disorder. There were also nonorganic sensory findings, other unusual involuntary movements, spontaneous improvement, and distractibility. Psychogenic facial spasm, manifest in these patients by a smirklike elevation of one corner of the mouth, is a rare but identifiable form of PMD.

Introduction: Differential diagnosis of chronic or recurrent facial spasm includes hemifacial spasm, blepharospasm, tics, and myokymia. Psychogenic movement disorders include dystonia, tremor, myoclonus, and parkinsonism. Psychogenic facial spasm is a subtype of psychogenic dystonia which has only rarely been reported (1). We describe three patients with psychogenic facial spasm who were referred to a movement disorders clinic within one year with a diagnosis of hemifacial spasm.

Case Reports: *Case 1.* A 28-year-old special education teacher presented with sudden onset of an irritated sensation in her right eye and subjective swelling of the right face. This was followed the next day by acute onset of persistent muscle twitching involving the right face. She reported hyperacussis in her right ear. She stopped working. Neurologic examination 3 months after onset showed an intermittent, smirklike elevation of the right corner of her mouth, inconsistent muscle twitching in midface, and absence of facial weakness. Seven months after onset, she had three brief episodes of flexion–extension movements of her right hand. EEG, MRI/MRA, and spinal fluid were normal. Botox on two occasions produced only a brief response. Examination 11 months after onset showed nearly constant upward deviation of the right corner of her mouth. This frequently disappeared while speaking or distracted. There was restricted movement of the left face when asked to smile or grimace. When asked to activate left facial muscles, the right upward deviation cleared. There was a small patch of reduced pin and light touch in the right cheek. There was no facial weakness or other findings. EMG showed intermittent activation of motor units concurrent with visible spasm without evidence of denervation or features of hemifacial spasm. There were no current signs of anxiety or depression, but there was a long prior history of anxiety and panic disorder treated with paroxetine. Following EMG, facial spasm became episodic and, for the first time, became associated with prodromal anxiety. Repeat examination one month later showed only narrowing of the right palpebral fissure. She was advised that her symptoms were due to anxiety, accepted this explanation, and remaining signs cleared.

Case 2. A 53-year-old writer was seen 10 months after acute onset of episodic upward pulling of the right corner of her mouth, followed later by lateral pulling of the left corner of her mouth. She reported a single episode of elevation of her right shoulder and "diaphragm spasms" several months earlier which cleared spontaneously. She joined a national support group for dystonia. Examination showed a constant smirklike elevation of the right corner of her mouth associated with lateral pulling of the left corner of her mouth, present only when not speaking and which repeatedly suppressed when distracted. There was occasional frontalis and procerus contraction producing a puzzled or frowning expression and intermittent right shoulder elevation accompanied by slight right-sided head tilt. There was generalized give-way weakness. Brain MRI was normal. Previous neurologic history included extensive negative evaluations over 14 years for unexplained episodes of generalized weakness, numbness, fatigue, dizziness, and speech arrests. Diagnosis was pseudoseizures versus complex partial seizures. A diagnosis of psychogenic facial spasm was made. Symptoms persisted and the patient was followed by her primary physician with a diagnosis of somatoform disorder.

Case 3. A 38-year-old customer service representative had acute onset of right facial droop, pain around the right eye, and involuntary blinking of the right eye one day following a motor vehicle accident (MVA) in which she suffered mild trauma to the right face. There was litigation and she stopped working. There had been a previous MVA 2 years earlier followed by chronic neck pain. All symptoms resolved over several months except for right eye blinking. Six months later there was acute onset of recurrent right facial spasm precipitated by eye closure together with face, head, and neck pain. Two months later she began to have involuntary blinking of her left eye. Botox in right frontalis relieved her pain but not the eye-blinking. Examination 9 months after onset showed continuous, bilateral blepharospasm in ambient light, eyelid fluttering in darkness, hesitation in opening her eyes, weakness of right eyelid closure, and reduced light touch in right face, scalp, and anterior neck. Vibration was increased in right scalp, forehead, and cheek. Brain MRI showed a small hypodensity in inferior left basal ganglia. Symptoms remitted dramatically, but transiently, following a first but not a second treatment with Botox, both of which were followed by transient myalgia, fever, and recurrent face pain. Blepharospasm later remitted for 3 months followed by acute recurrence of all symptoms, this time together with upward elevation of the right corner of her mouth. She was treated with paroxetine for pain and anxiety and referred for counseling where a diagnosis of anxiety was made which she accepted with gradual improvement of all facial symptoms.

Discussion: All three patients displayed features more closely resembling facial dystonia than hemifacial spasm. They displayed tonic, upward deviation of one corner of the mouth, which produced a smirklike facial expression different from the usual appearance of either facial dystonia or hemifacial spasm. There were other abnormal facial movements in each case. History and examination were characterized by features of psychogenicity in each patient (Table A11.1).

TABLE A11.1
FINDINGS SUGGESTING PSYCHOGENICITY IN THREE PATIENTS

History		Examination	
Acute onset	3	Inconsistent signs	2
Nonprogressive	3	Changing character of signs	2
Episodic	3	Other unusual facial movements	3
Other episodic symptoms	2	Distractibility	2
Other somatizations	2	Other psychogenic findings	3
Prior history of anxiety	2		
Stopped working	2		
Litigation	1		
Spontaneous remissions	1		

Dystonia may present with unusual clinical features, is typically unassociated with helpful laboratory or radiological studies, and is often incorrectly diagnosed as psychogenic (2). It is therefore necessary to be very careful before making the diagnosis of psychogenic dystonia. Useful criteria for the diagnosis of psychogenic movement disorder have been proposed by Fahn and Williams (3,4). They classify four levels of certainty: documented, clinically established, probable, and possible. Cases 1 and 3 met diagnostic criteria for documented psychogenic movement disorder in that symptoms completely remitted after the diagnosis of anxiety disorder was made; one after being advised of the diagnosis and the second after several months of counseling. Both had been symptomatic for less than one year. Case 2, with a previous history of treatment-resistant somatoform disorder, was also symptomatic for less than 1 year but failed to improve. She had a clinically established psychogenic movement disorder characterized by inconsistent and incongruent signs, distractibility, false weakness, multiple somatizations, and obvious psychiatric disorder.

Conclusion: Psychogenic facial spasm is a rare but identifiable manifestation of psychogenic dystonia.

1. Tan E, Jankovic J. Psychogenic facial spasm. *J Neuropsychiatry Clin Neurosci.* 2001;13:380–384.
2. Marsden CD, Harrison MJG. Idiopathic torsion dystonia. *Brain.* 1974; 97:793–810.
3. Fahn S, Williams DT. Psychogenic dystonia. *Adv Neurol.* 1988;50:431–455.
4. Fahn S. Psychogenic movement disorders. In: Marsden CD, Fahn S, eds. *Movement disorders 3.* London: Butterworth-Heineman, 1994:359–372.

ABSTRACT 12
Biofeedback Therapy for Psychogenic Movement Disorders

Joel K. Levy, Madhavi Thomas

Objective: This study was performed to study the effectiveness of biofeedback therapy in psychogenic movement disorders (PMD).

Background: Patients with PMD have abnormalities in the specific muscle groups in the affected areas which may in some cases act as trigger points for exacerbation of the PMD. Biofeedback therapy has been successfully used in management of several disorders including pain. Patients with PMD may benefit from targeted biofeedback therapy in addition to pharmacotherapy.

Methods: Patients with PMD were evaluated and diagnosis was confirmed by the movement disorders specialist (MT) at the Baylor College of Medicine. Some of these patients were referred for biofeedback therapy as part of our management and treatment plan. Patients were followed by the movement disorders clinic as well as the neuropsychologist (JKL) administering biofeedback therapy periodically. Surface EMG diagnostic protocol developed by Jeffrey Cram, Biofeedback Institute, Seattle, was used for analysis and treatment (1,2). Treatment protocol for biofeedback included evaluation using

muscle map localization techniques, based on the patient's report of the location of most intense symptoms. Once the muscle map is completed by the patient, surface electromyographic (EMG) screening is performed, including paraspinous muscle scan, to detect abnormalities and asymmetries in muscle movement and muscle tension. Biofeedback is performed with a J&J computer interface with two channels of EMG, and is specifically aimed at decreasing the amplitude of the stereotypy and activation of specific muscle groups. Maladaptive muscle tone is countered with relaxation training. Patient participation is essential throughout this period, and patients are trained to decrease specific muscle tension by aiming for a reduction in the amplitude of the surface EMG. Patients are trained for several sessions, and are given exercises to perform at home. Once patients are trained, they are discharged from biofeedback training, and they continue to follow up with the movement disorders specialist until recovery is achieved. Patient compliance is greatly encouraged through the process. Results are determined using a global clinical improvement scale (0, no improvement; 1, mild improvement; 2, moderate improvement; 3, marked improvement; and 4, complete resolution of symptoms).

Results: Fifteen patients with tremor (three), dystonia (six), stereotypy (two), myoclonus (three), and vocalizations with stereotypy (one) were treated. Eleven women and four men participated in this study (n = 15). Mean age was 42.58 ± 12.4 years, with mean duration of follow-up being 10.5 ± 13.2 months (1 week–48 months), and mean duration of symptoms was 23.25 ± 16.9 months (1 month–4 years). Of the 15 patients, three (20%) had tremor, three (20%) had myoclonus, two (13.3%) had stereotypic movement, and two (13.3%) had focal dystonia, while three (20%) had generalized dystonia, and one (6.7%) patient had vocalizations and dyskinesia. Underlying psychiatric disorder was present in seven patients (46.7%) with major depressive disorder in three patients (20%). Abnormalities on surface EMG scan were seen in six patients, and in five of these patients there was correlation between the location of PMD and the abnormality on the scan. The results of surface EMG scan are as shown in Table A12.1. Of the total number of patients, ten (67%) were treated with a combination of pharmacotherapy and biofeedback, one patient received biofeedback alone, one refused treatment, and three patients were noncompliant. Nine patients (60%) reported improvement, and three patients did not follow up, while three patients reported no improvement.

Conclusions: In this small study we have seen promising results with targeted biofeedback therapy. Patient compliance rate was very high. Improvement of the movement disorder was noted in 60% of patients. These results are very encouraging, considering the short duration of this protocol. Future studies with a larger number of patients will be more helpful.

1. Cram JR. Surface EMG recordings and pain-related disorders: a diagnostic framework. *Biofeedback Self Regul.* 1988;13:123–138.
2. Cram JR, Steger JC. EMG scanning in the diagnosis of chronic pain. *Biofeedback Self Regul.* 1983;8:229–241.

TABLE A12.1

SURFACE EMG FINDINGS AND CORRELATION OF LOCATION OF ABNORMALITY IN PATIENTS WITH PSYCHOGENIC MOVEMENT DISORDER

Patient Number	Location of Abnormality on Clinical Exam	Surface EMG Correlation (Seen as Increased Activity in Specified Areas)
1	Generalized dystonia with face and shoulder involvement	Facial musculature bilaterally, upper trapezius bilaterally
2	Segmental myoclonus involving upper back	Rhomboids, trapezius bilaterally, abnormal midthoracic and lumbar paraspinous
3	Generalized myoclonus	Abnormalities in upper, and lower paraspinous quadriceps, and left tibialis
4	Focal arm dystonia	Biceps and wrist flexors asymmetry in the T8, T10, L1, L3, L5 areas
5	Dystonia involving left leg, neck and forearm	Left finger flexors, left gastrocnemius
6	Gait disorder	Abnormal lumbar, and thoracic paraspinous with asymmetry on left side, abnormal left splenius

EMG, electromyographic.

ABSTRACT 13

Long-term Prognosis of Psychogenic Movement Disorders

Madhavi Thomas, Polo Alberto Banuelos, Kevin Dat Vuong, Joseph Jankovic

Objective: To assess the long-term prognosis of patients with psychogenic movement disorders (PMD), and to determine the prognostic indicators for recovery.

Methods: Patients evaluated in Baylor College of Medicine Movement Disorders Clinic and coded in the database with a diagnosis of PMD were selected for this study. A structured telephone interview was conducted with the patients whom we were able to contact. The telephone interview included administration of McMaster Health Index Questionnaire (1,2). Data collected from the interview (telephone follow-up) and detailed chart review (Visit 1) were entered into the database. The diagnosis of the PMD was categorized into documented, clinically established, probable, and possible, based on the Fahn and Williams criteria (3). Statistical analysis was performed using chi square, and Spearman's rho on ordinal and nominal variables; ANOVA was performed for continuous variables. Backward logistic regression analysis was performed to assess the relationship between probability of same/worst outcome, as the dependent variable and the various dependent variables.

Results: Out of a total of 12,625 patients seen in our movement disorders clinic, 517 patients (4.1%) satisfied the criteria for the diagnosis of PMD. Their predominant movement disorders were categorized as follows: 211 (40.8%) tremor, 208 (40.2%) dystonia, 88 (17.0%) myoclonus, 22 (4.3%) tics, 20 (3.9%) gait disorder, 16 (3.1%) parkinsonism, seven (1.4%) dyskinesia, and three (0.6%) chorea; 38 had more than one form of PMD. Totals of 228 out of 517 (44.1%) patients were included in this data analysis. Of these, 136 (59.6%) patients met the diagnostic criteria for clinically established PMD, while 44 (19.3%) were probable, 32 (14%) were documented PMD, and 16 (7%) patients met the criteria for possible PMD.

There was a marked female preponderance; 166 (72.8%) were women ($p < 0.0001$). The mean age was 42.3 ± 14.3, mean duration of symptoms was 4.7 ± 8.1, and mean duration of follow-up was 3.4 ± 2.8 years. The majority [187 (82.7%)] of patients had abrupt onset of symptoms ($p < 0.0001$). The most common precipitating event was personal life stress as noted by 76 patients (33.5%). The most common comorbid psychiatric illnesses were depression in 118 patients (51.8%) and anxiety in 50 patients (21.9%). Coexistent neurologic disorder was seen in 70 (30.7%) patients, while coexistent organic movement disorder was seen in 37 (16.2%) patients. Outcome was measurable reliably in 122 patients who completed the interview. Out of these, 69 (56.6%) reported an improvement, and 27 (22.1%) reported worsening, while 26 (21.3%) reported no change in clinical status. Logistic modeling suggests that poorer outcome was predicted reliably by a factor of 2.88 for those exhibiting inconsistent PMD movements, 5.35 for those with a positive history of smoking, 1.07 for every year of duration of PMD symptoms, and 4.90 for those reporting satisfactory social life perceptions. The proportion of patients with better outcome was greater than those with worse or same outcome ($p < 0.0001$). Smoking seemed to correlate with weaker physical health and negative social life perceptions ($p < 0.05$). Positive social life perception correlated with better McMaster Health Index ($p < 0.0001$). Perceived effective treatment by physician was associated with improved outcome ($p < 0.0001$). Patients with shorter duration of illness had a better outcome ($p < 0.012$). Stronger physical health and positive social life perceptions correlated with improved outcome ($p < 0.018$).

Conclusion: Poor prognostic indicators for PMD include presence of inconsistent movements, suggestibility, and dissatisfaction with the physician, positive history of smoking, and longer duration of illness. Good prognosis was associated with patients' perceptions of receiving effective treatment by physician, attribution of a specific medication, good physical health, positive social life perceptions, elimination of stressors, and comorbid anxiety disorder.

1. Chambers LW, Sackett DL, Goldsmith CH, et al. Development and application of an index of social function. *Health Serv Res.* 1976; 11:430–441.
2. Chambers LW, MacDonald LA, Tugwell P, et al. The McMaster Health Index Questionnaire as a measurement of quality of life for patients with rheumatoid disease. *J Rheumatol.* 1982;9:780–784.
3. Fahn S, Williams D. Psychogenic Dystonia. *Adv Neurol.* 1988;50:431–455.

ABSTRACT 14

Psychogenic Tremor: Clinical Characteristics and Long-term Progression

Madhavi Thomas, Kevin Dat Vuong, Joseph Jankovic

Objective: To evaluate clinical features of psychogenic tremor (PT) and to assess the long-term prognosis of PT.

Methods: Patients seen in the Baylor Movement Disorders Clinic with a diagnosis of psychogenic movement disorders (PMD) were selected for this study. Doctors contacted patients by telephone using existing contact information, Internet search engines, operator assistance, and people finder to obtain telephone numbers. Data collected from a structured interview (telephone follow-up) and detailed chart review (Visit 1) were entered into a database. Statistical analysis was performed using chi square and Spearman's rho on ordinal and nominal variables; ANOVA was performed for continuous variables. Backward logistic regression analysis was performed to assess the relationship between probability of same/worst outcome, as the dependent variable, and the various dependent variables. The tremor subset was analyzed, examining the characteristics as well as outcome of patients with tremor. Clinical features of the PMD were categorized using the Fahn and Williams criteria for diagnosis (1), the McMaster Health Index Questionnaire (2,3), treatment offered, and outcome measures including reason for improvement were recorded.

Results: The diagnosis of PMD was given in 4.1% (n = 517) of all patients evaluated in our movement disorders clinic between 1988 and 2002, with PT being the most common type, accounting for 40.8% of all patients with PMD. We were able to obtain follow-up information on 127 of 211 (60.2%) patients with PT, followed for a mean of 2.9 ± 2.7 years. Among them, 92 (72.4%) were women, the mean age at initial evaluation was 43.7 ± 14.1 years, and mean duration of symptoms was 4.6 ± 7.6 years. Despite a higher prevalence of PT in women (p <0.0001), no age differences were found between men and women with PT (p = 0.17). The following clinical features were considered to be characteristic of PT: abrupt onset (78.7%), distractibility (72.4%), variable amplitude, and frequency (62.2%), intermittent occurrence (35.4%), inconsistent movement (29.9%), and variable direction (17.3%). Most common location of tremor was in the hand(s). Precipitating events identified prior to the onset of tremor included personal life stress (33.9%), physical trauma (23.6%), major illness (13.4%), surgery (9.4%), and reaction to medical treatment or procedure (8.7%). Coexistent "organic" neurologic disorder was present in 37.0% of PT patients, while psychiatric comorbidities included depression (56.7%) and anxiety (30.7%). Evidence of secondary gain was present in 32.3%, including maintenance of a disability status (21.3%), pending compensation (10.2%), and litigation (9.4%). At last follow-up, 58.7% of patients having rated themselves "better" on a global rating scale and consistently scoring better on other outcome indicators were considered improved (p <0.0001). The strongest reason for improvement per the patient was perceived effective treatment by the physician.

Conclusions: In this largest series of PT patients, we have identified a variety of clinical features of tremor of which abrupt onset, distractibility, variable amplitude, and frequency are the predominant features. Women seem to be more affected than men, and depression is the most common psychiatric comorbidity. Improvement with time was noted in 57.9% patients, and there is a positive correlation between clinical improvement and perceived effective treatment. These features are consistent with those reported by other, smaller series (4–6).

1. Fahn S, Williams D. Psychogenic dystonia. *Adv Neurol.* 1988;50: 431–455.
2. Chambers LW, Sackett DL, Goldsmith CH, et al. Development and application of an index of social function. *Health Serv Res.* 1976;11: 430–441.
3. Chambers LW, MacDonald LA, Tugwell P, et al. The McMaster Health Index Questionnaire as a measurement of quality of life for patients with rheumatoid disease. *J Rheumatol.* 1982;9:780–784.
4. Koller WC, Lang AE, Vetere-Overfield B, et al. Psychogenic tremors. *Neurology.* 1989;39:1094–1099.
5. Deuschl G, Koster B, Lucking C, et al. Diagnostic and pathophysiological aspects of psychogenic tremors. *Mov Disord.* 1998;13:294–302.
6. Kim YJ, Anthony S, Pakiam I, et al. Historical and clinical features of psychogenic tremor: a review of 70 cases. *Can J Neurol Sci.* 1999;26: 190–195.

ABSTRACT 15

Underlying Psychiatric Conditions in Patients with Psychogenic Movement Disorders: Recognition and Effective Treatment

Madhavi Thomas, and H. Florence Kim

Objective: To develop an effective treatment protocol using a team approach for patients with psychogenic movement disorders (PMD).

Background: Often, psychodynamic issues may play a key role in the severity of movement disorder symptoms in patients with PMD. It is especially important to include psychiatric consultation in the comprehensive workup of psychogenic movement disorders, even if there is no clear psychiatric diagnosis apparent at first glance.

Methods: Patients with clinical diagnosis of PMD were selected for this protocol from the Movement Disorders Clinic. All patients seen by the movement disorders specialist (MT) are classified into a category of movement disorder based on clinical examination and using the Fahn and Williams criteria (1), and counseled regarding the diagnosis of psychogenic movement disorder (explained to the patient as a disorder resulting from underlying psychiatric or psychological condition). Patients were then referred to the psychiatrist (HFK) for evaluation and exploration of underlying psychiatric and psychosocial factors. The psychiatrist offered patients various forms of therapy including pharmacotherapy, psychotherapy, and in some cases biofeedback therapy. Patients are followed on a regular interval of every 1 to 2 months for reassessment, and progress is evaluated by a global improvement scale based on percentage of improvement as stated by the patient, and noted by the examiner (MT).

Results: Twenty-one patients (16 women and 5 men) aged between 25 and 78 (mean age 47.5 ± 12.5 years) were treated using the above clinical protocol. Mean duration of follow-up was 1 month to 48 months (mean 10.5 ± 13.2 months), and duration of symptoms varied from 1 month to 60 months (mean 14.7 ± 60 months). Seven patients (33.3%) had tremor, five (23.8%) had myoclonus, four (19.04%) had dystonia, four (19.04%) had a gait disorder, and one patient (4.75%) had stereotypic movements. A clear precipitating factor is identified in 12 patients (57.14%), and five (23.8%) patients had comorbid organic movement disorder. Underlying psychiatric conditions were diagnosed in 19 patients (90.47%). Major depressive disorder was diagnosed in four patients (19%), generalized anxiety disorder was diagnosed in four patients (19%), three patients (14.3%) had depression not otherwise specified, seven patients (33.3%) had anxiety not otherwise specified. Posttraumatic stress disorder was identified in two patients (9.5%), two patients (9.5%) had polysubstance abuse, two had dysthymia (9.5%), and two (9.5%) had pain disorder. Cognitive impairment was identified in three patients (14.3%), and panic disorder was diagnosed in one patient (4.8%). Treatment offered varied from pharmacotherapy in 19 patients (90.4%), supportive psychotherapy in ten (47.6%), more than one form of therapy was offered to 12 patients (57.1%), biofeedback therapy in four patients (19%), hypnotherapy in one patient (4.8%), systematic desensitization in one patient (4.8%), two patients (9.5%) were noncompliant, and one (4.8%) refused therapy. Pharmacotherapy included SSRI in 15 patients (71.4%), benzodiazepines in ten patients (47.6%), atypical antipsychotics in two patients (9.5%), and mirtazapine in one patient (4.8%). Twelve patients (57.14%) had improvement following the treatment protocol, one patient (4.8%) reported worsening, five patients (23.8%) remain unchanged, and three patients (14.3%) did not follow up with us. Patient compliance rate was very high using this team approach (80.95%).

Conclusion: In this small group of patients, we have identified a wide range of psychiatric problems including traumatic brain injury, generalized anxiety disorder, and major depressive disorder. Our current data suggest that some of the patients with psychogenic movement disorders can have a very quick recovery if the underlying condition is a clear stressor, or in the case of a less complex psychiatric problem. But patients with more severe anxiety disorder or major depressive disorder need prolonged periods of therapy, and also a team approach by the treating physicians. We have noted very encouraging results using this initial treatment protocol for a team approach to psychogenic movement disorders.

1. Fahn S, Williams D. Psychogenic dystonia. *Adv Neurol.* 1988;50: 431–455.

ABSTRACT 16
Psychogenic Palatal Tremor
David R. Williams

Palatal tremor is a rare disorder characterized by rhythmic movements of the soft palate. A case of probable psychogenic palatal tremor (PPT) is reported here.

Clinical Summary: A 44-year-old woman presented 3 years after developing an unusual "vibration in her throat." Its onset coincided with a period of substantial psychological stress, and around this time she became aware of a neighbor who developed true palatal tremor. Initially, it occurred only occasionally for short periods, and within 2 months it was happening daily. At that time she noticed a coincidental clicking sound in both ears. It was absent during sleep, and was not present on waking. Typically it would reoccur within 2 hours of waking, and would vary in frequency and intensity. It would disappear spontaneously for up to several hours during the day and was absent during mouth opening, swallowing, talking, and singing. She was being treated for a generalized anxiety disorder and previously suffered from postpartum depression. There is no history of childhood motor or vocal tics. There is a strong family history of psychiatric illness. Neurologic examination was normal except for an audible clicking sound that could be heard by the examiner; the frequency varied, and could be increased or decreased volitionally. The clicking was present only with the mouth closed. It was distractible and could be suppressed by pressing the tongue to the roof of the mouth, which produced feelings of anxiety that were relieved by re-emergence of the ear click. The palatal tremor did not spontaneously cease at anytime during clinical assessment. With the mouth open, only short periods of voluntary ear clicking were possible, with symmetrical elevation of the soft palate, but quickly fatigued. Video nasoendoscopy demonstrated intermittent, symmetrical movements of the soft palate only, which occurred with the mouth closed. MRI of the brain and inferior olives was normal. There has been no response to antidepressants and anxiolytics.

Discussion: The patient described here has rhythmic palatal movements that closely resemble essential palatal tremor (EPT). One quarter of patients with palatal tremor have no cause found and are classified as having EPT (1). However, several features in this case are unusual for EPT: (i) The mode of onset, with a sense of "vibration in the throat" described is not typical. While sensory phenomena preceding dystonia, parkinsonian tremor, and tic disorders are well-documented, they have not previously been reported in EPT. (ii) The intermittent bouts of clicking that start several hours after waking and last from minutes to hours are unusual for EPT, where the palatal hyperkinesias are continuous throughout the day and typically disappear during sleep and recur on, or soon after, waking (1). (iii) The extent of volitional control of palatal movements in this case is unusual for EPT and may represent the acquisition of special motor skills. Voluntary control of tensor veli palatini producing rhythmic palatal movements has been reported in one family (2) without EPT and following resolution of EPT in two other cases (3,4). (iv) Disappearance of ear click with mouth opening has been reported in few cases of EPT (5). In contrast to these reports, the palatal movements in this case were invariably absent during mouth opening, even slight opening, and the ear click returned on mouth closure after a latency of no less than 10 seconds. (v) Anecdotal observations of two patients with presumed psychogenic palatal tremor (PPT) have previously been made where both patients were aware of true palatal tremor in other patients (1). In the case presented here, the inconsistent character of the movements, the increase with attention, disappearance with distraction, and contact with a case of true palatal tremor around the time of symptom onset suggest a psychogenic etiology. While psychopathology is present, a causal relationship cannot be proved. The straightforward definitions of EPT (1) do not include several seemingly important clinical phenomena which may help to differentiate this condition from motor tics, voluntary palatal movements, and PPT.

1. Deuschl G, Wilms H. Palatal tremor: the clinical spectrum and physiology of a rhythmic movement disorder. In: Fahn S, Frucht SJ, Hallet M, et al., eds. *Myoclonus and paroxysmal dyskinesias. Advances in neurology.* Vol. 89. Philadelphia, PA: Lippincott Williams & Wilkins, 2002:115–130.
2. Klein C, Gehrking E, Vieregge P. Voluntary palatal tremor in two siblings. *Mov Disord.* 1998;13(3):545–548.
3. Lawrence L, Newman RP, Bozian D. Disappearing palatal myoclonus. *Neurol.* 1981;31:748–751.
4. Wakata N, Sugimoto H, Iguchi H, et al. A case of voluntary palatal myoclonus with ear click: relationship between palatal myoclonus and click. *Eur Neurol.* 2002;48:52–53.
5. Kadakia S, McAbee G. Volitional control or palatal myoclonus. *(Letter) Mov Disord.* 1990;5(2):182.

Index